Bill's Clinical Pharmacology *and* Therapeutics *for* Veterinary Technicians

Fifth Edition

Melinda Anderson, Pharm.D., FSVHP, BS, RVT
Veterinary Clinical Pharmacist
Assistant Professor
Department of Basic Medical Sciences
Purdue University Veterinary Teaching Hospital
West Lafayette, Indiana

ELSEVIER

Elsevier
3251 Riverport Lane
St. Louis, Missouri 63043

BILL'S CLINICAL PHARMACOLOGY AND THERAPEUTICS FOR VETERINARY
TECHNICIANS, FIFTH EDITION

ISBN: 978-0-323-88040-4

Notice

Practitioners and researchers must always rely on their own experience and knowledge in evaluating and
using any information, methods, compounds or experiments described herein. Because of rapid advances
in the medical sciences, in particular, independent verification of diagnoses and drug dosages should be
made. To the fullest extent of the law, no responsibility is assumed by Elsevier, authors, editors or contributors
for any injury and/or damage to persons or property as a matter of products liability, negligence or otherwise,
or from any use or operation of any methods, products, instructions, or ideas contained in the material herein.

Previous editions copyrighted 2017, 2006, 1997, 1993.

Content Strategist: Melissa Rawe
Content Development Manager: Ranjana Sharma
Senior Content Development Specialist: Vaishali Singh
Publishing Services Manager: Deepthi Unni
Project Manager: Nayagi Anandan
Designer: Margaret Reid

Printed in India

Last digit is the print number: 9   8   7   6   5   4   3   2   1

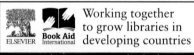

To all veterinary technology students, past, present, and future.

To Dr. Pete Bill, one of the greatest professors I was privileged to be taught and mentored by. He has graciously transferred authorship to me to be able to bring this edition to all veterinary technology students, past, present, and future.

REVIEWERS

Jim Budde, PharmD, FSVHP, DICVP
Pharmacy Manager, UW Veterinary Care
School of Veterinary Medicine University of
   Wisconsin-Madison
Madison, Wisconsin

Joseph G. Herman, BS, RVT
Veterinary Medical Writer
Moorpark, California

PREFACE

THE CHANGING ROLE OF VETERINARY TECHNICIANS

The expectations for today's veterinary technician in terms of the technician's level of performance, degree of medical understanding, and ability to make independent decisions are different from those for the technician we educated 10 or 15 years ago. When the profession began, the primary role of the veterinary technician was to be an extension of the veterinarian's hands; therefore, the technician was used primarily for completing manual procedures and tasks.

Today, with the increasing sophistication of veterinary care, contemporary veterinary practice has shifted toward utilizing the veterinary technician not only to complete nursing/surgical techniques quickly and efficiently but also to work more independently to assess and monitor patient status, to implement therapeutic protocols, and to obtain or perform needed diagnostic procedures. Today's well-utilized veterinary technician often works on a team with the veterinarian and the veterinary assistants and depends heavily on medical knowledge, problem-solving skills, management skills, and decision-making skills to carry out his or her responsibilities. Thus today's veterinary technician must *know and think* as well as "do."

A greater understanding of the medicine and science behind the diagnostics, therapeutics, and surgical interventions used in veterinary medicine is essential for today's veterinary technician to effectively assess his or her patient's current status, anticipate the patient's immediate medical and nursing needs, know what the veterinarian is likely to need next, and be one step ahead of the progression of the patient's condition. Knowledge of clinical pharmacology and therapeutics helps the veterinary technician function in this manner.

The breadth and depth of information in clinical pharmacology and therapeutics at the veterinary technician level have increased as the sophistication of veterinary medicine has advanced. When the first edition of this veterinary technician pharmacology text was published in 1993, it was the only one of its kind. Today there are many texts on pharmacology and therapeutics targeted toward veterinary technicians as well as regular features in the veterinary technician journals that present current information on drugs and therapeutic agents. Though this text was originally titled *Pharmacology for Veterinary Technicians,* the subsequent editions were appropriately retitled to reflect the need for *understanding* the clinical applications of these drugs.

Like its predecessors, this edition provides understandable explanations of the "how" and "why" behind drugs, their actions, their mechanisms, and their problems. In this fifth edition, all drug groups have been updated to reflect changes in both the therapeutic agents themselves and the medical philosophies that determine how these drugs are used in different species. The self-assessment test questions at the end of the chapters also provide an excellent review of pharmacology and therapeutic knowledge for certification examinations. A convenient answer key for all of the questions is included to assist in the reader's review of the content and for self-testing.

Instructors will find the "systems" organization of the chapters easy to follow and to modify as needed to fit their own curricula or program emphasis. The questions at the back of the chapters can readily be modified to create an examination for the classroom while still providing the students with a review of the content in each chapter.

My ultimate goal with this text is to help improve veterinary care, animal health, and patient well-being by helping veterinary technicians understand how and why drugs work the way they do. By using this text to understand how drugs can be safely used and how potential problems can be avoided, a veterinary technician will be able to provide better care for his or her patients as well as to help educate the owners who love these patients.

"As veterinary professionals, our education is not for our own benefit but for the benefit of all the patients we serve."

PETE BILL

I am very honored and humbled to take over authorship of this textbook. Dr. Pete Bill has a great passion for improving veterinary patient care through the education of veterinary technicians. I am dedicated to carrying on his legacy through providing important medication and regulation updates through each edition of this textbook moving forward. New medications are released more frequently than we can keep up with in this textbook; therefore, it is important that the veterinary technician build on the foundational principles attained from this textbook to understand the new medications discovered to use in their daily practice.

"Your patient depends on you to always practice at the top of your license regardless of what other distractions are on your mind. It is your responsibility to provide the right medication at the right dose, time, and frequency to the right patient every time."

MELINDA ANDERSON

CONTENTS

Veterinary Pharmacology and the Veterinary Technician: An Introduction to Understanding Therapeutic Applications

OBJECTIVES

After studying this chapter, the veterinary technician should be able to:

- Describe why a veterinary technician needs to know pharmacology to serve patients, clients, and the public.
- Explain the four crucial rules that should be used to guide safe drug usage.
- Recognize and explain the differences among the chemical, nonproprietary, generic, proprietary, trade, and brand names of drugs.
- Explain why, as a general rule, the original drug is almost always more expensive than the generic equivalent drug.
- Describe and explain the difference between an over-the-counter (OTC) drug and a legend drug.
- Recognize and describe the common solid, liquid, and semisolid dosage forms.
- Recognize and describe the purpose for the shape of caplets, the presence of enteric coating, and the sustained-release (SR) drugs.
- Describe the differences in physical composition and uses of drug suspensions vs solutions.

- Describe why some sugar-free syrups should not be used in dogs.
- Identify where a veterinary technician can find accurate and reliable drug information and the limitations inherent in each type of information source.
- Explain what extra-label or off-label means and why extra-label drug use (ELDU) needs to be controlled to protect the public.
- Explain what the drug information heading (including symbols) and each section or paragraph of a drug description tell about the drug.
- Explain and apply the meanings of precautions, warnings, and contraindications.
- List and describe the criteria for acceptable ELDU.
- Explain the difference between the types of drugs regulated by the FDA vs the Environmental Protection Agency (EPA).
- Describe the steps needed to report adverse drug reactions (ADRs).

KEY TERMS

active ingredient
adverse drug reaction (ADR)
Animal Medicinal Drug Use
    Clarification Act of 1994
    (AMDUCA)
ampules
aqueous solution
bioequivalence
black box warning
boxed warning
brand name
caplet
capsules
chemical name
clinical pharmacology
contraindications
controlled-release coatings
controlled substance
creams
depot forms
dosage form
drug formularies
drug insert
elixirs
emulsion
enteric coating
Environmental Protection Agency
    (EPA)
excipients

extract
extra-label drug use (ELDU)
Food and Drug Administration
    (FDA)
gel caps
gels
generic equivalent
generic name
implants
indication
inert ingredients
injectable dosage forms
insoluble
label information
legend drugs
liniments
liquid dosage forms
lotions
lozenge
medium
molded tablets
multidose vials
nonproprietary name
off-label use
ointments
over-the-counter (OTC)
package insert
pastes
pharmacology

precaution
proprietary name
repository dosage form
"Rx" symbol
schedule drug
semisolid dosage forms
side effect
single-dose vials
solid dosage form
soluble
solution
suppositories
suspension
sustained-release (SR) drugs
syrups
tablets
therapeutics.
tinctures.
trademark (™)
trade name
troche
United States Adopted Names (USAN)
    Council
United States Pharmacopeia (USP)
veterinarian-client-patient relationship
    (VCPR)
warning
withdrawal time/period
xylitol

ROLE AND RESPONSIBILITIES OF TODAY'S VETERINARY TECHNICIAN AND TECHNOLOGIST

"Today's veterinary technician is a professional and, as such, has the responsibility to understand the reasons and the expected outcomes for the treatments he or she performs. Today's veterinary technician is more than a skilled set of hands. Today's veterinary technician must know how to critically evaluate, problem solve, think, and adapt to his or her patient's needs."

Pete Bill, DVM, PhD, during a panel presentation on the topic of veterinary technician and paraprofessional utilization at the American Association of Veterinary Medical Colleges meeting, Washington, D.C.

Veterinary medicine as a whole continues to become more sophisticated in all aspects of diagnostics, mechanics of diseases, surgery, and therapeutics. Accordingly, veterinary technicians today must be much more sophisticated in their understanding of veterinary medicine than they were 10 years ago. Although technicians are still legally prohibited from making diagnoses, performing surgeries, rendering prognoses, and prescribing treatments, today's veterinary technician has the responsibility to understand why the diagnosis was made, why the surgery was performed, why the prognosis was rendered, and why the treatment was prescribed.

◉ MYTHS AND MISCONCEPTIONS

To be a great veterinary technician requires only being really good at technical skills.

False! To be a really great veterinary technician requires having good technical skills and a strong understanding of the science and medicine behind the nursing and technical skills.

WHY IS PHARMACOLOGY IMPORTANT FOR VETERINARY TECHNICIANS?

Pharmacology is the study of how drugs behave in the body. Applying pharmacology to specific treatments is called clinical pharmacology or therapeutics. To be effective as a contributing member of the veterinary team, veterinary technicians should know more than just the names of medications or the route by which the drugs are administered; they must understand the "why" behind the clinical pharmacology and therapeutics of the medications they are giving in order to better protect and serve the nursing needs of their patients.

Knowledge of how drugs change physiology, how the drug's beneficial effect alters the patient's clinical signs, and how adverse drug reactions (ADRs) will appear in patients is an important subset of veterinary nursing knowledge that distinguishes well-educated veterinary technicians and technologists from individuals who have largely learned their nursing skills through an apprenticeship model of education.

For example, a veterinary technician with in-depth knowledge of anesthetic drugs will be able to more accurately evaluate an anesthetized patient's status, determine whether there is an abnormal physiologic response to the anesthetic drug, and then appropriately correct the anesthetic administration to avert an anesthetic crisis. A veterinary technician with a good understanding of how antibiotics, anti-inflammatories, or other drugs affect the body's physiology can more quickly identify a potentially severe drug side effect in a hospitalized patient. Finally, a deeper understanding of pharmacology of dispensed medications will allow the veterinary technician to identify clues in a pet owner's casual comments that might indicate the early appearance of an unexpected change in the patient's response to the drug. By having a strong working knowledge of how drugs affect the body in all of these situations, the veterinary technician can alert the veterinarian to potential patient/drug problems at an earlier stage and thus increase the chances of successfully reversing or avoiding the drug's side effect.

Understanding veterinary pharmacology will also provide veterinary technicians with a more medically correct understanding of veterinary drug-related problems or animal-related issues that appear in the popular press, on television, or on the Internet. For example, the link between veterinary drug residues in livestock meat, milk, or eggs used for human consumption and the development of bacterial resistance to human antibiotics is often surrounded by a cloud of information that may not be entirely correct. Many television newscasts or Internet postings reduce these complex issues to audience-capturing sound bytes or headlines, resulting in public misinformation or fear. A veterinary technician who is well informed about the science behind the issue can be the voice of reason that counters the unfounded rumors or misconceptions with medical fact.

Thus, one of the primary goals of this textbook is to help veterinary technician and technology students become familiar with the "why" behind veterinary clinical pharmacology so they can better serve the needs of their patients, the veterinary team, and the general public.

FOUR RULES TO LIVE BY FOR SAFE DRUG USAGE

Rule #1: All Drugs Are Poisons

Every drug is a poison. Every drug administered has the potential to save a life or to take a life. The only difference between whether a drug kills or saves life is often the way in which the drug is administered. For example, arsenic is generally recognized as a deadly "poison." But small amounts of arsenic compounds are used to safely treat heartworm disease in dogs. Likewise, drugs that might otherwise devastate an animal's (or person's) bone marrow production of cells critical to life can also be used successfully to kill deadly cancer cells. Even common drugs found in almost every household can be beneficial or deadly depending on their administration. For example, the drug acetaminophen is safe for use in human beings, is moderately tolerated by dogs, but can easily kill a cat. Thus the selection, the amount, or the

method of administration of a medication can potentially determine whether a drug cures or kills.

Rule #2: No Drug Is a Silver Bullet

Drugs are not "silver bullets" that magically seek out and destroy a disease or miraculously correct a clinical condition. Drugs work by altering the normal physiology; every drug has physiologic effects on the body other than the intended beneficial effect for which the drug was used. Effective use of drugs involves knowing how to maximize the beneficial changes while minimizing the bad physiologic effects.

The drug alteration of normal physiology is often complicated by the physiology alterations caused by the disease process, the animal's gender, species, breed, or age. In other words, appropriate administration of drugs requires the veterinarian and the veterinary technician to understand the individual patient's particular physiology and its complex interactions among the drug effect, the disease effect, and the individual genetic or environmental variables. Thus no drug is a "silver bullet" that will always behave in the same way for the same disease in all animals.

Rule #3: All Doses Are Guesses

The dosage in the manufacturer's drug information is an estimation of the actual amount of drug a specific patient will need for a particular disease. Because of the physiologic variables stated in Rule #2, the dose calculated for any particular patient is actually a scientific guess based on how the population of animals is supposed to behave when given the drug.

Granted, the "guess" is probably a very good guess, because the dosage was determined from clinical trials done in large numbers of animals to represent the entire population of similar animals. Although the actual dosage constitutes the amount of drug needed for the majority of animals of that breed with that particular disease, if the individual patient has genetic characteristics, physiologic changes caused by disease or environmental factors that were not found in the majority of animals, the resulting dose could be too much or too little for this particular patient. Thus, the veterinary professional must always consider these factors and modify the dose as needed to match the specific physiologic needs of the patient.

MYTHS AND MISCONCEPTIONS

All drug dosages used in veterinary medicine are based on controlled scientific trials and medical evidence specifically for veterinary patients.

False! Although dosages approved by the FDA or other drug regulatory agencies in countries outside of the United States are based on clinical trials and protocols required for drug approval, many of the dosages reported in case studies or textbooks are based on the clinician's personal experience or generally accepted standards of treatment based in part on anecdotal evidence. With the increasing emphasis on "evidence-based medicine," many older drug dosages are being reexamined to determine whether there is a scientific validity for the recommended dosage. In some cases, this reexamination has led to changes in recommended dosages. The veterinary technician needs to keep up-to-date on current drug dosages to assure that the patient receiving the drug is receiving the appropriate amount of medication for the condition.

Rule #4: Complacency Kills

Veterinary practices often use the same relatively small group of drugs over and over on most of their patients. With repeated successful use of these drugs a natural complacency about the drug's potential to do harm can develop. Unfortunately, this expectation for safe and beneficial effects on 100% of the patients means that the veterinarian administering the drug or the veterinary technician monitoring the treated animal may forget rules #1, #2, and #3 mentioned earlier. When these rules are forgotten and vigilance for adverse effects decreases, the clinical signs of an adverse drug effect may be overlooked until significant damage to the patient has occurred.

Thus, by remembering that all drugs are poisons all the time, that no drug truly behaves exactly the same way in any two patients, and that all doses we give are approximations, complacency can be held in check and vigilance for adverse drug effects maintained.

LEARNING THE VOCABULARY: TERMINOLOGY USED TO DESCRIBE THERAPEUTIC AGENTS

Drug Names

Drugs are generally referred to by three different names (Fig. 1.1). The chemical name, such as "D(−)-α-amino-*p*-hydroxybenzyl-penicillin trihydrate," describes the chemical composition or molecular structure of a drug (in this case, amoxicillin) and is used by chemists and pharmacologists but is of little practical use for the veterinary professional.

The nonproprietary name, also called the generic name, is a more concise name given to the specific chemical compound. Examples of nonproprietary names include "aspirin," "acetaminophen," and "amoxicillin" and are compounds produced by many different drug manufacturers. The nonproprietary names are also listed as the active ingredients on drug labels.

In contrast to nonproprietary names, the proprietary name, trade name, or brand name is a unique name a manufacturer gives its particular brand of a drug. For example, one manufacturer may produce amoxicillin under the trade name Amoxi-Tabs, but another manufacturer produces its own brand as Amoxil.

Certain trade names are so well integrated into our veterinary/medical culture that they are often erroneously used to describe or represent medications produced by other drug companies. For example, it is common to hear the trade name Tylenol used for any acetaminophen product, the trade name Lasix used for furosemide products, and the trade name Valium for any diazepam tranquilizer.

Because trade names are proper nouns, their first letter is capitalized like other proper nouns (e.g., Mary, Indiana, or Chicago). The trade names are followed by the marks ® or ™ to signify that the trade name is a registered trademark and cannot legally be used by other manufacturers.

❓ ASK DR. BILL

Question:

Dr. Bill, how do they come up with all those strange names for drugs?

Answer:

When drug companies patent a new drug, they have to first come up with a generic name. There are some rules and conventions for naming generic drugs based on the drug group to which the drug belongs. A drug company with a new drug can submit up to three possible generic names to the United States Adopted Names (USAN) Council, which is the body that selects generic drug names. Any USAN Council name must be checked with the World Health Organization (WHO) to make sure the selected name is not too similar to another drug name used in another country. Estimates vary, but it is generally accepted that *thousands* of people are injured or die from the wrong drug being administered because the drug's name was too similar to another drug.

Trade names are created by marketing agencies but still have to be approved by the USAN Council and must be approved by the FDA's Office of Postmarketing Drug Risk Assessment to make sure that the trade name does not sound like any other trade name and that the trade name does not try to convey what the drug claims to do (thus there will be no Goze-to-Sleep sleep aid). Here are a couple of other points cited in an article from the *Stanford Medicine Magazine,* June 7, 2005.

- Generic drug names do not begin with letters "H," "J," "K," or "W" because those letters do not exist in some of the countries that use US generic names or have different sounds in different languages.
- The USAN Council will no longer approve generic names starting with "X" or "Z" because these letters sound alike when used at the beginning of drug names.
- Marketing agencies love the letter "X" in their drug trade names—it makes the drug name sound "technical."
- Marketing agencies feel that the letters "X," "F," "S," or "Z" are thought to convey speed. The letters "P," "T," or "D" imply power.

For additional information about the screening process by which the FDA reviews drug names, go to the FDA website (www.fda.gov) and use their search engine to find "drug names."

Source:

Ipaktchian S. Take two whatchamacollits and call me in the morning. *Stanford Medicine Magazine.* June 7, 2005.

CHEMICAL NAME	NONPROPRIETARY NAME	PROPRIETARY/TRADE NAME
D(-)-α-amino-*p*-hydroxybenzyl-penicillin trihydrate	amoxicillin	Amoxi-Drop® Biomox® Robamox-V®
[(3-phenoxyphenyl) methyl *cis-trans*-3-(2,2-dichloroethenyl)-2,2-dimethylcyclopropanecarboxylate)]	permethrin insecticide	Atroban® Defend® Flysect®
dl 2-(*o*-chlorophenyl)-2-(methylamino) cyclohexanone hydrochloride	ketamine hydrochloride	Ketaset® Vetalar®

Fig. 1.1 Types of drug names.

Note that some "generic brand" drugs do not have a specific trade name but simply use the nonproprietary name or the active ingredient on their label, as seen in Fig. 1.2. This is common with older drugs such as aspirin, penicillin, or prednisone, which have been produced by many drug manufacturers and for which a unique trade name provides no advantage in marketing the drug.

Generic Equivalents

When a drug company develops a new drug, obtains the patents, and completes all of the extensive testing required to obtain Food and Drug Administration (FDA) approval to market the new drug, that company has the exclusive rights to manufacture this drug for a number of years. During that time, no other drug manufacturer can produce the same drug. In the United States, this exclusive protection of manufacturing rights extends 20 years from when the patent of the drug was approved. However, the approval of the patent typically occurs several years before the drug actually reaches the market. Thus, the effective time for which the company has exclusive rights to manufacture the drug is typically 7–12 years after the drug has been released to market.[1] This period of exclusive manufacturing theoretically allows the original "parent" drug company to recover the costs of the research, development, and testing required to bring the drug to market.

After the exclusive manufacture rights expire, other companies are then permitted to produce the drug. Drugs produced or marketed by companies other than the original "brand" developer are called generic equivalent drugs because they have active ingredients equivalent to those of the original compound but are not produced by the original manufacturer. Generic equivalents are usually sold at a much lower price than the original manufacturer's product because the generic drug producer did not have to underwrite the original drug development, testing, and marketing costs of the parent or brand drug. Typically, when generic versions of drugs become available, the market economics drive down the cost for both the original brand drug and the generic versions.

Extracts

In addition to the drug names listed earlier, a drug may be called an extract, a term that describes where the drug came from. An extract is a therapeutic agent composed of specially prepared plant or animal parts rather than synthesized chemicals in a laboratory. Examples of extracts include thyroid supplements made from pig or cattle thyroid glands and pancreatic enzyme powder extract derived from prepared livestock pancreas. Many health food stores sell extracts of plants and plant materials for a wide variety of purposes.

The veterinary extract products made by major drug manufacturers must produce reasonably consistent effects from bottle

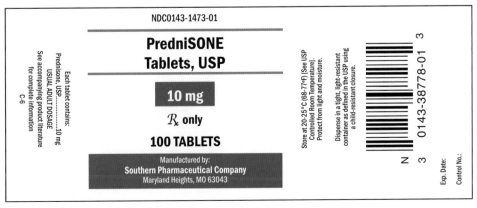

Fig. 1.2 The generic drug label.

to bottle of extract to be approved by the FDA. However, extracts marketed as "nutraceuticals" (nutritional supplements) are not required to be registered with the FDA, and the potency of different batches of drug extract may vary as a result of variation in amounts of extracted natural drug contained in the plant or animal part. Although extracts are often less expensive to purchase, they may not provide as consistent a clinical response to the active ingredient of the drug as a compound developed by conventional manufacturing processes.

Legend Drugs vs Over-the-Counter Drugs

A trip down the aisle at the drugstore reveals that drugs for headaches, coughs, colds, flu, or diarrhea are available for anyone to purchase without a prescription from a doctor or veterinarian. Such medications are referred to as over-the-counter (OTC), drugs. These drugs typically contain either an ingredient that is very safe to use or such low concentrations of an active ingredient that it is difficult to accidentally use the drug in a harmful way. Examples of OTC drugs in veterinary medicine include pet vitamins, flea products for use on the surface of the skin, and dietary supplements.

Most veterinary drugs used to treat or prevent disease are legend drugs, meaning that they are limited to dispensing by or on the order of a licensed prescriber (veterinarian or physician). Legend drugs contain ingredients that require greater control of dispensing either because of their toxic effects, potential to be abused or diverted as an illegal substance, or potential to do harm to the patient or the person handling the drug.

Each state or Canadian province regulates control over the prescription of legend drugs. Generally, however, legend drugs cannot be dispensed to a client or animal owner without a valid prescription written for an animal for which a valid veterinarian-client-patient relationship (VCPR) has been established. Legally, a VCPR means that the veterinarian has examined or has adequate medical knowledge of the patient and has agreed to assume responsibility for veterinary care of the patient. Thus, it is against the law for a veterinarian to prescribe medication for a patient he or she has not seen.

If the veterinarian orders legend medication to be dispensed from his or her own veterinary hospital, the veterinarian or veterinary technician may legally fill this drug order in that same hospital (it would not technically be called a prescription in this case). However, it is illegal for a veterinary technician or veterinarian to fill a prescription from another veterinary practice because that would be considered the definition of pharmacy practice and hence is limited to regulated pharmacies and registered pharmacists. More information on prescriptions and drug orders are in Chapter 2.

🔎 ASK DR. BILL

Question:
Dr. Bill, why is it that some veterinary products I get from my veterinarian, especially flea products, are also sold at grocery stores, farm supply stores, and drugstores as OTC products? Aren't they also legend products and hence only available by prescription?

Answer:
The FDA, as the name implies, is charged with regulating and maintaining the safety of food, food products, drugs, blood products, biologics (e.g., vaccines), and medical devices. The **Environmental Protection Agency (EPA)** has responsibility for pesticides as part of its charge to protect the environment. Flea and tick products applied to the surface of the skin and hair (applied topically) are considered pesticides and hence regulated by the EPA. EPA products do not require a prescription to be dispensed or obtained by the public (although stronger pesticides can only be used by certified pest control operators). Therefore, almost all of the flea powders, tick collars, insect dips, some spot-on applications, and other topically applied applications can be dispensed OTC and thus are found in your local grocery store. Many drug companies will only sell their veterinary topical OTC flea and tick medications to veterinarians to sell to their clients. This practice allows the veterinary staff to provide appropriate product education to the client for appropriate product utilization.

Note, however, that if an insecticide is administered internally (e.g., some orally administered heartworm preventatives like Heartgard™) or is applied topically and then absorbed into the body (e.g., topical deworming or heartworm medications like Revolution™), then this product would be considered a drug, it would be regulated by the FDA, and in most cases would be classified as a veterinary legend drug and thus only available by prescription from a licensed veterinarian.

Source:
https://www.fda.gov/animal-veterinary/unapproved-animal-drugs/how-can-i-tell-if-flea-and-tick-product-approved-fda-animal-drug-or-registered-epa-pesticide. Accessed 05.23.22.

THE DOSAGE FORM

Another way drugs are described is by their dosage form. A drug's dosage form is the description of its physical appearance and is typically included in the drug's description in the package insert and the drug label. Examples of dosage forms include solid dosage forms like tablets or capsules; liquid dosage forms like syrups, suspensions, or liniments; and a variety of semisolid dosage forms that do not easily fit the "solid" or "liquid" categories, such as gels, ointments, creams, and pastes.

Solid Dosage Forms

Tablets are created by compressing powdered active ingredients and other inert ingredients called excipients together to form disk-shaped dosage forms (Fig. 1.3). Excipients help the tablet

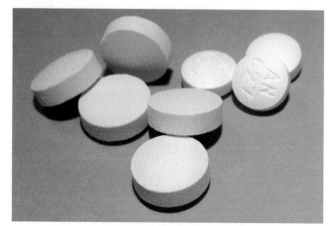

Fig. 1.3 Picture of typical tablets of compressed powdered drug. (Courtesy Robert Bill.)

perform as it is intended and may include binders (to hold the tablet together), disintegrants (to make the tablet break up more easily), diluents (to fill up the bulk of the tablet not occupied by the active ingredient), flavoring agents, or even colors to make the dosage form distinctive or identifiable (e.g., red tablets may be 100 mg of drug but blue tablets may be 200 mg of drug). Tablets are not the same as pills.

⊚ MYTHS AND MISCONCEPTIONS

The disk-shaped dosage forms commonly used as oral medications in veterinary medicine are pills.

False! Although tablets are commonly called pills by nonprofessionals, a pill describes an ancient dosage form made by rolling a soft mass of active ingredient(s) into a spherical shape. The veterinary technician should always use professional language when communicating dosage forms.

Sometimes tablets are pressed into an oblong or elongated dosage form roughly similar in shape to a capsule. Because these dosage forms are solid like a tablet but shaped like a capsule, this dosage form is referred to as a caplet. The idea behind the elongated form is to facilitate swallowing of the dosage form when it aligns with the esophagus at the back of the throat (Fig. 1.4).

Tablets or caplets may have a mark across them ("scoring") to help break the dosage form into halves or, less frequently, quarters. As a general rule, tablets used in veterinary medicine are rarely broken into anything less than halves unless a human formulation of drug is used in a small veterinary patient and requires quartering to provide the appropriate dose of the drug. Tablets or caplets without scoring should typically not be split.

Molded tablets are also called "chewable tablets" and consist of the active ingredient drug in powdered form mixed with lactose, sucrose, or dextrose and a flavoring agent to encourage the patient to chew the soft tablet. Examples of molded tablets include chewable vitamins, chewable heartworm preventives, and chewable antiinflammatory drugs (Fig. 1.5).

Tablet Coatings

Tablets are often coated after being compressed. Although sugar coating was commonly used in the past, today's coatings are

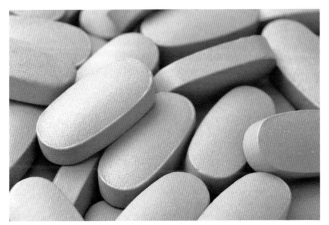

Fig. 1.4 Compressed powdered drug tablet in the shape of a capsule for easier swallowing; also called a caplet. (Copyright © iStock.com.)

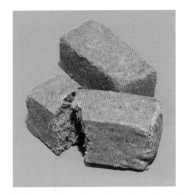

Fig. 1.5 Chewable tablet. (Courtesy Robert Bill.)

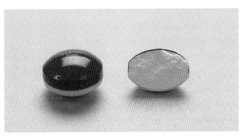

Fig. 1.6 Special enteric-coated tablet to protect drug from stomach acid. (From Klieger D. *Essentials of Medical Assisting*. 2nd ed. Maryland Heights: Saunders; 2010.)

more sophisticated polymers and complex sugar molecules and are used to protect the tablet from breaking apart during shipping or storage, to cover up an unpleasant taste of the active ingredient, to provide a smoother finish for easier swallowing, to protect the underlying tablet from disintegration from absorption of moisture, or even to protect light-sensitive drugs from degradation caused by light. The coloring of the tablet coating also allows drug manufacturers to make the tablet distinctive. The drug manufacturer may also print identification numbers or other markings on the tablet coating.

There are two special coatings: enteric coating and controlled-release coating. Enteric coating is designed to protect the active ingredient from the harsh acidic environment of the stomach by not allowing the tablet to dissolve until it reaches the more alkaline environment of the small intestine (Fig. 1.6).

Controlled-release coatings slow the rate at which the tablet dissolves as the tablet moves along the intestinal tract, resulting in a more gradual and sustained release of the active ingredient as opposed to being released all at once. Such controlled-release coated drugs are also referred to as sustained-release (SR) drugs. The SR properties of the drug may be a result of the coating, the construction of the entire solid dosage form, or a combination of both. SR drugs are sometimes identified in the proprietary trade name with an "SR" designation to distinguish the drug from the normal release dosage form. "Delayed-release" and "extended-release" are other controlled-release dosage forms.

Important note: Enteric coated or controlled-release coated tablets should not be split because this ruins the function of the special tablet coating.

One of the disadvantages of using a human SR tablet in a veterinary patient is that the human SR drug is designed to be released over the length of the human gastrointestinal (GI) tract and dog and cat GI tracts are shorter than the human GI tract. A medium-sized dog's tract is around 13 ft (3.9 m) long, and cat's tracts are typically about 5–6 ft (about 1.7 m) long, compared with 22 ft (7 m) for the average human GI tract.[2] Thus, SR tablets designed to dissolve in the longer human GI tract may not dissolve completely in a dog or cat before they pass out in the feces.

Gel caps or capsules are powdered drug surrounded by a capsule made of gelatin, modified starch, or cellulose (Fig. 1.7). Just like with tablets, the capsule itself can be modified to make it harder, softer, more stable, more readily dissolvable, colored, or lubricated for easier swallowing. Although popular for use in human patients, capsules are less popular with veterinary patients because they may stick to the surface of the mouth when administered, making it easier for the animal to spit out the capsule or chew it to release the powdered contents in the mouth.

The lozenge or troche (pronounced TROH´-key) dosage form incorporates the drug into a hard, candy-like tablet like those found in human cough drops, throat lozenges for sore throat, or some breath mints. Because veterinary patients never hold these dosage forms in their mouths long enough to receive the beneficial effect, they are not used in veterinary medicine.

Although most solid dosage forms are associated with oral administration of drugs, many forms are also formulated to be used as suppositories. Suppositories are dosage forms designed to be placed in the rectum where they dissolve and release drug that is then absorbed across the intestinal wall of the rectum. A common use for suppository drugs is in veterinary patients that are vomiting and cannot take medications by mouth. Suppositories containing anticonvulsant drugs (antiseizure drugs) may be used by dog owners at home to stop a pet's epileptic seizure.

Liquid Dosage Forms

Liquid dosage forms are classified as solutions or suspensions. A solution is a drug completely dissolved in a clear liquid medium. The liquid medium (equivalent in chemistry to the solvent) can be water, alcohol, or other liquid into which the drug is capable of dissolving.

In contrast to solutions, suspensions are often cloudy, opaque liquids in which the drug has been suspended (is "hanging" in the liquid medium) but has not been completely dissolved. Typically, the drug particles in the suspension will settle to the bottom of the drug bottle, requiring the bottle be shaken to resuspend the drug before the drug is withdrawn from the bottle or administered (Fig. 1.8). Failure to completely resuspend the drug will result in a greater concentration of drug near the bottom of the bottle than at the top and result in unpredictable amounts of the drug that are actually withdrawn with the liquid from the bottle.

Solutions and suspensions used in veterinary medicine are further characterized by the way the liquid dosage form is used and the liquid medium into which the drug has been dissolved or suspended. An aqueous solution has a water medium in which the drug has been dissolved. Often drug molecules are chemically modified by adding a sodium, potassium, or chloride molecule to the drug molecule to make the drug totally soluble (i.e., able to be dissolved) in the water medium (e.g., potassium ampicillin). Aqueous solutions are often used as intravenous (IV) injectable dosage forms.

Syrups are drugs dissolved in a liquid sugar solution (e.g., 65% sucrose solution). The sugar solution is designed to mask

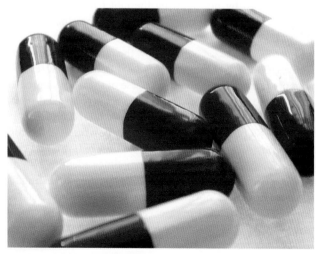

Fig. 1.7 Powdered drug enclosed in gelatin capsule. (Copyright © iStock.com.)

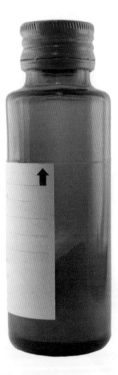

Fig. 1.8 Because drugs in suspension are not dissolved in the liquid, they precipitate out and the bottle must be shaken to resuspend the drug before administration. (Copyright © iStock.com.)

the unpleasant taste of the active ingredient and to act as a preservative. Diluting a syrup solution with water lowers the sugar concentration of the syrup, potentially making the solution an excellent nutrient base for growth of yeast and bacteria. Thus, dilution of syrups is not recommended.

Sugar-free syrups are aqueous solutions into which other sweet-tasting compounds like sorbitol or aspartame have been added. One artificial sweetener that should not be used with dogs is xylitol (pronounced ZI´-leh-tahl). Although xylitol is tolerated by humans and found in many sugar-free gums, candy, peanut butter and human oral solutions (ex: commercial gabapentin), xylitol in dogs causes a massive release of insulin. This insulin release is due to the absorption of xylitol into systemic circulation in dogs that does not occur in other species. In the dog, this results in a hypoglycemic (low blood sugar) crisis and/or damages the liver, possibly resulting in death. Thus, compounding pharmacies (where the pharmacist creates a dosage form) should never create xylitol-based syrups for use in dogs.[2]

! YOU NEED TO KNOW

Why Shouldn't "Sugar-Free" Human Syrups Be Used in Dogs?

Xylitol is an artificial sweetener found in many sugar-free gums, peanut butter and human prescriptions. In dogs, xylitol causes massive release of insulin, causing blood sugar to drop as the insulin moves the glucose from the blood into the tissues. In some cases, this drop in blood sugar (i.e., glucose) has resulted in a hypoglycemic crisis resulting in death. More recently, it has been shown that xylitol can also produce significant liver damage. Thus xylitol-based syrups should never be used in dogs.

Source:
Schmid RD, Hovda LR. Acute hepatic failure in a dog after xylitol ingestion. *J Med Toxicol.* 2016;12(2):201–205. doi: https://doi.org/10.1007/s13181-015-0531-7. PMID: 26691320; PMCID: PMC4880608.

Tinctures and elixirs are alcohol-based solutions used for oral or topical (on the surface of the skin) application. Many drugs are insoluble (unable to be dissolved) in water; thus, to create a true solution for these drugs, an alcohol medium may be required. In herbal medications, the active ingredients are often extracted from leaves or other plant parts using alcohol to form herbal tinctures. Although most tinctures are alcohol based, there are "nonalcoholic" tinctures where glycerin or vinegar is used in place of the alcohol.

Elixirs tend to have sweetening agents added to the alcohol to help mask the taste of the drug or the alcohol medium. Elixirs are typically associated with oral use, but tinctures can be used both orally and topically. Because the alcohol taste is often very strong with elixirs or tinctures, they are difficult to administer orally to veterinary patients. It is important to remember that topically applied tinctures have an alcohol medium and if they contact an open wound on the skin, the tincture will cause a great deal of pain. Although technically tinctures contain a higher percentage solution of ethanol (i.e., alcohol) than elixirs, the differences between these two dosage formulations are of little practical concern for the veterinary technician. Because alcohol and water do not mix, alcohol-based dosage forms should not be diluted with water.

An emulsion is a liquid suspension composed of two liquids that do not readily mix together. Thus, an emulsion can be thought of as one liquid suspended in a second liquid medium. Diet supplements that contain dietary oils suspended in water are an example of an emulsion. Propofol, a short-acting injectable anesthetic agent, is another example. Because one liquid (typically the drug or active ingredient) is suspended and not dissolved in the second liquid, an emulsion typically appears as an opaque or cloudy white- or tan-colored liquid and if left alone will usually settle into two distinct layers of liquid. Like any suspension, an emulsion should be stirred or shaken to resuspend the active ingredient before the emulsion is dispensed.

Many liquid lotions are emulsions of oil and water plus additional ingredients that help keep the two liquid layers from separating. Topically applied lotions include hand creams, antibiotic lotions, antifungal lotions, or antiseptic lotions.

Liniments are topically applied liquid dosage forms that may be an emulsion, a solution, or a suspension. The characteristic of a liniment is that it is always applied by rubbing it into the skin. Balms are an example of a liniment dosage form. Liniments are most commonly used in equine medicine to reduce muscle stiffness in race horses or as alcohol liniments used to cool horses through the evaporation of the alcohol component and the vasodilating effect of the liniment itself.

Other Dosage Forms Used in Veterinary Medicine

Semisolid dosage forms are those that are neither liquid nor solid and include dosage forms such as ointments, creams, pastes, and gels. Ointments and creams can be either suspensions or solutions that liquefy at body temperatures when applied topically to the skin, eye, ear, or mucous membranes (Fig. 1.9). By liquefying, the ointment or cream can more readily spread across or into an area such as the ear canal. In veterinary medicine, ointments are more commonly used than the thicker emulsion creams found in human cosmetic preparations.

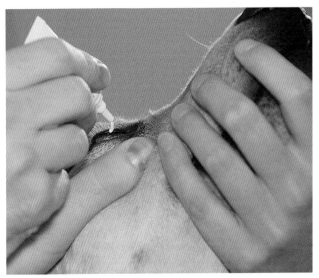

Fig. 1.9 Ointments are semisolid but liquefy at body temperature. (From Taylor S. *Small Animal Clinical Techniques.* 2nd ed. St. Louis: Elsevier; 2016.)

In contrast to semiliquid creams and ointments, pastes are semisolid, orally administered suspension dosage forms that tend to keep their semisolid form at body temperature. Pastes are commonly packaged in large plastic syringes for administering deworming medications orally to horses, cattle, sheep, and occasionally dogs. Gels are drugs suspended in a semisolid or jellylike form, such as toothpaste or certain human cosmetic preparations.

Injectable dosage forms are administered by a needle and syringe. Injectables are often referred to by the type of container in which the drug is supplied. For example, ampules are dosage forms in which the drug is contained within a small, airtight thin glass bottle that is opened by snapping the narrow neck of the ampule bottle (Fig. 1.10). Drugs contained within ampules typically do not have preservatives; therefore, the entire contents of the ampule are intended to be used at one time and must be filtered to remove glass particles created when the neck is snapped.

Vials are thicker glass bottles with rubber stoppers through which the drug is withdrawn with a sterile needle and syringe. Vials may be multidose vials, in which multiple doses can be withdrawn over time, or single-dose vials, in which all the drug is used at once. Most injectable drugs in veterinary medicine come in the multidose vial form. The single-dose vial is most commonly used with vaccines. The rubber stopper on multidose vials should be kept clean to prevent inserted needles from carrying bacteria or contaminants through the rubber stopper and into the vial.

In addition to the standard injectable dosage form, injectables can also be classified as *repository* or depot forms. This dosage form is formulated to allow a slow absorption of the drug from the administration site, providing more sustained drug concentrations in the body over time. Typically, depot injectables are oil-based injectables that do not readily dissolve in the water-based tissue fluid or are manufactured so that the active ingredient is formed into crystals that take longer to dissolve and release the active ingredient.

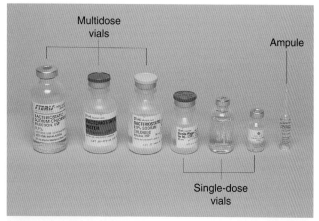

Fig. 1.10 The ampule is designed to be broken open and its contents used all at once. Single-dose vials are designed to have all of their contents withdrawn into a syringe all at one time. Multidose vials are designed to supply multiple doses of drug. (From Klieger D. *Essentials of Medical Assisting.* 2nd ed. Maryland Heights: Elsevier; 2010.)

Implants are a special type of injectable repository dosage form in which a solid object containing the drug is injected or inserted under the skin. Once in place, the implants are designed to dissolve or release medication over an extended period (weeks to months).

WHERE CAN A VETERINARY TECHNICIAN FIND ACCURATE DRUG INFORMATION?

With the advent of the Internet, a good deal of information on veterinary drugs can be obtained with a few keystrokes on the computer. However there also exists a great deal of misinformation regarding veterinary drugs. It is very important that veterinary professionals use only drug information that is supported by clinical research and extensive testing and regulated by the appropriate watchdog agencies (e.g., FDA).

Unfortunately, for many so-called minor species (e.g., sheep, goats, llamas, wildlife, zoo animals, and many laboratory animals), there is very little clinical trial information or solid medical evidence on the safe and effective use of veterinary drugs. In those species, much of the information is anecdotal or based on the experience of veterinarians working with these species. Although this anecdotal information is sometimes the only available information the veterinarian or veterinary technician has for a minor species, one must remember that this information has not undergone the rigorous testing or clinical research required to be an FDA-approved veterinary drug.

Label and Extra-Label Information

Generally, the most accurate drug information for a particular product, including the most recent changes in the drug formulation, dosages, or warnings/precautions, will be found in the drug insert or package insert, which is the manufacturer's documentation inserted into or attached to the side of each bottle, package, or box of medication. The drug insert will contain the information that is mandated by FDA regulations for veterinary drugs but will only contain that information for which the manufacturer has done the mandated testing or otherwise documented in compliance with FDA requirements. Thus, this information in the drug insert or package insert, and printed on the drug label, would be considered to be the label information.

Unfortunately, advances in clinical veterinary medicine typically occur much faster than a manufacturer can complete testing and receive a new drug use approval for an existing drug. Indeed, it is often not cost-effective for a drug manufacturer to spend the thousands to millions of dollars to get FDA approval for every new use, new means of administration, new species use, or new dose for their drug. Instead, veterinarians often use drugs in an *extra-label* manner, meaning they are using the drug in a manner other than the FDA-approved dose, route of administration, disease/condition, or species listed on the drug label.

Extra-label, or off-label, use of veterinary drugs is permissible by federal law under certain circumstances. However, because of the potential threat of veterinary drug residues finding their way into human food or food products, the FDA regulates how drugs can be legally used in an extra-label manner (see You Need to Know box "What Is the Big Deal About Extra-Label Drug Use?" and Boxes 1.1–1.3). Unfortunately, such extra-label uses will not appear on the manufacturer's drug insert, and the veterinary professional must use other medical sources such as veterinary journals or personal communication with other veterinary experts to obtain extra-label dosing or drug effect information.

BOX 1.1 Requirements for Permissible Extra-Label Drug Use

For a drug to be legally used in an extra-label manner in veterinary medicine, the following conditions must be met:

- A licensed veterinarian must order the drug.
- A valid veterinarian-client-patient relationship (VCPR) must exist.
- The health of the animal would be threatened if the drug is not used; the use of the drug to enhance production of food animals is strictly prohibited (e.g., growth promoters).
- No FDA-approved veterinary drug for the particular disease or condition can already exist; or, if such a drug exists, the veterinarian determines that for the particular patient in the VCPR the existing drug or its dosage form would be clinically ineffective.

There are additional requirements for ELDU in food animals that could potentially be used for human consumption:

- An extended withdrawal period or withdrawal time (i.e., time between last dose and when the animal can be slaughtered for meat or food products such as eggs or milk can be used) supported by scientific documentation (if available and applicable) must be used in any animal treated with the drug.
- The veterinarian must institute procedures to assure that the identity of the treated animal is maintained and that the prescribed withdrawal time is observed.
- If scientific information on the safety of this drug in human food is not available, the veterinarian is responsible for taking steps to assure that the treated animal or its food products do not enter the human food supply.

Source:
Food and Drug Administration. *Extra Label Use of FDA Approved Drugs in Animals (Website)*. https://www.ecfr.gov/current/title-21/chapter-I/subchapter-E/part-530/subpart-E/section-530.41. Accessed 07.6.22.

BOX 1.2 Information That Must Be on a Label for Veterinary or Human Drugs Used in an Approved or Extra-Label Manner in Veterinary Patients

Any drug that is used in an extra-label manner must contain the following information on the label of the container in which the drug is dispensed:

- Name and address of the prescribing veterinarian.
- Name of client, patient and species.
- Date of dispensing the drug.
- Established name of the active ingredient in the drug (not the trade name); if more than one ingredient is used, all ingredients must be listed.
- Drug strength and quantity prescribed.
- Number of authorized refills.
- Expiration date of prescription.

- Detailed information about how the drug is to be administered including the species on which it is to be used, the specific animals that are to be treated (identifications such as ear tag number), what dosage and frequency, the route by which the drug is to be administered, and the duration of therapy.
- Any cautionary statements from the veterinarian (e.g., warning of potential harm to person administering the drug, threat to environment if spilled).
- A specific withdrawal time (time between last dose and when animal can be sent to market) or discard time for milk, eggs, or any human food that might be derived from treated animals.

Source:
Food and Drug Administration. *Extra Label Use of FDA Approved Drugs in Animals* and Section 503(f) Food, Drug and Cosmetic Act (Website). https://www.ecfr.gov/current/title-21/chapter-I/subchapter-E/part-530. Accessed 07.6.22.

BOX 1.3 Drugs Never to Be Used in Food-Producing Animals

According to the FDA as of June 2022, these are some of the drugs that are never to be used in food-producing animals. A more extensive list can be found on the FDA's website: https://www.ecfr.gov/current/title-21/chapter-I/subchapter-E/part-530/subpart-E/section-530.41.

- Cephalosporins, not including cephapirin (antibiotic) in cattle, swine, chickens and turkeys:
    - (i) For disease prevention purposes;
    - (ii) At unapproved doses, frequencies, durations or routes of administration; or
    - (iii) If the drug is not approved for that species and production class.
- chloramphenicol (antibiotic),

- clenbuterol (bronchodilator used in horses with chronic obstructive pulmonary disease),
- diethylstilbestrol or DES (estrogen hormone),
- fluoroquinolones (antibiotic family that includes enrofloxacin and marbofloxacin),
- furazolidone except for approved topical uses (antibiotic),
- nitrofurazone except for approved topical uses (antibiotic),
- phenylbutazone in female dairy cattle 20 months of age or older (antiinflammatory), and
- sulfonamide drugs in lactating dairy cattle, except for few sulfas approved for this specific use (antibiotic).

Because extra-label drug use (ELDU) is such an important topic in veterinary medicine, the veterinary technician needs to be very familiar with the legal and professional obligations the law requires for ELDU under the Animal Medicinal Drug Use Clarification Act of 1994 (AMDUCA).

! YOU NEED TO KNOW

What Is the Big Deal About Extra-Label Drug Use?

"Extra-label use" is defined by the FDA on their website www.fda.gov as: *Actual use or intended use of a drug in an animal in a manner that is not in accordance with the approved labeling. This includes, but is not limited to, use in species not listed in the labeling, use for indications (disease and other conditions) not listed in the labeling, use at dosage levels, frequencies, or routes of administration other than those stated in the labeling, and deviation from labeled withdrawal time based on these different uses.*

Because there is the potential for drugs used in food animals to enter the human food supply, veterinary medical drugs are tightly regulated by the FDA, primarily for the benefit of the humans who consume animal products and less so for the animal. Until passing of the Animal Medicinal Drug Use Clarification Act of 1994 (AMDUCA), the Federal Food, Drug, and Cosmetic Act made it technically illegal for a veterinarian to use any human drug in veterinary patients or to use a veterinary drug in any manner other than the label use for which the drug was approved by the FDA. AMDUCA gives the veterinarian the opportunity for off-label or extra-label drug use (often abbreviated as "ELDU") under certain conditions. These conditions are listed in Box 1.1. An additional restriction on human drug use in veterinary patients is that it is still illegal to use a human-approved drug if a valid veterinary equivalent drug exists. All veterinary drugs prescribed in an extra-label manner must bear a label that contains information necessary for safe administration of the drug to reduce the chance of veterinary drug residues appearing in meat or food products intended for human consumption (see Box 1.2).

Because extra-label drug use in nonfood-producing animals (e.g., companion animals, sporting animals, exotic animals) does not ordinarily pose a threat to the public health through contamination of the human food supply, extra-label use of drugs is permitted in nonfood-producing species without any major restrictions except in those rare cases where the public health might be threatened by administration of the drug (e.g., unusual species being used for human food or food supplementation).

Limitations of the Information Found in Sources

Printed veterinary publications can be a good resource for general drug information and extra-label uses. However, there are limitations for each type of printed publication. Generally, textbooks or references from major veterinary medical publishers are fairly reliable sources of information because they are usually written by experts in the field or have been reviewed by other professionals. One advantage of these references over the information contained in the manufacturer's drug insert is that they are not constrained by the FDA to only approved uses or dosages for the drugs and can be good sources of extra-label information for minor species use or for uses beyond the disease or condition listed on the drug label.

Unfortunately, textbooks or print references are generally 4–6 months out of date by the time they are first released. With the rapid advancement of veterinary medical therapeutics, a textbook or similar print resource that is 2–3 years old is still reliable for general information but may be inappropriate for use for the most recent dosage or side effect information.

◎ MYTHS AND MISCONCEPTIONS

Animal doses for human medication can be reasonably extracted from human doses for the medication.

False! The physiology of animals is sufficiently different from that of humans that we can't think of cats or dogs as "little humans" when it comes to dosing drugs. Also the physiology between common species is different enough that we can't think of cats as being equivalent to "little dogs" for dosing or selection of drugs. Believing this myth can result in potentially disastrous outcomes for the veterinary patient.

Information for Use of Human Drugs in Veterinary Medicine

Human drugs are frequently used in veterinary patients. However, information on most human drugs is not contained in most veterinary text resources unless the drug use has been previously published in veterinary medical journals. Information about the effect of drugs in humans should never be extrapolated directly to veterinary patients because there are far too many physiologic differences between humans and common domestic animals.

However, human drug information references used by the human nursing or medical profession can be useful to identify the general class of a drug or the basic physiologic effect of a drug when a pet has been accidentally poisoned by ingestion of a human product. But human doses should never be applied proportionally to veterinary patients unless such use has been documented in the veterinary literature.

Veterinary Journals, Trade Publications, and Proceedings

Veterinary journals can be useful for case studies or clinical trials of new veterinary drugs or new doses for existing veterinary drugs. A peer-reviewed journal is one in which the article has been reviewed by another content expert before the article's acceptance by the journal. It is also important to remember that the studies or reports in peer-reviewed journals may still be on a relatively small number of animals and therefore clear conclusions of a safe dose or beneficial effects of the drug may be tentative until other studies can confirm or refute the conclusions made in the journal article.

Trade publications (these can be recognized by the large amounts of product advertisements), newsletters, and some journals may not be peer reviewed, which means the dosage or drug information in an article may represent only the opinion of the author with or without evidence to support the author's recommendation. Thus the usefulness of the drug information in an article must be interpreted based on the type of publication.

Proceedings from presentations made at major veterinary conferences often list dosages. It is important to remember that these proceedings may not be peer reviewed before publication and the dosages cited in the presentation proceedings may be the opinion of the presenter with or without supporting evidence based on published veterinary data. A check of the references cited by the author in the proceedings provides some insight into how widely supported the author's dosage recommendations are by clinical evidence.

The Internet: Good and Bad

As was mentioned at the beginning of this section, the Internet can be a wealth of information and a swamp of misinformation. For example, several of the citations and references for this chapter came from the FDA's official government website. Because the information from the FDA is heavily scrutinized and reviewed by experts, and the date the web page was updated is listed on the web page, the information posted can be reasonably relied on to be current and accurate. However, for every one legitimate site, there are probably dozens that have information that is old or incomplete, represents a hidden bias or opinion, or is plain wrong.

Remember that anyone, whether knowledgeable or not, can put up a website. Veterinary practices often have websites promoting their practices and providing client information. However, this web information may not be updated very frequently and could represent information that is incomplete or not current. Internet pharmacies and businesses that sell pet products, animal feeds, or other animal-related supplies typically have drug information about the products they sell. In some cases, the information posted on the retailer's website is copied directly from the drug's manufacturer, and, if the information posted is the label information from the FDA-regulated package or drug insert, this information is likely to be accurate. If the retailer's drug information on their website does not have a "last updated" date listed, the information may be outdated or not reflect the most recent information on the drug.

Here are some clues that a website is likely to be authoritative and a fairly reliable resource:

- The website has the author's name listed, the author's credentials, and ideally the means by which questions can be directed to the author or other credible authority.
- The website has a recent "website was last updated" date.
- The website cites references or has links for further information.
- The website has a .gov or .edu extension and is a website of a recognizable government or college/university entity.
  Warning signs of a questionable website:
- Misspellings or poor grammar.
- Cheap looking (no professional logo, fuzzy photographs, poorly organized, nonstandard fonts, broken links to other web pages, or poor navigation between pages or back to home page).
- Website sponsored by an organization with a mission statement that advances a singular point of view that might be predisposed to bias when presenting information.
- The use of many hyperboles ("great," "wonderful," "fantastic," "world's best").
- Advertisements for products not directly related to the website.

Major drug companies' websites typically have a section that contains the drug insert information about their legend products. Typically this technical information section can be recognized by its plain font, the presence of little color or other adornments, and very technical language. Because this information is likely to be the same information required by the FDA, it can be assumed to be accurate and free of marketing bias.

However, other parts of the same website that are designed by the drug company's marketing team will contain information targeted toward the public consumers with the intent of enticing the consumer to purchase the product. Thus, the information is likely to largely emphasize only the positive attributes of the product.

The bottom line in using veterinary resources is to understand the source of the information and the degree to which unbiased medical evidence is provided that supports the drug information.

A VETERINARY TECHNICIAN'S GUIDE TO UNDERSTANDING THE INFORMATION IN DRUG REFERENCES

As discussed in the previous section, knowing where to find drug information is the first step in being able to retrieve the information needed to help the veterinary patient. The second step is being able to translate the information listed in the resource. In most compiled drug references or drug formularies, there is a fairly standardized set of terms and symbols used to describe the drug characteristics. Understanding these terms and symbols is essential for accurately extracting the needed information.

The Heading

In most printed drug references, each drug description begins with a standard heading that contains several pieces of important information, as shown in Fig. 1.11. The boldface, capital letters with the circled R (®) indicate the name of the drug has been successfully registered with the US Patent and Trademark Office (e.g., Nembutal®). In some cases, the trademark symbol (™) is used, which indicates that the drug company asserts it owns that drug name, symbol, or icon but has not registered the name or symbol with the US Patent and Trademark Office (USPTO). Therefore, when the "TM" is used, the drug company does not necessarily have exclusive rights to use the name even though some federal and state laws can protect the unregistered trademark. The "TM" is often used when a company is in the process of obtaining registration for a ® with the USPTO.

What appears to be the letters "R" and "x" together and sometimes referred to as the "Rx" symbol, is actually a single symbol in the heading that indicates this product is a legend drug and hence is available only by prescription or on the order of a licensed veterinarian. Selling drugs with this designation as OTC drugs through grocery stores, feed stores, or discount stores is illegal.

NEMBUTAL® SODIUM SOLUTION

[*nêm'–bū–tal sō'–dĭ–um*]
(pentobarbital sodium injection, USP)
Ampules – Vials

℞ ⓒ

Fig. 1.11 An example of the information contained in the head of a drug description.

Controlled Substance or Schedule Designations

The "C" and "II" in the drug heading in Fig. 1.11 indicate that the drug is a federally controlled substance or schedule drug; this refers to the classification or "schedule" of the abuse potential for these drugs. The Roman numeral II indicates the general level of abuse potential for the drug and the required degree of regulatory control based on the level of risk for diversion of the drug into illicit or illegal drug sales. Categories, or schedules, of controlled substances range from a designation of C-I to C-V. The higher the value of the Roman numeral, the lesser the abuse potential of the drug. Drugs classified as C-I (and pronounced as the letter "C" and "one") have the highest potential for abuse; drugs classified as C-V ("C five") have the least. Controlled substance storage and use regulations are discussed in greater detail in Chapter 2.

A somewhat recent addition to the drug heading by some publishers has been the phonetic spelling of the drug, as shown in brackets below the trade name in Fig. 1.11. This is helpful for the veterinary professional when communicating the drug name to other veterinarians, veterinary technicians, physicians, or pharmacists.

The nonproprietary name (e.g., pentobarbital sodium) is printed in smaller type below the boldface name and phonetic spelling and usually includes a descriptor of the dosage form (e.g., tablets, syrup, or injectable). In the example in Fig. 1.11, the heading states that the drug form is for injectable use.

United States Pharmacopeia Designation

The "USP" designation in the nonproprietary name stands for the United States Pharmacopeia (USP). The USP is a nongovernmental organization that sets the standards for drug manufacturing quality, purity, and consistency for any drugs sold in the United States.[3] The USP designation provides some assurance that drug was produced in a manner that delivers predictably consistent effects and has been manufactured to the standards required for drugs manufactured in the United States.

Finally, the heading may have a separate line that conveys additional information about the drug. In the example in Fig. 1.11, the heading indicates that the dose form also comes in ampules and vials.

Active vs Inert Ingredients

The drug information in the paragraphs after the heading is organized into different categories for quick information access. Typically the first paragraph following the heading is the description, or composition statement, which describes the physical characteristics and ingredients of the drug or drug combination. The active ingredient, which is the part of the drug that produces the intended beneficial effect, is identified by the generic name of the drug. Any inert ingredients, such as any preservatives, stabilizers, liquid media, or other additives that make up the dosage form, should also be listed in the composition statement. Although the inert ingredient list is often not given much attention, veterinary professionals need to remember that some inert ingredients can produce adverse reactions in veterinary patients.

Indications

One of the next paragraphs or statements is the drug's indication. The indication is the approved reason for which the drug can be used. When a new drug is developed and tested for FDA approval, the manufacturer must state for what specific indication the drug is to be used. If approved, this approved indication will appear on the drug's label.

For example, a sulfonamide antibiotic might have an indication or be *indicated* for treating a urinary tract infection. Even though the sulfonamide antibiotic might also be effective in treating a skin infection, the drug manufacturer cannot list "treatment of skin infections" on the label unless the drug company specifically tested for, and received FDA approval for, this indication. Thus using the sulfonamide antibiotic to treat a skin infection would be considered an extra-label use and the veterinarian would be professionally liable for insuring that the drug would be used safely and the use meets governmental guidelines for extra-label drug use.

Adverse Drug Reaction Information

After the composition and indication statements, several sections of the drug listing are devoted to any undesirable effects of the drug. A side effect is any effect of the drug other than its intended beneficial effect that occurs when the drug concentrations are within the normal therapeutic range. Side effects for a drug can range from mildly annoying to potentially fatal. Occasionally a drug is used for its side effect, such as the immune system suppression drug cyclosporin, which is used for its side effect of stimulating tear production in patients with dry eyes.

ADR is a broader term that includes any adverse reaction either within the therapeutic range (side effect) or as the result of a toxic accumulation of drug. ADRs include any unwanted patient response to the chemical or physical properties of the drug.[4]

The information on side effects or ADRs are further broken down into precautions, warnings, and contraindications for the drug. If a drug has a history of a particularly risky side effect, the drug may also have a separate section (sometimes surrounded with a black box and referred to as a "boxed warning") on the specific adverse reaction.

Precautions

Generally, a precaution either describes a mild adverse reaction, some predictable change in clinical state or the patient's condition, or some other effect that typically doesn't require much medical intervention. A precaution may also contain information that is provided to consumers for their own information. For example, stomach upset caused by ingesting aspirin is considered a mild side effect in humans and is included under the precaution heading. Other precautions include "do not drive while taking this medication," "drink plenty of water when taking this medication," or "this medication may change the color of the urine."

In most cases, precautions need to be communicated to clients when dispensing the medication for their pet or animal or noted on the patient's record as information to the hospital staff monitoring the patient. The veterinarian is obligated to use his or her clinical judgment to decide whether the benefits of the drug outweigh the potential side effects listed under the precautions.

For some drugs, the listing of precautions can be extensive and include clinical signs or adverse effects that are rarely observed in clinical patients. However, by listing all of the precautions (including even the mild side effects), the drug manufacturer has legally informed the veterinarian of the potential side effects or adverse reactions and placed the responsibility for administering the drug on the veterinary professional.

Warnings

Warnings are more serious or frequent side effects than those found in the precautions section and constitute adverse drug effects that could potentially do significant harm to the patient. Some resources group both precautions and warnings together because it is difficult sometimes to clearly differentiate when a side effect becomes severe enough to warrant being classified as a warning instead of a precaution.

Examples of warnings might include the potential for a severe drop in blood pressure from certain heart medications, the inflammation and skin sloughing that can result if an IV-administered drug is accidentally administered outside of the vein, or the development of neurologic side effects from high-dose administration of the drug. Because many of the adverse reactions in the warnings section are clinically significant and potentially life threatening, veterinary professionals have a moral and ethical obligation to thoroughly understand the key points of warnings and to inform the client or owner of the potential problems that may arise. Drugs that have warnings are still able to be given if the veterinarian feels the potential benefit outweighs the risk.

Black Box Warnings

A "black box warning," "black label warning," or "boxed warning" is the strongest warning the FDA can require a drug manufacturer to include in their drug information. The information is, as the term implies, surrounded by a black box so that the contained information is clearly visible to the reader of the drug insert. Black box warnings typically contain adverse effects that have a significant risk for severe or life-threatening effects. Examples of this would be the boxed warning that certain antidepressants can cause suicidal tendencies in adolescents or administration of some blood thinners can cause fatal hemorrhage.

Contraindications

Contraindications are circumstances or conditions in which the drug should not be used. For example, a patient's severe and life-threatening allergy to penicillin is a contraindication for giving the drug. A contraindication can also be a situation in which there is a high risk for permanent damage to the patient and for which the drug manufacturer feels that the risk for injury is too great to leave the use of the drug to the discretion of the veterinarian. An example of this would be the way enrofloxacin, an antibiotic commonly used in veterinary

medicine, is contraindicated in young, rapidly growing dogs because of the risk for malformation of developing joint cartilage and subsequent development of arthritis as the dog ages.

If the veterinarian or veterinary technician fails to heed a known drug contraindication and the animals suffers injury or dies as a result of administration of the medication, the veterinary professional may have little defense against a claim of malpractice.[5]

Dosage and Administration

Only the FDA-approved dosage and method of drug administration will be listed under the dosage and administration section of most references unless the reference also cites additional extra-label dosages or administration methods taken from the veterinary scientific literature. As mentioned previously, this FDA-approved dosage and route of administration should achieve drug concentrations in the body that produce the intended beneficial effect with minimal toxicity in the majority of patients. However, as stated by Rule #3 earlier, these official FDA-approved dosages are meant to be the starting place for calculating the dose a particular patient actually needs given the disease state and the physiologic state of the patient's body.

When applicable, information on treatment for drug overdose, withdrawal times, or other relevant information meant to inform the veterinarian or protect the manufacturer from litigation will also be listed in the drug information.

The FDA and individual drug manufacturers want to know when an adverse reaction is observed with a veterinary drug. Thus veterinarians and veterinary technicians are encouraged to report detailed information surrounding suspected adverse events to the FDA or the drug manufacturer. See You Need to Know box "How to Report Adverse Drug Effects" for information on how to report such suspected adverse drug events.

! YOU NEED TO KNOW

How to Report Adverse Drug Effects

The FDA's toll-free phone number for reporting adverse drug reactions (1-888-FDA-VETS) is available from 7:00 a.m. to 4:00 p.m. EST, with next-day callback service available after hours.

The FDA website has an online form that can be completed and submitted to report an adverse drug effect: www.fda.gov/AnimalVeterinary/SafetyHealth/ReportAProblem

A written letter can also be sent to the FDA at the following address:

ADE Reporting System
Center for Veterinary Medicine
U.S. Food & Drug Administration
7500 Standish Place
Rockville, MD 20855-2773

Most drug manufacturers have technical service veterinarians to accept reports of drug reactions or discuss problems or concerns with their drugs. These phone numbers or other means of contacting these companies can be found by typing in the company name plus "adverse drug event" into almost any web search engine.

The United States Pharmacopeia (USP)'s Veterinary Practitioner's Reporting Program for reporting adverse reactions as mentioned in the third edition of this textbook is no longer available.

REFERENCES

1. Food and Drug Administration. Generic Drugs: Questions and Answers (Website). www.fda.gov/Drugs/ResourcesForYou/Consumers/QuestionsAnswers/ucm100100.htm. Accessed 06.06.22.
2. Schmid RD, Hovda LR. Acute hepatic failure in a dog after xylitol ingestion. *J Med Toxicol.* 2016;12(2):201–205. https://doi.org/10.1007/s13181-015-0531-7. PMID: 26691320; PMCID: PMC4880608.
3. The United States Pharmacopeia. About USP (Website). www.usp.org/about-usp. Accessed 06.06.22.
4. Boothe DM. Drug induced diseases. In: Boothe DM, ed. *Small Animal Clinical Pharmacology and Therapeutics.* St. Louis: Saunders; 2012.
5. Food and Drug Administration. Guidance for Industry—Warnings and Precautions, Contraindications, and Boxed Warning Sections of Labeling for Human Prescription Drug and Biological Products (Website). https://www.fda.gov/regulatory-information/search-fda-guidance-documents/warnings-and-precautions-contraindications-and-boxed-warning-sections-labeling-human-prescription. Retrieved 01.07.15.

SELF-ASSESSMENT

1. Fill in the following blanks with the correct item from the Key Terms list.

    A. _____ This term means the application of pharmacology to specific treatments.

    B. _____ This name of a drug is often written as a description of the drug's molecular formula.

    C. _____ This name of a drug is an approved name for the active ingredient and is not owned by one particular drug manufacturer or company.

    D. _____ This is the component of the drug's composition that performs the beneficial effect. It is often the same as the generic name.

    E. _____ This is the name of the drug that is owned specifically by one particular drug company. It is trademarked or copyrighted by that drug company.

    F. _____ This is the governmental regulatory agency in the United States that controls drug approval.

    G. _____ This describes a drug that is manufactured by another drug company other than the original manufacturer.

    H. _____ This describes a therapeutic agent that is created from specially prepared plant or animal parts.

    I. _____ This is a type of drug that can be legally obtained without a prescription.

    J. _____ This describes a group of drugs that can only be obtained through dispensing by or on the order of a licensed prescriber.

    K. _____ This is the legal term for the arrangement for treatment that exists between a veterinarian, an animal owner, and the animal.

    L. _____ This term is a description of the physical appearance of the drug.

    M. _____ This is the solid dosage form created by compressing powdered active ingredients and other inert ingredients together to form disk-shaped dosage forms.

    N. _____ This term describes the inert ingredients in a solid dosage form that may include binders, disintegrants, diluents, or flavoring/coloring agents.

    O. _____ This describes a solid dosage form made from powdered drug and compressed into an oblong shape for easier swallowing.

    P. _____ This is powdered drug mixed with lactose or other sugars and made into a dosage form that is chewable.

    Q. _____ This type of tablet covering prevents a tablet from dissolving in the acidic environment of the stomach.

    R. _____ This is a solid dosage form in which the dose form slowly dissolves to allow for a more gradual release of active ingredient over a longer period of time.

    S. _____ This is powdered drug surrounded by a capsule made of gelatin, modified starch, or cellulose.

    T. _____ This describes a dosage form wherein the drug is incorporated into a hard, candy-like tablet and is meant to be held in the mouth until dissolved.

    U. _____ This is a dosage form administered by being placed in the rectum.

    V. _____ This term describes the liquid into which a drug is suspended or dissolved.

    W. _____ This is any type of liquid dosage form in which the drug is floating in an undissolved state.

    X. _____ This is any type of liquid dosage form in which the drug has been dissolved.

    Y. _____ This is any type of liquid drug solution in which the medium is water.

    Z. _____ This is any liquid dosage solution in which the medium is a sugar solution.

    AA. _____ This is an artificial sweetener sometimes included in sugar-free syrups but should never be given to dogs.

    AB. _____ These are alcohol-based solutions used for oral or topical application.

    AC. _____ This term means the drug is unable to be dissolved in the liquid medium.

    AD. _____ This is a type of suspension formed from two liquids that do not readily mix.

AE. _____ This is a topically applied liquid dosage form that is rubbed into the skin to produce its beneficial effect.

AF. _____ This is a semisolid dosage form that liquifies at body temperature.

AG. _____ This is a semisolid dosage form that retains its shape at body temperature.

AH. _____ This is an injectable dosage form contained within a small glass vial that is opened by snapping the vial apart at the narrow neck of the vial.

AI. _____ This is an injectable dosage form that is formulated to be absorbed over a prolonged period of time.

AJ. _____ This is a special injectable dosage form that is solid, but is injected under the skin and releases medication over weeks to months.

AK. _____ This is the term that describes the manufacturer's drug information and is either inserted into each drug container or attached to the drug bottle.

AL. _____ This is the information on any drug that describes the specific use and administration of the drug that has been approved by the Food and Drug Administration (FDA).

AM. _____ This term describes any use of a drug in a manner other than the use or manner that has been approved by the FDA.

AN. _____ Those drugs with the potential for abuse that are more tightly regulated by the government.

AO. _____ This is the nongovernmental US organization that sets the standards required for all drugs manufactured in the United States.

AP. _____ These are the ingredients in the drug compound that include preservatives, stabilizers, or other additives other than the active ingredient.

AQ. _____ This is the term that means the label-approved use for the drug.

AR. _____ This term describes any effect other than the intended effect of a drug that occurs within the normal therapeutic range.

AS. _____ This term describes a mild adverse reaction or some predictable side effect that does not typically require medical intervention.

AT. _____ This term describes more serious or frequent side effects that could potentially do harm to the patient but are not severe enough to preclude the drug from being used.

AU. _____ This term describes the strongest warning the FDA can require a drug manufacturer to include on a drug label.

AV. _____ This term describes circumstances in which the drug should not be used.

AW. _____ This organization is responsible for approving drug names in the United States.

AX. _____ This is the term used by the FDA to determine whether generic drugs are equivalent to the parent drug.

AY. _____ This is the legislation that gives veterinarians the right to prescribe drugs for extra-label use in veterinary patients.

AZ. _____ This is the period of time between the last dose and when the animal can be slaughtered for human food or its food products can be sold.

2. Identify the meaning of the following acronyms.
   ADR
   AMDUCA
   ELDU
   EPA
   FDA
   OTC
   SR
   USAN
   USP
   VCPR

3. Indicate whether the following statements are TRUE or FALSE.
   A. Veterinarians can legally use drugs in an extra-label manner to treat animals that will be used as human food.
   B. The® symbol indicates that the drug is restricted to use only by a veterinarian.
   C. Legend drugs are to be dispensed only with a prescription or on the order of the veterinarian.
   D. Flea treatments applied to the animal's skin but that require absorption into the body to work would typically be regulated by the EPA and not the FDA.
   E. Veterinary journals usually have more recent information than veterinary textbooks.
   F. Websites with .gov are probably reliable websites for veterinary drug information.
   G. A controlled substance with a schedule III would have greater abuse potential than a schedule II drug.
   H. The following statement would be considered a warning: "Do not administer this drug if the patient is allergic to it."

4. You are speaking at a local high school about the veterinary technology profession. As you are contrasting the education required to become a credentialed veterinary technician vs a veterinarian, one of the students raises his hand and asks, "Why do veterinary technicians have to learn about drugs even though veterinary technicians can't prescribe drugs?" How might you address this legitimate question?

5. The veterinarian has given a client a prescription. On the prescription is marked "generic drug can be substituted." After the veterinarian has left, the client has several questions for you: What is a generic drug? How is it different from a regular drug? Why are generic forms of drugs so much less expensive than trade name drugs? Are generic drugs as good as the better known drugs?

6. An owner reports an unusual side effect for a drug the veterinarian prescribed. How should such information be reported?

7. Mrs. Jones is a well-informed client. She dutifully researches the information on medications for her pet. When she asks you, "What is the reason for having an enteric coating on a tablet?" for a medication her pet is taking, what should you tell her?

8. Mr. Smith has some respiratory medication for himself that is very similar to the medication his dog is prescribed. But his dog's medication is marked SR for "sustained release." Mr. Smith wants to know how a sustained-release tablet is different from a regular tablet. How do you respond?

9. Why can't an enteric-coated or SR tablet be halved to provide a more accurate dosing of the medication?

10. Why are sugar-free syrup medications with xylitol dangerous to dogs?

11. Which liquid formulation of a drug can be safely given intravenously, as a solution, or as a suspension? Which needs to be shaken before administration?

12. If a standard injectable form of a drug is given every 12 h, would the repository form of the same drug be more likely to be given every 6 h or every 48 h? Would it be the same for a depot drug?

13. Mr. Jones found a compound for treating his dog's hypothyroidism (low levels of thyroid hormone) on the Internet. It is listed as an extract and it is much less expensive than the other drug formulations the veterinarian has prescribed for treating his dog's condition. He wants to know what an extract is, how it is different from a regular drug, and why it is so much cheaper than the drug the veterinarian is prescribing for treating the same medical problem. How might you respond to Mr. Jones's questions?

14. A pet owner is passing through town and stops by your veterinary clinic to see whether she can pick up some car sickness tablets for her dog. The owner is on a cross-country car trip and has no more of the motion sickness medication that was dispensed by her veterinarian. The doctor is not in the clinic at the moment. Is it legal to dispense the medication if you first telephone the doctor to obtain permission?

15. Explain whether each of the following situations is considered an appropriate or inappropriate use of drugs in an extra-label manner according to FDA requirements.
    A. The owner of a cow telephones to describe the clinical signs that the cow is showing. The veterinarian dispenses an extra-label drug for the cow that has been used to treat other cattle on adjoining farms.
    B. The veterinarian dispenses an off-label drug because it is as effective as the FDA-approved drug but its cost is half the price.
    C. After making a farm call, the veterinarian leaves a bottle of medication with a livestock producer to use on any other livestock showing similar signs, thus saving the producer the cost of multiple farm calls.
    D. The veterinarian uses an off-label injectable drug on a producing dairy cow that he has examined and tells the dairy farmer not to worry about a milk discard time because there is nothing on the drug insert that mentions a withdrawal time.
    E. The veterinarian examines a goat and dispenses a medication used in calves because veterinary journals have published studies showing the drug is effective in goats.
    F. The veterinarian examines a heifer, determines that an off-label drug for which there is no FDA-approved alternative would be the best drug to treat the condition, informs the livestock producer of the withdrawal times according to FDA guidelines on similar drugs in cattle, writes the information into the record, and then dispenses it in a bottle with the cow's ID tag number and the drug name on it.

16. List the four rules to live by for safe drug usage.

Pharmacy Procedures and Dosage Calculations

CHAPTER OUTLINE

OBJECTIVES

After studying this chapter, the veterinary technician should be able to:

- Describe the difference between pharmacy and pharmacology.
- Describe the requirements for properly written prescriptions and drug labels.
- Describe and know how to comply with storage, logging, and dispensing of controlled substances (schedule drugs).
- Accurately read and write abbreviations commonly used in drug orders.
- Identify and avoid the common errors made in writing drug orders.
- Accurately translate between equivalent amounts in the metric, apothecary, and household systems.
- Accurately calculate the amount of drug mass needed by the individual patient.

- Accurately calculate the amount of dosage form needed for the individual dose.
- Accurately perform calculations using percentage solutions (weight by volume [w/v], weight by weight [w/w], volume by volume [v/v]).
- Accurately calculate the number of dosage forms that must be dispensed to fulfill the need of the drug order.
- Describe the legal requirements for allowable compounding and the restrictions that are necessary to achieve these legal requirements.
- Describe the requirements for a label and type of container that must be used for any dispensed veterinary medication.
- Describe special storage and handling requirements for cytotoxic and hazardous drugs.

KEY TERMS

Animal Medicinal Drug Use Clarification Act (AMDUCA)
apothecary system
carcinogenic effects
compounding
concentration

controlled substances
cytotoxic drugs
dosage
dosage form
dosage range
dosage regimen

dose
dose interval
Drug Enforcement Administration (DEA)
drug order
Extra-Label Drug Use (ELDU)
Federal Food, Drug, and Cosmetic Act (FFDCA)

Food and Drug Administration (FDA)	percentage solution	teratogenic
household measurement system	pharmacology	veterinarian-client-patient relationship (VCPR)
material safety data sheet (MSDS)	pharmacy	volume by volume (v/v) percentage solution
metric system	Poison Prevention Packaging Act of 1970	weight by volume (w/v) percentage solution
mutagenic	prescription	weight by weight (w/w) percentage solution
Occupational Safety and Health Administration (OSHA)	schedule drugs	withdrawal time
	strength of the dosage form	

It is a misconception that the practice of pharmacy and the study of pharmacology are the same thing. They are not. Pharmacy is the art and science of preparing and dispensing medications. Pharmacology is the study of how drugs work. Veterinary technicians need pharmacy skills to be able to understand and accurately fill drug orders, handle medications safely, and deliver the appropriate amount of drug or therapy. As described in the previous chapter, veterinary technicians need pharmacology knowledge to understand how drugs they are administering affect the body. Although both skill sets are needed, they are different, but related, skill sets.

◎ MYTHS AND MISCONCEPTIONS

Pharmacy is the same as pharmacology

> **False!** Pharmacology is the study of how drugs work. Pharmacy practice is the preparation and dispensing of drugs. Pharmacologists are not the same as pharmacists. Well-educated veterinary technicians understand both the pharmacy practice and the pharmacology behind the treatments they are administering.

Pharmacy skills are typically covered in greater detail in veterinary technology nursing textbooks and medical mathematics/dose calculation resources. This chapter will introduce the basic pharmaceutical skills needed for veterinary nursing with the understanding that if the student needs additional information, other resources should be consulted.

THE GOAL: THE CORRECT DOSE ADMINISTERED IN THE CORRECT WAY

According to a publication released in the *International Journal of General Medicine* in December of 2020, "Medication Administration Errors and Associated Factors Among Nurses," an estimated 7000 human patients die annually from potentially preventable adverse drug events resulting from misadministration, inadequate monitoring of medications and inappropriate training.[1] These deaths resulted from a breakdown at some point in the chain of communication between the prescriber of the medication (the human physician) and the actual administration of the drug to the patient (performed by the nurse). To avoid similar mistakes in veterinary nursing and successfully administer medications, each of the following steps must be accurately completed:

1. The veterinarian must accurately transcribe his or her intention to administer a drug, either onto a drug order form or medical record for internal use by a veterinary technician in the veterinary hospital or onto a prescription for transmission to a registered pharmacist.
2. The drug order or prescription must be read and accurately interpreted by the veterinary technician (for the drug order) or the pharmacist (for the prescription).
3. The veterinary technician must be able to accurately calculate the mass of drug (typically mg of drug) needed for the specific patient.
4. The veterinary technician must identify the appropriate dosage form (liquid, solid, tablet, ointment, or other form) described in the drug order and must convert the prescribed mass of drug (e.g., milligrams of drug) into the appropriate number of units of the dosage form (e.g., number of milliliters, tablets, cc) for the specific patient's dose.
5. The veterinary technician must administer the medication to the <u>right</u> patient in the <u>right</u> amount, by the <u>right</u> route of administration, at the <u>right</u> time and repeated doses must be given at the <u>right</u> dose interval (five rights of medication administration).
6. For dispensed medication the veterinary technician must be able to calculate the total amount of dosage forms (e.g., tablets) needed to complete the entire duration of the dosage regimen (e.g., 20 tablets for 10 days, 15 mL for 1 week).
7. For dispensed medications, the veterinary technician must be able to communicate the drug order to the animal owner or caretaker in a way that the person administering the drug knows exactly what he or she must do.

A failure to complete any of these steps can lead to the inappropriate administration of a drug and a potentially severe adverse drug effect.

UNDERSTANDING THE PRESCRIPTION VS THE DRUG ORDER

In Chapter 1, the concept of legend or prescription drugs vs over-the-counter (OTC) drugs was introduced. Veterinary legend drugs are prescription drugs that carry the notice: "Caution:

Federal law restricts this drug to use by or on the order of a licensed veterinarian." Though the focus of this chapter will be on pharmacy aspects of prescription drug orders, much of this information also applies to OTC drugs.

The Drug Order

A drug order is a request by a veterinarian to dispense or administer a drug within a hospital. In many states, the term "drug order" is defined in much greater detail by pharmacy law, but for purposes of this textbook we will use "drug order" in its simpler form as being an internal order for dispensing or administration of a drug by a veterinary technician.

The drug order is typically made by writing the order in the patient's medical record, completing a drug order request form, or verbally communicating the drug order to a veterinary technician. In the case of the verbal orders or a separate drug order request form, it is important that the veterinary technician ensure that the drug order has also been recorded in the patient's permanent medical record.

The Prescription

The prescription is a drug order sent from a licensed professional (the veterinarian in this case) to a separate dispensing facility (the pharmacy), where it is filled by another licensed professional (the pharmacist). As noted in Chapter 1, veterinarians and veterinary technicians can fill drug orders from within their own veterinary hospital, but they cannot legally fill prescriptions or drug orders from other veterinary practices. This practice would put the veterinary hospital in the role of the "dispensing facility" and the person filling the drug order or prescription would be acting as a pharmacist. In most state or provincial law, only a pharmacist can legally fill, or direct to be filled, a submitted prescription. Thus, for another veterinary practice to fill a drug order or prescription would be a violation of pharmacy law.

The prescription is a legal document, and the information that must be included is primarily mandated by the state or provincial pharmacy law (Fig. 2.1). In general, the following items must be included on a prescription[2]:
- Name of the veterinary hospital or veterinarian issuing the prescription
- The address and telephone number of the prescribing professional
- Date on which the prescription was written
- Client's (owner's) name and address
- Species of animal (animal's name optional but recommended)
- Rx symbol (from the Latin, meaning *take thou of*)
- Drug name, concentration/strength, and number of units to be dispensed
- Whether refills are allowed; if so, how many
- Sig (from the Latin *signa,* meaning *write* or *label*), which indicates directions for the treatment of the animal
- Signature of the veterinarian (may be an electronic signature in most states/provinces)

Although pharmacy law typically does not require identification of the animal, AMDUCA requires that any extra-label drug dispensed by a pharmacist must include some identification of the patient (name, ear tag number, etc.). The weight of the animal is not required by regulation or law to be included on a prescription. However, many practices will include this information to allow a pharmacist familiar with veterinary drugs and their use to double check the dose prescribed.

Controlled Substances Have Special Requirements

Controlled substances are drugs like narcotics, strong sedatives, analgesics, or hallucinogenic drugs that have the potential for abuse. In the United States, regulation of the use of potential abuse drugs is the primary responsibility of the

---

HOMETOWN VETERINARY ASSOCIATES
2000 West Chelsea Ave., Brookside, PA 13233
(324) 555-0214

Date: *November 22, 2017*

Patient: *Cricket*   Species: *Canine*

Owner: *Kathy Gagnier*   Phone: *555-0127*

Address: *2000 Christopher Ln,*
West Brookside, PA 13235

℞ *Amoxicillin tablets 100 mg #30 tabs*
Sig: 1 tab q8h PO PRN until gone

Robert L. Bill D.V.M.

Fig. 2.1 A properly written prescription.

Drug Enforcement Administration (DEA). In Canada, laws governing potential abuse drugs are regulated by the federal government's Department of Justice with the Royal Canadian Mounted Police having primary enforcement powers over abuse of controlled drugs.

In the United States, controlled substances are also called "schedule drugs" and are identified on their box or bottle with a "C" and a Roman numeral. In the United States, the veterinarian cannot legally prescribe any controlled substances without being registered with the DEA and the states own controlled substances registry. If the veterinarian prescribes a controlled substance, the prescription must also include the veterinarian's DEA registration number.[2]

Controlled substances are rated on their potential abuse by the "C" scale of I–V (1–5), with a C-I drug having the most potential for abuse. The C-II rating is the highest level of potential abuse drugs for which veterinarians may legally write prescriptions. To write a C-II drug prescription, additional information or a different prescription form may have to be used. Even with a DEA permit, a veterinarian cannot prescribe C-I drugs, which include heroin, lysergic acid diethylamide (LSD), and other hallucinogenic or abuse drugs that do not have any clear medical use.

Dispensed controlled substances must be placed in childproof containers and include the following warning on the label: "Caution: Federal law prohibits the transfer of this drug to any person other than the [client and] patient for whom it was prescribed."

It is generally recommended that veterinary practices keep only a minimum of controlled substances to reduce the risk of being a target for theft or diversion of drugs from their intended use. Human pharmacies are generally more secure and better suited for storage of highly attractive abuse drugs than the typical veterinary practice. Still, certain analgesics, anti-seizure medications, anesthetics, or tranquilizers must be kept readily available in most veterinary practices to insure smooth running of the anesthesia service and emergency/trauma services. For those drugs used and stored within a veterinary hospital, detailed and accurate records must track every unit (mL, tablet, capsule) of the controlled substance from the time it arrives in the veterinary hospital until it is administered to a specific patient or leaves with a specific client.

The Controlled Substances Log

The DEA requires that all records of the controlled substance inventory and their use be maintained and readily available for inspection for a minimum of 2 years.[3] States have the option of requiring a longer period for retaining these records; thus, veterinary technicians should check their local laws to make sure the veterinary practice is in compliance with both federal and regional or local laws. An example of a drug log is shown in Fig. 2.2.

DRUG: Butorphanol

Drug	Inventory ID	Lot Number	Starting Volume Number	Patient ID	Spec.	Client	Date	Amount	Purpose	Disp. by	Amount Balance
Butorphanol 0.5 mg/mL FD	031-MW-RB-071210	2343-AAB	10 mL	"Casey" 042523	C	P. Williams	7/15/10	1.2 mL	Pre-anes	JW	8.8 mL
				"Reese" 032125	C	P. Pennington	7/16/10	2.3 mL	Pre-anes	ML	6.5 mL
				"Abbey" 032511	F	S. Salisbury	7/17/10	0.8 mL	Analgesic	ML	5.7 mL
				"Cooper" 032214	C	M. Landon	7/23/10	2.5 mL	Pre-anes	JW	3.2 mL
				"Flyer" 029911	C	D. Welsh	7/23/10	2.8 mL	Pre-anes	JW	0.5 mL
				"Clare" 030022	C	C. Anning	7/24/10	0.5 mL	Analgesic	ML	0 mL
Butorphanol 0.5 mg/mL FD	032-MW-RB-071210	2343-AAB	10 mL	"Clare" 030022	C	C. Anning	7/24/10	0.6 mL	Analgesic	ML	9.4 mL

Drug: Drug active ingredient, concentration or strength (0.5 mg/mL), manufacturer (FD = Fort Dodge)

Inventory ID: Number that goes on bottle (001), purchased from (MW = Midwest Veterinary Supply), veterinarian whose DEA number was used to order the drug (RB = Robert Bill), date bottle received (071210 = July 12th, 2010)

Fig. 2.2 Example of a controlled substances drug log.

Computer logs of controlled substances can be considered legitimate record keeping if the software allows only minor editing of medical entries and generates an uneditable log of any such record edits. Many states require keeping a hard copy (paper) of the log in addition to the computer record and may require that an auxiliary record-keeping system be established in the event that the computer documentation becomes inoperable. As with all aspects of controlled substance regulation, the state may have additional requirements for computer-kept logs to be considered valid documentation.

Because the veterinary technician is often designated to record the in-hospital use of medications, and because improper logging of controlled substances can have serious consequences for the veterinarian, the veterinary technician must be familiar with the documentation process and with the legal requirements for recording controlled substance use.

The declaration of the opioid crisis as a public health emergency by President Trump in 2017 has brought light to veterinary clinics being targeted by drug abusers. There is documented evidence to support the fact that drug abusers will use their pets to obtain drugs of abuse from their veterinarians, and/or are breaking into veterinary clinics to obtain opioids. In an effort to prevent abusers from obtaining illegitimate opioid prescriptions from veterinarians, many states are now mandating veterinarians report the controlled substances they dispense into a prescription drug monitoring program (PDMP). The prescriber must register with their state PDMP, however, the veterinarian, in most states, can delegate a veterinary technician to log controlled substances dispensed, as well as search the database for patterns of abuse. This is a state mandate, so it is the veterinary technician's responsibility to learn the controlled substance reporting laws for the state in which they practice.

See the You Need to Know boxes "Controlled Substances," "Documentation and Inventory of Controlled Substances," and "Storage of Controlled Substances" for important information every veterinary technician should know about controlled substances.

! YOU NEED TO KNOW

Controlled Substances

A capital C followed by a Roman numeral I, II, III, IV, or V on a drug label indicates that the drug is considered a controlled substance or *schedule drug*. A controlled substance is defined by law as a substance that has the potential for physical addiction, psychological addiction, and/or abuse. The Roman numeral denotes the drug's theoretic potential for abuse.

C-I: Has an extreme potential for abuse and no approved medicinal purpose in the United States; includes such drugs as heroin, lysergic acid diethylamide (LSD), and nonmedical marijuana. These drugs are not available by prescription written by veterinarians or physicians (for humans), although in some states, the state law allows physicians to prescribe medical marijuana for a limited number of specific medical conditions.

C-II: These are drugs that can be prescribed by a veterinarian but have the highest potential for abuse that may lead to severe physical or psychological dependence; includes such drugs as opium, fentanyl, oxycodone, oxymorphone, pentobarbital, morphine, and wild-animal restraint drugs such as etorphine hydrochloride. Surprisingly cocaine, which was used many years ago as a local anesthetic in the eye and is currently used topically for its vasoconstrictive properties in human nasal surgeries, is classified as a C-II and not a C-I drug. Stimulants such as Adderall™ (amphetamine and dextroamphetamine) and Ritalin™ (methylphenidate hydrochloride), two human drugs used to treat attention deficit hyperactivity disorder (ADHD), are also in this category (C-II) for their potentially addictive properties. Ordering of any of these drugs requires special forms (DEA 222 form).

C-III: These drugs have some potential for abuse but less than that of C-II drugs; may lead to low to moderate physical dependence or high psychological dependence; includes ultrashort-acting barbiturates, ketamine, Telazol (zolazepam and tiletamine), and drugs with limited amounts of narcotics (e.g., Tylenol plus codeine). Anabolic steroids sometimes used by athletes to increase muscle mass are classified as C-III because of their relatively high level for abuse.

C-IV: These drugs generally have a low potential for abuse but use may lead to limited physical or psychological dependence; includes such drugs as butorphanol and diazepam (Valium).

C-V: These drugs are subject to state and local regulations and restrictions but have a low potential for abuse. Gabapentin is now in this category in many states due to its abuse potential when combined with other addictive drugs.

A complete listing of DEA Controlled Substances can be found at the DEA's website: https://www.deadiversion.usdoj.gov/schedules/.

NOTE: By federal law, prescriptions for C-II controlled substances cannot be written with refills; prescriptions for C-III and C-IV can have up to five refills within 6 months; C-V prescriptions may be refilled as often as authorized by the veterinarian. Each state has the ability to make a medication a controlled substance or place it in a lower schedule than the DEA. Due to this variability, it is your responsibility to know the scheduled medications in the state you are practicing in.

Sources:

Controlled Substance Schedules; US Department of Justice, Drug Enforcement Administration; https://www.deadiversion.usdoj.gov/schedules/orangebook/orangebook.pdf.
Riviere JE, Papich MG, eds. *Veterinary Pharmacology and Therapeutics.* 10th ed. Ames, Iowa: Wiley-Blackwell; 2018.
Title 21 Code of Federal Regulations; Part 1306—Prescriptions; US Department of Justice, Drug Enforcement Administration; www.ecfr.gov/current/title-21/chapter-II/part-1306?toc=1.

! YOU NEED TO KNOW

Documentation and Inventory of Controlled Substances

Documentation of any dispensed controlled substance is required by law, and in many states require documentation in a prescription drug monitoring program (PDMP). This documentation helps decrease the diversion of abuse drugs from their intended use into illegal or illicit use. Veterinarians are not required by law to document prescriptions written for controlled substances to be dispensed by a licensed pharmacy by a registered pharmacist. However, it is still good practice to document every prescription of controlled substances in the patient's medical record in the event that a question is raised about whether or not the animal's owner is "shopping" different veterinarians or veterinary hospitals to obtain a series of controlled substance prescriptions to fill for diversion to other uses.

Also, stealing prescription pads or individual prescription sheets and subsequently forging a prescription are also a common way by which abuse drugs may be illegally obtained. Some practices keep photocopies of written prescriptions so that in the event a suspicious prescription appears, the suspected prescription can be compared with those prescriptions actually written by the veterinarian or practice.

Documentation is required by law for those controlled substances purchased, stored, used/administered, and discarded (as with expired drugs) by a veterinary hospital. The DEA requires such records be maintained and readily available for review for a minimum of 2 years. Individual states can require longer storage requirements. The dispensing or administration of any controlled substance must be documented in the individual patient record because each use of these drugs are restricted to one particular patient that meets the requirement for a valid veterinarian-client-patient relationship (VCPR). For purposes of tracking the purchase, use, and disposal of controlled substances, it is highly recommended that a separate controlled substance dispensing record be maintained in addition to (but not substituting for) the recorded information in the individual patient's medical record. Such a log book (in paper or secure electronic form) would make producing documentation much easier should the DEA or state agency make a sudden visit to the veterinary facility to check on records.

NOTE: Although not required specifically by law, if a paper system of a controlled substance log book is being used, practices are strongly advised against using a three-ring binder type notebook or any other paper recording method by which a page could be removed and replaced by another page containing false information. A better method is to have a bound laboratory-style notebook with numbers imprinted sequentially on each page by the notebook manufacturer so no page can be removed without the record obviously being altered.

Although specific recommendations on how best to inventory controlled substances in veterinary practices will vary somewhat, here are some basic principles to follow:

1. When a new shipment of controlled substances arrives, number the individual bottles or vials and log them into the controlled substances log book; keep the invoices sent with the shipment. Best practice is to have two people receive the new shipment and sign the log book for verification of receipt.
2. As any controlled substance is used or dispensed, make sure it is logged into the individual patient record and the controlled substances log book; perhaps keep the controlled substances log book near the surgery/anesthesia induction area for convenient accessibility.
3. Whenever a controlled substance is used or dispensed have a second individual verify appropriate drug, strength and quantity with an initial in the logbook.
4. Whenever a controlled substance is used or dispensed, make sure the individual bottle number (assigned when the product arrived) is recorded so that an individual bottle volume or pill count can be matched against the amount of drug actually dispensed or used. A discrepancy between the numbers dispensed and the numbers in the log book is a warning flag for either poor record keeping, inaccurate dosing/dispensing, or potential diversion of the hospital's controlled substances.
5. Inventory and verify the amount of controlled substance drugs used against the amount left in the bottles or vials at least once a month and every time inventory is received or dispensed. Being able to identify the cause for discrepancies in inventory of controlled substances becomes much harder beyond that time.
6. Rotate who is in charge of the controlled substance log book, or require the monthly inventory be completed by at least two individuals performing independent log/inventory verifications.
7. Best practice would be to require a signature and driver's license number for all controlled substances and gabapentin (if not controlled in your state) being picked up for use at home.

Remember that ultimately the control of these abuse drugs is the responsibility of the veterinarian whose DEA number appears on the purchase order for the drugs. When marking purchased bottles or vials of controlled substances with their unique in-house tracking number, the tracking number might include an indicator code for the person whose DEA number was used to order the drug (e.g., use "B" for Dr. Bill in the tracking code: 2016/07-003-B).

To see other methods by which abuse drugs are illegally obtained and the methods to prevent this diversion, the AVMA and CDC websites have credible and up to date information for your reference.

Sources:

US Department of Justice, Drug Enforcement Administration, Office of Diversion Control. https://www.deadiversion.usdoj.gov/pubs/index.html.

Riviere JE, Papich MG, eds. *Veterinary Pharmacology and Therapeutics*. 10th ed. Ames, Iowa: Wiley-Blackwell; 2018. https://www.deadiversion.usdoj.gov/schedules/orangebook/orangebook.pdf.

! YOU NEED TO KNOW

Storage of Controlled Substances

According to the DEA's *Practitioner's Manual*, practitioners (veterinarians) are required to store all C-II to C-V drugs in a "securely locked" and "substantially constructed" cabinet with limited access (meaning few have a key or know the combination to the lock). Beyond additional storage requirements for certain high-potency narcotic drugs, these phrases constitute the extent of the specific requirements for storage of controlled substances. Thus the actual storage of controlled substances is left up to interpretation by the veterinarian. However, in the event of a break-in or theft from the cabinet, the facility veterinarian will be required to prove to the DEA that he or she took appropriate security steps to minimize the risk for loss of the controlled substances. The following are bad examples of controlled substance storage:

- Controlled substances stored in a locked fishing tackle box hidden behind cleaning supplies in a closet.

    Why this is bad: Tackle box can simply be lifted and taken. Hiding the drug storage container is not sufficient security.

WRITING THE DRUG ORDER: THE DOSAGE REGIMEN

The dosage regimen is the complete information needed to determine the mass of drug to be given to the animal, the route by which the drug is to be given, how often it is to be given, and for how long the drug is to be administered. The amount of drug to be given to a specific patient is the dose, and the time between doses (e.g., every 12 hours) or the number of times per day is referred to as the dose interval. Box 2.1 shows examples of dosage regimens.

Dose vs Dosage

Before there can be a discussion about the dosage regimen, the terms dose and dosage must be clarified. Often these terms are used interchangeably in veterinary medicine, but they do have different meanings (Box 2.2). The dosage is the description of the mass of drug needed per unit of weight of animal for use in any animal. "10 mg/kg" or "2 mg/lb" would be examples of

dosages. In contrast, the dose is the specific number of dosage forms or mass of the drug that has been calculated for administration one time to a specific patient. "50 mg" or "10 grams" would be examples of doses. The dosage form is the physical form of the drug to be administered. "1 tablet" or "1 mL of solution" would be examples of dosage forms.

Thus, an antibiotic might have a dosage for any dog of 5 mg/kg, but a 10-kg dog would receive a dose of 50 mg (5 mg/kg × 10 kg = 50 mg). The 50 mg could be a dosage form of one 50-mg tablet or 1 mL of a 50-mg/mL solution.

Dosage Range

Occasionally instead of a single dosage being listed for a drug (e.g., 5 mg/kg), a dosage range may be listed (e.g., 5–10 mg/kg). Recall Rule #3, which states that all doses are guesses and doses must be adjusted to compensate for the patient's disease severity or physiologic condition. Dosage ranges allow the veterinarian to have some latitude in deciding whether to use the top end of the approved dosage range or a lower part of the dosage range.

A dosage range also allows the veterinary technician to tailor the dose to the available dosage forms. For example, if the prescribed medication's dosage form comes only in 100-mg tablets, the veterinary technician should be able to find an acceptable dosage within that dosage range that allows the medication to be dispensed as whole tablets so the owner doesn't have to split the tablets.

Abbreviations: The Language of the Drug Order

Generally the abbreviations used for writing prescriptions sent to a pharmacy are the same as those used for filling in-house drug orders and recording treatments in the patient's medical record. These abbreviations constitute a standardized form of communication between veterinary professionals and other health professionals involved in the delivery of animal health care. Veterinary technicians should commit these abbreviations to memory so they may be able to accurately translate a drug order given to them or be able to communicate drug dosing information to others. A list of the most common abbreviations and their meanings is provided in Table 2.1.

BOX 2.1 Examples of Dosage Regimens

Mass + route + dose interval + duration of treatment
- 5 mg IM q8h for 10 days
- 10 mg PO qd for 5 days
- 10 mL of the 5-mg/mL solution PO q12h for 2 weeks
- 2 of the 500-mg tablets PO s.i.d. for 10 days
- 0.5 gr (grains) PO q6h PRN (as needed)

BOX 2.2 Dose vs Dosage

A dose is for ONE particular patient:
- The 25-lb dog gets 250 mg
- The 5-kg cat gets 20 mg
- The estimated 1000-lb horse gets 4 grams

A dosage is for ANY patient:
- Dogs get 10 mg/lb
- Cats get 4 mg/kg
- Horses get 1 gram for every 250 lb

TABLE 2.1 Abbreviations Commonly Used in Prescriptions

b.i.d.	twice a day
cc	cubic centimeter
disp	dispense
g (or gm)	gram
gr	grain
gtt	drop
h (or hr)	hour
IM	intramuscular
IP	intraperitoneal
IV	intravenous
L	liter
lb	pound
mg	milligram
mL (or ml)	milliliter
OD	right eye
OS	left eye
OU	both eyes
oz	ounce
PO	by mouth
PRN	as needed
q	every
q4h	every 4 hours
q8h	every 8 hours
qd	every day (daily)
qh	every hour
q.i.d.	four times daily
q.o.d.	every other day
s.i.d.	once a day
SQ (or SC)	subcutaneous
stat	immediately
TBL or Tbsp	tablespoon
t.i.d.	three times daily
tsp	teaspoon

The standard format for most of these Latin abbreviations is to print the letters in lowercase with a period after each letter. However, the standard format is frequently ignored and these abbreviations may be used in all-capitalized form and may or may not use periods after each letter. For example, drug routes of administration like IV, IM, and PO are most often written as all-capitalized letters without periods. Regardless, the underlying principle is that each abbreviation must be written clearly and legibly so there is no doubt as to the dosing information being conveyed.

Note that pharmacists for human medicine are not trained to recognize the abbreviation "SID" or "s.i.d." used commonly in veterinary medicine to indicate "once daily." Therefore, in communicating a once-daily dose to a human pharmacist, "per day" should be used.

Common Medication Errors

The following rules from the National Coordinating Council for Medication Error and Reporting are useful to avoid writing ambiguous or confusing drug orders or dosing information.[4]

1. Avoid the use of trailing zeros after the decimal point (e.g., use 5 mL, not 5.0 mL). If the decimal point is overlooked, the number could be interpreted to be much higher (e.g., thought to be 50 mL instead of 5 mL).

2. Always put a zero in front of any decimal number less than zero (e.g., use 0.5 mL, not .5 mL). If the decimal point is overlooked, the number could be interpreted to be much higher (e.g., thought to be 5 mL instead of .5 mL).

3. Use "mL" (milliliter) instead of "cc" (cubic centimeter or "cm^3") even though they are equivalent. "cc," when poorly written in script handwriting, can look like a "u."

4. Avoid using teaspoon ("tsp." or "t.") and tablespoon ("tbsp." or "T") measurements because they are very close to each other in spelling and could easily be confused. Also, there are different acceptable equivalent metric volumes (mLs) for teaspoons and tablespoons depending on the country. In the United States, 1 US teaspoon = 4.93 mL and 1 US tablespoon = 14.79 mL, whereas in the United Kingdom 1 UK teaspoon = 3.55 mL, 1 UK tablespoon = 14.2 mL. In addition, tablespoon and teaspoon volumes in the metric system have volumes that are rounded to the nearest mL: 1 metric teaspoon = 5 mL, 1 metric tablespoon = 15 mL. In the United States, this last equivalency is the most commonly used equivalency in veterinary medicine. To avoid confusion, it is recommended best pharmacy practice to use the metric equivalents in place of the teaspoon or tablespoon units (i.e., 1 teaspoon = 5 mL; 1 tablespoon = 15 mL).

5. Write out "grains" instead of using the abbreviation "gr" because that can be confused with the abbreviation for "grams," which is "g" or "gm." Grains are an older unit of measurement still used with some medications like phenobarbital or aspirin. 1 grain = 64.799 milligrams (usually rounded to 65 mg), and confusing grains with grams will result in a significant miscalculation. To add to the confusion, 1 grain is also sometimes listed as being equivalent to the rounded amount of 60 mg instead of 64.8 mg so that 60 mg = 1 grain can be more evenly divided into half-grain (30 mg) and quarter-grain (15 mg) amounts.

6. Use "mcg" for micrograms (1×10^{-6} grams) instead of using the micron mu symbol "μ" as in "μg" or instead of the lowercase letter "U" with a "g" as in "ug." When handwritten or hand-printed, the mu "μ" can look like an "m," resulting in the microgram "μg" being interpreted as milligram "mg" (1×10^{-3} grams) and resulting in a 1000-fold miscalculation.

7. Be very clear in writing "a.u.," "a.d.," or "a.s." (both ears, right ear, left ear) to make sure it is readily differentiated from "o.u.," "o.d.," or "o.s." (both eyes, right eye, left eye). Ear medications inadvertently administered in the eye can be very damaging to the eye.

8. Never use "o.d." to mean "once daily" as it actually means "right eye."

9. Recognize that "s.i.d." (once daily) is not universally used outside of the veterinary profession. Hence "q.d." should be used for "every day" instead of "s.i.d."

10. It is preferable to use "q12h" (every 12 hours) instead of "b.i.d." (twice daily) because a client may not understand that the medication needs to be given in equally spaced dose intervals 12 hours apart. "q8h" (every 8 hours) should be used in place

of "t.i.d." (three times daily), and "q6h" (every 6 hours) should be used in place of "q.i.d." (four times daily).

11. Take extra care to differentiate "q.d." (every day) from "q.i.d." (four times daily) when writing or reading drug orders. Confusion between "q.d." and "q.i.d." can be avoided by writing out "every day" in place of "q.d." Also, do not use "q1d" (every 1 day) because it is far too easy to confuse with "q.i.d." (four times daily).

12. Write out the word "units" (e.g., "2 units of insulin") instead of using the "units" abbreviation "U." When poorly written, a "4U" can look like a "40." The abbreviation for "International Units" ("IU") used to quantify the unit of activity of some antibiotics and other drugs can look like "IV" (intravenous) unless clearly written.

Finally, if there is any doubt on how to write a drug order or if one's handwriting is sometimes marginally legible, always write out the complete information instead of using the abbreviations.

⊚ MYTHS AND MISCONCEPTIONS

"b.i.d." and "t.i.d." are the same as q12h and q8h

False! Although as veterinary professionals we think of "b.i.d." as equivalent to "every 12 hours" and "t.i.d." as "every 8 hours," literally b.i.d. and t.i.d. only mean to give the medication twice and three times daily, respectively. Thus, the pet owner may give the drug at 8:00 a.m. and 4:00 p.m. because those are the times most convenient for the owner. Because only 8 hours elapsed between 8:00 a.m. and 4:00 p.m. instead of the intended 12 hours a b.i.d. dose interval should have, the animal is going to have higher drug concentrations at the 4:00 p.m. dose than the concentrations at the 8:00 a.m. dose administration the next morning that occurs at the end of the 16-hour dose interval. Thus the veterinary technician should use the "q12h," "q8h," and "q6h" abbreviations instead of the "b.i.d.," "t.i.d.," and "q.i.d.," and animal owners should be instructed to give the medication "every 12 hours" instead of "twice daily."

If any question exists about the interpretation of the written information on a drug order, the veterinary technician is always obligated to check with the veterinarian for verification before administering the drug. Taking a few moments to ask for clarification is always better than making an incorrect guess and harming the patient. As Dr. Bill says, "When in doubt, check it out." "When in doubt, write it out." "It is always better to risk asking a silly question than to make a foolish mistake."

THE NEXT STEP: DETERMINING THE AMOUNT OF DRUG NEEDED

Now that the information of the drug order has been accurately conveyed from the veterinarian to the veterinary technician, the veterinary technician must translate the order into the dose the particular patient needs.

The Metric, Apothecary, and Household Measurement Systems

To understand how to calculate drug doses, the veterinary technician first needs to understand the different measurement systems used in veterinary medicine. Each system typically has

TABLE 2.2	Common Prefixes Used in the Metric System	
kilo (k)	multiplies by 1000	$\times 10^3$
hecto	multiplies by 100	$\times 10^2$
deka	multiplies by 10	$\times 10$
deci (d)	multiplies by 1/10	$\times 10^{-1}$
centi (c)	multiplies by 1/100	$\times 10^{-2}$
milli (m)	multiplies by 1/1000	$\times 10^{-3}$
micro (μ or mc)*	multiplies by 1/1,000,000	$\times 10^{-6}$
nano (n)	multiplies by 1/1,000,000,000	$\times 10^{-9}$

*Micro- is typically noted by the Greek letter mu. However, when "μ" is handwritten, it can look similar to a script letter "m" or printed letter "u." Therefore "mc" is becoming more commonly used in handwritten dosing orders, although "μ" is still often seen in typewritten text.

units to describe mass (weight), volume, and length. The metric system is the measurement system most commonly used today in veterinary medicine; however, some units of the apothecary system and the household measurement system can still be found in the veterinary literature.

The metric system uses different prefixes attached to a basic metric unit to designate 1000 ("kilo-"), 1/100 ("centi-"), or 1/1000 ("milli-") units. The basic metric unit of mass to which the prefix is attached is the *gram* (e.g., kilograms, milligrams); the basic metric unit of volume is the *liter* (e.g., kiloliters, milliliters); and the basic metric unit of length is the *meter* (e.g., kilometers, centimeters, millimeters). Conversion within the metric system from one unit to another equivalent unit (e.g., centimeters to millimeters) is much easier than within the other systems because all conversions are multiples of 10 (e.g., 1, 10, 100, 1000). See Table 2.2 for the common prefixes of the metric system used in veterinary medicine.

The apothecary system, which is a much older system than the metric system, is not used much in veterinary medicine. However, some volumes are still occasionally measured as "fluid ounces" ("fl oz") or "minims" (seen on the side of some syringes as a "℥" symbol) and mass is sometimes represented in "grains" ("gr"). Tablet strengths of aspirin, phenobarbital, and some OTC (over-the-counter) antiinflammatory drugs are listed in "grains" instead of the metric system milligrams; 1 grain = 60 milligrams.

⊚ MYTHS AND MISCONCEPTIONS

"Ounces" and "fluid ounces" really mean the same thing

False! An "ounce," appropriately named the "avoirdupois ounce" is a unit of *weight*. In fact "avoirdupois" is French for "goods of weight." A "fluid ounce" is a unit of *volume*. Thus a cup of water or any liquid *holds* 8 fluid ounces (8 fl. oz.), whereas a cup of water *weighs* 8.3 ounces (8.3 oz.) and a cup of honey *weighs* 12 ounces (12 oz.). Unless the word "ounce" is preceded by "fluid," assume that the "ounce" refers to a unit of weight or mass.

The household system, as the name implies, is based on common household units of measurement, such as the teaspoon, tablespoon, cup, pint, gallon, and pound. OTC liquid medications such as cold, flu, or pain relief medications are sometimes dispensed with directions stated in household measurements (e.g., "Give 1 teaspoon twice daily"). Because a pet owner may choose to literally use a utensil teaspoon vs a cooking measurement teaspoon, the more precise unit of "milliliter" is preferred for describing the amount of liquid oral drug formulations; 1 teaspoon is equivalent to 5 milliliters, and 1 tablespoon is equivalent to 15 milliliters.

Because these three systems of measurement are still used in human and veterinary medicine, the veterinary professional must be able to readily convert from a unit in the apothecary or household system to its equivalent metric unit. Additionally the veterinary technician must be able to reliably convert from one metric unit to another equivalent metric unit (e.g., from liters to milliliters). The equivalent conversions most commonly used in veterinary medicine are shown in Tables 2.3 and 2.4.

❓ ASK DR. BILL

Question:

My autocorrect software keeps correcting my spelling of "liter" to "litre." Which spelling is correct?

Answer:

Both are correct. However, the spelling "litre" is the spelling recognized by the International Bureau of Weights and Measures and the International System of Units (abbreviated "SI" for the French "Système International d'Unités"). The official SI spelling of "litre" is the spelling used in most English-speaking countries. However, in American English the spelling switches the "e" and "r" to the more phonetic spelling of "liter." Thus, if you are using a scientific or medical dictionary as your dictionary in your autocorrect software, it is likely using the SI spelling because that is the spelling version most accepted worldwide.

The Steps for Calculating the Drug Mass Needed

To calculate the dose for a particular patient, there are two pieces of information needed:
1. The weight of the animal
2. The dosage (in mass of drug per unit of weight or mass of animal)

   Given the animal's weight in pounds (lb), kilograms (kg), or grams (g) and the dosage in milligrams of drug per kilogram of

TABLE 2.3 Equivalent Units of Weight or Mass in the Metric, Apothecary, and Household Systems

Weight or Mass		
1 kilogram (kg)	=	2.2 pounds (lb)
1 kilogram (kg)	=	1000 grams (g)
1 kilogram (kg)	=	1,000,000 milligrams (mg)
1 gram (g)	=	1000 milligrams (mg)
1 gram (g)	=	0.001 kilogram (kg)
1 milligram (mg)	=	0.001 gram (g)
1 milligram (mg)	=	1000 micrograms (µg or mcg)
1 pound (lb)	=	0.454 kilogram (kg)
1 pound (lb)	=	16 ounces (oz)
1 grain (gr)	=	64.8 milligrams (mg) (household system)
1 grain (gr)	=	60 milligrams (mg) (apothecary)

TABLE 2.4 Equivalent Units of Volume in the Metric, Apothecary, and Household Systems

Volume		
1 liter (L)	=	1000 milliliters (mL)
1 liter (L)	=	10 deciliters (dL)
1 milliliter (mL)	=	1 cubic centimeter (cc)
1 milliliter (mL)	=	1000 microliters (µL or mcL)
1 tablespoon (TBL or Tbsp)	=	3 teaspoons (tsp)
1 tablespoon (TBL or Tbsp)	=	15 milliliters (mL)
1 teaspoon (tsp)	=	5 milliliters (mL)
1 gallon (gal)	=	3.786 liters (L)
1 gallon (gal)	=	4 quarts (qt)
1 gallon (gal)	=	8 pints (pt)
1 pint (pt)	=	2 cups (c)
1 pint (pt)	=	16 fluid ounces (fl oz)
1 pint (pt)	=	473 milliliters (mL)

body weight (mg/kg) or milligrams of drug per pound of body weight (mg/lb), this calculation will yield the mass of drug needed for this particular patient in milligrams, grams, or kilograms of drug. Note that the dosage of the drug is not usually expressed as liquid volumes, such as milliliters, cc, or liters, because the amount of drug contained within a volume of liquid may be 10 mg, 100 mg, 1000 mg, etc. The same is true for solid dosage forms such as tablets, capsules, or powders, because a tablet may have 5 mg or 50 mg of drug. The dose should always be expressed as mass (mg, grams) of drug.

The dose calculation method that will be demonstrated in this text is the method sometimes referred to as "dimensional analysis" or the "cancel-out" method. A brief description of the principles of this method is shown in the You Need to Know box "An Explanation of Dimensional Analysis or the Cancel-Out Method of Dose Calculation."

❗ YOU NEED TO KNOW

An Explanation of Dimensional Analysis or the Cancel-Out Method of Dose Calculation

Dimensional analysis (sometimes called the "cancel-out method") is a calculation method used extensively in human nursing and has been largely adopted by veterinary professionals. Once the concept of dimensional analysis is understood, it can be applied to any number of calculations used in veterinary nursing.

In a dimensional analysis problem, a Known Value (e.g., weight of the animal) and the units of that known entity (e.g., pounds) are multiplied by a Conversion Factor (e.g., the dose expressed in units of in mg/lb) to produce the answer in the units required (e.g., mg of drug the animal needs).

KNOWN VALUE × CONVERSION FACTOR = ANSWER

As stated previously, the Conversion Factor is typically expressed as a fraction of two different units with one unit in the numerator (top part) of the fraction and the other unit in the denominator (bottom part) of the fraction (e.g., 10 mg/lb, 4 mL/kg, 5 tablets/dose).

How the units of the Known Value, the Conversion Factor, and the answer are arranged determines whether or not the correct answer will be calculated using dimensional analysis. The equation must be set up so that the Known Value unit (e.g., kg, lb, and mg) must be the same as the unit in the bottom part of the fraction, or denominator, of the Conversion Factor fraction (e.g., for "10 mg/kg" the bottom denominator unit would be "kg"). In this way, the unit of the Known Value "cancels" with the denominator unit of the Conversion Factor, eliminating this unit from the equation (hence the name "cancel-out method"). If the equation has been set up correctly, the only remaining unit on the left side of the equal sign after all similar units have been canceled out will be the same unit wanted for the answer. The next example shows this concept:

$$KNOWN\ VALUE \times CONVERSION\ FACTOR = ANSWER$$

$$5\ kg \times \frac{10\ mg}{kg} = ?\ mg$$

$$5\ \cancel{kg} \times \frac{10\ mg}{\cancel{kg}} = ?\ mg\ \P$$

$$5 \times \frac{10\ mg}{1} = ?\ mg$$

$$5 \times 10\ mg = 50\ mg$$

Dimensional Analysis Rules:
1. A unit in the numerator (top part) of any fraction in the equation can cancel with the denominator (bottom part) unit of any other fraction, thus removing that unit from the equation. Note that the whole number "5 kg" is the same value as the fraction "5 kg/1" and thus the kg in "5 kg" can be canceled out with a kg unit in the denominator of another fraction.
2. After all other units are canceled out, the unit used in the answer ("mg" in the previous example) must always be found in the top (numerator) part of some fraction.
3. The individual components of the equation (Known Values and Conversion Factors) need to be moved, manipulated, or inverted (flipped) until all the units on the left side of the equation cancel out with the exception of the unit(s) in which the answer is to be expressed.
4. Once the equation units have been appropriately canceled, the solution is determined by simple multiplication of the equation.

The Known Value (the "given value") in this equation is the body weight of the animal; the Conversion Factor is the dosage (mass of drug per unit of body weight); and the desired answer is the drug dose (mass of drug) needed for this particular animal.

$$KNOWN\ VALUE \times CONVERSION\ FACTOR = ANSWER$$

$$BODY\ WEIGHT \times \frac{MASS\ OF\ DRUG}{UNIT\ OF\ WEIGHT} = DRUG\ DOSE$$

$$BODY\ WEIGHT \times DOSAGE = DRUG\ DOSE$$

If the animal weighs 20 pounds (lb) and the dosage of a drug listed by the drug manufacturer is 5 mg of drug per pound of body weight (5 mg/lb), then we can plug these values into the equation and multiply to determine the dose.

When the problem is set up, the fraction for the Conversion Factor (the 5-mg/lb dosage) is arranged so that the "lb" unit is placed in the denominator to "cancel" the "lb" unit in the body weight, leaving only the unit "mg" in the numerator (top) of the Conversion Factor fraction on the left side of the equal sign. "mg" is the unit needed in the answer, and that unit is in the numerator on the left side of the equation, thus meeting the criteria for correctly setting up the equation as described in the

Need to Know box "An Explanation of Dimensional Analysis or the Cancel-Out Method of Dose Calculation." Multiplying the equation gives the answer.

$$20\ lb \times \frac{5\ mg\ drug}{lb\ body\ weight} = DRUG\ DOSE\ (mg)$$

$$20\ \cancel{lb} \times \frac{5\ mg\ drug}{\cancel{lb\ body\ weight}} = DRUG\ DOSE\ (mg)$$

$$20 \times \frac{5\ mg\ drug}{1} = DRUG\ DOSE\ (mg)$$

$$20 \times 5\ mg\ drug = 100\ (mg)$$

The 100 mg is the mass of drug needed for this particular 20-pound animal and hence constitutes the specific dose for this animal derived from the dosage of 5 mg/lb.

Pounds and Kilogram Conversion

With the integration of the metric system into the US medical system it is common to have the drug dosage listed in the metric system (e.g., 10 mg/kg) but still have the animal's weight listed in pounds. The animal may also be weighed on a metric scale and the weight listed in kilograms but the dosage is listed as milligrams of drug per pound of body weight. Either way, for dimensional analysis to work all of the units on the left side of the equation must cancel out, leaving just the answer unit intact on the left side of the equation. Because pounds and kilograms are not the same, they cannot directly cancel each other out. However, if we convert pounds to kilograms or kilograms to pounds using the Conversion Factor of 2.2 lb/kg or 1 kg/2.2 lb, we can arrange the problem to cancel out all the units, leaving just "mg" for the answer, thus meeting the criteria for correctly setting up a dimensional analysis problem.

GIVEN: 10-kg dog and a dosage of 5 mg/lb, what is the dose in mg?

$$KNOWN\ VALUE \times CONVERSION\ FACTOR$$
$$\times CONVERSION\ FACTOR = ANSWER$$

$$BODY\ WEIGHT \times LB\ TO\ KG\ CONVERSION\ FACTOR$$
$$\times DOSAGE = DOSE\ (mg)$$

$$10\ kg \times \frac{2.2\ lb}{1\ kg} \times \frac{5\ mg}{lb} = DOSE\ (mg)$$

$$10\ \cancel{kg} \times \frac{2.2\ lb}{1\ \cancel{kg}} \times \frac{5\ mg}{lb} = DOSE\ (mg)$$

$$10 \times \frac{2.2\ lb}{1} \times \frac{5\ mg}{lb} = DOSE\ (mg)$$

$$10 \times \frac{2.2\ \cancel{lb}}{1} \times \frac{5\ mg}{\cancel{lb}} = DOSE\ (mg)$$

$$10 \times \frac{2.2}{1} \times \frac{5\ mg}{1} = DOSE\ (mg)$$

$$10 \times 2.2 \times 5\ mg = 110\ mg$$

Know Your Metrics and How to Convert to Different Equivalent Units

Because weights of animals may be expressed as kilograms, grams, or pounds, the veterinary technician needs to commit to memory the prefixes used in the metric system (Table 2.2) and the basic equivalents between the metric system units and the apothecary and the household measurement system units still commonly used in veterinary medicine (Tables 2.3 and 2.4). A summary of how to mathematically convert from one unit to the equivalent unit is summarized in the You Need to Know box "Making Any Conversion From One Unit to the Equivalent Unit."

! YOU NEED TO KNOW

Making Any Conversion From One Unit to the Equivalent Unit

Conversion of one unit to another equivalent unit (e.g., X number of mg to corresponding number of grams) is one of the most commonly used medical mathematical functions performed by the veterinary technician. To do so is simple with dimensional analysis. The same basic formula involving the Known Value and Conversion Factor is used; for this example we will convert 1500 mg to the corresponding value in grams.

$$KNOWN\ VALUE \times CONVERSION\ FACTOR = ANSWER$$

In this case, the Known Value is the 1500 mg that needs to be converted, the Conversion Factor is the ratio of equivalency between milligrams and grams expressed as a fraction (e.g., 1000 mg = 1 gram is expressed mathematically as the fraction 1000 mg/gram or 1 gram/1000 mg), and the answer needs to be in the units of grams. For this problem, the equation would be set up as:

$$1500\ mg \times \frac{1\ gram}{1000\ mg} = ?\ grams$$

Note how the Conversion Factor is arranged so that the milligram unit on the bottom of the fraction can cancel with the milligram unit of the Known Value, leaving the answer unit of grams in the top part of the fraction on the left side of the equation. This meets the criteria for correctly setting up a dimensional analysis problem.

$$1500\ \cancel{mg} \times \frac{1\ gram}{1000\ \cancel{mg}} = ?\ grams$$

$$1500 \times \frac{1\ gram}{1000} = ?\ grams$$

$$\frac{1500\ grams}{1000} = ?\ grams$$

$$1.5\ grams = ?\ grams$$

Using the same technique, any value expressed as one type of unit can be converted to the equivalent value in another unit either within the metric system or between the metric and the other measurement systems.

A Variation in the Dosage: Milligram of Drug per Square Meter (mg/m²)

Occasionally a dosage is listed as milligram of drug per square meter of the patient's body surface area instead of the more familiar mg/kg body weight or mg/lb body weight. This method of dosage tends to be more accurate for animals that are significantly larger or smaller than the typical "average sized" animal upon which development of the dosage was based. This degree of accuracy typically is not needed with most drugs but for certain toxic drugs (e.g., cancer chemotherapy agents, certain toxic cardiac drugs) the margin between the beneficial dose and a dose that produces significant toxicity can be very close, thus necessitating a more accurate dosing method for significantly smaller or larger patients.

The square meter body surface area (m^2) of an animal is determined using a mathematical formula that takes into account the patient's body weight and length (height) and is most commonly determined using a table in a veterinary drug reference. Thus if a dose for a drug is given in mg/m^2, then the patient's weight and length must be converted into square meters (m^2) of body surface area to solve the problem. Once this conversion is made, the exact same equation is used for calculating a mg/lb or mg/kg dose, except that in place of lb or kg, m^2 is used instead.

$$2\ m^2 \times \frac{5\ mg\ drug}{m^2\ surface\ area} = DRUG\ DOSE\ (mg)$$

Understanding the Language to Adjust the Dose

Sometimes an animal requires a greater or lesser amount of the dose based upon the physiologic condition of the animal. For example, an animal in renal failure administered a drug that is normally excreted by the kidneys would require a decreased drug dose compared with a normal dog. When writing drug orders a veterinary technician may be told to adjust a dose by a particular fraction or percentage. Therefore it is important to understand the wording because slight changes in how these drug orders are expressed can mean completely different prescribed orders.

If a veterinarian says to "decrease the dose by 25%," this means that the veterinary technician must determine what constitutes 25% of the total calculated dose and subtract that from the total. For example, a veterinarian ordered that a patient needed 25% less of the normal 100-mg dose for that size of patient. To determine what constituted a 25% decrease, the veterinary technician multiplied 100 mg × 25%. Remember that any percent number "XX%" is the same as the decimal number "0.XX." Thus, 100 mg × 0.25 = 25 mg. To decrease the dose by 25%, the veterinary technician subtracted 25 mg from the total calculated dose of 100 mg to arrive at the new adjusted dose of 75 mg.

If the veterinarian had said to "decrease the dose to 25% of its original dose" the veterinarian was saying that the dose was going to be reduced to a size of that percentage. If the calculated dose for a normal animal was 100 mg, a reduction to 25% would mean multiplying the 100 mg × 0.25 = 25 mg. In this case, the calculated percentage is not being subtracted from the original dose: the percentage is the new adjusted dose. Thus it is very important to clearly understand what is being communicated in these drug orders.

A similar situation would occur if the veterinarian said to "increase the dose by 40%." In this case, the veterinarian is saying to determine what 40% of the normal calculated dose is, then add that to the normal calculated dose. If the normal calculated dose was 100 mg, then 40% of the 100 mg would be 100 mg × 0.40 = 40 mg, and the 40 mg would be added to the 100 mg to give 140 mg for the new adjusted dose.

If the veterinarian orders the dose to be increased to 150% of its original, the veterinary technician needs to ignore the fact that mathematically percentages can't go higher than 100% and instead multiply the original dose by the percentage to produce the new adjusted dose. If 100 mg was the original dose, then 100 mg × 1.50 = 150 mg is the new adjusted increased dose.

Because subtle changes in language can produce very different changes in dose, the veterinary technician should always confirm that the change in dose calculated by the veterinary technician is what the veterinarian had actually intended. When it comes to patient care, there is no excuse for not clarifying a question on drug orders before administering the drug.

CALCULATING THE AMOUNT OF DOSAGE FORM NEEDED

Now that the mass (dose) of the drug has been determined for the patient, the next step is to determine how many dosage units are needed to deliver the dose of drug.

The same general formula used for determining the dose using dimensional analysis can be used for determining the number of dosage form units needed.

KNOWN VALUE × CONVERSION FACTOR = ANSWER

In this case, the Known Value is the dose calculated previously for the patient (typically expressed in milligrams of drug), the Conversion Factor is the concentration or strength of the dosage form, and the answer is the number of dosage form units.

The Conversion Factor for liquid dosage forms is the drug concentration in the liquid typically expressed as milligrams of drug per unit of volume of the liquid dosage form (e.g., 15 mg of drug for each mL of dosage form liquid would be a concentration of 15 mg/mL). The Conversion Factor for solid dosage forms would be the milligrams or mass of drug found in each tablet, caplet, or capsule but is more commonly referred to as the dose form's "strength." A 100-mg tablet or a 50-mg capsule contains 100 mg of drug in each tablet or 50 mg of drug in each capsule.

The following example applies this basic dimensional analysis formula to determine the number of dosage forms needed to deliver the required drug dose for a patient. Assume that a drug order calls for a patient to receive 100 mg of drug in liquid dosage form via injection. The veterinary hospital carries the injectable drug in bottles of 25-mg/mL concentration. Given the calculated dose of 100 mg needed for the patient, the veterinary technician needs to determine the volume (mL) of the 25-mg/mL liquid needed to deliver 100 mg of drug to this patient. Because the answer must be in milliliters (mL), the equation must be set up so that the units of "mg" cancel out, leaving only the unit of "mL" in the numerator (upper) part of the fraction. Here is how the equation was set up:

KNOWN VALUE × CONVERSION FACTOR = ANSWER

DOSE × CONCENTRATION = VOLUME OF FLUID

$$100 \text{ mg} \times \frac{1 \text{ mL}}{25 \text{ mg}} = \text{VOLUME OF FLUID (mL)}$$

Notice how the concentration of 25 mg/mL was inverted to 1 mL/25 mg to comply with the rule in dimensional analysis

that requires canceling out all units except the answer unit. The milligram (mg) unit in the numerator of the fraction 100 mg/1, which is the same value as 100 mg, is canceled with the matching milligram (mg) unit in the denominator in the 1 mL/25 mg fraction. If the concentration had been set up as 25 mg/mL instead of 1 mL/25 mg, the "mg" units would not have been able to cancel each other because they both would have been in the numerator of their fractions.

Because the equation is set up so the milligram (mg) units can cancel out, leaving just the mL unit in the numerator, we know we have set up the equation correctly and can proceed with multiplying to find the answer.

$$100 \text{ mg} \times \frac{1 \text{ mL}}{25 \text{ mg}} = \text{VOLUME OF FLUID (mL)}$$

$$100 \times \frac{1 \text{ mL}}{25} = \text{VOLUME OF FLUID (mL)}$$

$$\frac{100 \text{ mL}}{25} = \text{VOLUME OF FLUID (mL)}$$

$$4 \text{ mL} = \text{VOLUME OF FLUID (mL)}$$

Thus to deliver 100 mg of drug to the patient, 4 mL of the 25-mg/mL concentration of the drug must be injected into the animal.

The same method is used to determine the number of tablets a patient would need to take orally to deliver the appropriate dose of drug. The tablet strength would take the place of the liquid concentration for the Conversion Factor in the previous example. Here is an example where the number of tablets a patient needs has been determined from a calculated patient dose of 200 mg and the tablet strength of 50 mg per tablet.

KNOWN VALUE × CONVERSION FACTOR = ANSWER

DOSE × TABLET STRENGTH = NUMBER OF TABLETS

$$200 \text{ mg} \times \frac{1 \text{ tablet}}{50 \text{ mg}} = \text{NUMBER OF TABLETS}$$

$$20 \text{ mg} \times \frac{1 \text{ tablet}}{50 \text{ mg}} = \text{NUMBER OF TABLETS}$$

$$200 \times \frac{1 \text{ tablet}}{50} = \text{NUMBER OF TABLETS}$$

$$\frac{200 \text{ tablets}}{50} = \text{NUMBER OF TABLETS}$$

$$4 \text{ tablets} = \text{NUMBER OF TABLETS}$$

Important note: The number of tablets in the answers of these calculations rarely comes out to a whole tablet for the dose. More frequently the answer is something like "1.245 tablets" or "0.665 tablets." As a general rule, tablets should only be dispensed as whole or half tablets. Thus when the number of tablets per dose appears as a decimal fraction, it must be rounded to the nearest whole or half tablet. This may require rounding the dose down to the nearest half or whole if the calculated number of tablets is closer to a half or whole by rounding down than rounding up. The examples illustrate this rounding principle.

0.65 tablets rounds to 0.5 tablet
0.85 tablets rounds to 1 tablet
1.2 tablets rounds to 1 tablet
1.3 tablets rounds to 1.5 tablets
5.2367 tablets round to 5 tablets
5.6666 tablets rounds to 5.5 tablets
5.7777 tablets rounds to 6 tablets

One of the most common mistakes in calculating the total number of tablets to be dispensed is failing to round the number of tablets per dose to the nearest half or whole tablet before determining the total number of tablets to be dispensed. This will be discussed more in the section that shows how to determine the total number of tablets needed to be dispensed for the dosage regimen time span.

Percentage Solutions: A Variation in the Typical Liquid Drug Concentration

One day a veterinary technician completed a dose calculation for a patient, determined the patient needed 800 mg of injectable drug, and retrieved the bottle to withdraw the appropriate volume of liquid to deliver the 800 mg. She was surprised to find the drug concentration listed on the bottle as "10% solution" instead of some "mg/mL" and thus did not know how to proceed. Solving this problem requires knowing the definition for what constitutes a "percentage solution."

A percentage solution is most commonly used in liquid dosage forms as the number of grams of drug (not mg) per 100 mL of liquid. This percentage solution is referred to as a weight by volume percentage solution because it is a weight (grams) of drug in a volume (100 mL) of medium. Percentage solutions can also be volume by volume, representing the number of milliliters (mL) of drug per 100 mL of total liquid medium (e.g., volume of liquid drug mixed with volume liquid medium) or, less frequently, weight by weight, representing the number of grams of drug per 100 grams of drug and medium (e.g., mass of powdered drug mixed with powdered filler medium or mass of drug mixed with mass of liquid medium). The different percentage solutions are often abbreviated as "w/v," "v/v," or "w/w" to represent weight by volume, volume by volume, or weight by weight, respectively. Table 2.5 shows examples of percentage solutions with their corresponding concentrations in each of these three formats.

Regardless of the nature of the percentage solution, the percentage solution needs to be converted into its w/v, w/w, or v/v

equivalent to determine the number of dosage forms to be used to meet the dose requirements. In the example earlier, the 10% percentage solution is a w/v equivalent of 10 grams of drug per 100 mL of liquid in the bottle. To determine the volume of drug needed to deliver the 800 mg of drug, the 10 grams/100 mL should be converted to the equivalent milligrams per milliliter (mg/mL) and then plugged into the equation as was shown previously for determining the volume of dosage form needed. To make this conversion, the grams in the 10 grams/100 mL must be converted to milligrams and the fraction reduced.

Using the dimensional analysis format, the 10 grams/100 mL becomes the Known Value and the Conversion Factor is the relationship of "1000 milligrams = 1 gram" expressed as "1000 mg/1 g." Notice in the following steps how the equation is set up so the gram units are appropriately positioned on the top or bottom of the fractions to cancel out, leaving the mg unit in the numerator (top) part of the fraction and the mL unit in the denominator (bottom) part of the fraction.

$$\text{KNOWN VALUE} \times \text{CONVERSION FACTOR} = \text{ANSWER}$$

$$10\% \text{ solution} \times \frac{1000 \text{ mg}}{1 \text{ gram}} = ?\frac{\text{mg}}{\text{mL}}$$

$$\frac{10 \text{ grams}}{100 \text{ mL}} \times \frac{1000 \text{ mg}}{1 \text{ gram}} = ?\frac{\text{mg}}{\text{mL}}$$

$$\frac{10 \ \cancel{\text{grams}}}{100 \text{ mL}} \times \frac{1000 \text{ mg}}{1 \ \cancel{\text{grams}}} = ?\frac{\text{mg}}{\text{mL}}$$

$$\frac{10}{100 \text{ mL}} \times \frac{1000 \text{ mg}}{1} = ?\frac{\text{mg}}{\text{mL}}$$

$$\frac{10000 \text{ mg}}{100 \text{ mL}} = ?\frac{\text{mg}}{\text{mL}}$$

$$\frac{100 \text{ mg}}{1 \text{ mL}} = ?\frac{\text{mg}}{\text{mL}}$$

$$\frac{100 \text{ mg}}{\text{mL}} = ?\frac{\text{mg}}{\text{mL}}$$

Now that the 10% concentration has been converted into the 100 mg/mL format, the calculation for the number of milliliters (mL) of the dosage form can be completed like the calculations previously shown.

TABLE 2.5 Definitions of Different Percentage Solutions			
Type of Percentage Solution	X% Solution Equals	Example 5% Solution	Formula
weight by volume (w/v)	X grams drug dissolved in 100 mL liquid medium	5% = 5 grams drug/100 mL liquid = 50 mg/mL	Solid drug dissolves in liquid medium so doesn't add to the volume
volume by volume (v/v)	X mL liquid drug in 100 mL of liquid drug + liquid medium (total volume)	5% = 5 mL drug/100 mL total liquid volume drug + medium	Liquid drug doesn't dissolve into liquid medium so total volume = drug volume + medium volume
weight by weight (w/w)	X grams drug in 100 grams of drug + powder medium (total weight)	5% = 5 grams drug/100 grams total weight drug + medium	Powdered drug doesn't dissolve into powdered medium so total weight = powdered drug weight + powdered medium weight

12 grams of drug dissolved in 100 mL of water = 12 g/100 mL = 12% w/v solution.
50 g of powdered drug mixed with 100 g powdered medium = 50 g/150 g = 33% w/w solution.
15 mL drug mixed with 35 mL water = 15 mL/50 mL = 30% v/v solution.

The **dilution equation** ($C_1V_1 = C_2V_2$) can also be used to calculate percent solutions. This equation is especially helpful when making a percent solution such as 2.5% dextrose. To create a 2.5% dextrose solution you must know the following information:

1. What percent dextrose do you have (C_1)?
2. What percent solution do you want to make (C_2)?
3. What total volume of fluid are you making your percent solution into (V_2)?
4. All units must match (e.g., All mass units in mg and all volume units in mL)
5. Solve for V_1, amount of C_1 you need to make the desired percent solution.

For example, the veterinarian asks you to make a 2.5% dextrose solution in 1000 mL of the prescribed fluids. Your dextrose stock solution is 50%. This is how you would solve this problem using the dilution equation.

1. You have 50% dextrose, C_1 (convert to mg/mL = 500 mg/mL)
2. You want to make 2.5% dextrose solution, C_2 (convert to mg/mL = 25 mg/mL)

3. The total volume you are making is 1000 mL (V_2)
4. All units match
5. Solve for V_1

(500 mg/mL)(V_1) = (25 mg/mL)(1000 mL) solve the equation for V_1 and be sure to cancel units as you go. If you have done this correctly you will be left with $V_1 = 50$ mL. We now know to make the 2.5% dextrose solution, we need to add 50 mL of the 50% dextrose to the 1000 mL bag of fluids. To make an exact 2.5% solution, you would remove 50 mL of fluids from the bag before adding the 50 mL of 50% dextrose to the bag. Many practices will not remove the fluid as long as the volume added is less than 10% of the total volume in the bag. It is important that the veterinary technician know the preference of the veterinarian they are working with when making percent solutions for their patients.

Percentage solutions are used in a variety of nursing settings in veterinary medicine. Therefore it is important that the veterinary technician be able to calculate percentage solutions to compound powdered drugs into liquid formulations, dilute concentrations of liquid drugs, or add drugs to intravenous fluids to achieve the appropriate concentration.

! YOU NEED TO KNOW

Using Weight by Volume (w/v) Percentage Solutions

A weight by volume (w/v) solution is one in which a dry mass of drug (the "weight") is added to, and dissolves in, a liquid medium (the "volume"). For example, a veterinary technician has been given a drug order to create 200 mL of a 4% solution (4 grams of drug per 100 mL of medium) using drug in powdered form and sterile saline for the liquid medium. The Known Value is total volume of the final drug solution (200 mL), the Conversion Factor is the 4% solution concentration (this converts mL of volume to grams of dry drug needed to be put into the liquid), and the answer is the number of dry grams of drug needed to make a 4% solution.

KNOWN VALUE × CONVERSION FACTOR = ANSWER

$$200 \text{ mL} \times 4\% \text{ solution} = ? \text{ grams}$$

$$200 \text{ mL} \times \frac{4 \text{ grams}}{100 \text{ mL}} = ? \text{ grams}$$

$$200 \text{ mL} \times \frac{4 \text{ grams}}{100 \text{ mL}} = ? \text{ grams}$$

$$\frac{800 \text{ grams}}{100} = ? \text{ grams}$$

$$8 \text{ grams} = ? \text{ grams}$$

Or with the dilution equation ($C_1V_1 = C_2V_2$): The concentration we have is 100% of the power and want a 4% solution in 200 mL. This is how you could solve this equation with this method, making sure all of your units match:

$$(100 \text{ g}/100 \text{ mL})(X) = (4 \text{ grams}/100 \text{ mL})(200 \text{ mL})$$

Solve for X to get 8 grams of the 100% powder to add to the 200 mL of sterile saline liquid medium to produce a 4% solution required by the drug order.

Thus 8 grams of powdered drug must be dissolved in 200 mL This same basic formula can be rearranged to accommodate variations in this type of question. For example, if the veterinary technician is given 8 grams of drug and asked to make a 4% solution by dissolving it in sterile saline, the volume of sterile saline can be determined as shown:

KNOWN VALUE × CONVERSION FACTOR = ANSWER

$$8 \text{ grams} \times 4\% \text{ solution} = ? \text{ mL}$$

$$8 \text{ grams} \times \frac{100 \text{ mL}}{4 \text{ grams}} = ? \text{ mL}$$

$$8 \times \frac{100 \text{ mL}}{4} = ? \text{ mL}$$

$$\frac{800 \text{ mL}}{4} = ? \text{ mL}$$

$$200 \text{ mL} = ? \text{ mL}$$

If the veterinary technician is told that 8 grams of drug was added to 200 mL of liquid and asked the percentage solution that resulted, a dimensional analysis is not required. A w/v percentage solution is defined as the number of grams over 100 mL of liquid. In this problem, it was stated that 8 grams of drug are in 200 mL of liquid, so it is merely a matter of reducing the 8 grams/200 mL to X grams/100 mL. In other words, this question asks what fraction of "X grams/100 mL" is equivalent to 8 grams/200 mL. Because we are asking for the equivalent fraction to 8 grams/200 mL, the problem is set up as an equation:

$$\frac{8 \text{ grams}}{200 \text{ mL}} = \frac{X \text{ grams}}{100 \text{ mL}}$$

The problem just needs to be solved for "X" using simple algebraic cross-multiplying to isolate the unknown X on the right of the equal sign. For help in how to cross-multiply algebraically, see a medical math textbook.

$$\frac{8 \text{ grams}}{200 \text{ mL}} = \frac{X \text{ grams}}{100 \text{ mL}}$$

$$\frac{8 \text{ grams}}{200 \text{ mL}} \times 100 \text{ mL} = \frac{X \text{ grams}}{100 \text{ mL}} \times 100 \text{ mL}$$

$$\frac{8 \text{ grams}}{200 \text{ mL}} \times 100 \text{ mL} = \frac{X \text{ grams}}{100 \text{ mL}} \times 100 \text{ mL}$$

$$\frac{800 \text{ grams}}{200} = X \text{ grams}$$

$$4 \text{ grams} = X \text{ grams}$$

Plug the "4 grams" into the "X grams" to get 4 grams/100 mL, which is a 4% solution. Thus 8 grams dissolved in 200 mL of liquid yields a 4% solution.

Calculations involving percentage solutions using weight by weight (w/w) or volume by volume (v/v) require an additional calculation step because in these mixtures the volume or mass of the drug added to the medium increases the volume or mass of the final mixture. This is in contrast to w/v percentage solutions where the drug simply dissolves into the liquid medium without adding any volume or mass to the final drug form. See the You Need to Know box "Calculating Dosage Forms Using Weight/Weight (w/w) and Volume/Volume (v/v) of Percentage Solutions" for how to modify the steps in the calculation of percentage solution when using weight by weight or volume by volume percentage solutions.

❗ YOU NEED TO KNOW

Calculating Dosage Forms Using Weight/Weight (w/w) and Volume/Volume (v/v) of Percentage Solutions

Using volume by volume (v/v) or weight by weight (w/w) percentage solutions requires one step added to the method used to determine weight by volume (w/v) percentage solutions as described in the You Need to Know box "Using Weight by Volume (w/v) Percentage Solutions." This additional step is required because unlike the weight by volume (w/v) where the dry drug powder is dissolved in the liquid volume and does not add to the final volume of the liquid, a volume by volume or weight by weight problem adds to the volume or mass of the total mixture.

For example, a 2% v/v solution would be 2 mL of drug in a TOTAL of 100 mL of fluid that is composed of 2 mL of solution plus 98 mL of the original liquid medium (e.g., water, sterile saline, alcohol) to which the solution was added.

The same concept applies to the weight by weight (w/w) percentage mixtures where a 2% w/w solution would be composed of 2 grams of drug powder mixed with 98 grams of filler (medium) powder to equal a total of 100 grams of the mixture (2 grams of drug in 100 total grams of mixed powder = 2%). Or a 2% w/w might be 2 grams of liquid drug added to 98 grams of a liquid medium (2 grams of liquid drug in 100 total grams of mixed liquids).

Therefore, in a w/w or v/v percentage solution, the weight or volume of drug calculated as the answer must be subtracted from the TOTAL weight or volume of the final mixture to determine the weight or volume of medium needed for the final mixture. As previously mentioned, many institutions will not pull out the liquid for the additive unless it is greater than 10% of the total volume. This is something that is dependent on the veterinary facility you are working in, and understanding you are not creating the exact percent solution ordered. The following example illustrates this difference.

A veterinary technician has been given the drug order to create 200 grams of a 4% w/w mixture of powdered drug using powdered sugar as the medium or filler. Using the general dimensional analysis equation previously described, the Known Value component is the final mass of the total mixture (200 grams) and the Conversion Factor would be the 4% w/w solution. A 4% solution in w/w would be 4 grams/100 grams of TOTAL mixture. The answer will be expressed as the number of grams of drug needed to make the total 200 grams of the final mixture. From that answer the number of grams of filler can also be calculated.

KNOWN VALUE × CONVERSION FACTOR = ANSWER

200 grams (total weight) × 4% solution (w/w) = ?grams (drug)

$$200 \text{ grams (total weight)} \times \frac{4 \text{ grams (drug weight 4\% solution)}}{100 \text{ grams}}$$
$$= ? \text{ grams (drug)}$$
$$200 \times \frac{4 \text{ grams}}{100} = ? \text{ grams}$$
$$\frac{800 \text{ grams}}{100} = ? \text{ grams}$$
$$8 \text{ grams} = ? \text{ grams}$$

8 grams is the total weight (mass) of drug that is found in the total mixture of 200 grams of a 4% solution (w/w). But if we weigh out 8 grams of drug, how many grams of the powdered sugar filler need to be added to the 8 grams of drug to complete the compilation of 200 mg of 4% solution (w/w)? This is where the additional step comes in for w/w and v/v percentage solutions.

If the total weight of the final mixture of the 4% solution is 200 grams, then 200 grams minus the drug weight will equal how much of the filler medium is needed:

200 grams (total weight) − 8 grams (drug weight)
= X grams (filler medium weight)

192 grams = X grams (filler medium weight)

The same basic procedure is done for v/v percentage solution problems, substituting units of volume for units of mass from the previous example. In this case, the final volume to be administered to the patient is 200 mL of a 4% solution (v/v). The Known Value component is the 200 mL and the Conversion Factor is the 4% solution (v/v). A 4% solution (v/v) is 4 mL of drug in 100 mL of the final mixture of liquid drug and liquid medium.

KNOWN VALUE × CONVERSION FACTOR = ANSWER

$$200 \text{ mL (total volume)} \times \frac{4 \text{ mL (drug volume 4\% solution)}}{100 \text{ mL}}$$
$$= ? \text{ mL (drug)}$$
$$200 \times \frac{4 \text{ mL}}{100} = ? \text{ mL}$$
$$\frac{800 \text{ mL}}{100} = ? \text{ mL}$$
$$8 \text{ mL} = ? \text{ mL}$$

If 8 mL of the 200 mL total mixture volume gives the required 4% solution of drug, then the 192 mL of total mixture volume must be liquid medium (200 mL − 8 mL = 192 mL).

Determining the Total Number of Dosage Units to Be Dispensed to Fill a Drug Order

Once the number of dosage forms (e.g., tablets, capsules, milliliters) has been determined for one dose, the total number of dosage forms to be dispensed for the whole dosage regimen must be calculated. The number of dosage forms needed for one dose is the Known Value and the relationship between number of doses needed per day and the number of days in the dosage regimen as the Conversion Factors.

Continuing with the previous example, the veterinary technician correctly calculated that the patient needed four tablets per dose. If the drug order was written to dispense enough drug for "q8h for 10 days," the Known Value in the dimensional analysis equation would be the four tablets per dose, and the Conversion Factors would be "dose/day" ("q8h" is equivalent to three doses daily) and "days/total dosage regimen" ("10 days").

KNOWN VALUE × CONVERSION FACTOR = ANSWER

$$\frac{4 \text{ tablets}}{\text{dose}} \times \frac{3 \text{ doses}}{\text{day}} \times \frac{10 \text{ days}}{\text{dosage regimen}} = ?\frac{\text{tablets}}{\text{dosage regimen}}$$

$$\frac{4 \text{ tablets}}{\cancel{\text{dose}}} \times \frac{3 \cancel{\text{doses}}}{\cancel{\text{day}}} \times \frac{10 \cancel{\text{days}}}{\text{dosage regimen}} = ?\frac{\text{tablets}}{\text{dosage regimen}}$$

$$\frac{4 \text{ tablets}}{} \times \frac{3}{} \times \frac{10}{\text{dosage regimen}} = ?\frac{\text{tablets}}{\text{dosage regimen}}$$

$$\frac{120 \text{ tablets}}{\text{dosage regimen}} = ?\frac{\text{tablets}}{\text{dosage regimen}}$$

Thus, 120 tablets must be dispensed to fulfill the drug order for the entire 10 days.

The Dosage Regimen Calculation Short Cut: Using Long Equations

Once the veterinary technician is comfortable calculating the individual steps to convert the patient's weight units to pounds or kilograms as needed, the dosage to the patient's dose, and the patient's dose to the number of dosage forms to be dispensed, many veterinary technicians find it easier to combine several of these individual steps into a single longer calculation using dimensional analysis rules. The following is an example of how this is done.

The veterinarian writes the following drug order for tablets to be administered to a 44-pound dog: "Dispense 2 mg/kg q12h for 10 days using the 50-mg tablets." The first calculation steps determine the number of tablets in one dose for this patient, and then the second calculation steps determine the total number of units (tablets) needed to fulfill the dose order.

The Known Value in the dimensional analysis formula equation would be the weight of the dog (44 pounds), and the Conversion Factors would include the pound-to-kilogram conversion for body weight, the dosage of 2 mg/kg to convert body weight to mass of drug needed, and the tablet strength of 1 tablet/50 mg to convert mass of drug needed into number of tablets needed. The veterinary technician knows the problem is set up correctly because all of the units on the left side of the equation cancel out, leaving only the number of tablets in the top part of a fraction for the answer. The answer for the first steps in the equation should be the number of tablets needed per dose.

KNOWN VALUE × CONVERSION FACTOR = ANSWER

WEIGHT × WEIGHT CONVERSION × DOSAGE × TABLET STRENGTH = ANSWER

$$44 \text{ lb} \times \frac{1 \text{ kg}}{2.2 \text{ lb}} \times \frac{2 \text{ mg}}{\text{kg}} \times \frac{1 \text{ tablet}}{50 \text{ mg}} = ?\text{tablets}$$

$$44 \cancel{\text{lb}} \times \frac{1 \cancel{\text{kg}}}{2.2 \cancel{\text{lb}}} \times \frac{2 \cancel{\text{mg}}}{\cancel{\text{kg}}} \times \frac{1 \text{ tablet}}{50 \cancel{\text{mg}}} = ?\text{ tablets}$$

$$44 \times \frac{1}{2.2} \times \frac{2}{} \times \frac{1 \text{ tablet}}{50} = ?\text{ tablets}$$

$$\frac{88 \text{ tablets}}{110} = ?\text{ tablets}$$

$$0.8 \text{ tablets} = ?\text{ tablets}$$

It is important to round the calculated dose to the nearest half or whole tablet before proceeding. In this case, the 0.8 tablet per dose is rounded to 1 tablet per dose. Had this not been done, the wrong number of total tablets would have been calculated. After rounding, the total number of tablets dispensed q12h (2 doses per day) for 10 days can be calculated with the second equation.

$$\frac{1 \text{ tablet}}{\text{dose}} \times \frac{2 \text{ doses}}{\text{day}} \times \frac{10 \text{ days}}{\text{dosage regimen}} = ?\frac{\text{tablets}}{\text{dosage regimen}}$$

$$\frac{1 \text{ tablet}}{\cancel{\text{dose}}} \times \frac{2 \cancel{\text{doses}}}{\cancel{\text{day}}} \times \frac{10 \cancel{\text{days}}}{\text{dosage regimen}} = ?\frac{\text{tablets}}{\text{dosage regimen}}$$

$$\frac{1 \text{ tablet}}{} \times \frac{2}{} \times \frac{10}{\text{dosage regimen}} = ?\frac{\text{tablets}}{\text{dosage regimen}}$$

$$\frac{20 \text{ tablets}}{\text{dosage regimen}} = ?\frac{\text{tablets}}{\text{dosage regimen}}$$

So 20 tablets would need to be dispensed to cover the 10 days of the dosage regimen.

The Most Common Mistake When Calculating Total Tablets to Be Dispensed

In the problem just shown, if one continuous equation had been used instead of two calculations with a rounding step from 0.8 tablet to 1 tablet for the individual tablet dose, the veterinary technician would have incorrectly calculated that 16 tablets needed to be dispensed for the whole dosage regimen.

$$\frac{0.8 \text{ tablet}}{\text{dose}} \times \frac{2 \text{ doses}}{\text{day}} \times \frac{10 \text{ days}}{\text{dosage regimen}} = \frac{16 \text{ tablets}}{\text{dosage regimen}}$$

However, 16 tablets cannot be evenly divided to the nearest whole or half tablet over the 20 doses given during the dosage regimen (2 doses per day for 10 days). Thus the tablet per dose needs to be determined and rounded to the nearest half or whole tablet per dose before determining the total number to be dispensed.

A similar problem would have occurred if the veterinary technician had determined the entire mass of drug (mg of drug) needed for the full 10 days and then divided that total mass into tablet sizes. Using another example to show this, let's say it was determined that a patient needed 23 mg of drug per dose and there were two doses per day for 8 days.

Thus the total mg of drug needed for the full 8-day dosage regimen would be determined by multiplying 23 mg × 2 × 8 to yield a total of 368 mg. If the tablet size to be used in this example was 50 mg, the veterinary technician would logically have divided the total 368 mg of drug by 50 mg/tablet to determine a need for 7.36 tablets. The 7.36 tablets would have been rounded up to the nearest whole or half tablet, giving 7.5 tablets for the 8-day regimen. However, given that the dosage regimen requires twice daily dosing for 8 days, this means there are 16 doses that must be administered. It is clear that 7.5 tablets are not going to go evenly into 16 doses. The error the technician made was determining the total mass of drug needed for the full dosage regimen instead of determining the number of tablets per dose after the mg (mass) of drug per dose was calculated.

Therefore, the individual number of tablets per dose must always be determined and rounded to the nearest half or whole tablet before calculating the total number of tablets to be dispensed.

Volume of Liquid Dosage Forms to Be Dispensed

Liquid dosing calculations for the total amount of drug to be dispensed over a dosage regimen can be done in the same way as tablets except the rounding of tablets to the nearest whole or half tablet is replaced by the rounding of the liquid dosage volume to the smallest volume unit that can be accurately delivered by the syringe.

For example, if the total volume of drug to be administered per dose was calculated to be 1.376 mL, then the dose would probably be administered in a typical 3-cc (3-mL) syringe, which is marked in 1/10-mL increments. Thus, for administering this drug with a 3-cc syringe, the 1.376 mL needs to be rounded to the nearest 1/10, which in this example would be 1.4 mL.

If, however, the total dose volume was calculated as 38.456 mL, a much larger syringe would be required to administer this volume of drug and the smallest practical unit for delivering the drug dose would most likely be to the nearest 1 mL. In this case, the dose would be rounded from 38.456 mL down to 38 mL because 38.456 mL is closer to 38 mL than it is to 39 mL.

Determining the Cost of the Dispensed Medication

When the total number of dosage form units for dispensing has been determined, the cost for the dispensed medication requires one additional step. In this case, the Known Value is the total number of units to be dispensed, the Conversion Factor is the cost per unit, and the answer is the cost for the entire dispensed medication. An example is shown here for a dispensed medication order of 30 tablets at the cost of 25 cents or $0.25 apiece. Notice again how the factors are set up so the units cancel, leaving only the unit of the answer ($).

KNOWN VALUE × CONVERSION FACTORS = ANSWER

$$30 \text{ tablets} \times \frac{\$0.25}{1 \text{ tablet}} = ?\$ \text{ total}$$

$$30 \text{ } \cancel{\text{tablets}} \times \frac{\$0.25}{1 \text{ } \cancel{\text{tablet}}} = ?\$ \text{ total}$$

$$30 \times \frac{\$0.25}{1} = ?\$ \text{ total}$$

$$30 \times \$0.25 = \$7.50$$

Sometimes a dispensing fee is attached to the cost of any medication to cover the cost of preparing the medication, the cost of the tablet vial, and the label. This additional fee would simply be added to the final calculated cost.

If the cost of the individual dosage unit is not known (e.g., the cost of the total bottle from which the drug form will be dispensed is known, but the individual unit price is not known), the individual unit cost can be determined by taking the total cost of the entire bottle of tablets or vial of liquid and dividing that cost by the number of individual units within the bottle or vial.

A $50 bottle of 100 tablets calculates to $0.50 or 50 cents per tablet with the following equation:

$$\frac{\$50.00}{100 \text{ tablets}} = \frac{\$?}{\text{tablet}}$$

A similar calculation can be used to determine the cost per milliliter if given the cost of a full bottle of liquid drug.

COMPOUNDING DRUGS

Because veterinary patients have different medical needs from those of human patients, the human dosage formulations available to veterinarians may not always meet the veterinary patient's need. For example, adding fish or beef flavoring to oral medications may facilitate the owner administering the dispensed drugs to the reluctant patient. Or if a patient more readily takes liquid medication orally than tablets, a liquid suspension can sometimes (depends on the medication, not all medications can be crushed) be made by crushing the tablet into liquid. These dosage form alterations to facilitate drug administration are examples of compounding.

Compounding is defined by the Federal Food, Drug, and Cosmetic Act (FFDCA) as any manipulation of a drug product to produce a different dosage form other than what is approved by the Food and Drug Administration (FDA). Veterinary professionals in practice often compound drugs without being aware that they are creating an unapproved drug according to the law. For example, the practice of creating "anesthetic cocktails" by combining a tranquilizer drug with an analgesic drug in the same syringe is an example of compounding. Other examples of compounding include diluting commercially prepared drugs with saline, another drug, or glycerol; crushing a tablet or emptying a capsule into a liquid to create a suspension or solution; or mixing two or more powdered drugs into the same solution.

Any manipulation or alteration of the drug dosage form or formulation means that the drug may not behave in the way the original drug performed in the clinical trials that were required for the drug's approval. Thus, the drug could end up persisting in the body longer than normal, could be absorbed more erratically, or could distribute to tissues in higher concentrations than expected, resulting in a stronger drug effect or unacceptably high drug residues in the tissue.

Compounding laws were designed primarily to protect the public by preventing drug residues in meat and food products like eggs and milk, and hence they have a greater impact on the practice of food animal medicine. However, the compounding laws also apply to small animal medicine and compounding is allowed only if it is performed in a way that complies with the Federal Food, Drug and Cosmetic Act (FFDCA), the Extra-Label Drug Use (ELDU) regulations, and the Animal Medicinal Drug Use Clarification Act of 1994 (AMDUCA). These criteria include[5,6]:

1. A valid veterinarian-client-patient relationship (VCPR) must exist. The compounding must be done with an intent to use the compounded material on a specific patient belonging to a specific client/owner for which the veterinarian has agreed to deliver care.

2. The animal's health will be threatened, the animal will suffer, or the animal will die without the use of the compounded drug. There must be a justification for the drug that relates to the specific patient's immediate health care need.

3. No FDA-approved veterinary drug in a medically appropriate dosage formulation exists. If an FDA-approved formulation exists, it must be used instead of the compounded formulation.

4. The compounded drug is made only from an FDA-approved veterinary or human drug(s).

5. Only a licensed veterinarian or a licensed pharmacist working on the order of a licensed veterinarian may compound the drug. The veterinarian will determine whether the compounding requires the use of a pharmacist. Veterinary technicians are not legally allowed to compound drugs; however, this is still commonly done in practice under the close supervision of the veterinarian.

6. The compounded drug must be safe and effective. The compounded drug must be consistent with pharmaceutical and pharmacologic standards for safety and effectiveness and not pose a danger to the patient, client, or public.

7. If the compounded drug is to be used in food-producing animals, the veterinarian must establish a withdrawal time between the last administration of the drug and the time when the animal can be sent to market or the food products (eggs and milk) can be used. Because a compounded drug is a "new" drug without any testing to determine a withdrawal time, the veterinarian is required to use his or her judgment and experience to determine a "safe" withdrawal time for the compounded product. No drug may be compounded if it violates drug residue laws or poses a threat to public health.

8. No drug can be compounded from the FDA list of prohibited drugs that pose a threat to the public health.

9. All compounds must be labeled with the following information: name and address of the attending veterinarian, date on which the drug was dispensed and date of expiration (expiration date not to exceed the length of prescribed treatment), medically active ingredients, identity of treated animals, directions for use, cautionary statements if applicable, withdrawal times if needed, and the condition or disease for which the compound is being used.

10. Compounding must comply with all local and state laws.

Several human pharmacies now offer compounding services for veterinarians. Examples of compounding done by pharmacies include the following:

- Formulating drugs with flavored compounds (e.g., fish, beef) so they are more readily accepted by a dog or a cat
- Formulating raw drug into capsules or tablets for those human drugs used in veterinary medicine that are no longer available (e.g., diethylstilbestrol for urinary incontinence in dogs, cisapride for cats with megacolon)
- Formulating drugs into different forms (e.g., gels, pastes, dermal patches, rectal suppositories) to facilitate administration
- Formulating a raw chemical into a drug dosage form for administration to animals (e.g., putting potassium bromide reagent into a syrup or elixir formulation for use as a veterinary anticonvulsant)

A legal distinction is made between compounding a medication for use in the veterinary practice and compounding a product for sale or use outside the veterinary practice. The former is considered compounding if it follows the legal requirements listed earlier. However, the latter is considered illegal drug *manufacturing* because a veterinary practice may not legally compound for another veterinary practice for resale to a patient/client for which it does not have a valid VCPR. In this example, the compounding veterinarian would be compounding on the order of another veterinarian in a separate practice and therefore would be illegally acting as a pharmacist.

Even within a practice, compounding is only legal if it is done on an "as needed" basis for a specific client/patient. For example, repackaging bulk powdered drug into smaller bottles of liquid for sale would also be considered illegal compounding or drug manufacture because there is no specific patient for whom the drug is being compounded.

The government and public are much more aware of the potential negative effect of drug residues in meat or animal food products, and compounding poses a potential threat for creating such drug residues if misused. Veterinary professionals must be aware of, and comply with, the regulations governing safe compounding of drugs in veterinary practices. Failure to comply with compounding regulations could result in threats to public safety from drug residues, litigation or fines against the veterinarian who orders the compounding or the veterinary technician who compounds on the order of the veterinarian, and ultimately a further restriction by federal governmental agencies over veterinary drugs available to treat animals.

THE DISPENSING LABEL AND CONTAINER

Pharmacies are required by pharmacy law to provide specific information on the label of every drug that is dispensed from the pharmacy. Similarly there are state and federal laws that

Pietre Veterinary Hospital, Inc.
2300 South State Street
Gracie, MO 55555
Phone: (555) 555-5555

Patient: "Michy" Frisco   Species: Canine

Address: 545 North 5th Street
                Newton, MO 55551

Give 1 tablet by mouth every day for 10 days

PREDNISOLONE 5 MG TABLET #10
Date: 11/22/2015
Expires: 4/22/2016   Refills: 2
Dispensing Veterinarian: Dr. Robert L. Bill

FOR VETERINARY USE ONLY
KEEP OUT OF REACH OF CHILDREN

Fig. 2.3 Information that must be included on the label of dispensed medication.

regulate the information that should appear on the label of dispensed medications from facilities, including veterinary hospitals. The information required on a label of dispensed drug from a veterinary hospital is shown in Fig. 2.3.

The Poison Prevention Packaging Act of 1970 enabled the FDA to require special packaging for drugs that may be dangerous to children. However, current packaging regulations apply to drug manufacturers and pharmacists but not necessarily veterinarians.[1] Therefore although it is not technically illegal to dispense veterinary medication in paper "pill envelopes" or other non-childproof containers, if the dispensed medication were to be ingested by a child and suffer harm, the veterinarian could theoretically be held liable for negligence and placing the child at risk.

Sometimes dispensing medication in non-childproof containers is necessary, such as for elderly clients with arthritic hands. In these circumstances, veterinarians are justified giving these clients medications packaged in easy-opening dispensing vials with lids that are not childproof. Nevertheless, veterinary professionals are morally and ethically obligated to inform clients when the dispensed containers are not childproof and should advise them to keep medication out of the reach of children. Best practice would be to have the client sign an informed consent form that they understand the risk, and approve the non-childproof containers for their pets medication. This form could be kept in the permanent medical record for future reference if needed.

STORAGE OF DRUGS IN THE VETERINARY FACILITY

Techniques for storage and inventory control of drugs and other supplies are often taught in conjunction with other business management concepts in veterinary professional programs. However, there are medical and legal reasons for proper storage and handling of drugs. For example, drugs that are not stored at the proper temperature or amount of light exposure can degenerate or otherwise become inactivated. Drugs that remain on the pharmacy shelf after the listed expiration date may have lost some of their potency, may be less effective, and in some cases could actually become unsafe. As discussed previously in this chapter, controlled substances, such as narcotics, have additional legal requirements for storage and inventory control. Thus the veterinary technician needs to know the specific storage needs for each of the drugs in the pharmacy inventory and to comply with storage and handling requirements to maintain the quality and effectiveness of the drugs.

Environmental Concerns for Proper Storage

Drugs should be stored at their optimal temperature according to their label specifications to prevent damage or inactivation. Temperatures for drug storage are as follows:

Cold: not exceeding 8°C (46°F)
Cool: 8–15°C (46–59°F)
Room temperature: 15–30°C (59–86°F)
Warm: 30–40°C (86–104°F)
Excessive heat: greater than 40°C (104°F)

Note that "cold" temperatures may include those temperatures below freezing. Unless the package or label states "Do not freeze," drugs classified as needing to be stored in "cold" temperatures are probably safe to freeze.

Large animal practitioners must be especially aware of environmental conditions because of the tendency to forget about drugs stored in the practice vehicle. Drugs stored in the practice truck that is parked unprotected outside may be subjected to wide variations in temperature, changing the physical composition of the drug and reducing the effectiveness of the drug. When frozen, some drugs physically change from small molecules into larger crystalline formations that are harder to keep in suspension or cause pain when injected. Overheated drugs can be denatured, damaged, or inactivated, rendering an otherwise effective drug product useless.

Drugs that are sensitive to light are usually kept in dark amber containers and their labels usually contain instructions that the drug is not to be exposed to light. Light-sensitive liquid drugs should only be dispensed in dark amber dispensing bottles.

Tablets and powders are sensitive to moisture so their original containers usually contain silica packets or other desiccation packets designed to absorb moisture and keep the drug dry. Some binders and other inert ingredients used in the dosage form may make the tablets sensitive to humidity, resulting in the tablets becoming soggy or breaking apart if exposed to the moisture in the air. Capsules (gel caps) are especially sensitive to humidity and may stick together in humid or overly warm environments. Among the other threats to stored drugs are ionizing radiation, such as from X-ray scatter, or physical vibrations that can break apart complex drug molecules.

A veterinarian thought he was doing his elderly clients a favor when he instructed his technician to unwrap each foil-wrapped tablet he was going to dispense and put them conveniently in a pill vial. His reasoning was that it would be easier for his clients to give the medication to their pet because they would not have to open the individual foil wrapping.

Unfortunately, what the veterinarian failed to consider was the hygroscopic (water absorbing) nature of the dose form, which is why the manufacturer sealed each individual tablet in foil in the first place. After 2 days the tablets turned into mushy crumbles inside the pill vial. The clients returned the tablets and received replacement tablets (in their foil wrapping). The veterinarian learned, at some loss of profit to his practice, that his good intentions failed to consider the physical makeup of the medication.

What should be learned from this situation: The manufacturer knows best how to store its medications. Tampering with the environmental or physical storage properties of a medication or failing to follow the manufacturer's guidelines for storage of the drug can result in the drug becoming useless. Always read and follow the manufacturer's guidelines for storage and dispensing of medications. All drug package inserts can be found at dailymed.com if the paper copy is not available.

Drugs that must be reconstituted before use (e.g., a powder in a vial to which a liquid is added) often do not contain preservative agents to prevent bacterial growth should the container become contaminated after reconstitution. Repeated insertion of needles increases the risk for contaminating vials. Reconstituted products may be chemically unstable once reconstituted and have a very short period of time in which they can be used. The manufacturer's label will list the length of time in which the drug is considered to be effective after reconstitution. Therefore in spite of the money-saving incentive, it is inappropriate to keep reconstituted drugs for several days with the intent of using all of the contents on several animals. Labeling the bottle with the new "beyond use date" will help all employees know when to discard the medication. This is also important to note on multi dose vials (i.e., insulin) that are only guaranteed for a certain number of days after opening.

Storing and Handling Cytotoxic and Hazardous Drugs

As has been emphasized, all drugs need to be stored and handled in a way that is safe for the patient, client, and any veterinary professional or assistant treating the animal. The concern for safe handling and storage becomes even more important when cytotoxic drugs are being used. Cytotoxic ("cell poison") drugs can be especially poisonous to mammalian cells and include *antineoplastic agents* used to treat cancer and some antimycotic agents used to treat fungal infections.

In 1986, the US Department of Labor's Occupational Safety and Health Administration (OSHA) developed and published guidelines for safe storage, use, and disposal of hazardous chemicals and drugs. These guidelines can be found online in Section VI of the OSHA Technical Manual at www.osha.gov/dts/osta/otm/otm_toc.html. More recently OSHA has made the *Veterinary OSHA Manual* available for a fee; this is targeted specifically for use in veterinary hospitals (www.oshamanual.com/vet_OSHA.html). Veterinary oncology texts and human nursing textbooks also typically contain guidelines and procedures for safe administration of antineoplastic agents.

Cytotoxic drugs and hazardous compounds should be stored separately from other drugs, with particular attention paid to environmental requirements, such as temperature and exposure to light. Every compound must be clearly labeled with easily-read information that clearly identifies the compound, the hazards that it poses, and any additional precautionary information required or recommended by OSHA or other regulatory laws.

Improper handling of cytotoxic and hazardous drugs can result in accidental exposure, inhalation, or ingestion of the drug and can potentially cause birth defects (teratogenic or mutagenic *effects*) in the fetus of a pregnant veterinary professional or increase the risk for development of cancer or preneoplastic changes (carcinogenic effects) in animals and human beings. Because little is known about the long-term effects of many of these cytotoxic drugs, the veterinary professional must handle mutagenic and carcinogenic drugs with great care.

As a Veterinary Technician, Set an Example for Staff

Unfortunately, veterinarians and veterinary technicians sometimes contribute to their exposure risk by acting complacent about proper use of common-sense hygiene practices. Veterinarian and technician lunches are sometimes stored in the same refrigerator as a specimen jar containing formalin, a container with a fecal sample, or a vial of antineoplastic medication. In a busy practice, veterinary professionals often quickly eat lunch between procedures and may briefly place food on a countertop that has been contaminated with cytotoxic medication.

These poor practices may be mimicked by staff who have less understanding of the consequences of unhygienic practices or how to protect themselves from exposure to hazardous drugs or chemicals. Therefore veterinary professionals have an ethical responsibility to model safe practices and behaviors for staff to help reduce the risk for exposure to cytotoxic or hazardous drugs.

Training and the Material Safety Data Sheet (MSDS) Notebook

In addition to being aware of potential exposure situations and modeling good practice procedures and hygiene, the veterinary facility should take responsibility to educate all involved personnel on the safe handling and storage of hazardous drugs. Training may be conducted as in-house seminars or may be obtained through workshops offered by human nursing or physician groups, or state/federal regulatory agencies. Safety training should be periodically repeated to emphasize the importance of safe handling and serve as a refresher for staff members. Depending on the state, regulations from the state OSHA may dictate what training is required based on the type of institution or facility, the types of hazardous materials the staff are likely to encounter, or the type of work that is performed in the facility.

Training should include educating the staff and employees on where to find necessary information about any potentially hazardous material used within the facility. Information on all cytotoxic agents or hazardous compounds should be compiled into a readily accessible and clearly marked notebook in a location known to all staff members and employees. This notebook should include the following items:

- A material safety data sheet (MSDS) for every cytotoxic agent or hazardous compound used in the practice. The MSDS must contain guidelines for protective precautions, cleanup procedures, and first aid for accidental exposure.
- A package insert for every drug used in the practice.
- Hospital policies and descriptions of procedures for handling a cytotoxic or hazardous drug spill or exposure and procedures for routine disposal of drugs, contaminated syringes or equipment, and empty vials (based on manufacturer's recommendations in the MSDS and package insert).

Accidental Exposure to Cytotoxic Drugs and How to Reduce the Risk

The first step in protecting oneself from exposure to hazardous or cytotoxic drugs is to understand how accidental exposure can occur. Veterinary professionals and staff most commonly expose themselves to toxic drugs during routine procedures such as[7]:

- Drug absorption through the skin from drug spilled from a syringe or drug vial or contact with a surface contaminated with spilled drug
- Inhalation of an aerosolized drug as the needle is withdrawn from a vial that has been pressurized by the technician injecting air into the vial to facilitate drug removal
- Ingestion of food contaminated with drug by aerosolization, direct contact, or contact with surfaces contaminated with cytotoxic drug
- Inhalation of aerosolized drug powder resulting from crushing or breaking tablets of cytotoxic drugs
- Drug absorption or inhalation when opening glass ampules containing cytotoxic drugs

Fortunately, adhering to the following general guidelines and steps for safe preparation, administration, and disposal of toxic drugs should reduce the risk for inadvertent exposure[8,9]:

1. If reconstitution of the cytotoxic drug requires mixing dry drug with liquid diluent, the reconstitution should be done just before the actual administration of the drug to decrease the risk of spilling or otherwise contaminating the treatment area with the active prepared drug.
2. Prepare and administer toxic drugs in a low-traffic, well-ventilated area. A ventilated hood is preferred.
3. Wear proper protective attire when preparing or administering the drug. Such attire should include the following:
   - A high-efficiency filter mask (surgical masks do not protect against inhalation of aerosols)
   - Some form of gloves, either two pairs of surgical-quality latex gloves (all latex gloves are porous to some degree), commercially available heavy-weight gloves for use with cytotoxic agents, or latex gloves with large animal obstetric sleeves to protect the arms
   - A long-sleeved, nonporous gown with close-fitting cuffs over which the gloves are worn
   - Goggles to protect the eyes from aerosol exposure

4. Use syringes and intravenous lines with screw-on attachments to prevent spillage or accidental blow-off of the needle hub.
5. Recheck the calculated dose just before administration of the drug.
6. Confirm that the catheter is correctly placed within the vein and is still patent just before administration of the drug.
7. Immediately after completion of the administration, place all syringes, intravenous lines, catheters, and discarded vials in sealable plastic bags.
8. Place all bagged items in a leak-proof, puncture-proof container designed for and labeled as hazardous waste.
9. Trained veterinary professionals should properly clean and decontaminate the treatment area rather than depend on the lay staff to do so.

In any veterinary facility that uses hazardous chemicals or cytotoxic drugs, a chemotherapy spill kit should be stocked and readily available in the event that a significant spill of these compounds occurs. Just like the MSDS notebook, the spill kit's location should be known to every staff member in the hospital. This kit should include a complete set of protective clothing as outlined earlier, several absorbent pads with nonporous backing for cleaning up any spilled liquid, a "sharps" container for needles, broken glass, or other sharp objects, and a hazardous materials disposal bag.

REFERENCES

1. US Consumer Product Safety Division. Child-Resistant Closures and Veterinary Drugs Dispensed by Veterinarians to the Consumer; 2010. CPSC Document #5104. http://permanent.access.gpo.gov/gpo1293/5104.pdf.
2. US Department of Justice. Drug Enforcement Administration, Office of Diversion Control. In: *Practitioner's Manual, Section V—Valid Prescription Requirements*; 2008.
3. Sommars J. How to keep the DEA happy. *AAHA Trends Magazine*. 2011;(May/June):65–69.
4. National Coordinating Council for Medication Error and Reporting. *Recommendations to Enhance Accuracy of Prescription Writing* (Website). www.nccmerp.org/recommendations-enhance-accuracy-prescription-writing. Accessed 06.12.22.
5. American Veterinary Medical Association. *Veterinary Compounding* (Website). www.avma.org/KB/Policies/Pages/Compounding.aspx. Accessed 06.12.2022.
6. United States Food and Drug Administration. *The Animal Medicinal Drug Use Clarification Act (AMDUCA) of 1994* (Website). http://www.fda.gov/AnimalVeterinary/GuidanceComplianceEnforcement/ActsRulesRegulations/ucm085377.htm. Accessed 06.12.22.
7. Hohenhaus AE. Chemotherapy administration: protecting your chemotherapy nurse, your staff and your patients. In: *Proceedings of the 2008 Atlantic Coast Veterinary Conference, Atlantic City*; October 2008.
8. Brook K. Chemotherapy considerations: safety and handling. In: *Proceedings of the 2008 British Small Animal Veterinary Congress, Birmingham*; April 2008.
9. Tsegaye D, Alem G, Tessema Z, Alebachew W. Medication administration errors and associated factors among nurses. *Int J Gen Med*. 2020;13:1621–1632. https://doi.org/10.2147/IJGM.S289452. PMID: 33376387; PMCID: PMC7764714.

WEB RESOURCES

www.osha.gov
The official site of OSHA, a division of the US Department of Labor, contains a large amount of information regarding OSHA standards, news, issues, events, and related resources.

www.fda.gov/search.html
This site, sponsored by the US Food and Drug Administration, has a search feature that uses key words (e.g., "compounding") to locate relevant articles and documents.

www.usp.org
The United States Pharmacopeia is an organization that sets standards that manufacturers must meet to sell their products in the United States. The USP home page provides links to veterinary drug information, quality standards, and the Veterinary Practitioner's Reporting (VPR) Program.

SELF-ASSESSMENT

1. Fill in the following blanks with the correct item from the Key Terms list.
   A. _____ This is the art and science of preparing and dispensing medications.
   B. _____ This is the study of how drugs work.
   C. _____ This is a request by a veterinarian to dispense or administer a drug within a veterinary hospital.
   D. _____ This is a drug order from a veterinarian to a licensed pharmacist.
   E. _____ This is a set of drugs that includes narcotics, analgesics, or other drugs that have the potential for abuse.
   F. _____ This is the agency in the United States that is charged with regulating potentially abusive drugs.
   G. _____ This is another term for controlled substance drugs.
   H. _____ This is the term that describes how a drug is to be administered including what mass of drug, what route, how often it is to be administered, and for how long.
   I. _____ This is the term that describes the mass of drug to be administered to a specific patient.
   J. _____ This is the term that describes the amount of time between doses.
   K. _____ This is the term that describes the mass of drug needed per unit of weight of animal for any animal.
   L. _____ This is the description of the physical form of the drug to be administered.
   M. _____ This is a range of mass per unit of body weights that can be used to determine the specific mass of drug needed for a specific patient (e.g., 15–30 mg/lb).
   N. _____ This is the system of measurement that uses grams, liters, and meters as the basic elements of weight, volume, and length.
   O. _____ This is the system of measurement that uses grains and minims.
   P. _____ This is the system of measurement that uses teaspoons, tablespoons, and cups.
   Q. _____ This is a description of the mass or amount of drug in a tablet, capsule, or volume unit of the dosage form.
   R. _____ This is defined as the number of grams of drug per 100 mL of liquid.
   S. _____ This is defined as the number of milliliters of drug per milliliter of combined liquid medium and drug.
   T. _____ This is defined as the mass of drug, expressed in grams, found within 100 grams of combined drug and medium.
   U. _____ This is defined by the Federal food, Drug, and Cosmetic Act as any manipulation of a drug product to produce a different dosage form other than what is approved by the FDA.
   V. _____ This term describes a legal relationship between the animal, the animal's owner, and the attending veterinarian.
   W. _____ This law requires pharmacists and human hospitals to use childproof containers.
   X. _____ This term means that the drug is "poisonous to cells" and primarily meant to refer to mammalian cells.
   Y. _____ This agency in the United States is responsible for, among other things, establishing and enforcing guidelines for safe storage, use, and disposal of hazardous chemicals and drugs.
   Z. _____ These two terms are used to describe drugs that potentially cause birth defects.
   AA. _____ This term means a drug has the potential to cause cancer.
   BB. _____ This contains information on any hazardous compound in the veterinary practice including precautions, cleanup procedures, and first aid in case of accidental exposure.

2. What do the following abbreviations stand for?
   DEA
   ELDU
   FFDCA
   FDA
   MSDS
   OSHA
   VCPR

3. What do the following abbreviations from drug orders stand for?
   b.i.d.
   q.i.d.

t.i.d.
q12h
PO
OD/OS/OU
IM
IP
IV

SQ
PRN
TBL

4. Why is it incorrect to state that the act of filling a drug order for the veterinarian is pharmacology?
5. How is a veterinary legend drug identified on its label?
6. What is the difference between a drug order and a prescription in terms of who can legally fill the order?

7. What is missing from the following prescription?

Johnstown Veterinary Hospital, INC
3526 E. Caroline Ave SW
Johnstown, IA 74214-2441
(315) 521-2151

August 21ˢᵗ, 2016

Mr. James Morrisi "Felix" (feline)

215 Boxwood Apt. 3a, Johnstown 523-4111

℞ *Amoxitabs #24*

SIG: 1 tablet q12h PO for 12 days

Dr. Lucenda Morgenstine

---

8. What is the schedule of the most potential abuse drugs for which a veterinarian may legally write a prescription (what Roman numeral)?
9. What label must be included on the container of dispensed controlled substances?
10. In the controlled substances log, is it sufficient to list the drug name, the amount, and the client's name?
11. A veterinary practice uses a three-ring binder notebook for keeping the hospital's controlled substances log book. Is this appropriate?
12. The veterinarian stores his controlled substances in a 1-cubic-foot metal tool box with a heavy-duty padlock. Is this adequate storage for schedule drugs? What about a wooden cabinet with a lock?
13. What is a reverse distributor and what does it have to do with controlled substances or schedule drugs?
14. The Drug Enforcement Agency requires controlled substances records be maintained for how long?

15. Arrange the following schedule drug classifications in order from most potential for abuse to least potential for abuse: C-III, C-IV, C-I, C-V, C-II.
16. Translate the following drug orders
    50 mg q8h 3d
    100 mg PO PRN for pain
    0.5 mg/lb IV stat
    3 gtt OD q2h
17. Why do we prefer to use q12h and q8h instead of b.i.d. and t.i.d.?
18. Make the following conversions:

2 g = _____ mg		0.00043 kg = _____ mg	
5 mg = _____ g		25,488 mg = _____ lb	
14 lb = _____ kg		0.0092 lb = _____ mg	
23 kg = _____ lb		25 mL = _____ L	
83 kg = _____ mg		43 cc = _____ mL	
65 kg = _____ lb		1.5 L = _____ mL	
0.4 kg = _____ g		800 cc = _____ L	
0.003 lb = _____ mg		0.055 L = _____ mL	
15 lb = _____ g		0.65 mL = _____ L	

19. Given the dosage, determine the dose for the patient:
    10 mg/lb for a 20-lb dog
    2.2 mg/kg for a 35-lb dog
    6 mg/lb for a 15-kg dog
    0.8 mg/kg for a 5-kg cat
    15 mg/kg for a 900-lb horse
    0.75 mg/lb for a 350-kg steer
    10 mg/m² for a 1.2-m² dog

20. Given the dosage, the animal's weight, and the dosage formulation, calculate the number of dosage units needed. No tablet may be cut into anything smaller than a half tablet (no quarter tablets, third tablets).
    10 mg/kg, 22-lb dog, 20-mg tablets = ? tablets
    5 mg/lb, 44-kg pig, 250-mg/mL liquid = ? mL liquid
    50 mg/kg, 1-gram rat, 0.01-mg/mL liquid = ? mL liquid
    2.5 mg/lb, 5-kg cat, 25-mg tablets = 1.1 tablet = ? tablets
    3 mg/kg, 897-lb horse, 250-mg tablets = 4.89 tablets = ? tablets
    45 mg/kg, 8.1-lb cat, 50-mg tablets = 3.31 tablets = ? tablets

21. Complete the following table of conversions of percentage solutions (w/v, w/w, v/v) and the number of milligrams or milliliters of drug per unit of medium.

Percentage Solution	Milligrams or Milliliters per Unit of Medium
5% solution w/v	___ grams/100 mL = ___ mg/100 mL = ___ mg/mL
10% solution w/w	___ grams drug/100 grams drug + medium
15% solution v/v	___ mL drug/100 mL drug + medium
20% solution w/v	___ grams/100 mL = ___ mg/100 mL = ___ mg/mL
25% solution w/w	___ mg drug/100 mg drug + medium
___% solution w/v	300 mg/mL
___% solution w/v	4000 mg/100 mL
___% solution w/v	160 mg/2 mL
___% solution w/v	36 grams/300 mL

22. The veterinarian asks you to prepare a dose of ketamine sufficient to restrain a 15-lb cat. The drug formulary recommends using 15 mg/kg intravenously or intramuscularly. The concentration of ketamine in the vial is 100 mg/mL. What volume of ketamine is required for this cat?

23. The veterinarian asks you to fill a prescription for butorphanol for a coughing dog, dispensing sufficient tablets for 5 days of treatment. The dog weighs 55 lb. The recommended dose is 0.08 mg/kg. The tablets are available in 1-, 5-, and 10-mg sizes. The charge is $0.35 per tablet. How many tablets are required for a single dose? If the dosage specifies using the calculated dose q6h, how many tablets are required for each day of treatment? How many tablets should you dispense for the total 5 days of treatment? What is the charge for the dispensed medication?

24. The veterinarian wants to medicate a 16-lb Chihuahua, a 27-lb terrier, and a 66-lb collie. The recommended dosage is 3–5 mg/kg given once daily. You are to dispense enough medication to last each dog 180 days (6 months). The 50-mg tablets cost $0.03 each, the 100-mg tablets cost $0.05 each, and the 200-mg tablets cost $0.07 each. What are the minimal and maximal daily doses (in milligrams) for each dog based on the recommended dosage range? How many tablets and what strength are required for each dog each day? How much does the medication for the 180 days of treatment cost for each dog?

25. The veterinarian asks you to dispense a medication for a client's dog. The recommended dose is 0.22 mg/m², with m² being the number of square meters of body surface area. The dog's body surface area is 0.8 m². The medication elixir is available in a concentration of 0.15 mg/mL. To prevent overdosing, the doctor instructs you to use 60% of the calculated normal dose for this dog. How many milliliters of this medication should this dog receive for each dose?

26. You were calculating the total number of tablets to be dispensed and somehow came up with an unusable answer. The dog weighs 42 lb (19.1 kg). The dose is 10 mg/kg t.i.d. for 10 days and the tablet size is 50 mg. You calculated the dose by multiplying 19.1 kg by 10 mg/kg to get 191 mg per dose. You wanted to determine the total milligrams needed for the 10 days, so you took the 191 mg per dose and multiplied it by three doses per day (t.i.d.) to get 573 mg and then multiplied that by 10 days to get 5730 mg total for 10 days. The 5730 mg total comes out to 114.6 of the 50-mg tablets that you rounded to 115 tablets to cover the 10 days. But when you attempt to determine how many tablets the owner needs to give the dog with each dose, the number of tablets per dose does not make sense. Determine how many tablets this animal should get per dose based on this calculation of total milligrams of drug needed for the 10 days and determine where the mistake in logic was made in doing this calculation.

27. A client wants to buy $10 worth of vitamins for his dog. The doctor asks you to dispense the medication but not to exceed the $10 value. The dog weighs 8 lb. The recommended dosage is 8 mg/kg given once daily. The medication is supplied as 15-mg tablets. A bottle of 1000 tablets costs $130. How many days' worth of tablets can you dispense for $10?

28. True or False. Adding acepromazine tranquilizer to a bottle of ketamine is not considered compounding as long as it is not sold to another practice.

29. The veterinarian wants to have a compounding pharmacy compound an antidiarrheal drug because the compounded drug will be far cheaper than the FDA-approved version. Is this legal?

30. What additional instruction for use of a compounded drug in food-producing animals (meat, milk, eggs) must be included in the client instructions that is not required in small animal compounded drugs?

31. Why is it illegal for a veterinarian to buy a large bulk-order size of drug and repackage it into multiple smaller units for resale within the practice?

32. A veterinarian in another practice sees that there is a market for the "blue goo" concoction that he compounded as a teat dip to prevent mastitis. Can the doctor legally sell this product to your practice if he applies a label to each bottle stating "For use by or on the order of a licensed veterinarian"?

33. True or False. The use of pill vial caps that are not child-proof is illegal in veterinary medicine because they violate the Poison Prevention Packaging Act of 1970.

34. True or False. If a drug is labeled as "store at room temperature," then keeping it cool in a refrigerator is acceptable.

35. Is it acceptable to freeze a drug that is to be stored at "cold temperatures"?

36. True or False. Because the MSDS notebook contains information about drugs, including controlled substances, it must be kept locked away in a restricted access area.

37. A fellow staff member routinely uses a surgical mask and a single pair of latex surgical gloves during preparation and administration of antineoplastic drugs. Is this adequate protection?

Pharmacokinetics and Pharmacodynamics: The Principles of How Drugs Work

CHAPTER OUTLINE

OBJECTIVES

After studying this chapter, the veterinary technician should be able to:

- Apply the bucket analogy to dosing scenarios and predict the outcome of changes in drug absorption, distribution, metabolism, or excretion/elimination.
- Describe when a loading dose is appropriate for clinical use.
- Calculate a total daily dose and be able to change a dosage regimen to another regimen that has an equivalent total daily dose.
- Describe and explain the differences in the drug concentrations achieved by the parenteral routes of administration.
- Describe the differences, advantages, and disadvantages between the passive and active transport mechanisms by which drugs move around.

- Describe what constitutes a lipophilic or hydrophilic drug, how lipophilic or hydrophilic properties affect absorption of drugs, and what environmental factors can change the hydrophilic or lipophilic nature of drug molecules.
- Define and describe the four components of pharmacokinetics (A.D.M.E.).
- Describe why the bioavailability varies among intravenous (IV), oral (PO), intramuscular (IM), and subcutaneous (SQ) routes of administration.
- Describe the effect hydrophilic and lipophilic properties of drugs have on absorption.
- Define and describe the roles of P-glycoprotein (P-gp) and cytochrome P-450 (CYP P-450) in the absorption, distribution, metabolism, and elimination of drugs.

- Describe how dissolution and gastrointestinal (GI) motility affect absorption.
- Define and describe how the first-pass effect affects absorption of drugs in one particular route of administration.
- Define and describe the blood-brain barrier; discuss why it is a barrier; and explain to what kinds of drugs it is a barrier.
- List other tissues that have a drug barrier to distribution.
- Describe how tissue perfusion affects distribution of a drug.
- Define and describe how protein binding affects drug distribution and how conditions such as hypoproteinemia affect this distribution.
- Define and use the concept of volume of distribution (V_d).
- Describe the receptor concept for pharmacodynamics.
- Describe how affinity and intrinsic activity are involved with the definition of agonists, antagonists, reversal agents, and blockers.
- Describe the difference between competitive and noncompetitive antagonists.
- Define and apply the definition of partial agonist/partial antagonists to uses such as anesthesia.

- Describe how induction of metabolism occurs, where it occurs, what makes it occur, and what effect induction has on clinical effects of drugs.
- Describe species and age differences in the metabolism of drugs.
- Describe the primary routes of elimination and the factors that reduce or enhance elimination through those routes.
- Describe how filtration, active secretion, and reabsorption all contribute to the rate at which a drug is renally excreted, where these occur, and how they can be altered by physiology or disease.
- Define and describe clearance and half-life; be able to apply these concepts to adjust doses of patients with altered clearance or half-lives.
- Predict the half-life of elimination given plasma drug concentration data (time postinjection and concentration at that time).
- Predict the time to reach steady state given the elimination half-life.
- Describe why withdrawal times are a public health issue and what factors influence food product producers complying with withdrawal times.

KEY TERMS

active secretion (renal)
active transport
aerosol administration
afferent renal arteriole
affinity
agonist
antagonist
aqueous medium
biliary excretion
bioavailability
biotransformation
blockers
blood-brain barrier
Bowman's capsule
chelators
clearance
competitive, reversible, surmountable
    antagonism
concentration gradient
conjugation
constant rate infusion (CRI)
cytochrome P-450 (CYP)
dissolution
distal convoluted tubule
distribution
elimination
endocytosis
enterohepatic circulation
excretion
extracellular fluid
extravascular injection
facilitated diffusion
fenestrations

filtration
first-pass effect
free form
gastric motility
glomerulus
half-life of elimination
hepatic excretion
hepatic portal system
hepatocytes
hydrophilic
induced metabolism/induction
inducible enzymes
inhibitors
intestinal motility
intraarterial (IA) injection
intradermal (ID) injection
intramuscular
intraperitoneal (IP) injection
intravenous (IV)
intravenous (IV) bolus
intravenous (IV) infusion
intrinsic activity
ionized/nonionized
lipophilic
loading dose
loop of Henle
maintenance dose
maximum effective concentration
metabolism
metabolite
minimum effective concentration
narrow therapeutic index
narrow therapeutic range

noncompetitive, irreversible, or
    insurmountable antagonism
non–receptor-mediated drug reaction
P-glycoprotein (P-gp)
parenterally administered drugs
partial agonist
partial antagonist
passive diffusion
peak concentration
perfusion
peritubular capillaries
perivascular injection
per os (PO)
per rectum
phagocytosis
pharmacodynamics
pharmacokinetics
pinocytosis
polarized/nonpolarized
prodrug
protein-bound drug
proximal convoluted tubule
reabsorption
receptor
redistribution
renal excretion
reversal agent
route of administration
saturated
sinusoids (hepatic)
steady state/plateau
subcutaneous (SC or SQ)
subtherapeutic concentrations

therapeutic range/window
t-max (transportation maximum)
tolerance
topically administered drugs

total daily dose
trough concentration
unbound fraction
vasoconstriction

vasodilation
volume of distribution (V_d)
withdrawal time
xenobiotics

Pharmacokinetics is the study of how a drug moves into, through, and out of the body. Pharmacodynamics is the study of how the drug produces its effects on the body. This chapter, when combined with the information in the previous two chapters, provides the veterinary technician with an explanation for how administered drugs behave inside the body.

THE THERAPEUTIC GOAL: DRUG CONCENTRATIONS WITHIN THE THERAPEUTIC RANGE

As stated in Chapter 1, Rule #1 for safe drug usage states that all drugs are poisons. Giving too much of a truly beneficial drug can injure or kill a patient. In contrast, a small dose of a deadly poison may not produce clinical signs of toxicity or death. Or if a deadly poison is applied to the skin of an animal, the animal may not show signs of toxicity as long as the poison is not absorbed into the body. Ultimately, it is the concentration of the drug inside the animal that determines whether a drug will produce a beneficial effect or a deadly/toxic effect.

Generally, there is an acceptable range of concentrations a drug needs to achieve inside the body to produce the beneficial effects without causing significant toxic or side effects. This desirable range of drug concentrations is referred to as the therapeutic range, or therapeutic window.

The top concentration of the normal therapeutic range is called the maximum effective concentration and represents the border between those concentrations that are beneficial and those concentrations at which signs of toxicity are likely to develop (Fig. 3.1).

If insufficient drug is administered or the patient's physiology prevents the drug from achieving adequate concentrations inside the body, the drug will not produce the intended beneficial drug effect. The bottom concentration of the normal therapeutic range below which the drugs will not work sufficiently is called the minimum effective concentration. Drug concentrations below the minimum effective concentration are said to be subtherapeutic concentrations.

As discussed in Chapter 1, administering the drug according to the manufacturer's approved drug dosage should result in concentrations within the therapeutic range for the majority of the animals to which the drug is administered. However, Rule #3 for safe drug usage states that "all doses are guesses," reminding us that every patient responds individually to a dose based upon the physiologic state at the time. Disease can change a patient's physiology and thus the drug's pharmacokinetic behavior, potentially resulting in an excessive accumulation of drug within the body and producing toxic side effects. Even if the physiology of the patient is normal, a small percentage of the patients may be especially sensitive or responsive to the drug, meaning a "normal" dose produces a much greater response than it does in most other patients. Patients can also be far less responsive to the drug meaning, that a "normal" dose produces a far weaker response than expected.[1] Thus it is important to remember Rule #3 and to treat each patient as an individual when dosing a drug.

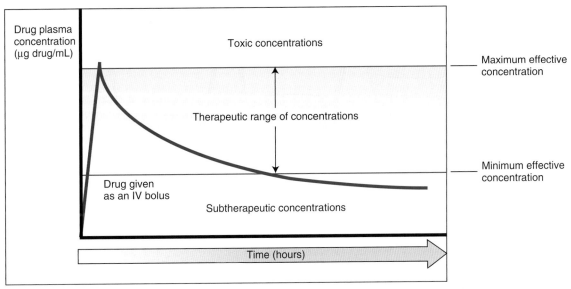

Fig. 3.1 The therapeutic range of concentrations of an intravenous (IV) drug in the plasma.

Balancing Inflow With Outflow

To maintain drug concentrations within the therapeutic range of concentrations, the amount of drug entering the body must equal the rate at which the body removes the drug. This would be achieved by giving an appropriate drug dose for "inflow" into the body and balancing it against the body's physiologic ability to eliminate the drug, or the "outflow." If balanced appropriately, the body accumulates just enough drug to achieve the ideal therapeutic concentrations.

A simple analogy may help explain this concept. Think of the body as a bucket with a small leaky hole in the bottom (Fig. 3.2). Think of a dose of a drug as being an amount of water poured into the top of the bucket. When the "dose" of water is poured into the bucket, some level of water is achieved in the bucket. For this example, let us assume the water "dose" produces a half-filled bucket of water. At the same time, the bucket is being filled with the dose, the hole in the bottom of the bucket is allowing water to drain out. Thus, if the bucket is to be kept at the halfway mark after the initial water is added, more water will have to be continually added at a rate that matches the rate at which the water leaks out.

The rate at which water is added to the bucket represents the dose of drug added to the body (mass of drug given at a particular dose interval). The water leaking through the hole in the bottom of the bucket represents the rate at which the body removes the drug by elimination or metabolism. The halfway mark on the bucket represents the ideal therapeutic range or desired drug concentration within the body.

As shown in Fig. 3.2, if the hole in the bottom of the bucket were to become smaller but the amount of water poured in remained the same, the accumulating water in the bucket would rise above the halfway mark and eventually overflow the bucket.

Applying this analogy to the body, if the route by which a drug is eliminated or metabolized is adversely affected by disease or a change in physiology, the rate at which the drug is removed from the body can be slowed. Because the liver and kidneys are the primary organs involved in removing drugs from the body, damage to these organs from disease or impaired function reduces the elimination or metabolism and "makes the hole smaller." Unless the drug dose (the amount of water added to the bucket) or the frequency of administration of the drug dose (how often water is added) is reduced, the drug will accumulate to toxic concentrations (the bucket will overflow).

In another example, if the amount of water added to the bucket is decreased but the hole in the bottom is still the original size, the water level would drop below the halfway mark. Similarly, if a drug is underdosed, the drug concentrations achieved in the body will be below the normal therapeutic range (i.e., subtherapeutic concentrations) and the desired effect will not be attained.

A similar water level decrease would occur if the hole in the bottom of the bucket were enlarged. Similarly, a drug's concentration will decrease more quickly if elimination is enhanced by increasing the rate by which the drug leaves the body via the kidney or liver. Renal excretion can be enhanced by the use of intravenous (IV) fluids to increase the filtration of renally excreted drugs from the blood into the urine. The same thing can occur if the liver metabolizes a drug at an accelerated rate.

If the elimination or metabolism rate is increased and it is desirable to keep the drug concentration at the same level, an increased dose would need to be added, much as additional water would need to be added to keep the water level at the halfway mark should the hole in the bucket become larger.

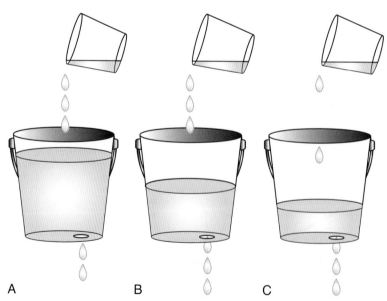

Fig. 3.2 The bucket analogy for understanding the effect of pharmacokinetics on therapeutic concentrations. (A) If the rate at which water is poured into a bucket (drug dose administered) is greater than the rate at which it is leaving (drug excreted from the body), the water level will rise. (B) If the rate at which water is poured into a bucket is equal to the rate at which it is leaving, the water level will remain stable. (C) If the rate at which water is poured into a bucket is less than the rate at which it is leaving, the water level will fall.

The point of this analogy is to illustrate that any factors that affect absorption of a drug (pouring water into the bucket), its metabolism to an inactive form, or its elimination (hole in the bottom of the bucket) can alter the expected drug concentrations achieved in the body for a given dose. Unless the veterinarian and veterinary technician understand and correct for these changes, the patient can end up being overdosed or underdosed.

THE DOSAGE REGIMEN AND ROUTES OF ADMINISTRATION

Chapter 2 introduced the concept of the dosage regimen. The dosage regimen included the calculated dose, the dose interval between doses, and the duration of the dosing. Typically included in the dosage regimen is the route of administration by which the drug dose is to be administered. An effective dosage regimen achieves therapeutic concentrations only if the appropriate dose, interval, and duration are chosen and if the dose is administered by a route that successfully allows the drug to enter the body.

Loading Dose and Maintenance Dose

Some dosage regimens begin with a large initial dose followed by smaller doses. For example, an animal with an infection may initially receive 2000 mg of an antibiotic by IM injection followed by 100 mg tablets every 8 h for the next 10 days. The reason for these two doses (2000 and 100 mg) can be explained with the bucket analogy.

At first, the bucket is empty of water. To establish the water level at the halfway mark, a fairly large amount of water needs to be added to establish the water level at the halfway mark. However, once the adequate water level has been established, only smaller amounts of water are added at a rate that matches the rate the water leaks out from the bottom of the bucket to maintain the established water level. Likewise, when the patient is started on a drug, the patient's system is empty like the bucket and must be given a larger initial dose to establish drug concentrations within the therapeutic range. This larger dose is called the loading dose because it "loads" the body with sufficient drug to establish therapeutic concentrations. As the body removes or inactivates the drug by elimination or metabolism, the concentrations drop and must be replaced by additional drug. However, unlike the initial loading dose, the maintenance dose is smaller and is given at an amount and rate that matches the amount eliminated by the body. If properly dosed, the maintenance dose should maintain the drug concentrations within the normal therapeutic range.

Total Daily Dose

The combined amount of drug (mass) times the number of doses administered in a given day (dose interval) is referred to as the total daily dose. For example, a 100-mg tablet given four times daily results in a total daily dose of 400 mg. Veterinary professionals may use the total daily dose concept to adjust the dosage interval and dose of the drug to increase client compliance (the owner's willingness to administer the medication as directed) or to provide more consistent therapeutic concentrations.

For example, the following dosage regimens provide equivalent total daily doses of 480 mg:

$$480\,\text{mg s.i.d.} = 480\,\text{mg} \times 1\,\text{time a day} = 480\,\text{mg}$$
$$240\,\text{mg b.i.d.} = 240\,\text{mg} \times 2\,\text{times a day} = 480\,\text{mg}$$
$$160\,\text{mg q8h} = 160\,\text{mg} \times 3\,\text{times a day} = 480\,\text{mg}$$
$$120\,\text{mg q6h} = 120\,\text{mg} \times 4\,\text{times a day} = 480\,\text{mg}$$
$$80\,\text{mg q4h} = 80\,\text{mg} \times 6\,\text{times a day} = 480\,\text{mg}$$

Generally, an owner is more likely to consistently and reliably administer a once-daily dosage regimen (dosage interval of 24 h) than a dosage regimen that requires administration three times a day. So if client compliance is more likely with a once-daily administration, why aren't all dosage regimens prescribed once daily?

Unfortunately, the greater the interval between doses, the wider the swings between the high peak concentrations and the low trough concentration. In the leaky bucket analogy, the only way to maintain the water level exactly at the halfway mark would be to continuously trickle in water at a rate that matches the rate at which the water leaks from the bottom. For drugs, this would be equivalent to a drug given as a constant rate intravenous infusion.

However, if additional water is only added once every 30 s, it would be impossible to hold the water level exactly at the halfway mark because the water level would fall for 30 s before being brought back up to its "peak" when additional water was added. Instead, the best that can be accomplished is to average the high water level and the low water level so that on average the water level is at the halfway mark over the 30-s interval between additional water doses. To do this successfully, the amount of water added every 30 s would need to exactly match the amount of water lost every 30 s.

If the interval between additional water were increased to every 3 min, each water "dose" would have to be even larger than the 30-s interval dose to compensate for the greater amount of water that would be lost over the 3 min. Thus, water levels in the bucket would drop farther than when the 30-s interval was used, and correspondingly the peak of the water level would also be higher. Thus, the swing between high water level and low water level becomes greater and greater as the interval between water doses increases.

Similarly if a patient has a dose changed from every 6 h to every 12 h, the swing between the peak concentration (highest drug concentration) to the trough concentration (lowest drug concentration) will be greater with the 12-h dosage regimen. The danger in the wider swings is that the concentrations at the peak concentration point could exceed the therapeutic range (producing toxicity) or the trough concentrations could fall below the normal therapeutic range (subtherapeutic concentrations and insufficient drug effect).

Drugs that have a maximum effective dose and the minimal effective dose very close to each other have a narrow therapeutic range and are said to have a narrow therapeutic index. Because the dose that produces the minimal beneficial effect is not that far from the dose that produces toxicity, these drugs should not be dosed in such a way that causes wide swings between the peak and the trough concentrations. For these drugs, extending the dosage interval but keeping the same total daily dose is not advised.

Although client compliance may be enhanced by decreasing the number of times a day a drug dose has to be administered to the patient, the potential problems from the larger concentration swings may outweigh any benefit from client compliance.

Parenteral Routes of Drug Administration

As stated previously, the route of administration is the route by which the drug is given and the pathway by which the drug enters the body. Each route of administration has its own limitations and advantages, as will be discussed later in this chapter under the principles of absorption.

Fig. 3.3 shows the routes of administration that are performed using a syringe and needle. Drugs given by injection are said to be parenterally administered drugs. The word "parenteral" breaks down to "para-" meaning "beside, beyond, or apart from," and "enteral" which refers to the intestines. Thus, a parenterally administered drug enters the body via the space between the outside of the intestinal tract and the surface of the skin.

As shown in Fig. 3.3, parenteral administration of drugs is further divided into specific routes described by the location in which the drug is deposited by the needle. Intravenous (IV) administration means the drug is injected directly into a vein. IV injections can be given as a single large volume at one time, called an IV bolus, or slowly injected or "dripped" into a vein over a period of several seconds, minutes, or even hours as an IV infusion or constant rate infusion (CRI). As shown in Fig. 3.4, a constant rate IV infusion results in a steady accumulation of drug concentrations in the body until the drug concentration reaches a plateau or steady state. In the bucket analogy, an IV bolus would be comparable to dumping all the water dose into the bucket at once, while in contrast an IV infusion is comparable to dribbling water into the bucket at a faster rate than it leaks out, resulting in an accumulation of water in the bucket (Fig. 3.2).

IV drug administration may be used to safely administer a drug that would otherwise be irritating or painful if injected into the muscle or beneath the skin. The accidental injection of an IV drug outside the vein is called an extravascular injection or perivascular injection because the drug has been deposited outside (extra-) or around (peri-) the blood vessel. Some drugs injected extravascularly can cause extreme tissue inflammation, tissue necrosis (tissue death), and sloughing of the skin over the injection site.

! YOU NEED TO KNOW

Common Word Roots and Prefixes Used in Pharmacology

The veterinary technician needs to be familiar with the commonly used prefixes in scientific literature to understand what the term says about the drug. Some of the common prefixes used in pharmacology are shown here.

Word Root, Prefix	Meaning	Example
aero-	air	aerosol = solution in air
anti-	against	antimicrobial = drug against microbes
arteri-	of the artery	intraarterial = within the artery
cardio-	heart	cardiovascular drugs = drugs affecting heart and vessels
chem-	chemical	chemotherapy = chemical therapy
contra-	against	contraindication = against an indication (do not use)
cyto-	cell	cytotoxic = poisonous to cells
derm-	skin	intradermal = within the skin
enter-	intestine	enteric = of the intestine
epi-	above	epidermis = above the dermis layer
erythro-	red	erythrocyte = red blood cell
extra-	outside	extravascular = outside the vessel
gastric	stomach	gastric acid = acid in the stomach
hypo-	below, less	hypothyroidism = lesser functioning thyroid disease
hyper-	above, more	hyperglycemia = higher than normal blood glucose
inter-	between	intercellular fluid = fluid between the cells
intra-	within	intravenous = within the vein
nephro-	kidney	nephrolith = stone in the kidney
per	through	per os = through the opening
peri-	around	perivascular = around the blood vessel
ur-	of urine	urolithiasis = condition of stones in the urine
vascu-	vessels	vasculitis = inflammation of the blood vessels
venous	of the vein	intravenous = within the vein

Although blood samples to evaluate blood oxygen levels are taken from arteries, drugs are not typically administered by intraarterial (IA) injection. Injecting a drug into an artery would deliver the full dose of the drug to a specific organ or tissue supplied by the artery and would expose that organ or tissue to very high and potentially toxic concentrations of the drug. Intravenously administered drugs do not share this problem because drugs administered IV are carried back to the heart, where they are mixed and diluted with blood before returning to the rest of the body tissues and organs.

Because large arteries and veins lie close to each other in many parts of the body, intraarterial injection can sometimes occur accidentally while attempting an intravenous injection, particularly in the large jugular vein in the horse neck, which lies next to the carotid artery. If, for example, an injectable IV

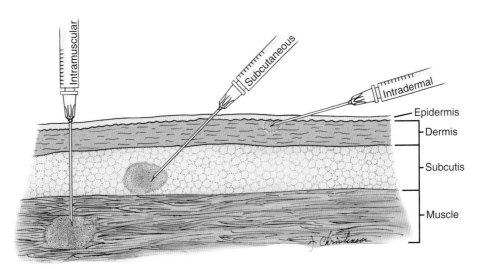

Fig. 3.3 The placement of drug with the intramuscular (IM), subcutaneous (SQ), and intradermal (ID) routes of parenteral administration. (From Christenson D. *Veterinary Medical Technology*. 2nd ed. St. Louis: Elsevier; 2009.)

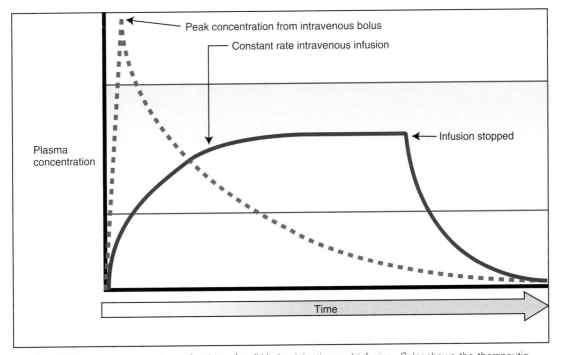

Fig. 3.4 Plasma concentrations of a drug after IV bolus injection and infusion. *Color* shows the therapeutic range.

anesthetic drug was accidentally administered into the equine carotid artery, the entire dose of anesthetic drug would reach the brain as a bolus, producing an overdose of the drug in the brain and resulting in seizures or collapse.

Intramuscular administration (IM) is a parenteral route of administration in which the drug is placed into the skeletal muscle. The prefix "intra-" means "within," so an intramuscularly administered medication is put "within the muscle." **Subcutaneous (SC or SQ)** injections are administered "sub-"

or "beneath" the "cutaneous tissue" or skin but not so deep as to be injected into the underlying muscle.

Intradermal (ID) injections use very small needles to place the drug into, but not below, the narrow layers of the skin. The intradermal route is usually reserved for special diagnostic procedures in which a small amount of a potentially reactive compound is injected into the layers of the skin and the degree of the body's reaction to the injected compound is measured. Intradermal skin testing for tuberculosis testing or evaluating a patient's sensitivity to allergenic substances are examples of ID drug administration.

Intraperitoneal (IP) injections are administered into the abdominal body cavity and are sometimes used when IV or IM injections are not practical (as in injecting some drugs into small laboratory animals) or when large volumes of solution must be administered for rapid absorption.

Nonparenteral Routes of Drug Administration

Drugs given by mouth are said to be given per os (PO), meaning "via a body opening." At the other end of the GI tract, drug suppositories are administered per rectum where they can be well absorbed from the terminal end of the colon. As mentioned previously with this dosage form, suppositories are sometimes used to administer drugs that pets cannot take orally because they are vomiting or having seizures and unable to swallow a medication PO without risk of aspirating the drug into the lungs. Drugs that are applied onto the surface of the skin, such as lotions and liniments, are called topically administered drugs. Aerosol administration means the drug is delivered into the lungs by "air or gas solution." Gas anesthesia or antibiotics given as an inhaled mist are examples of aerosol administered drugs.

Each route of drug administration has different absorption effectiveness (total amount of drug given that is successfully absorbed) and different absorption rates (how fast the drug is absorbed). The effectiveness or rate of absorption can be altered significantly by altered physiology or disease, requiring the dose be adjusted to compensate. By understanding how disease or physiologic changes alter the absorption effectiveness or rate, the veterinary technician can understand why a change in route of administration might be indicated or the dose increased or decreased to compensate.

HOW DRUGS MOVE IN THE BODY

Part of the variability of drug absorption by the different routes of administration is because of the way drug molecules move from one location in a fluid compartment to another location or how the molecules get across a cellular membrane. Drug molecules generally move from location A to location B in the body by four different mechanisms: passive diffusion, facilitated diffusion, active transport, and pinocytosis/phagocytosis.

Passive Diffusion

The majority of drug molecules moves throughout tissue fluid or across cellular membrane barriers by passive diffusion. Passive diffusion is the random movement of drug molecules "down the concentration gradient" from an area of high concentration of drug to an area of lower concentration. For example, if a colored liquid is poured into a pitcher of water, the color spreads, or diffuses, from the center of the pitcher to all parts of the water until the color is evenly distributed throughout the water. Similarly, when a drug is injected into the body, it passively diffuses "down the concentration gradient" from the high concentration at the injection site to the lower concentrations in the surrounding tissues, eventually reaching a blood capillary and entering the systemic circulation.

This process is called "passive" because no active cellular energy is expended by the body to move the drug molecules, and any drug molecule movement is based solely on the inherent molecular vibrations of drug molecules bouncing into each other.

The concept of passive diffusion of substances throughout a liquid medium is easy to understand because it is observed every day in life (e.g., mixing sugar in iced tea, adding milk to coffee). However, passive diffusion is also involved in the drug molecule movement through biological barriers like cell membranes. A drug may pass through a cell membrane by passive diffusion if the drug is able to dissolve in the membrane and then move by random molecular vibrations to the opposite side of the membrane. Although some drugs may be able to pass passively through a cell membrane via a special channel or aqueous pore (aquaporin), most passive diffusion across the membrane is simply by the molecule dissolving into and passing directly through the membrane itself.[1]

As shown in Fig. 3.5, the cell membranes, on a molecular level, are not solid structures. Instead, the cell membranes are composed primarily of two layers of phospholipid molecules arranged head-to-head. The phospholipid molecules give the cell membrane an outer layer of phosphate groups that can interact with water-soluble, or hydrophilic molecules ("water loving"), and an inner core (like the meat inside a sandwich) of fatty acids that are fat soluble, or lipophilic ("fat loving").[2] The lipophilic inner layer of fatty acids behaves like a fat or oil barrier and constitutes the major barrier to passive diffusion of many drug molecules through the membrane. Therefore, for a drug molecule to passively diffuse from one side of the cell membrane to the other, it must be *lipophilic* like a fat or oil molecule and thus capable of dissolving in, and passing through, the inner lipophilic core. Hydrophilic drug molecules will not be able to dissolve in and pass through the lipid core of the membrane and hence will be unable to passively diffuse through the cell membrane barrier.

In passive diffusion the drug molecules continue to pass from an area of higher concentration to an area of lower concentration until the drug molecules are equally distributed and the movement of drug molecules is said to be at *equilibrium*. At equilibrium, the number of molecules moving from point A to B is the same as the number of molecules moving from point B to A. Hence, even though the individual molecules continue to move around their space randomly, there is no net direction of drug molecule movement when the drug molecules are at equilibrium.

Facilitated Diffusion

Facilitated diffusion is considered a passive transport mechanism across cell membranes because it does not require the cell to expend energy to move the molecule. However, facilitated diffusion differs from passive diffusion in that facilitated diffusion uses a special "carrier molecule" located in the cellular membrane to move the drug molecule across the membrane. The carrier molecule, usually a protein floating among the phospholipid molecules in the cell membrane, has a specific site to which a drug molecule can attach. When a drug molecule combines with

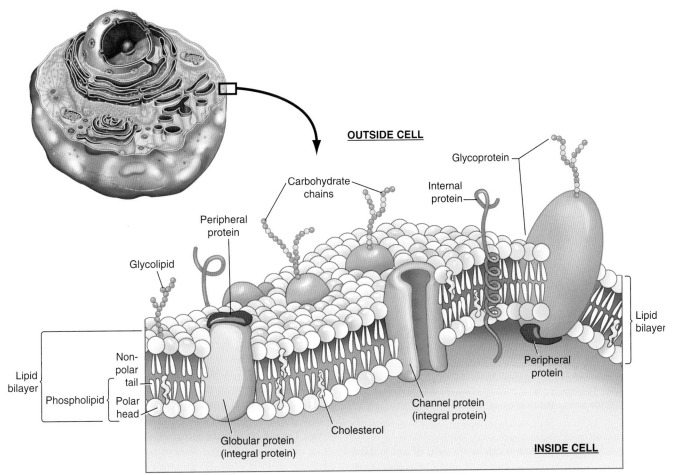

OUTSIDE CELL

Glycoprotein

Carbohydrate chains

Internal protein

Peripheral protein

Glycolipid

Lipid bilayer

Lipid bilayer

Phospholipid

Non-polar tail

Polar head

Globular protein (integral protein)

Cholesterol

Channel protein (integral protein)

Peripheral protein

INSIDE CELL

Fig. 3.5 Cellular membrane structure. (*Top left*: Modified from Patton KT, Thibodeau GA. *Anatomy & Physiology*. 9th ed. St. Louis: Mosby; 2016. Colville T. *Clinical Anatomy and Physiology for Veterinary Technicians*. 3rd ed. St. Louis: Elsevier; 2016. *Bottom*: From Colville T. *Clinical Anatomy and Physiology for Veterinary Technicians*. 3rd ed. St. Louis: Elsevier; 2016.)

the carrier, the carrier molecule changes its configuration or shape, allowing the drug molecule to be carried through the cell membrane without having to dissolve into the cell membrane like those molecules that cross the membrane by passive diffusion (Fig. 3.6). Because facilitated diffusion is still a passive process requiring no cellular energy, the carrier only moves drug molecules in the direction determined by the concentration gradient. Once equilibrium is attained, the number of drug molecules crossing the membrane via the carrier is equal in either direction.

Facilitated diffusion can be thought of as functioning in the same way that a passive revolving door allows people to move through a wall. The people (drug molecules) provide the "push" that moves the revolving door (the carrier molecule) and eventually transports the person to the other side of the wall (the drug molecule to the other side of the membrane). People or drug molecules can move either way through the wall or membrane, but neither the building nor the cell expends energy to transport the people or the drug molecule through the barrier.

Active Transport

Active transport is a less common method for drug molecule movement than diffusion. However, active transport plays a very important role in explaining why some drugs produce toxicity when others do not. As with facilitated diffusion, active transport of drug molecules involves a specialized carrier molecule. However, in active transport the cell expends energy to either move the drug molecule across the cell membrane or to "reset" the carrier molecule after transport is completed so that the carrier molecule can transport again.

Unlike passive or facilitated diffusion, in which drug molecules can move either way across the membrane and the net direction of drug movement is determined by the concentration gradient, active transport occurs in only one direction and can actually move drug molecules against the concentration gradient. Thus, drug molecules can be moved from areas of lower concentration to areas of higher concentration, and the net direction of drug molecule movement does not stop when equilibrium is reached.

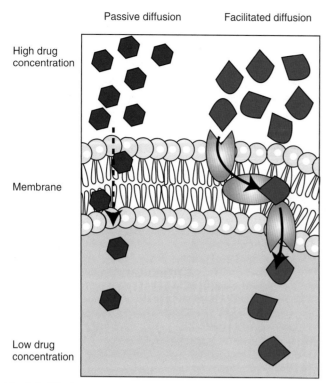

Passive diffusion   Facilitated diffusion

High drug concentration

Membrane

Low drug concentration

Fig. 3.6 Diffusion across a membrane. Passive diffusion through the cellular membrane. Facilitated diffusion using a carrier molecule that moves the drug molecule across the membrane.

Although facilitated diffusion can be thought of as a passive revolving door, active transport can be thought of as an electrically powered pump. Although an electrical pump requires energy to operate, it can also move tremendous quantities of water from one area to another without any consideration of how much water has already been pumped into the receiving area. As long as there is water available to pump, the electric pump will pump it to the other side. Likewise, in active transport, the cellular energy continues to move drug molecules across the membrane regardless of the amount already transported; this can sometimes result in toxicosis from very high accumulations of drug molecules accumulating inside a cell or body compartment.

Pinocytosis and Phagocytosis

Pinocytosis and phagocytosis are less common forms of an active transport process that involves a cell's membrane physically engulfing the drug molecule (Fig. 3.7A and B). Pinocytosis (meaning "cell drinking") is sometimes also called endocytosis and involves a small invagination forming in the cell membrane that surrounds the drug molecule and brings it into the cell. Vitamin B_{12} is brought into the body via pinocytosis in the GI tract, and aminoglycoside antibiotics are taken from the blood into kidney cells by pinocytosis.[1]

Phagocytosis (meaning "cell eating") is a process in which much of the entire cell surrounds the molecule, forming a vesicle large enough to contain the phagocytized molecule or object. Both processes obviously require cellular energy, but they are relatively rare methods by which drugs are moved across

membranes. Phagocytosis is required to move large antibody protein molecules intact across the intestinal tract cell and is crucial for newborn animals to absorb antibodies from the mother's colostrum milk within the first few hours of life.

Factors That Affect Rate of Drug Molecule Movement

It takes time for drug molecules to move through a liquid by passive diffusion or to cross a cellular membrane by facilitated diffusion, active transport, or pinocytosis/phagocytosis. When drug molecule transportation across a cell membrane is dependent on a carrier molecule, the rate at which drug molecules can pass across the membrane is dependent on how quickly the carrier molecule can move the drug molecule and then reset to receive the next drug molecule. The overall rate of transport across a membrane would also be limited by the number of carrier molecules that exists in the cellular membrane. If all the carrier molecules are continuously occupied with transporting drug molecules across the membrane, there are no "open" carrier proteins available to transport another drug molecule and the transport system is said to be saturated. When the transport system is saturated, the transport system is working at its maximum speed and is said to be operating at its transportation maximum, or t-max. A saturated carrier transport system operating at its t-max is similar to a crowded toll road when cars back up at the toll booths. If all the toll booths are continuously occupied, the toll booths are saturated and the rate at which the cars can move through the toll booths is operating at t-max. Saturated transport systems can affect how quickly drug molecules may be distributed to tissues, metabolized to other compounds, or eliminated from the body.

In contrast to carrier transport systems, passive diffusion only requires the drug molecules to dissolve into and pass through any part of the cell membrane; therefore, the rate of transport is not limited by the number of available carrier molecules or how quickly they work/reset. However, the rate at which drug molecules diffuse across the membrane can be influenced by the following factors:

- The difference in concentration gradient on either side of the membrane: The greater the concentration gradient, the faster the net rate at which molecules move across. Individual molecules don't pass faster, but a larger number of molecules will move across the membrane down the concentration gradient than will move back across against the gradient; thus the net movement of molecules from higher to lower concentrations is greater when the drug concentration differences are larger on either side of the membrane.
- The drug molecule size: The smaller the drug molecule size, the more readily the molecule can move across a membrane.
- The lipophilic ("fat-loving") nature of the molecule: The more a drug molecule can dissolve into the phospholipids of the cell membranes, the more readily it will diffuse across the membrane to the other side.
- The temperature of the cellular environment: Generally, the lower the temperature, the slower the molecular movements and the slower the passive diffusion.

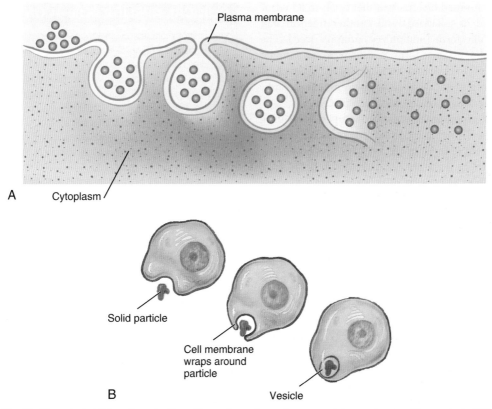

Fig. 3.7 Pinocytosis (A) is an invagination of the cell membrane to surround drug molecules. Phagocytosis (B) is the cell surrounding the large molecule to bring it into the cell. (Panel [A]: From Nix S. *Williams' Basic Nutrition and Diet Therapy*. 4th ed. St. Louis: Elsevier; 2013. Panel [B]: From Applegate E. *The Anatomy and Physiology Learning System*. 4th ed. St. Louis: Elsevier; 2011.)

- The thickness of the membrane: The thicker the membrane, the slower the diffusion across it.

Thus, the maximal rate of drug molecule passive diffusion across a cellular membrane occurs when a large concentration gradient is present, the drug molecule is small and lipophilic, the temperature at the cellular membrane is increased, and the membrane is quite thin.

Effect of a Drug's Lipophilic or Hydrophilic Nature on Drug Molecule Movement

As stated previously, for drugs to be able to move by passive diffusion across a cell membrane, they must dissolve, or be soluble, in the membrane. Biological membranes are largely composed of phospholipids, which have chemical properties similar to fats. Therefore, to move across a membrane, drug molecules must be in a lipophilic ("fat-loving") form that is capable of dissolving in fat or oil.

However, not all molecules readily dissolve in fat. For example, when fat or oil is mixed with water, the fat will separate into distinct globules that appear to clump together into a layer separate from water. This can be observed when oily salad dressings, gravy, or grease are mixed with water. Molecules that do not readily dissolve in fat or oil are said to be hydrophilic, meaning "water loving." Technically, these molecules should be referred to as lipophobic, meaning "fat fearing"; however, a drug molecule that does not dissolve readily in fats or oils is assumed to dissolve readily in water and is therefore called hydrophilic.

Because membranes are largely phospholipids and have a lipophilic nature, drug molecules that have a hydrophilic chemical nature have a difficult time dissolving in and passing through the cellular membranes by passive diffusion. Therefore, hydrophilic drug molecules are dependent on carrier-mediated transport mechanisms to be transported across membranes.

Conversely, lipophilic drugs dissolve readily in fat but do not readily dissolve in water and if introduced into an aqueous medium (water-based medium), the lipophilic drug molecules will clump together and not readily disperse throughout the medium.

What makes a drug molecule hydrophilic or lipophilic? Hydrophilic drugs are either polarized, meaning they contain positive and negative charges at the ends of the molecule, or they are ionized, meaning they contain a net positive or a net negative charge such as HCO_3^- or NH_4^+. The charged nature allows the drug molecule to dissolve more readily in water but prevents it from passing through lipophilic cellular membranes. In contrast, lipophilic drug molecules tend to be **nonpolarized** and **nonionized** molecules.

An important point in understanding the lipophilic/hydrophilic nature of drugs is that when a mass of drug molecules is introduced into the body, all of the molecules do not become exclusively hydrophilic or lipophilic. More typically the drug molecules will be composed of a fraction that exists in a hydrophilic form (ionized or polarized) and another fraction that exists in the lipophilic form (nonionized, nonpolarized). The number of molecules in each form is usually a set ratio of hydrophilic molecules to lipophilic molecules based upon characteristics of the drug molecule and the environmental conditions into which the drug molecule has been placed.

For example, the group of molecules from a particular drug may exist predominantly in the lipophilic drug molecule form in the acidic environment of the stomach but exist predominantly in a hydrophilic form in the more alkaline environment of the small intestine. These changes in drug form from predominantly hydrophilic to lipophilic and vice versa change the overall ability of the drug to penetrate a cell membrane or disperse within an aqueous medium, thus affecting the drug's ability to move into and throughout the body. The effect of the lipophilic and hydrophilic forms is discussed in greater detail later in the context of absorption, distribution, and excretion from the body.

CLINICAL APPLICATION

Nephrotoxicosis From Drug Accumulation

An older, intact female dog was presented to a veterinary hospital with a history of lethargy, not eating, and discharge from the vulva. The veterinarian determined that the dog had a pyometra, an infection of the uterus in which a great deal of pus is produced. The veterinarian recommended surgery to remove the infected uterus and the ovaries (ovariohysterectomy). During removal of the infected uterus, the surgical site was contaminated (bacteria were introduced into the site). The veterinarian chose to use gentamicin, a potent antibiotic, to combat the infection introduced into the abdomen during surgery. Because of his concern over the potentially serious nature of the infection, he chose to give the dog a high-dose IV every 12 h.

Over the next 2 days the dog became feverish, continued to be lethargic, was not interested in eating, and seemed to have pain in the abdomen. By day 3, however, the fever started to decrease and the dog seemed more alert. To be safe, the veterinarian continued to hospitalize the animal and administer gentamicin for an additional 7 days (9 days total). On day 10, the veterinarian was going to send the dog home. A blood test and urinalysis suggested that the animal had laboratory signs consistent with kidney damage or disease. Fearing an effect from the gentamicin antibiotic, the veterinarian stopped the gentamicin and hospitalized the dog for an additional 3 days on IV fluids. After that time, the blood tests and urinalysis indicated that renal function had improved. The dog was sent home and recovered uneventfully.

How did drug molecule transport of gentamicin molecules possibly cause kidney damage?

In this case, the veterinarian was using an antibiotic that is known to be potentially damaging to the kidney. When laboratory signs of kidney damage appeared, he stopped the drug and provided supportive care for kidney injury. In this case, the dog recovered.

Gentamicin and other aminoglycoside antibiotics (e.g., amikacin, neomycin, streptomycin) are potentially nephrotoxic drugs, meaning they have the ability to be poisonous to the kidney (nephro, pertaining to the kidney). These drugs are nephrotoxic because they are actively transported into the kidney cells from the blood by pinocytosis and can accumulate at high enough concentrations within the kidney cells to poison the kidney cell, producing a condition called nephrotoxicosis.

Gentamicin is actively transported into the kidney cell by pinocytosis but has no active transport mechanism to move back out of the cell. Thus, movement of

CLINICAL APPLICATION—CONT'D

drug is mostly into the cell. In addition, gentamicin is mostly ionized (hydrophilic) at the body pH of 7.4, and therefore passive diffusion back out through the kidney cell's membrane is slow. Because passive diffusion relies on a concentration gradient, gentamicin will only leave the kidney cell if blood concentrations outside the cell drop low enough to facilitate passive diffusion. By stopping the gentamicin administration, the concentrations in the blood dropped quickly and established a concentration that favored the gentamicin moving back out of the cell, thus decreasing the concentration of the gentamicin within the cell before it could do permanent damage to too much of the kidney.

What should be learned from this situation: Active transport mechanisms of drugs can be beneficial for veterinary patients if the active transport of an antibiotic is into a site of infection. However, active transport of drugs into other areas of the body may result in accumulated drug concentrations that exceed the therapeutic range and become toxic, resulting in the death of normal, healthy cells. Thus knowing which specific drugs are transported in this manner and understanding how that transportation causes toxicity allow us to take steps to prevent the local toxicity from occurring.

PHARMACOKINETICS: ABSORPTION—GETTING DRUGS INTO THE BODY

Pharmacokinetics is the study of how drugs move into, through, and out of the body and is affected by the characteristics of the drug and the physiology of the body. The pharmacokinetics of drugs is usually described in four basic steps: absorption, distribution, metabolism, and excretion (or elimination). These four steps are often abbreviated as *A.D.M.E.* Drug dosages on a drug label "should" achieve normal therapeutic range drug concentrations in the average patient that possesses a similar degree of health and physiologic state as those animals upon whom the drug was tested and approved. However, each of these four A.D.M.E. pharmacokinetic steps can be altered by disease or changes in physiologic conditions. Therefore, the veterinarian and veterinary technician must recognize when these changed conditions occur, how such changes may potentially alter the pharmacokinetics, and in what manner the drug dose may have to be changed to achieve or maintain the drug concentrations within the therapeutic range.

⊚ MYTHS AND MISCONCEPTIONS

Absorption and distribution of drugs are essentially the same thing.

False! Many veterinary technician students confuse these two steps in pharmacokinetics. Absorption is the movement of drug *from* the location where the drug was administered (e.g., the skeletal muscle for an IM injection) *to* the systemic circulation (the blood vessel). Once the drug arrives at the blood vessel it is considered to be absorbed. Distribution is the movement of the drug *from* the blood vessel *to* all tissues. Both absorption and distribution must occur for a drug to be effective, but they are two different steps in the pharmacokinetic process.

Drug Absorption and Bioavailability

After a drug has been ingested, injected, inhaled, or applied to the skin, it must be absorbed into the blood and travel to the body areas (i.e., target tissues) where it will have its intended effect. Absorption of a drug is defined as the movement of drug molecules from the site of administration to the systemic circulation. Thus absorption of an IM injected drug would be the movement of the drug from the skeletal muscle injection site into the adjacent capillaries.

Generally, a drug is useless until it is absorbed into systemic circulation. Exceptions to this are drugs designed to work only where they are applied, such as local anesthetics, topical insecticides for killing fleas, topical antibiotics, and drugs that are intended to work within the lumen of the intestine. With the exception of these locally acting medications, rapid, total absorption of the drug into the blood is desirable.

As previously mentioned, the degree to which any route of administration is effective in getting all of the drug into systemic circulation varies. Many drugs are not completely absorbed unless they are placed directly into the blood via IV injection. After being administered by a non-IV route, the drug molecule may be metabolized by the liver before it reaches the blood, it may be inactivated by enzymes in the tissues through which it passes on the way to the blood, or it may be in a form that does not readily move through cellular barriers.

How much of an administered drug is ultimately absorbed is referred to as its bioavailability. Bioavailability is the percentage of drug administered that actually makes it into systemic circulation. On most drug descriptions, bioavailability is indicated by a decimal number from 0 to 1.0 and the letter "f" or "F." Thus, if 100% of the drug administered makes it to systemic circulation, the drug is said to have a bioavailability of 100%, or 1.0 (the decimal equivalent of 100%) and may be listed as "$f = 1.0$" or "$F = 100\%$." A drug that is only half absorbed would be listed as "$f = 0.5$" or "$F = 50\%$," and a drug only 25% successfully absorbed would have an "$f = 0.25$" or "$F = 25\%$."[3]

Effect of Route of Administration on Absorption

The route of drug administration (e.g., PO, IM, and SQ) directly affects the drug's bioavailability. The IV route of administration places the drug directly into the vein; hence the drug has no absorption phase (it is already in systemic circulation) and has a bioavailability of 1.0.

Drugs administered IM into actively moving skeletal muscle are usually placed close to capillaries and thus are rapidly and almost completely absorbed. Because of this, IM administered drugs have a bioavailability only slightly less than drugs administered IV. PO and SQ administered drugs must overcome several barriers to be absorbed and are more susceptible to inactivation, metabolism, or removal before they reach systemic circulation; therefore, they may have a bioavailability significantly less than 1.0.

In addition to affecting the overall bioavailability of the drug, the rate at which a drug is absorbed into systemic circulation is affected by the route of administration. The curves that represent the absorption of drug by different routes are shown in Fig. 3.8.

As mentioned previously under the section about total daily dose, the peak concentration of the drug is the highest concentration achieved during a dose interval, and the trough concentration is the lowest concentration between doses. Fig. 3.8 illustrates how intravenously administered drugs almost instantly achieve their peak concentration after administration. As soon as the IV drug enters the systemic circulation, it begins

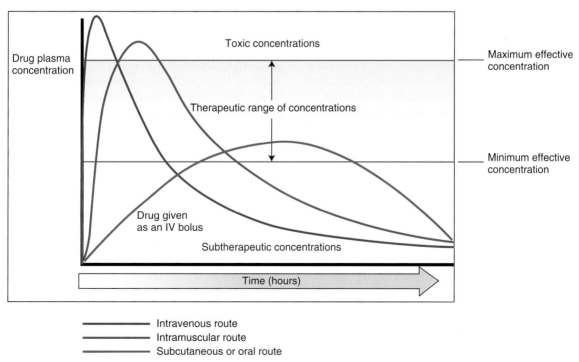

Fig. 3.8 Plasma drug concentrations attained after IV, IM, SQ, and PO administration.

to be excreted from the body and the drug concentrations begin to fall immediately after the peak until the entire drug has been excreted.

Drugs given intramuscularly show a similar pattern to IV administered drugs because they are rapidly, but not instantaneously, absorbed from the injection site. Fig. 3.8 shows a rapid increase in drug concentrations between the time of injection and attainment of the peak plasma concentration a few minutes later. Because IM absorption is spread out over a slightly longer time than the instantaneous peak from IV administration, the IM peak plasma concentration attained is similar to, but not quite as high as, the peak from using the IV route of administration.

If an IM drug is injected into skeletal muscle of an animal that is comatose, recumbent, or anesthetized, the drug absorption will be slower than if the drug were injected into the same muscle site of a conscious animal that is actively using the muscle. The absorption is quicker in the active skeletal muscle because more capillaries are open and have greater blood flow than inactive muscle. Thus, the IM injected drug does not have to travel as far before it reaches an open, flowing capillary.

In Fig. 3.8, it is seen that drugs given PO or SQ take much longer to reach their peak plasma concentrations and the peak concentration is much lower than the concentration achieved with the same dose of IM or IV administered drug. Even if the bioavailability of the SQ or PO administered drug is 100%, the absorption rate is much slower and is spread out over a longer period of time during which the drug is also being excreted from the blood.

SQ administered drugs typically must diffuse a greater distance to reach an open capillary and systemic circulation than an IM injected drug because SQ tissue generally has a poorer blood supply than muscle. (Think about which bleeds more when cut by a scalpel in surgery: the tissue under the skin or skeletal muscle. Muscle bleeds much more freely.)

PO drugs must move along the intestinal tract until they dissolve, pass across the intestinal tract wall, and enter into another capillary system that takes them to the liver before they gain access to systemic circulation. All these steps cause a delay after PO drug administration before plasma drug concentrations can be seen to increase. The slow absorption also spreads out the absorption over a much longer time, producing a much lower peak concentration than IM injected drugs and a more gently sloped concentration curve.

In emergency situations or in clinical circumstances for which the beneficial drug effect is needed "stat," the IV route is preferred over all the other routes. With the IV route the drug is able to attain therapeutic concentrations in the blood almost immediately, thus hastening the distribution of the drug to the target tissues.

Even though the IV route of administration has many advantages, the rapid, high peak concentration achieved immediately after an IV bolus dose is given may for a short period (minutes) result in plasma drug concentrations that could exceed the therapeutic range. To avoid such a high peak and potential toxicity from an IV bolus, the IV drug administration could be given slowly over several minutes as an IV infusion or IV "drip."

Drugs with a risk for toxicity from rapid IV bolus administration have a warning or caution label that states that the drug is "not to be given as a bolus" or it should be "infused slowly."

It is vital that veterinary technicians be aware that suspensions or drugs dissolved in media that is not appropriate for IV administration must not be given intravenously. Unless the drug label states specifically that the drug is for IV use, it should not be given by that route of administration.

Some IV drugs require dilution before administration. Failure to do so could result in a severe inflammation of the vein into which the concentrated drug is administered, or it could produce a severe systemic reaction in the patient. Some IV drugs can cause a very severe inflammation of the vein (i.e., vasculitis) and surrounding tissue if the drug is accidentally given outside of the vein. If such drugs are accidentally injected perivascularly, they should be diluted with sterile IV fluids and the area given additional heat or cold treatment as appropriate for the particular tissue reaction.

Finally, IV administered drugs are often added into IV fluid bags or diluted with IV fluids. However, some IV drugs are not compatible with certain intravenous fluids and the mixture can cause the drug to precipitate out of solution or to mix unevenly within the IV fluid. The veterinary technician must always check the drug insert or information to determine if the drug can be safely mixed with intravenous fluids.

Effect of the Drug's Chemical Properties on Absorption: Lipophilic and Hydrophilic Drugs

As mentioned previously, drug molecules can exist in hydrophilic (water-loving) or lipophilic (fat-loving) forms when put into the body, and these forms can affect the drug molecule's ability to dissolve in water or pass through a cellular membrane. Whether a drug exists predominantly in a lipophilic or hydrophilic state is dependent on the chemical nature of the drug and the pH of the environment into which the drug is placed.

The route of administration dictates whether the hydrophilic drug molecules or the lipophilic drug molecules are going to be successfully absorbed. For example, drugs injected subcutaneously or intramuscularly are deposited into the extracellular fluid (fluid/water outside the cells) and must diffuse through that fluid to reach the capillaries and be absorbed into systemic circulation. Because extracellular fluid is an aqueous medium, drug molecules in the hydrophilic form will diffuse more readily through the fluid than will molecules in the lipophilic form. Thus, a drug with molecules predominantly in the hydrophilic form will be more rapidly absorbed via the IM or SQ route of administration than drugs that exist primarily in the lipophilic form.

In contrast to drugs given by the SQ and IM route, drugs given by mouth must pass through cellular membranes lining the GI tract to be absorbed. Unlike the more loosely organized cells of the muscle or connective tissue where IM or SQ administered drug molecules can pass in the tissue fluid between cells, the cells lining the intestinal tract are tightly adhered to their neighboring cells and form a continuous cellular barrier that separates the contents of the intestinal tract from the rest of the body. Therefore, drugs given by mouth must be in a lipophilic form to dissolve in, and pass through, the cellular membrane barrier of the intestinal tract wall and be absorbed. Drugs that exist primarily in the hydrophilic form at the pH found in the small intestine are poorly absorbed from the gut and may largely remain in the intestinal tract to be expelled with the feces.

In some cases, a drug is purposely formulated to exist in a form that is not well absorbed. For example, deworming agents or antibiotics intended to work within the lumen (inner space) of the intestine are chemically formulated to exist primarily in the hydrophilic form to prevent their absorption from the intestine. Similarly, some drugs that are injected IM or SQ are formulated to exist predominantly in a lipophilic form so that absorption of the drug will be slowed and occur over hours to days. Some injectable antibiotics or hormone drugs are manufactured in this manner to provide concentrations of drug for several days after the drug is injected.

To summarize, for a drug to be rapidly absorbed by the SQ or IM route, the drug molecules need to be mostly in the hydrophilic form. To be rapidly absorbed by the PO route, the drug molecules need to be predominantly in the lipophilic form. An IV administered drug has no such requirements because the drug is absorbed 100% by directly depositing the drug into the blood regardless of the hydrophilic or lipophilic nature of the drug molecules.

P-Glycoprotein and Drug Absorption From the Gastrointestinal Tract

The body has many mechanisms for keeping "poisonous" compounds out of the body, and some of these affect the drugs used in veterinary medicine. One such mechanism is an active transport pump found most notably in the epithelium of the intestinal tract wall, blood-brain barrier and in the liver called P-glycoprotein and sometimes abbreviated **P-gp**. The purpose of the active transport pump is to actively transport selected molecules back into circulation for excretion. P-glycoprotein is found in other cellular barriers in the body and plays a role in what is known as "multiple drug resistance." Thus a lipophilic drug molecule may be able to move from circulation into the cells lining the intestinal tract, blood-brain barrier and liver, only to be grabbed by the P-glycoprotein and ejected back into the intestinal lumen or circulation for excretion.[1] P-glycoprotein will be discussed throughout this text to explain the pharmacokinetic behavior of certain drugs used in veterinary medicine such as ivermectin, opioid antidiarrheals, and some antifungal drugs.

Cytochrome P-450 and Drug Absorption From the Gastrointestinal Tract

When drug metabolism is discussed later in this chapter, the focus will be on enzymes located in the liver. These enzymes break down or alter the drug's molecular structure, either inactivating the drug, decreasing the drug's activity, or in some cases increasing the drug's activity. The intestinal tract also has enzymes located in the cells of the intestinal wall that can inactivate drugs that successfully move across the cell membrane barrier lining the GI tract. These enzymes belong to a family of enzymes called cytochrome P-450 enzymes and are often abbreviated as *CYP*.

Cytochrome P-450 subtype 3A, called *CYP 3A*, is the CYP that accounts for most of the drug effect in the intestinal tract. CYP 3A tends to metabolize the same drugs that P-glycoprotein removes from the cell. Thus a combined effect of CYP 3A and P-gp can be a formidable barrier to prevent the absorption of some lipophilic drugs.

During drug development, any effect of the intestinal enterocyte CYP enzyme to reduce the absorption of the drug is reflected in the dosage recommended by the drug's manufacturer. Remember, the dosage is based upon the amount of drug that has to be administered so that the drug's concentration in the body reaches the therapeutic range. Thus if some percentage of the drug is destroyed by the cytochrome P-450 enzymes before it reaches systemic circulation or rejected by P-glycoprotein, a greater amount of drug would have to be administered in the recommended dose.

Drugs or disease may inhibit the function of CYP enzymes or P-glycoprotein. Any inhibition of these intestinal CYP enzymes or P-glycoprotein would mean that a "correct" dose would deliver a larger than normal quantity of drug dose into the body, resulting in higher plasma drug concentrations and possible toxicity. If both the CYP 3A and the P-glycoprotein have been inactivated (as occurs with some drugs), the dose of any drug normally excluded from the body by these mechanisms would have to be decreased significantly to avoid achieving very high and possibly toxic concentrations. CYP will be discussed in greater detail with selected drugs in the following chapters.

Effect of Dissolution and Gastrointestinal Motility on Absorption of Orally Administered Drugs

Drugs given by mouth must be in the lipophilic form to penetrate the gastrointestinal (GI) mucosa and be absorbed. However, before any tablet, caplet, powdered drug, or granular drug can diffuse across the membrane barrier, it must be broken apart into particles small enough to pass through the cellular membrane of the GI tract wall. This process of breaking down dosage forms to the individual molecules is called dissolution or dissolving and is a critical step for drug absorption of PO administered drugs (Fig. 3.9).

Drugs in liquid dose form, such as solutions and elixirs, do not have a dissolution step because the drug already exists in a dissolved state within the liquid medium of the drug. Drugs that do not have to go through a dissolution phase are usually more rapidly absorbed by the oral route, attain therapeutic concentrations more rapidly, and often have greater bioavailability than the equivalent solid dosage forms such as tablets or caplets.

As previously described, sustained-release (SR) medications dissolve slowly or otherwise release their drug over minutes to hours, thus spreading out the amount of drug to be absorbed over a longer period of time. Although SR oral medications have the advantage of reducing the number of times the patient must be medicated per day, the disadvantage is that the concentrations achieved in the body tend to have a lower peak

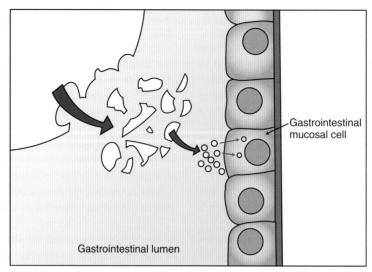

Fig. 3.9 Drugs administered in solid dosage form must completely dissolve to the molecular level before they can be absorbed across a cellular membrane by passive diffusion.

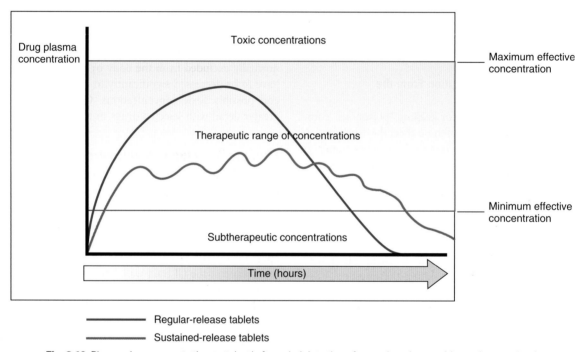

Regular-release tablets
Sustained-release tablets

Fig. 3.10 Plasma drug concentrations attained after administration of a regular-release tablet and a sustained-release (SR) tablet. The variability of the SR tablet reflects the variability in rate at which the tablet dissolves over time and the availability of dissolved drug for absorption.

concentration than the standard-release formulations, and the overall concentrations during the course of the dose interval are more variable. A hypothetical example of plasma drug concentrations for an SR tablet vs a regular-release tablet is shown in Fig. 3.10.

As described in Chapter 2, an additional disadvantage of using SR human oral medications in domestic animals is that the dosage form may not completely dissolve in the domestic animal's intestinal tract before it has moved beyond the small intestine, which is the site of greatest drug absorption into the body. Therefore, human oral SR medications may have a lower overall bioavailability than the same oral drug used in a regular-release dosage form because of the slower rate at which SR drugs are released.

Alteration of the normal motility of the stomach and intestinal tract can affect how much time the solid dose form has to dissolve and be absorbed and may alter the drug's bioavailability or how quickly a drug begins to work. Gastric motility refers to stomach contractions that mix stomach contents and move the contents from the stomach into the small intestine. Because the small intestine is the site of greatest drug absorption, any conditions, drugs, or diseases that decrease gastric motility can delay the movement of drug from the stomach into the intestine and therefore delay the absorption and onset of action of the drug. This would not necessarily be true for drugs absorbed from the stomach, but relatively few drugs are absorbed primarily in the stomach. Similarly, a spasm of the pylorus, the muscular ring controlling outflow of stomach contents into the duodenum, can also decrease gastric emptying, delaying drug absorption in the intestine. Conversely, increased gastric motility may result in the drug being absorbed sooner than normal.

Intestinal motility is defined as the mixing and peristaltic contractions of the intestine. Increased propulsion of intestinal contents, as in some forms of diarrhea, may move the orally administered tablet past the small intestine before it has completely dissolved, resulting in much of the drug passing out of the body in the feces and being unabsorbed. In contrast, decreased intestinal motility, such as occurs with constipation or some antidiarrheal treatments, can result in complete absorption of a drug, including those drugs that are not necessarily intended to be absorbed (e.g., antibiotics intended to work within the lumen of the intestine). When motility modifier drugs or disease alter GI motility, the veterinary professional has to consider the possible effect the motility change might have on orally administered medications.

The First-Pass Effect

Even if a drug in solid form has dissolved into small lipophilic molecules capable of diffusing readily across the GI tract wall, one final barrier separates the drug from the systemic circulation. All the blood supply from the stomach, small intestine, and proximal part of the large intestine passes first to the liver before it reenters the systemic circulation. The hepatic portal system is the system of blood vessels that conducts the blood from the capillaries of the GI tract to the capillaries of the liver and allows the liver to remove poisons, toxins, and other potentially dangerous substances absorbed from the GI tract before they reach systemic circulation. The liver recognizes many drugs as foreign substances (xenobiotics) or "poisons" and may remove certain drugs that successfully diffused across the GI tract wall. In dogs, for example, the tranquilizer diazepam is removed so extensively by the liver after "absorption" from the intestine that little of the tranquilizer makes it to the body to actually produce tranquilization. The phenomenon by which the liver removes so much of the drug that little reaches the systemic circulation is called the first-pass effect. Drugs that have an extensive first-pass effect are usually not recommended for PO administration.

Effect of Perfusion on Absorption of Parenterally Administered Drugs

As previously stated, when drugs are injected subcutaneously or intramuscularly they are placed in an aqueous extracellular fluid

between cells and must move by passive diffusion within this aqueous environment to an open blood capillary to reach systemic circulation. If there are few open capillaries in the tissues where the drug is injected, the distance from the injection site to an open capillary will be greater and it will take longer for the drug molecules to diffuse to the capillary. Or if capillaries in the area of the injection site have little or sluggish blood flow through them, the drug molecules may diffuse into and then back out of the capillary before the blood has had a chance to carry the drug molecule away from the injection site area. Thus the degree to which a tissue has a rich blood supply influences the rate at which an SQ or IM injected drug will be absorbed.

The extent to which a tissue is supplied with blood is called the tissue perfusion. Tissues that are well perfused with blood will absorb injected drugs much more quickly than tissues that are poorly perfused. Fat is a tissue that is poorly perfused (notice in surgery how little fat bleeds when it is cut); therefore, drugs injected into a fatty area or fat pad may remain there for an extended period without being absorbed. Skeletal muscle is usually much better perfused than SQ tissue; therefore, drugs injected IM are absorbed more quickly than those drugs injected SQ. This was illustrated previously in Fig. 3.8.

Tissue perfusion can vary with physiologic conditions. For example, an inactive muscle is not as well perfused as an active muscle; consequently, drugs injected into inactive muscles (e.g., in an animal not moving because of anesthesia or a comatose state) will be absorbed at a slower rate than those injected into a muscle that is moving.

Changes in environmental temperature can affect the perfusion of the subcutaneous tissue, resulting in changes in absorption of drugs administered SQ. Cold environmental temperatures cause the precapillary sphincters (circular rings of smooth muscle located at the entrance of the capillary) in the subcutaneous capillaries to contract, thereby reducing blood flow to the area (vasoconstriction). This constriction of superficial blood vessels protects the body from cold by shunting warm blood away from the body's surface. However, this same process of vasoconstriction also reduces perfusion of subcutaneous tissues and would decrease the rate of absorption of SQ drugs injected under these conditions.

Vasodilation (dilation of blood vessels) enhances perfusion of tissues and therefore increases drug absorption in subcutaneous tissue and skeletal muscle. Vasodilation in the subcutaneous tissues is initiated by increased body temperature (such as from warm, ambient temperatures or exercise) or drugs (such as alcohol). Vasodilation of skeletal muscles occurs when the muscle is exercising or the animal is under "emergency" conditions of "fight or flight" (sympathetic nervous system effect). Although fight-or-flight conditions increase the perfusion of skeletal muscles and hence increase absorption of IM injections, the same sympathetic nervous system stimulation causes vessels in superficial tissues, such as subcutaneous tissue, to become vasoconstricted, reducing absorption of SQ administered drugs. Understanding how the physiology or disease state affects tissue perfusion is necessary to insure that an administered drug is successfully absorbed.

CLINICAL APPLICATION

Lidocaine With and Without Epinephrine

Preparations of the local anesthetic lidocaine come in two versions: lidocaine alone and lidocaine plus epinephrine. Lidocaine by itself is the drug of choice for controlling irregular ventricular rhythms, especially sudden ventricular arrhythmias that occur during surgery. Because lidocaine also prevents nerves from firing, lidocaine is also used as a local anesthetic to anesthetize selected areas of skin or other superficial tissues for surgical procedures. The local anesthetic version of lidocaine incorporates epinephrine, which is a strong stimulator of heart rate and is a potent vasoconstrictor of peripheral superficial blood vessels.

So why would a heart-stimulating and vasoconstricting drug like epinephrine be added to a local anesthetic like lidocaine?

The epinephrine is used for its vasoconstricting activity. When lidocaine plus epinephrine is injected into subcutaneous tissue, the epinephrine causes the small blood vessels in the area to vasoconstrict, reducing perfusion of blood into the area where the local anesthetic had been injected. By decreasing the perfusion in the area, the local anesthetic lidocaine is not absorbed into the blood as readily and hence remains in the local area to produce anesthesia for a longer period of time.

Clinics typically keep both versions of lidocaine in stock: lidocaine alone for use to treat cardiac arrhythmias and lidocaine with epinephrine for use as a local anesthetic. It is important not to confuse these drugs as the epinephrine in the local anesthetic lidocaine if given to a patient with sudden ventricular arrhythmias could further stimulate the heart and potentially worsen the arrhythmia. To avoid someone picking up the wrong lidocaine bottle during a cardiac emergency, clinics often mark the two different forms of lidocaine with bright tape of different colors so the differences are immediately obvious at a glance. In the case of these two versions of lidocaine, what is good for a local anesthetic is not very good for a cardiac arrhythmia.

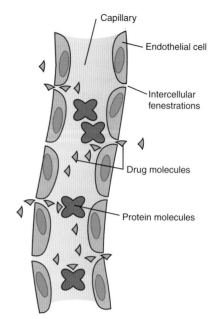

Fig. 3.11 Drug molecules are small enough to pass into and out of the capillary through fenestrations in the capillary wall, but the larger protein molecules cannot. Thus drugs do not have to be in the lipophilic form to move in or out of the blood to the tissues in most capillaries in the body. The exception is illustrated in Fig. 3.12.

PHARMACOKINETICS: DRUG DISTRIBUTION

Once absorbed, most drugs are not beneficial unless they reach the target tissue for which they are intended. If a cardiac drug cannot reach the myocardium (heart muscle), it will not benefit the patient. If a tranquilizer is unable to reach the brain, the patient will not become tranquilized. This movement of a drug from the systemic circulation into tissues is called **distribution**.

Barriers to Drug Distribution

Just as barriers to drug absorption exist, so do barriers to distribution. To distribute from blood to the tissues, drugs enter and leave the bloodstream through the thin-walled capillaries. Although capillaries conceptually may seem to be small, solid-walled "pipes" through which blood flows, in actuality they are more like leaky pipes. In most parts of the body, capillary walls are one cell thick and have small holes, or **fenestrations** ("windows"), within the cell that allow water and small drug molecules to move readily back and forth between the blood and the surrounding tissue while keeping larger molecules, proteins, and red blood cells within the capillary (Fig. 3.11). Distribution of the drug to the tissue occurs through these fenestrations.

Capillaries in the brain are different from capillaries in other tissues because the endothelial cells abut closely with each other to form tight junctions similar to the alignment of the cells lining the intestinal tract and the capillaries are "continuous," meaning they don't have fenestrations through which drug molecules can pass (Fig. 3.12). In addition to the continuous

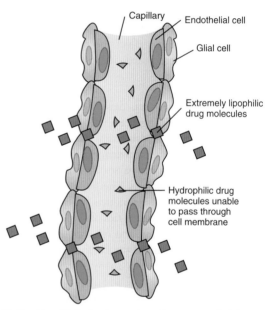

Fig. 3.12 The blood-brain barrier to drugs is composed of tightly aligned capillary cells, glial cells that surround the capillary, and P-glycoprotein (P-gp) active pumps that move drug molecules back into the blood. Only lipophilic drug molecules that do not get transported by the P-glycoprotein are able to move from the blood into the brain tissue.

capillary wall, structural cells in the brain called astrocytes and glial cells surround the capillaries, providing additional membrane barriers through which drugs would have to pass to distribute successfully from blood to brain.

In addition to the physical membrane barrier that blocks hydrophilic or ionized drug molecules, P-glycoprotein (P-gp) mentioned previously with GI tract absorption, is also associated with the cells of the brain capillaries. The P-glycoprotein of the brain capillaries actively pumps some passively diffusing lipophilic drug or poison molecules back into the blood, preventing them from reaching action sites on the brain cells. Thus even though some drug molecules like ivermectin are lipophilic and readily pass through cell membrane barriers, the P-glycoprotein keeps the drug molecule from actually reaching the brain tissue.

The combination of continuous capillary cell wall, the membranes of the supporting cells surrounding the capillaries, and the P-glycoprotein active transport molecules forms the blood-brain barrier (Fig. 3.12). The blood-brain barrier provides an excellent defense against many poisons, but unfortunately it also prevents distribution of beneficial drugs to the brain or central nervous system.

Similar barriers to drug distribution occur in the prostate gland, the globe of the eye, testicular tissue, and the synovial tissue surrounding joints, which explains why only selected antibiotics are effective for treating prostate infections and why many drugs meant to act within the globe of the eye must be injected directly into the globe itself.

Although the placenta is commonly thought of as being a protective barrier that guards the fetus against toxins or other damaging compounds, the capillaries in the placenta have fenestrations and allow most drugs to pass easily from maternal to fetal circulation. However, despite these "leaky" capillaries, a P-glycoprotein pump is also present in the placenta capillaries that moves a few selected drug molecules back into the maternal blood, thus decreasing the distribution of some drugs to the fetus. Still, the veterinary professional should always be aware of the potential for overdosing the fetus when giving drugs to the mother. Some drugs administered to the mother can disrupt normal fetal development, result in fetal malformation or cause fetal death and spontaneous abortion. Therefore, unless proven otherwise, it is best to assume that a drug given to the mother animal will also be distributed to the fetus.

Effect of Tissue Perfusion on Drug Distribution

Just as well-perfused tissues absorb drugs more quickly from the site of administration into systemic circulation, well-perfused tissues such as the brain, the liver, kidneys, and active skeletal muscle distribute drugs more rapidly and effectively. In contrast, inactive skeletal muscle and adipose (fat) tissue are relatively poorly perfused, so drug delivery to these tissues is delayed or less efficient.

The clinical effect of this difference in tissue perfusion and distribution can be seen with some IV injectable anesthetics like propofol and thiobarbiturates. When propofol is given intravenously as a bolus, all of the drug is deposited directly into the bloodstream (systemic circulation) and most quickly and effectively distributes into highly perfused tissues such as the brain. The effect of this rapid distribution is an almost immediate onset of anesthesia.

However, within just a few minutes after the anesthetic drug is given, the anesthetic depth decreases and the animal begins to move or exhibit signs of lessening anesthesia. This suggests that the propofol concentration in the brain has decreased. Indeed, the drug that entered the brain so rapidly is now decreasing at a much quicker rate than can be explained by the body breaking down or eliminating the drug. The reason for the decreased drug concentration in the brain is not caused by elimination of the

drug but from *redistribution* of the propofol from the brain to other tissues in the body. How does this occur?

Although the majority of the initial propofol dose distributed to well-perfused tissues like the brain and produced the immediate anesthetic state, the more poorly perfused tissues, like fat, were also receiving the drug via distribution but at a much slower rate. As the first few minutes passed after the anesthetic induction, propofol in the blood continues to enter fat tissue, and the propofol concentration in the blood slowly falls. As the drug blood concentration falls, the concentration gradient and direction of propofol movement from blood to brain reverse, and propofol begins to move down the concentration gradient from the higher concentration in the brain back toward the lower concentration in the blood. As concentrations in the brain slowly fall, the animal begins to wake up.

Thus, the lessening of anesthetic effect seen shortly after the initial bolus or quick IV infusion of propofol is due to *redistribution* of drug molecules from the brain back into the blood and then into lesser perfused tissues like the fat, as opposed to being eliminated from the body.

In many cases of propofol anesthesia, the initial dose produces too profound an anesthetic effect and the animal will stop breathing because the anesthetic drug is depressing the brainstem where respiratory centers are located. However, this apnea (cessation of breathing) reverses within a few short minutes because of redistribution of propofol to poorer perfused tissues and therefore does not require emergency interventions.

The redistribution effect is going to be most noticeable on animals that are obese. It is important to remember that when an animal is weighed for a dose of propofol, the animal is being dosed on its entire body mass including the poorly perfused fat. Thus, if a 60-lb obese dog receives a full 60-lb worth of propofol, the brain is going to be "overdosed" by receiving the majority of the drug that is normally intended to be equally distributed through the whole 60-lb animal. Therefore, it is important to dose such drugs on the basis of the estimated "lean" body weight of the animal instead of the total body weight, which includes weight contributed by poorly perfused fat. It should also be understood, however, that an obese animal's fat will continue to "fill up" with anesthetic drug over a longer period of time. Therefore, if a lower dose of drug is initially used to dose just the "lean" animal, multiple repeat doses may be needed until propofol has redistributed or distributed into all of the poorly perfused fat tissue and the fat has concentrations of propofol that are at equilibrium with the propofol blood concentrations.

Because drug redistributed into poorly perfused fat tissue goes in slowly, it will also come back out and reenter the blood slowly, meaning that the fat will act as a depot of propofol that will leech back into the blood long after the anesthetic levels in the brain have dropped below surgical anesthetic levels. Thus obese animals may have lingering low-level effects of the anesthetic drug (are groggy, ataxic, not very alert but awake) for a much longer period of time than the lean animal of the same weight.

Effect of Plasma Protein Binding on Drug Distribution

The plasma of blood contains circulating proteins such as albumin and other proteins capable of reversibly binding to specific hormones or compounds in the body. These proteins are too large to pass through the small capillary fenestrations and therefore remain in the systemic circulation and under normal conditions do not distribute into tissue (Fig. 3.11).

The molecular structure of some drugs predisposes these drug molecules to attach or bind to these large circulating blood proteins, resulting in some percentage of the administered dose being "stuck" in the blood and unable to distribute to the tissues. Those drug molecules attached to the blood protein are said to be *protein bound* and those molecules not attached are said to be the free form or the unbound fraction of the drug molecules. Drugs that are considered to be highly protein bound have greater than 80% of their administered dose bound to the proteins in the blood.[1] Only that percentage of the administered drug dose that is free and unbound from the blood protein can distribute to the tissues and produce the intended effect. Fig. 3.13 illustrates this concept.

The ratio of protein-bound molecules to the free molecules in the blood remains mostly constant so that when a free drug molecule leaves the blood to go into the tissue (distributes), some protein-bound molecules will dissociate from the protein to become free and thus maintain the same free to bound ratio. Thus even highly protein-bound drugs will eventually be able to distribute to the tissues, but the distribution occurs at a much slower rate than drugs that are less protein bound.

Some drugs are intentionally formulated to bind to blood protein to create a "depotlike" effect wherein the drug is slowly distributed into the tissue over a more extended period of time. Similarly, once drugs are distributed, some may bind to tissue proteins, preventing the drug from leaving the tissue and prolonging the drug's effect in that tissue. Both of these mechanisms can be found in some veterinary drugs that have long dose intervals between doses.

The FDA-approved manufacturer's dose for highly bound protein drugs takes into consideration that some amount of drug will be bound to blood protein and unavailable for immediate distribution to the target tissues. Thus anything that decreases the amount of blood protein (hypoproteinemia) or decreases the ability of the drug molecule to bind to the available blood protein will result in more drug molecules being distributed to the tissue, producing a greater-than-normal tissue concentration and drug effect. Theoretically this enhanced drug distribution could result in overdose or toxicity in the target tissue. Therefore, significantly decreased blood protein concentrations or conditions that decrease drug binding may require decreasing the highly protein-bound drug's dose to compensate for the enhanced drug distribution.

CLINICAL APPLICATION

Highly Protein-Bound Drugs

A 5-year-old, terrier-X, male, castrated dog was presented for a diagnostic workup for chronic diarrhea. The dog was diagnosed as having small intestinal disease that resulted in poor absorption of food and loss of protein through the gastrointestinal (GI) tract (protein-losing enteropathy). As a result of the chronic protein loss, the concentration of total blood proteins was below normal.

The dog was to be anesthetized with a highly protein-bound (90%–95%) injectable anesthetic drug to perform an endoscopic procedure to take an intestinal biopsy. The veterinary technician calculated the correct dose for the weight of the animal and administered the dose IV according to the manufacturer's recommendations.

Anesthesia was induced, but the dog stopped breathing, which is not unusual if this drug is given more rapidly than recommended. However, the apnea (cessation of breathing) continued for longer than normal, requiring the veterinary technician to artificially ventilate the patient to maintain oxygenation. After several minutes, the dog began breathing spontaneously on its own.

The veterinarian checked the technician's calculations and found them to be correct. Why did the dog become so profoundly anesthetized to the point of having apnea for so long?

This anesthetic drug was listed as being 90%–95% protein bound. The drug normally binds to albumin in the blood at such high levels that the dose is based upon the smaller 5%–10% free form of the drug that is available to distribute to the brain to produce anesthesia. However, in this case the dog had a low blood albumin level because of the loss of protein through the GI tract. Because the plasma albumin level was low, more administered anesthetic drug was available in the free form than normal and therefore more drug distributed to the brain. The result was higher than normal drug concentrations in the brain and a more profound effect on the central nervous system (including the respiratory control centers). Thus a normal, correctly calculated dose produced an overdose effect.

What should be learned from this situation: Although no formula can predict how much a dose of a highly protein-bound drug should be reduced in an animal with hypoproteinemia ("low protein in the blood"), the veterinary professional should err on the low-dose side in selecting doses of highly protein-bound drugs in hypoproteinemic animals. In this case, a reduction in protein binding could result in an additional 5% of administered drug being in the free form and available to distribute to the brain. That additional 5% would increase the free form available for distribution from the normal 5%–10% of the total dose to an increased 10%–15% of the total dose, constituting a 33%–50% increase in available drug over normal. That large of an increase in the drug accounts for the overdose signs seen in this dog.

As a general rule, the dose of highly protein-bound drugs should be reduced in animals with liver disease, protein-losing enteropathy (intestinal disease), protein-losing nephropathy (kidney disease), or any other condition that reduces protein-binding capacity.

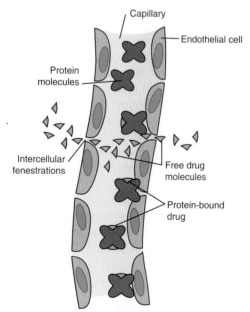

Fig. 3.13 Protein-bound drug molecules cannot distribute to tissues because the protein molecules are too large to pass through the capillary fenestrations. Free or unbound drug molecules are the only portion of the drug dose that can distribute to the tissue and produce an effect.

Volume of Distribution

The volume of distribution (V_d) is a pharmacokinetic value that provides an approximation of the extent to which a drug is distributed throughout the body. The V_d is determined by looking at the concentration of a drug in the blood shortly after an IV bolus is given and assumes that the drug concentration in the blood equals the concentration of the drug equally distributed throughout every compartment of the body.

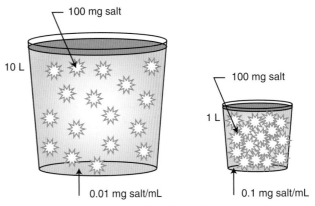

Fig. 3.14 The larger the volume of liquid in which the salt is dissolved, the more dilute the concentration of the salt. Therefore, the larger the volume of distribution (V_d) of a drug, the more tissue fluid the drug is distributed/dissolved in, and the lower the concentration of the drug in the tissue fluid and blood.

◎ MYTHS AND MISCONCEPTIONS

When it comes to drug distribution or movement, the body acts like one giant bag of fluid through which the drug molecules move.

False! The body has different compartments that have different barriers or rates at which drugs move into and out of the compartment. When an IV drug is deposited into the systemic circulation, the drug will distribute first to organs or tissues that are well perfused with blood supply and for which there are no significant cellular barriers. The drug will distribute much more slowly to less perfused tissues such as fat. Tissues like the brain, prostate, or globe of the eye have cellular barriers, and some drugs will penetrate into those tissues readily (lipophilic drug forms), whereas other drugs will be excluded from these tissues (hydrophilic drug forms). Thus, the body is actually like a series of different compartments into which drugs may or may not distribute, or on how fast they distribute into a compartment.

Generally, the larger the apparent volume of a drug's distribution, the more tissues and body compartments the drug appears to penetrate. So a drug with a V_d of 4 L would be considered to penetrate more body compartments and hence be distributed into a larger volume of body water than a drug with a V_d of 2 L.

At the same time, a larger volume of distribution usually means the concentration of the drug is diluted more and hence the drug blood concentration (drug mass per volume of blood) and drug tissue concentration (drug mass per mass of tissue) is lower. As shown in Fig. 3.14, 100 mg of salt is placed in a 1-L container of water and another 100 mg placed in a second container of water with a volume of 10 L. The 10-L container represents a larger volume of distribution for the salt than the 1-L container. As expected, the larger volume of fluid would result in a more dilute salt solution with a lower concentration of salt. In a similar manner, if a drug penetrates more body compartments and is distributed into a larger volume of tissue fluid and blood (a larger V_d), the drug solution will become more dilute and the concentration will be lower than the same amount of another drug that is distributed far less and has a lower volume of distribution.

A change in volume of distribution can require a change in a dose to compensate. If a drug has a greater distribution than normal, the drug concentrations may fall below the normal therapeutic range, resulting in subtherapeutic concentrations and loss of drug effectiveness. If body water is retained or accumulates as edema or ascites (fluid in the abdomen), the V_d for a drug may be increased and dilute the drug's concentration. By the same measure, clinically significant dehydration can decrease the body water into which a drug distributes and reduce the V_d, potentially increasing the drug concentration. In most cases, these changes will be detected by a change in body weight; thus daily weighing of a patient in the hospital and monitoring the patient's hydration status or fluid accumulation can help estimate how drug doses may need to be changed to compensate for an altered V_d.

PHARMACODYNAMICS: THE WAY DRUGS EXERT THEIR EFFECTS

Pharmacodynamics is the study of how drugs interact with the body to produce their effects. If a drug is well absorbed and readily distributed so that it achieves therapeutic concentrations in all areas of the body, the drug should theoretically have an effect on every tissue in the body. In reality, this is not the case. Generally, for cells to respond to a drug molecule, the drug has to combine with a specifically shaped protein located on the cell's surface or within the cell. This specific protein is called a receptor.

The Drug Is the Key, the Receptor Is the Lock

Each receptor has a unique shape so that only certain drugs can combine with the receptor and produce a response. This concept may be compared with a key and lock. The receptor is the lock into which only the correct key (the drug) will fit, and there are only a limited number of locks that can be opened by any key.

Receptors constitute a fairly broad range of proteins that, when activated by the drug, cause the cell to respond. Cellular responses may include the triggering of new protein production by the cell, the opening of a channel in a membrane to allow ions to pass, or activation of another "second messenger" that sets off a cascade of events to produce a cellular response.

If tissues do not have receptors to which a drug can combine, the tissue will not respond to the drug. For example, a drug may be able to combine with receptors on the smooth muscle cells of the small bronchioles in the lungs, causing the smooth muscle to relax and opening the bronchiolar airways. However, this same drug might achieve significant concentrations in the smooth muscle of the small intestine, but because there are no receptors for this drug on the intestinal smooth muscle, the intestinal smooth muscle cells does not respond to the presence of this drug.

As shown in Fig. 3.15, typically multiple types of receptors, each capable of combining with different drug molecules and producing a different cell response, will be found on a cell's surface or on organelles within the cell, such as the nucleus or lysosomes. For example, if Drug A combines with the Drug A receptor on the cell surface, it may stimulate the cell to begin secreting some protein. However, if Drug B combines with the Drug B receptor on the same cell, it may cause the cell to stop secreting proteins, or perhaps to secrete a different kind of protein, or maybe even stimulate the cell to divide. Hence, a single organ or tissue will typically have many different receptors, with each producing a different cellular effect when stimulated by a drug.

Affinity, Intrinsic Activity, Agonists, Antagonists, Reversal Agents, and Blockers

Tissues with a high density of one type of receptor are generally more sensitive to, or capable of responding to, drugs that fit into those receptors than tissues with fewer receptors. However,

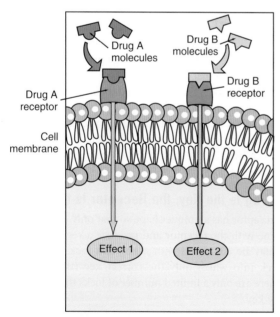

Fig. 3.15 Drug molecules have specific shapes that allow them to combine with specific receptors on the cell membrane surface to produce an effect. Drug A molecules combined with Drug A receptors produce Effect 1. A differently shaped Drug B molecule would not fit the Drug A receptor but can combine with the Drug B receptor to produce Effect 2.

there are many other factors that also contribute to a tissue's or organ's overall ability to respond to a drug.

First, a drug molecule has to possess the right shape and sometimes charge to be able to fit into a receptor in a way that stimulates a cellular response. This ability to bind or fit with the receptor is referred to as the drug's affinity for that receptor. A drug molecule that readily combines or binds strongly with a receptor is said to have a strong affinity.

It is important to remember that drug molecules do not combine with a receptor, produce an effect, and then just sit there. They typically combine, pop off, and may recombine multiple times. And each time the drug molecule recombines, it can stimulate the cell to respond. If a drug molecule binds readily to the receptor or tightly adheres to the receptor site once attached, this increased affinity can potentially translate into a greater effect by that drug molecule than another molecule with less affinity.

Even if a drug molecule combines with a receptor well, it may or may not actually produce a cellular response. Some molecules may cause a very strong cellular response, some a weak cellular response, and some no response at all. The ability of a drug molecule to produce a cellular effect when it combines with the receptor is called the drug's intrinsic activity.

A drug with both a good affinity for the receptor and the ability to produce intrinsic activity is called an agonist. A drug with good affinity, but little or no intrinsic activity, is called an antagonist drug. An antagonist drug occupies the receptor site and blocks, or antagonizes, the effect of any other agonist drug that might try to stimulate this receptor to produce a cellular effect (Fig. 3.16). In anesthesia, a drug that produces anesthesia in the animal would be the agonist drug, and the drug given to reverse the anesthetic effect and wake up the animal would be the antagonist.

Reversal agents and blockers are both antagonist types of drug molecules, but the terms refer to different types of compounds that are antagonized by these drugs. Reversal agents, or inhibitors, are drugs that are capable of combining with a receptor and blocking the receptor site from exogenous (from outside the body) agonist drugs, thus "reversing" or nullifying the effect of the agonist drug. Naloxone is an anesthetic reversal agent or inhibitor because it reverses the effect of strong narcotic anesthetic agonist drugs. In contrast, blockers are antagonist drugs that occupy a receptor and prevent endogenous (from within the body) agonist compounds, like hormones and neurotransmitters, from combining with the receptor and stimulating the cell. Thus, propranolol is called a "beta blocker" because it occupies beta receptors on the heart and prevents the endogenous neurotransmitter norepinephrine (the agonist) from combining with the beta receptor and speeding up the heart rate.

Competitive and Noncompetitive Antagonists

An antagonist drug can be a competitive or noncompetitive antagonist against other drugs or endogenous compounds that use the same receptor. A competitive antagonist drug is a drug

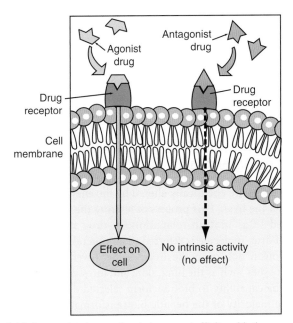

Fig. 3.16 An agonist drug molecule has good affinity with the receptor, and when it combines with the receptor, the drug molecule produces a cellular effect (has intrinsic activity). The antagonist drug is shaped much like the agonist drug molecule and has similar affinity for the receptor, but when it occupies the receptor site it does not produce an effect (no intrinsic activity). When the antagonist drug molecule is occupying the receptor site, it blocks the agonist molecules from combining with the receptor site and hence blocks a cellular response to the agonist drug.

that nearly equally competes for the receptor site with the agonist drug, and whichever drug succeeds in occupying the receptor site is mostly determined by which drug is present in the greater amounts. Take as an example an agonist drug Drug A plus a competitive antagonist drug Drug B, both of which compete for the same receptor on the heart. Drug A increases the heart rate when it combines with the receptor on the heart, and Drug B has equal affinity for the same receptor but has no intrinsic activity and so produces no effect. Because Drug A and Drug B have equal affinity for the receptor, they have equal opportunity to combine with the receptor. If Drug A is present in a larger amount than Drug B, Drug A will be more likely to occupy the receptor and the heart rate will increase. If, however, more Drug B is administered and the amount of Drug B at the receptor site increases, then the odds of Drug B occupying the receptor and preventing Drug A from combining with the receptor increase. The net effect after increasing the amount of Drug B is the heart returns to its resting heart rate. Should another dose of Drug A be given to increase Drug A's concentrations higher than Drug B, the heart rate would increase again, reflecting Drug A's dominance.

In this example, the agonist (Drug A) and the antagonist (Drug B) had equal opportunity to occupy the receptor site and the observed effect on the heart was determined by the quantity of each drug molecule present at the receptor site. This equal opportunity between two drugs to exert their effects on a receptor is the key characteristic of a **competitive antagonist** drug relationship. Because the effect of antagonist Drug B can be reversed by giving more of Drug A, this competitive antagonism is also called **reversible antagonism** or **surmountable antagonism**. The word "inhibition" can be substituted for the word "antagonism" when the effect of the antagonist drug stops the cellular effect of another agonist drug. Thus in the example earlier, Drug B would be a competitive inhibitor of Drug A because it inhibited or stopped the accelerated heart rate caused by Drug A.

A noncompetitive antagonist is a drug that either combines with a receptor very tightly (the drug has a high affinity for the receptor site), preventing other drug molecules from accessing the receptor site, or the noncompetitive antagonist drug somehow modifies the receptor so the agonist drug can no longer dock with the receptor (the drug decreases the receptor affinity for the agonist drug). A noncompetitive antagonist is defined as having some advantage over the other competing drugs so that just adding more of the competing drugs will not reverse the effect of the noncompetitive antagonist. Noncompetitive antagonism is also called **irreversible** or **insurmountable antagonism**. In most cases, the antagonism caused by the noncompetitive antagonist drug is not truly irreversible or insurmountable, but the reversal occurs very slowly (e.g., the antagonist molecule slowly dissociates from the receptor and allows the agonist to combine), giving the impression of being irreversible.

Partial Agonists/Partial Antagonists

As mentioned previously, the degree to which a drug has intrinsic activity varies with the drug molecule characteristics. For example, a drug's intrinsic activity when attached to the heart receptor might increase the heart rate 50% above baseline, whereas a second drug acting on the same receptor only increases the heart rate by 25%. Both drugs in this situation would be considered agonists because they both have intrinsic activity (they produce a cellular effect) when they combine with the receptor, but the degree of total effect for each drug is different. In this situation, the weaker drug that produces a 25% increase in heart rate would be called a partial agonist, because compared with the drug with the 50% increase response, it is not as strong an agonist as the other drug and produces only a partial agonist effect. The weaker agonist drug is also referred to as a partial antagonist, because if the stronger 50% increased response drug is given first and the weaker 25% increased response drug given second, the weaker agonist drug would appear to partially (but not completely) reverse or inhibit the accelerated heart rate of the first drug, dropping the heart rate from 50% increased down to 25%. Thus drugs that partially reverse the effect of a stronger drug but have some weaker effect of their own are called partial agonists/partial antagonists.

Agonists, Antagonists, and Partial Agonists/Partial Antagonists in Anesthesia

A dog undergoes a painful surgical procedure to remove a front limb that has osteosarcoma, a serious cancer of the bone. The surgeon wants the dog to be comfortable after surgery, so she prescribes a strong narcotic analgesic (pain reliever). She injects the narcotic analgesic at the completion of surgery to smooth the dog's anesthetic recovery. Because the drug produces cellular changes that result in analgesia when it combines with its receptor, the narcotic analgesic acts as an agonist.

As the dog recovers from the anesthesia the veterinarian notices that the dog appears to be resting comfortably without much pain but is a bit more sedated than desirable and has some respiratory depression as a side effect of the narcotic analgesic. The veterinarian wants to reverse the respiratory depression and have the animal a bit less sedated, but she does not want to lose the beneficial analgesic effect.

Instead of using the competitive narcotic antagonist drug to reverse the effect of narcotic analgesic completely, she chooses to use a partial agonist/partial antagonist drug. The partial agonist/partial antagonist drug is a competitive antagonist of the potent narcotic analgesic given initially, and given in sufficient quantities it will be able to displace the potent analgesic from the receptor site, ending its analgesia, sedation, and respiratory depression.

However, this partial agonist/partial antagonist has some intrinsic activity of its own and is capable of producing some degree of analgesia but less analgesia than the more potent narcotic analgesic given initially. The fact that the partial agonist/partial antagonist produces a cellular effect (mild degree of analgesia) makes it an agonist. However, when it is given after the potent narcotic analgesic, it partially reverses the analgesic, sedative, and respiratory effect and therefore also acts as a partial antagonist.

What should be learned from this situation: Drugs don't all produce the same level of effect. Therefore, by understanding the degree to which a drug is an agonist, antagonist, or partial agonist/partial antagonist, the appropriate drug can be selected to deliver the desired level of effect. By understanding how to apply these concepts, medical therapies can be tailored more effectively to the specific need and degree of need of the veterinary patient.

Non–Receptor-Mediated Reactions

Some drugs produce an effect on the body without combining with receptors. For example, mannitol is a sugar compound drug that is filtered out of the blood and into the urine by the kidney, drawing water from the body into the urine and causing diuresis (additional production of urine) by this osmotic effect. The mannitol does not attach to any cellular receptor to produce this diuretic effect, and hence this type of effect is referred to as a non–receptor-mediated drug reaction.

Chelators are another type of chemical that produce a biological effect by non–receptor-mediated actions. Chelators combine with ions (e.g., calcium, chloride, magnesium) or other specific compounds to produce their clinical effects but don't require a receptor to mediate the activity. For example, penicillamine is a chelator drug that is used to treat lead toxicosis. By combining with lead in the blood and causing the lead to precipitate out, the chelated lead/penicillamine combination is readily excreted into the urine. Ethylenediaminetetraacetic acid (EDTA) is a non–receptor-mediated calcium chelator found in lavender-topped blood collection tubes that prevents collected blood from clotting.

Another non–receptor-mediated action occurs when calcium, aluminum, or magnesium antacid drugs (e.g., Tums, Rolaids) combine with the strong hydrochloric acid in the stomach to form a much weaker acid, thereby reducing stomach irritation. These antacids do not combine with any cellular receptors in the stomach but directly combine with the acid itself to produce the intended effect.

PHARMACOKINETICS: BIOTRANSFORMATION AND DRUG METABOLISM

Many drugs are chemically altered by the enzymes as they pass through the liver. This process of altering the drug structure is referred to as biotransformation, or drug **metabolism**. The altered drug molecule is referred to as a metabolite. Most drug metabolism occurs in the hepatocytes (liver cells), although other tissues such as the lung, skin, and intestinal tract may also have the capability to biotransform selected drug molecules.[1,2]

The majority of the hepatic biotransformation enzymes are *mixed function oxidase enzymes* and specifically members of the cytochrome P-450 (CYP) family of enzymes. This is the same family of enzymes that was involved in enzymatic breakdown of drug molecules during absorption of drugs from the GI tract.

Biotransformation in the liver is usually a two-step enzymatic process. In phase I metabolism, the original drug molecule is structurally transformed by chemical processes that add or remove oxygen, hydrogen, or other key molecules. After phase I is complete, the resulting metabolite is typically less biologically active.

However, sometimes phase I biotransformation yields a drug metabolite that has more biological activity than the original drug molecule. Prodrugs are drugs that are biotransformed into a more active form. For example, prednisone is a commonly used antiinflammatory drug that is biotransformed by liver enzymes to its more active metabolite, prednisolone. Hence, prednisone is a prodrug for prednisolone. The prodrug form may be the preferred molecular configuration for administration because it is more readily absorbed than the biotransformed active drug molecule. Some insecticides are administered in a harmless, easily absorbed prodrug form that, once absorbed, is biotransformed by the insect's own enzymes into the active insecticidal form.

In phase II metabolism, the metabolite from phase I, or the original drug form, is chemically combined to another molecule such as glucuronic acid, sulfate, or glycine in a process called conjugation (meaning "to come together"). The conjugated molecule is usually more water soluble (hydrophilic) and therefore more readily excreted via the urine because the hydrophilic molecule will not reabsorb across the renal tubule walls back into the body. See the concept on ion trapping previously presented in this chapter for a further explanation of why a hydrophilic molecule is more readily excreted in the urine.

Drug Interactions Affecting Biotransformation

Animals with severe disease commonly receive multiple drugs to treat or control physiologic abnormalities in different body systems. Unfortunately, some drugs can alter the metabolism of other drugs, resulting in variable drug concentrations or adverse effects.

The liver's CYP enzymes are called inducible enzymes because when these enzymes are repeatedly exposed to and metabolize certain drug molecules, the cell is stimulated to produce additional CYP enzymes to increase the rate and efficiency with which these drug molecules can be metabolized. When the metabolism of a drug is sped up by this process, the drug metabolism is said to be induced, and when drug molecules have induced metabolism, they are typically inactivated at a faster rate than usual. Thus to produce the same degree of drug effect on the body after metabolic **induction** has occurred, the drug dose must be increased by either increasing the amount (dose) or by giving the drug more frequently (shortening the dose interval).

This induced enzymatic adaptation to the drug exposure and the subsequent need for a higher dose is one of the major mechanisms by which drug tolerance occurs. This type of drug tolerance explains why barbiturates or narcotics pain-relief medications often require an increased dose after a few treatments to achieve the same degree of beneficial effect. This induced metabolism tolerance effect is also seen with the repeated ingestion of alcohol and caffeine and helps explain why alcoholics or people who seem to be "addicted" to coffee require much higher doses to produce their desired effect than the "dose" required when they first started drinking alcohol or coffee.

When the CYP enzyme system has been induced by exposure to a particular drug, often more than one type of cytochrome enzyme is increased. Thus, any other drug normally biotransformed by the induced CYP enzymes will also have its own metabolism induced, resulting in a quicker drop of active drug concentrations and a shortened duration of clinical effect.

For example, repeated daily use of phenobarbital to control epileptic seizures in dogs will induce phenobarbital's cytochrome P-450 enzymatic metabolism and the rate of biotransformation of other drugs such as phenylbutazone, digitoxin, estrogens, dipyrone, and glucocorticoids. The dose of any other drug affected by phenobarbital's metabolic enzyme induction must also be increased to compensate for the increased biotransformation.

Species and Age Differences in Drug Biotransformation

Drugs vary significantly in how well they are biotransformed from species to species. As a general rule, cats have a more limited capacity to metabolize many drugs compared with dogs and horses and hence cats do not break down those drugs as quickly and are more prone to overdose toxicity if drug dosages (mg/kg) appropriate for the dog or horse are used in the cat. The cat's limited biotransformation capacity is because of deficiencies in the enzymes involved in phase I metabolism and enzymes that conjugate drug molecules with other molecules in phase II metabolism. This difference in biotransformation is another reason why dosages appropriate for one species cannot be assumed to be appropriate for another species.

CLINICAL APPLICATION
Cats Are Not Little Dogs

A client has an old German shepherd dog with long-standing degenerative hip disease (hip dysplasia) that has caused painful arthritic changes in the hip joint. Fortunately the discomfort is controlled with a daily dose of two regular-strength aspirin tablets given with the dog's food.

When this client's 8-year-old cat developed a swollen paw, most likely caused by infection from a cat fight, she decided to administer aspirin to relieve his discomfort. Realizing that the cat weighed approximately one fifth of the weight of the dog, she decided to give half of an aspirin tablet daily to relieve the cat's discomfort (approximately one fourth of the dog's total daily dose).

After 4 days, the swelling of the paw had decreased, but the cat was vomiting and acting lethargic. She took the cat to the veterinarian. On hearing the history, the veterinarian suspected aspirin toxicosis and began supportive therapy. The cat recovered and went home 3 days later with an owner who had learned an important lesson that "cats are not little dogs."

Why did the cat not tolerate a dose of aspirin that seemed close to a tolerable dose based on the dose that was working well in the dog?

Cats have a reduced ability to biotransform certain drugs; thus conversion to inactive metabolites and subsequent drug elimination occur more slowly in cats than in other species. One of the most important phase II biotransformations in mammals involves the conjugation (combining) of a molecule of the phase I drug metabolite with a molecule of glucuronic acid. This combination makes the drug hydrophilic and more readily eliminated by the kidney or liver.

Unfortunately cats have a reduced ability to synthesize glucuronic acid, and therefore, drugs like aspirin or other salicylates (bismuth subsalicylate in Pepto-Bismol and Kaopectate) that are normally metabolized by this conjugation pathway are shunted to other, less efficient metabolic pathways, requiring more time for the drug to be metabolized and subsequently eliminated. In the bucket analogy, the hole in the bottom of the bucket represents the combined metabolism and subsequent elimination of salicylates and thus is smaller for cats than it is for other species.

Even though metabolism is slower for cats, it does not mean that aspirin should never be used in cats. Cats can still metabolize aspirin and other salicylate drugs; however, they must be given smaller doses than dogs, with longer dose intervals to allow more time for the drug to be biotransformed between doses.

What should be learned from this situation: First, cats are not little dogs. Second, a dose of a drug in one species cannot necessarily be safely extrapolated to another species because of differences in species' ability to metabolize and excrete certain drugs. Drugs that do not depend on extensive biotransformation and conjugation by liver enzymes for elimination may be better tolerated by cats. However, whenever any doubt exists, the veterinary technician should always read the drug package insert closely, consult a drug reference, or ask the veterinarian.

Common domestic animal species also biotransform drugs quite differently from humans and this explains one of the reasons why veterinary patient drug dosages cannot be readily be extrapolated from human dosages. For example, although humans tolerate over-the-counter (OTC) antiinflammatory drugs like ibuprofen (e.g., Motrin, Advil) and naproxen (Aleve) very well, wide metabolic variability in the dog makes it difficult to predict if a dose of these drugs will produce a beneficial effect or a toxic effect in dogs. "Safe" dosages of these drugs have produced significant side effects in dogs including perforated ulcers of the stomach and duodenum.

Very young animals, and to a lesser extent older animals, also have a decreased ability to biotransform drugs. The liver of neonates (newborn animals) or pediatric veterinary patients may not be fully functional for several days to weeks after birth, depending on the animal species. Thus the significantly reduced metabolic breakdown of a drug in these young animals may require a decreased dose or require that the drug be avoided completely. As a general rule of thumb, always double-check any drug given to an animal only a few weeks old to determine whether the drug is safe to give or if the dose of the drug needs to be reduced to compensate for the poorer metabolism.

In older animals, the number of functional hepatocytes in the liver decreases as does the number of cytochrome P-450 enzymes within the remaining hepatocytes. The net effect is a decreased ability of the liver to metabolize drugs. Just like with pediatric patients, the geriatric patient's dose should be double-checked to determine whether or not the dose needs to be reduced to avoid excessive drug accumulation and subsequent toxicity.

PHARMACOKINETICS: DRUG ELIMINATION OR EXCRETION

The final step in pharmacokinetics is drug elimination or excretion. Drug excretion is the movement of drug molecules out of the body, most typically into the feces or urine. In the bucket analogy, elimination is the hole in the bottom of the bucket, and as such, changes in elimination have the potential to markedly change the dose needed to achieve therapeutic concentrations. The rate of drug elimination can decrease with dehydration, age-related degeneration of the kidney or liver, and a variety of other physiologic and pathologic (disease) conditions that affect function of the kidney or liver. By understanding the factors affecting drug elimination, the veterinary professional can anticipate how the drug dose needs to be adjusted to avoid causing drug toxicity.

Routes of Drug Elimination

The two major routes of elimination are by the kidney (renal excretion into the urine) and the liver (hepatic excretion or biliary excretion into the liver's bile duct and subsequently

the feces). Inhalant anesthetics and other volatile agents that exist in a gaseous state are mostly eliminated by the lungs. Other less common routes of elimination include saliva, milk (in lactating animals), and sweat. Certain drugs or elements like arsenic can be incorporated into the keratin of the hair, nails, and hooves. Because of the concern about residues of drugs in milk, the veterinary professional needs to be aware of the route of elimination for any drug used in lactating dairy animals because milk into which any drug has been excreted must be discarded.

Renal Elimination of Drugs

In the kidney, circulating drugs are renally eliminated by a combination of filtration, active secretion, and *reabsorption*. These three processes occur at different parts of the kidney's *nephron*, the functional unit of the kidney shown in Fig. 3.17.

Filtration is a passive diffusion process that occurs as the blood flows from the afferent renal arteriole (the incoming renal arteriole) into the specialized tuft of capillaries in the kidney called the glomerulus (*glow-MARE-u-luss*). The flow of blood into the glomerulus is regulated primarily by constriction or dilation of the smooth muscle surrounding the renal afferent arteriole. The *efferent arteriole*, which carries blood away from the glomerulus, is slightly smaller than the afferent arteriole. The difference in size between the afferent and efferent arteriole causes pressure to build up in the glomerulus, forcing water and small molecules through narrow capillary fenestrations into the first part of the nephron, the Bowman's capsule.

By constricting or dilating the smooth muscles surrounding the afferent arteriole, the kidney regulates the amount of blood flowing into the glomerulus and thus regulates the pressure in the glomerulus, the amount of filtration, and the volume of urine formation. When the body experiences low arterial blood pressure (hypotension) from causes such as dehydration, blood loss, or shock, the body responds by increasing the activity of the sympathetic nervous system ("fight or flight" part of the nervous system), causing vasoconstriction of blood flow to nonessential organs and tissues such as the skin, the GI tract, and the kidney. The sympathetic nervous system's vasoconstriction of the afferent renal arteriole decreases blood flow entering the glomerulus, decreases filtration pressure within the glomerulus, and thus decreases the force for moving water and small molecules into the Bowman's capsule. Therefore, filtration and elimination of renally excreted drugs and urine formation are decreased under conditions of systemic arterial hypotension.

Conversely, the administration of IV fluids or the use of drugs that dilate the afferent renal arteriole smooth muscle will increase blood flow into the glomerulus, increase glomerular filtration into the Bowman's capsule, and cause a more rapid filtration of drug molecules from circulation.

The capillary fenestrations and the openings in the Bowman's capsule are small enough that blood cells and larger protein molecules are not filtered out of the blood. Because proteins are too large to be filtered into the Bowman's capsule, any drugs bound to plasma/blood proteins will remain in circulation and not be filtered into the urine. If, however, blood protein levels decrease because of chronic liver disease, loss of protein through

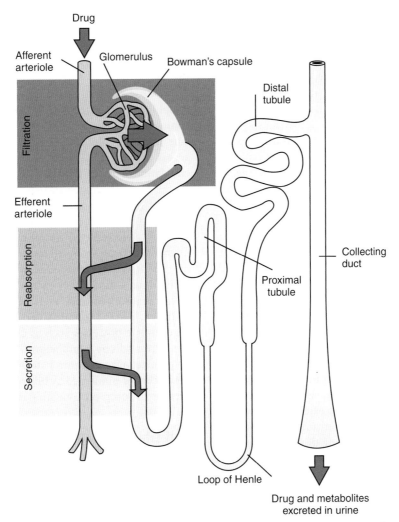

Fig. 3.17 Filtration, active secretion, and reabsorption. Drugs entering the kidney through the afferent arteriole (incoming arteriole) may be filtered out of the blood from the glomerulus (tuft of capillaries) into the first segment of the nephron (the Bowman's capsule). Drug molecules may also be actively transported from the blood in the peritubular capillaries into the proximal convoluted tubule by active secretion. If a drug molecule in the urine is lipophilic, it may passively diffuse back out of the urine into the peritubular capillaries at any point in the renal tubules and be reabsorbed into the blood. Those drug molecules remaining in the urine after the distal convoluted tubule are passed into the collecting duct, the ureter, and eventually the bladder, where they are then excreted from the body in the urine.

the kidney or GI tract, or other causes of hypoalbuminemia (low albumin protein in the blood), there will be more drug molecules free and unattached to protein that can pass into the Bowman's capsule. Thus, hypoalbuminemia or hypoproteinemia (low blood protein) can allow otherwise highly protein-bound drugs to be more rapidly filtered out of the blood into the Bowman's capsule and the drug to be more quickly eliminated.

After the glomerular filtrate of water, drugs, ions, and other small molecules has been filtered into the Bowman's capsule, the newly formed filtrate flows into the proximal convoluted tubule segment of the nephron. The proximal convoluted tubule of the nephron is a twisted (convoluted) tubular segment that contains many active transport mechanisms for moving electrolytes, glucose, selected drug molecules, and other

essential molecules back and forth between the urine and the renal tubular cell and the renal tubular cell and the peritubular capillaries that surround the renal tubule. The peritubular capillaries are the continuation of the efferent renal arteriole by which blood exits the glomerulus.

In the proximal convoluted tubule, some drug molecules are actively transported from the peritubular capillaries into the urine by a process called active secretion. Active secretion is an energy-requiring transport carrier mechanism, and as such the drug movement from the peritubular capillaries into the urine does not depend on the concentration gradient. The active transport process can result in very high drug concentrations in the urine. Penicillin antibiotic is an example of a drug actively secreted into the urine at very high concentrations, which helps explain why penicillin antibiotics are often used to treat bacterial infections located in the urinary tract.

Unlike the renal filtration process in the glomerulus, plasma protein binding of drugs does not interfere with active secretion of drugs. If the affinity, or attraction, between a plasma protein-bound drug molecule in the blood and the transport molecule in the cell membrane is very high, the drug molecule will separate from the plasma protein, combine with the active transport carrier, and be actively transported into the urine of the proximal convoluted tubule. If the protein-bound drug molecule has only a weak affinity for the membrane's carrier molecule, the drug molecule will most likely remain attached to the protein in the blood and not be excreted by this process.

From the proximal convoluted tubule, the filtrate flows along the nephron into the loop of Henle where some of the drug molecules may passively diffuse from the urine through the renal tubular wall and back into blood of the peritubular capillaries. This process is called *reabsorption* (as opposed to "absorption") because the drug previously "eliminated" into the urine by glomerular filtration or active secretion is now being reabsorbed back into the body.

Because reabsorption occurs by passive diffusion through the cell membranes of the renal tubule wall, the drug molecules must be in the lipophilic (nonionized) form. Hydrophilic (ionized) forms of drug molecules remain trapped in the urine and cannot be reabsorbed to any significant extent. As previously mentioned, urinary acidifying or alkalinizing drugs can alter the pH of the renal tubule filtrate, causing drug or poison molecules to shift from their easily reabsorbed lipophilic (nonionized) form to the hydrophilic (ionized) form, which is unable to be reabsorbed across the renal tubule cell membranes. By preventing reabsorption of a filtered or actively secreted drug, the drug is more effectively eliminated in the urine.

Beyond the loop of Henle, the urine water and electrolyte composition is altered by the body, but drug concentrations in the urine do not change significantly. Although some lipophilic molecules may continue to pass out of the urine by passive reabsorption after the loop of Henle or even through the wall of the urinary bladder, by the time the urine filtrate moves beyond the loop of Henle through the distal convoluted tubule, into the collecting ducts, and finally to the renal pelvis and ureter, the drug is considered to have been eliminated or excreted from the body (Fig. 3.11).

Hepatic Elimination of Drugs

Elimination of drugs by the liver is called biliary excretion or hepatic excretion. Biliary excretion refers to the liver's bile ducts. These bile ducts carry drugs removed from the blood and bile to the small intestine. Compared with renal elimination, biliary excretion is a slower and less clinically significant route of elimination.[1]

The liver has a very rich blood supply and not only removes poisons or drugs from the systemic circulation but as mentioned with PO absorption of drugs, also removes poisons or drugs brought from the GI tract to the liver by the hepatic portal system. As the drugs from the GI tract enter the liver, they pass into specialized liver blood cavities called sinusoids and then move by passive diffusion into the hepatocytes (i.e., liver cells) where they are either actively transported directly into the bile unchanged or metabolized first and then actively secreted into the bile.

If a drug excreted by the liver arrives in the duodenum in a lipophilic form, or the bacteria in the intestinal tract remove a conjugated molecule from the drug, making the drug molecule more lipophilic, the drug molecule can be reabsorbed across the intestinal wall, transported by the hepatic portal circulation back to the liver and then either excreted again by the liver or reenter systemic circulation. This movement of drug from liver excreted into intestinal tract, reabsorbed back into systemic circulation, and eliminated again by the liver is referred to as enterohepatic circulation. An unchanged drug excreted and reabsorbed in this way has the potential to exert its effect on the body for a much longer period than a drug either excreted as a hydrophilic metabolite or not reabsorbed once excreted.

If the liver is compromised by acute disease or chronic degenerative processes such as cirrhosis (replacement of functional liver cells by nonfunctional fibrous tissue), the liver's ability to metabolize and eliminate drugs is reduced. Therefore, the dose of drugs eliminated by biliary excretion must be reduced to prevent the drug accumulating to toxic concentrations.

Half-Life and Clearance: Measures of Drug Elimination Rates

The rate at which drugs leave the body is expressed as the drug's clearance and measured by the half-life of elimination. Drug plasma clearance is the measure of how fast a volume of blood is cleared of the drug by renal excretion, hepatic metabolism, biliary excretion, or a combination of these processes. Clearance is typically expressed as a volume of blood cleared over time, such as "liters (of blood/plasma) per hour." A drug that is "rapidly cleared" means that it is quickly eliminated from the body. Decreased function of either the kidney or liver will result in decreased clearance of a drug and hence decreased elimination from the body.

A drug's half-life of elimination is a time value that describes how long it takes for the drug concentration, usually measured in the blood or plasma, to decrease by 50%. Fig. 3.18 shows how a drug's blood (plasma) concentration does not decrease in a straight line but decreases over time in a predictable curve. In the example shown, the drug concentrations drop by half every 2 h until the drug is eliminated from the body. Therefore, this drug in this patient has a half-life of 2 h.

A drug's half-life may also reflect how efficiently the clearance organs are functioning. If the kidney is damaged by disease or is not well perfused because of a drop in systemic arterial blood pressure, the half-life of a drug excreted by the kidney increases (the time for concentrations to drop by 50% takes longer). Similarly, a drug that is very dependent on the liver for metabolism or elimination will have a longer half-life if the liver is diseased or less functional.

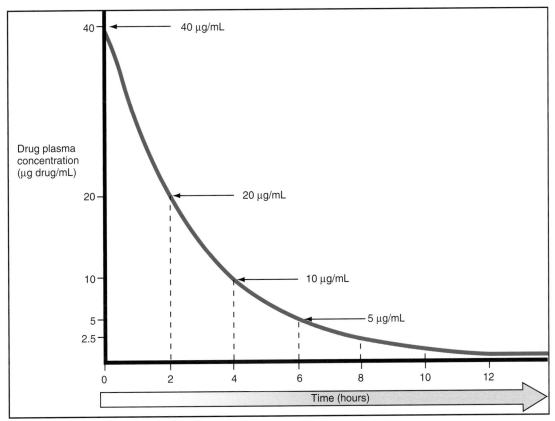

Fig. 3.18 This drug has been given as an IV bolus at time zero. The half-life of this drug is 2 h because every 2 h the concentration drops by half. Right after the IV bolus is completed, the blood concentration is 40 μg of drug per milliliter of drug (40 μg/mL). Two hours later the drug concentration in the blood has dropped by half to 20 μg/mL. Another 2 h later the drug concentration has again dropped by half to 10 μg/mL. The half-life of 2 h is constant so the concentrations continue to drop by half every 2 h until the drug is eliminated.

If kidney function is impaired, the half-life of drugs excreted mostly by the liver would not change significantly because the process of hepatic elimination is not dependent on renal function. Therefore, in an animal with renal disease, the veterinarian would prefer to use drugs that are primarily excreted through the liver, and drugs excreted by the kidney would be selected for use in animals with liver disease. This point emphasizes why veterinary professionals need to know if the drug is metabolized and by which route a drug is excreted when selecting a drug or modifying a dosage regimen for animals with liver or kidney disease.

Relation of Half-Life to Steady-State Concentrations

When a drug dose is administered, drug is added to the body, resulting in a corresponding increase in drug plasma/blood concentrations. As shown in Fig. 3.19, after the first drug dose is given, the second dose is typically given before the drug concentration from the first dose has been totally eliminated. Therefore, the peak concentration of the second dose is the result of the amount of drug left in the body from the first dose, plus the additional drug from the second dose. A similar pattern of accumulation is seen with subsequent drug doses.

Notice that the accumulating drug concentrations do not increase in a straight line but appear to form a curve or arc. This reflects the fact that as concentrations of drug increase in the blood, they are also eliminated at a faster rate, as shown by the curve in Fig. 3.18. Thus as the drug concentrations from repeated dosage administrations accumulate, drug elimination proceeds more rapidly and is reflected in the steeper downward slope seen at higher concentrations on the curve in Fig. 3.18.

Eventually, repeated doses produce drug concentrations where the accumulated amount of drug coming into the body with each dose is balanced against the more rapid elimination of drug seen with higher concentrations of drugs. At that point, the drug peak (high) concentrations and trough (low) concentrations will no longer increase but will reach the same consistent concentrations from dose to dose. At this point, where the peak and trough concentrations don't change with subsequent doses, the drug concentrations are said to be at *steady state* or a *plateau* (Fig. 3.19).

Because this steady state is associated with the balance between the drug amount given and the rate at which the drug is eliminated, how quickly steady state is achieved after starting drug therapy can be estimated using the drug's elimination

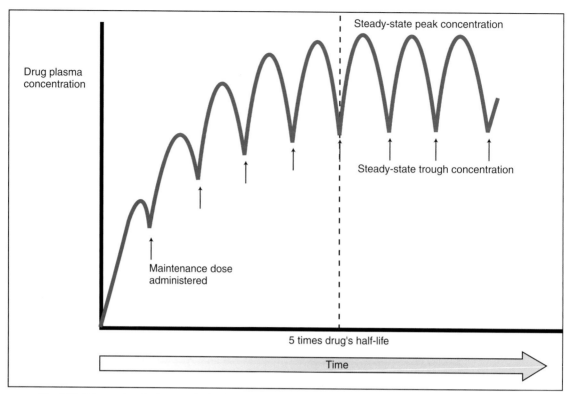

Fig. 3.19 When a drug is given, typically the next dose is given before the drug has been totally eliminated. The next dose will then have a higher peak concentration because the drug given in the next dose will be added to the drug left over from the first dose. However, as drug concentrations increase, elimination of the drug becomes faster. Eventually the accumulation of drug with each dose is offset by the faster rate of elimination, resulting in a plateau or steady state. Typically the time it takes to reach steady state is equal to five times the half-life of elimination for the drug. Thus, if the half-life for this drug were 5 h, it would take approximately 25 h to reach a steady state where all peak and trough concentrations are no longer accumulating.

half-life. In a drug given as a constant rate IV infusion or as repeated doses, it takes approximately 5 elimination half-lives to reach this steady state (steady state = 5 × half-life). If a drug has an elimination half-life of 8 h, the drug will achieve plateau or steady-state concentrations 40 h after the dosage regimen is started.

It is assumed that following the FDA-approved manufacturer's recommended drug dosage regimen should achieve steady-state concentrations within the therapeutic range for the patient. Therefore, the time to achieve steady state is important in determining how long it might take for the drug to begin to have its beneficial clinical effects. For example, if an antibiotic with a typically short half-life of 2 h is given in repeated doses or constant rate IV infusion, the time to reach steady state will be five times 2 h, or 10 h after the infusion has started. However, if the drug given is phenobarbital, which has a 30-h half-life in dogs, it will take five times 30 h, or 150 h, or more than 6 days for the drug concentrations to reach steady state after the dosage regimen has begun. The long time to reach steady state in the therapeutic range means a longer lag time between when the dosage regimen is started and when the beneficial effect of the drug begins.

For drugs with a long half-life, and hence a longer time to reach steady state, loading doses are often given to boost the concentrations close to steady state, after which the concentrations are maintained by the regular dosage regimen (the maintenance dose).

Remember that the time to reach steady state is predictable given the drug's elimination half-life. However, whether or not that steady state ends up being within the therapeutic range is dependent on all of the physiologic factors discussed so far in this chapter that can affect either absorption, distribution, rate of metabolism, or elimination.

❓ ASK DR. BILL

Question:
Can a drug be forced to reach steady state more quickly by giving a larger maintenance dose (e.g., giving 100 mg q12h instead of 50 mg q12h)?

Answer:
Although this would seem to be a logical result, the answer is no. How quickly a drug reaches its steady state still depends on time as expressed by the half-life of elimination—not the amount of drug given. The half-life for 100 mg of a drug is the same as 50 mg of that same drug in that the concentration of drug in the body will decrease by half regardless of which dose is used. Therefore, an increased dose will still achieve steady state in the same amount of time (5 × the half-life) for both doses, but the peak and trough concentrations at steady state will be higher for the increased dose than the peak and trough concentrations of the lower dose.

CLINICAL APPLICATION

Young Animals Are Special Cases

Three 5-day-old Springer Spaniel mix puppies presented with enlarged mandibular lymph nodes caused by a severe localized bacterial infection ("puppy strangles"). The veterinarian's challenge was to select an antibiotic and an appropriate dose form that young puppies could take and tolerate. Why is selecting drugs for neonates (newborns) and very young animals often a challenge for the veterinary professional?

From birth to approximately 1 month of age, deficiencies in the neonatal liver metabolism slow the rate of drug biotransformation. Drugs that in a mature animal are normally oxidized, reduced, or conjugated with glucuronic acid as part of the biotransformation and excretion process will accumulate more readily in a young animal's liver because these metabolic pathways are more limited than in the adult liver, resulting in slower breakdown and elimination of drugs. For that reason, ultra-short-acting barbiturates, some sulfonamide antibacterials, opioids, aspirin-like compounds (salicylates), some anticonvulsants, and local anesthetics (e.g., procaine) must be used with caution in neonates and very young animals. By 5 weeks of age, the liver of most neonates functions near adult capacity. The exception is young foals, which appear to develop important enzymes in their livers within a few days of birth.

Drug distribution is also different in young animals and can affect the selection of a drug and its dose. The blood-brain barrier in very young animals is more permeable to drugs than it is in adults. For this reason drug doses that normally do not produce therapeutic concentrations in adults may produce significant concentrations in a young animal's brain. The same is true for some toxic agents. For example, ingestion of even small amounts of lead can result in significant accumulations within the neonate or young animal's brain, leading to developmental problems in the central nervous system.

Plasma albumin levels are relatively low during the first 2–3 weeks of life. Therefore, less protein is available to bind with highly protein-bound drugs, and more free drug molecules are available for distribution to tissues. Doses of drugs that are normally highly protein bound must be reduced to compensate for a larger percentage of drug molecules free to distribute into the tissue.

The body composition of neonates and young animals contains a much higher ratio of water to fat than in adult animals. Therefore, when a drug that normally distributes to the extracellular fluid (water) is administered to a young animal, it is diluted in a larger volume of water than the same amount of drug in the same-sized older animal. Hence, a 10-mg dose produces lower concentrations in a young animal than the same 10-mg dose in an adult animal of the same weight.

Most drugs given by mouth to newborn ruminants (mammals with four-chambered stomachs) are absorbed in much the same way as in monogastric (single-stomach) animals. Therefore, absorption patterns of drugs change over the 4–6-week period as the GI tract develops from a monogastric GI tract to a functional ruminant GI tract. A functional rumen environment (fermentation vat) may degrade some orally administered drugs. The increasingly acidic pH in the abomasum may alter the ratio of ionized to nonionized drug molecules, reducing an alkaline drug's ability to readily absorb across the abomasal wall.

Because of these factors, veterinary professionals must review the package insert and other drug information closely before administering drugs to a neonate or young animal. The veterinary professional must remember that a young animal often cannot tolerate the same dose that an adult can because of differences in neonatal drug absorption, distribution, or biotransformation.

Drug Withdrawal Times

The presence of chemical or drug residues in beef, pork, lamb, chicken, and fish or egg and milk products used for human consumption is a growing public health concern. Because of this, all drugs approved for use in food animals have mandated withdrawal times. The withdrawal time (usually expressed as days) is the amount of time that must pass from the last drug administration until the animal can be sent to market for slaughter as human food or the eggs or milk can be safely used for human consumption.

Withdrawal times are based on the elimination half-lives of drugs. However, because drug half-lives are measured in the blood and not in the meat tissues, milk, or eggs, drug may remain in the meat or fat tissues for longer than is reflected by the half-life of elimination from the blood. This slower movement of drug from meat or fat tissues back into the blood means the drug may be incorporated into newly formed milk or eggs for a longer period of time. Thus, some drug withdrawal times may be quite long if the drug is normally sequestered (taken up and stored) by food animal tissues that are likely to enter the human food chain.

Withdrawal times cause additional expense for the food animal producers because the treated animal cannot be sent to market or the animal products (such as milk or eggs) cannot be sold during this time even though the producer must continue to pay to feed and house the animal. For that reason, some producers may be tempted to cut corners by sending the animals, milk, or eggs to market sooner than allowed by the required withdrawal time, hoping that the carcass or products will not be checked for antibiotic residues.

The government imposes fines and penalties on producers who attempt to sneak meat, milk, or egg products into the food chain that are contaminated with drug residues. For example, if it is discovered that a dairy producer sent antibiotic-contaminated milk to market and that contaminated milk was mixed into a holding tank with milk from several dairies, that offending producer will be required to "purchase" the entire tank of discarded contaminated milk.

The bottom line is that although a producer might consider cheating on withdrawal times for economic reasons, the economic penalty and potential effect on society (e.g., development of antibiotic resistance) far outweigh any marginal cost savings. Veterinary technicians play an important role in helping educate and reinforce the intent of withdrawal times so that food animal producers view regulations pertaining to withdrawal times as directly related to public health and not as arbitrary government interference.

USING CONCEPTS OF PHARMACOKINETICS AND PHARMACODYNAMICS

This chapter discussed the factors that influence the movement of drugs into, through, and out of the body and how drugs interact with a receptor to produce a cellular effect. By remembering the leaky bucket analogy and the fact that the amount of drug entering the body must balance the amount of drug leaving the body, veterinary professionals should be able to understand how these factors affect the daily care and treatment of veterinary patients. As the principles underlying good veterinary care become more familiar, it will become more readily apparent in which situations the normal dose of a drug may not be safe or effective for a particular patient. A vigilant veterinary technician can help the veterinarian prevent animal illness or death from inappropriate administration of a drug.

REFERENCES

1.. Boothe DM. Principles of Drug Therapy in Small Animal Clinical Pharmacology and Therapeutics. Philadelphia: Elsevier Saunders; 2012.
2.. Riviere J. Absorption, distribution, metabolism, and elimination. In: Riviere J, Papich M, eds. *Veterinary Pharmacology and*

Therapeutics. 10th ed. Ames, Iowa: Wiley-Blackwell Publishing; 2018.
3.. Rowland M, Tozer TN. Clinical Pharmacokinetics and Pharmacodynamics: Concepts and Applications. 5th ed. Philadelphia: Lippincott, Williams & Wilkins; 2011.

SELF-ASSESSMENT

1. Fill in the following blanks with the correct item from the Key Terms list.

    A. _____ This term means the study of how drugs move into, through, and out of the body.

    B. _____ This term means the study of how drugs produce their effects on the body.

    C. _____ This term describes the ideal drug concentrations that produce the drug's beneficial effect with minimal toxic or side effects.

    D. _____ IM, SQ, PO, and IV would be different examples defined by this term.

    E. _____ This is a larger than normal dose that is given initially to a patient to establish drug concentrations within the therapeutic range.

    F. _____ The highest concentration attained during a dose interval is called this.

    G. _____ If a drug's effective dose is very near the dose that produces toxicity, the drug is said to have this term.

    H. _____ This term describes any route of administration in which a needle is used; drug administered by these routes are placed "beside" or "apart from" the intestinal tract.

    I. _____ This is a drug dose administered IV or in an IV line over several minutes to hours and is designed to maintain drug concentrations continuously in the therapeutic range.

    J. _____ This is the point after a drug infusion is started or a drug has been administered multiple times that the drug concentrations will no longer increase.

    K. _____ This is the administration of an IV drug outside of the vein.

    L. _____ This route of administration administers the drug just under the layers of the skin.

    M. _____ This route of administration requires the use of very small needles so the drug can be placed within the narrow layers of the skin.

    N. _____ This route injects drug into the abdominal cavity.

    O. _____ This route of administration is given by mouth.

    P. _____ Drugs applied to the surface of the skin are said to be given by this route of administration.

    Q. _____ Drugs administered by this route of administration are breathed in as a gas or a mist.

    R. _____ This means of moving drug molecules from point A to point B is driven exclusively by concentration gradient and involves no carrier and no energy from the cell.

    S. _____ This method of moving drug molecules across a cell membrane involves a carrier molecule but does not require any energy expenditure by the cell.

    T. _____ This method of moving drug molecules across a cell membrane involves a carrier molecule and requires the cell to expend energy; the drug can be moved against a concentration gradient with this method of movement.

    U. _____ This describes the pharmacokinetic phase where the drug moves from its site of administration to the blood.

    V. _____ This term describes the percentage of drug administered that actually makes it to systemic circulation.

    W. _____ This route of administration always has an $F = 100\%$.

    X. _____ This route of administration achieves almost as high peak concentrations as an IV bolus owing to the high perfusion of the tissue into which the drug has been injected.

    Y. _____ This is the movement of an excreted drug molecule from the urine or the feces back into the body and systemic circulation.

    Z. _____ This special protein is an active transport pump that is found in the cells lining the GI tract where it pumps drugs that have crossed the cell membrane back across the cell membrane into the GI tract again.

    AA. _____ This is a family of enzymes found in the GI tract and liver that inactivate drug molecules. These enzymes are abbreviated as "CYP."

    AB. _____ This is the process by which a tablet physically breaks down into smaller particles in the GI tract until the particles are small enough to pass through the GI tract cell membranes.

    AC. _____ This describes the movement of the stomach.

    AD. _____ This describes the movement of the small intestine.

    AE. _____ This blood transport system carries drugs absorbed from the GI tract to the capillaries of the liver.

AF. _____ This is the phenomenon where a drug makes it across the GI tract wall, gets into the hepatic portal system, travels to the liver, but is almost totally removed by the liver before the drug reaches systemic circulation.

AG. _____ This term describes the extent to which tissue is supplied with blood.

AH. _____ This is the pharmacokinetic process by which drug moves from systemic circulation to tissue.

AI. _____ These are the small gaps in the wall of the capillaries through which water, ions, and small drug molecules pass.

AJ. _____ This specialized protein is part of the blood-brain barrier and actively transports molecules that diffuse across the barrier back into the blood.

AK. _____ This term describes the movement of drug that has been distributed back into the systemic circulation and then distributed to a second tissue.

AL. _____ This term describes a pharmacokinetic calculated value that is a rough measure of the degree to which a drug can penetrate tissues and be distributed throughout the body.

AM. _____ A drug molecule combines with this structure to produce an effect or block an effect in a cell.

AN. _____ This term describes the ability of a drug molecule to combine with a receptor.

AO. _____ This term describes the ability of a drug molecule to cause an effect on a cell once it has combined with the cell's receptor.

AP. _____ This term describes a drug that produces intrinsic activity when it combines with a receptor.

AQ. _____ This term describes a drug that has affinity for a receptor but has no intrinsic activity when combined with the receptor.

AR. _____ This type of antagonist can be reversed by another drug with the same affinity for the receptor but present in a larger amount.

AS. _____ A term to describe a drug that can reverse the effect of a previously given stronger agonist but still provides some intrinsic activity of its own when it combines with the receptor.

AT. _____ This is the pharmacokinetic process by which a drug molecule is broken down by enzymes like the cytochrome P-450 enzymes.

AU. _____ This term means that the rate of metabolism of a drug has been sped up.

AV. _____ This is the pharmacokinetic activity in which the drug leaves the body.

AW. _____ This is the part of renal elimination in which the drug moves from the blood into the Bowman's capsule.

AX. _____ This is the part of the renal elimination in which the drug molecule is actively transported from the blood of the peritubular capillaries into the urine of the proximal convoluted tubule.

AY. _____ This is the tuft of capillaries into which blood from the afferent renal arteriole flows and drug molecules are filtered into the Bowman's capsule.

AZ. _____ This is the repeating cycle where a drug is eliminated by the liver into the GI tract, is reabsorbed back into the body, circulates in the blood, and is eliminated again by the liver.

BA. _____ This term describes the amount of time it takes for the concentration of drug in the blood to fall by 50%.

BB. _____ This term describes the volume of blood from which all drug can be eliminated in a period of time.

BC. _____ This is the point in time after a constant rate infusion (CRI) has begun or a dosage regimen has been initiated that the resulting concentrations no longer increase.

BD. _____ This is the period of time between when the last dose of drug has been given and when an animal can be slaughtered for food production, or food products (eggs, milk) can be used for human consumption.

2. Indicate whether each statement is describing a lipophilic or hydrophilic drug molecule by writing in the appropriate term for each statement.

A. _____ Nonionized form of drug molecule.

B. _____ Ionized form of drug molecule.

C. _____ Form of drug molecule that readily passes through cell membrane by passive diffusion.

D. _____ Form of drug molecule that readily diffuses through cellular fluid.

E. _____ Form of the drug required to be absorbed from GI tract.

F. _____ Form of the drug required to be absorbed best from IM or SQ routes of administration.

3. Identify whether each of the following statements is true or false.

A. An acidic pH environment has more free hydrogen ions (H+) than an alkaline environment.

B. If the environment in which an acid drug is dissolved moves one pH unit toward the alkaline end of the pH scale, the ratio of ionized to nonionized molecules will shift $10\times$ greater in the direction of more nonionized molecules.

C. Generally, an alkaline drug in an alkaline pH environment would be expected to be more in the nonionized form than the ionized form.

D. A base drug with a pK_a of 7 would be expected to have an ionized to nonionized ratio of drug molecules of 100:1 at a pH of 5.

E. If a number of drug molecules enter a compartment of the body that has a different pH and the molecules become ionized, the drug molecules will all be trapped within that department forever.

F. Active skeletal muscle is less perfused than fat tissue.

G. A drug that is highly protein bound will be more readily distributed to tissue than a drug that is less protein bound.

H. A drug with a large volume of distribution is more likely to penetrate more tissues and be more widely distributed than a drug with a lesser volume of distribution.

I. If a drug has had its metabolism induced, the dose of the drug should be increased to compensate.

J. As a general rule, cats metabolize drugs better than dogs.

K. Biliary excretion is via the kidney.

L. Highly protein-bound drug molecules are not filtered into the Bowman's capsule very well but may be actively transported into the proximal convoluted tubule.

M. If a drug's half-life increases, the rate at which it is leaving the body has slowed and the dose of the drug would need to be decreased to compensate.

4. Which one of the following drugs is absorbed in the greatest amount (greatest number of mg)?

A. 100 mg of drug administered, bioavailability 0.7

B. 150 mg of drug administered, bioavailability 0.5

C. 200 mg of drug administered, bioavailability 0.4

D. 250 mg of drug administered, bioavailability 0.2

5. For each situation or condition, state whether the dose should be *increased* or *decreased* to compensate for the condition and still achieve therapeutic concentrations in the body.

A. The half-life for a drug is longer than normal.

B. The metabolism of a drug has been accelerated by exposure to phenobarbital.

C. A hypoproteinemic animal is given a drug that is normally highly protein bound.

D. The volume of distribution for a drug is decreased from normal.

E. The clearance of a drug has been decreased.

F. The blood flow to the glomerulus has been decreased (for a renally excreted drug).

6. A drug is injected as an IV bolus at time zero. Blood samples are taken at 1, 2, and 5 h after the injection and the plasma drug concentration determined. The data are shown here. Answer the following questions using the drug data listed.

Time After IV Injection	Drug Concentration (Plasma)
0 h	—
1 h	160 µg/mL
2 h	100 µg/mL
3 h	—
4 h	—
5 h	40 µg/mL
6 h	—
7 h	—

A. What is the half-life of this drug?

B. What was the drug plasma concentration at the 4-h postinjection point?

C. What was the concentration at 7 h postinjection?

D. What is the estimated peak concentration that occurred shortly after the IV bolus was given?

E. How long would it take multiple maintenance doses to reach a steady state for this drug?

7. The veterinarian is reviewing a brochure for a new drug that says: "Our drug reaches concentrations of 40 µg/mL within 2 h of administration where our competitor only reaches 25 µg/mL." The veterinarian comments that the drug concentration by itself does not indicate how effective the drug is. What is the reason for this comment, and what information is necessary to better assess the usefulness of this new drug?

8. A dosage regimen specifies 15 mg/kg IV for the loading dose followed by a maintenance dose of 5 mg/kg q12h PO. What is the advantage of using a loading dose?

9. The veterinarian wants to adjust a dosage regimen to increase a drug's dose interval. Using the equivalent total daily dose, the veterinarian switches from the 50 mg q6h PO to 100 mg q12h PO. What will happen to the amount of swing between the peak (high) concentration and the trough (low) concentration when the interval is switched from q6h to q12h? Why might this be of concern?

10. You are tired of fighting with a nasty stallion to give his IM injections every 8 h. Why not put the medication in a slurry of sweet molasses and give it to him PO to eat on his own?

11. The manufacturer of an antibiotic claims that the enteric coating on the product enhances the drug's effectiveness compared with products without enteric coating. How might this be possible?

12. Why would an orally administered antibiotic tablet not be well absorbed in an animal with diarrhea?

13. Why are some toxic materials not very toxic when ingested but extremely lethal if accidentally injected?

14. Why are SQ injected drugs absorbed more slowly on a cold day than on a hot day?

15. Diabetic animals are often overweight. Why should you be careful not to accidentally inject insulin (for control of diabetes mellitus) into the fat?

16. How can an antibiotic be effective for killing a strain of bacteria in many parts of the body but be ineffective against the exact same bacterial strain in the brain?

17. Which drug would probably better penetrate tissues: Drug A with a V_d of 1 L, or Drug B with a V_d of 3 L? If equal amounts of Drug A and Drug B were given to an animal, which would be present in greater concentrations in the plasma?

18. A dog is hospitalized because of insecticide poisoning. The veterinarian is concerned and says, "We can't use an antidote to reverse the insecticide effect because the insecticide has a strong affinity and is a noncompetitive agonist." What does this comment mean?

19. What effect would a partial narcotic agonist/partial narcotic antagonist such as butorphanol have on an animal if it was given after administration of a strong narcotic, such as hydromorphone? How would butorphanol's effect be different from that of a true narcotic antagonist, such as naloxone?

20. How can a chelating drug produce its physiologic effect when placed in a cell-free test tube of serum or within the lumen of the intestine where no cells, and hence no cellular receptors, are present for the drug to attach to?

21. Why must veterinary professionals be concerned about using hepatically biotransformed drugs in young animals and cats? Should they have similar concerns about administering drugs that are excreted unchanged through the kidneys?

22. A dog is being treated with phenobarbital to control epileptic seizures. Why must the dosage be adjusted 2–3 weeks after therapy begins? Is the dose likely to be increased or decreased at that time and why?

23. A particular dose of penicillin is quite effective against a specific bacterium when it is found in the urine. However, when the same bacterial strain is found in other tissues in the body, the same dose of penicillin is not nearly as effective. Based on what you know about penicillin from this chapter and how it is eliminated in the kidney, explain why penicillin works in the urine but not the rest of the body.

24. An animal has ingested a poison and the veterinarian gives the animal activated charcoal PO to make the poison in the GI tract stick to the charcoal and be excreted from the body with the feces. Because this particular poison has enterohepatic circulation, the charcoal must be administered many times over the next 24 h to keep the animal from continuing to get sick from the poison. Why does enterohepatic circulation require giving the charcoal repeatedly rather than only once or twice?

25. Why is a loading dose more necessary with a drug that has a long half-life than with a drug that has a short half-life?

26. Which food animal drug would require a longer withdrawal time: Drug A with a half-life of 30 min or Drug B with a half-life of 5 h?

Drugs Affecting the Gastrointestinal Tract

CHAPTER OUTLINE

OBJECTIVES

After studying this chapter, the veterinary technician should be able to:

- Describe the autonomic nervous system control on the gastrointestinal (GI) tract function.
- Describe how vomiting is stimulated and what receptors are used by drugs to induce or control emesis.
- Describe how diarrhea occurs and by what mechanisms drugs are used to control diarrhea.

- Describe how laxative, cathartics, and purgatives produce their effects.
- Describe how stomach acid production is controlled and how antacids and antiulcer drugs work on those mechanisms.
- Describe how drugs are used to maintain rumen health.
- Describe the appropriate role of antimicrobials (antibiotics) in GI tract disease.

KEY TERMS

adjunct drug
adsorbents
alpha (α) adrenergic receptors
antacids: systemic, nonsystemic
antibloat medications
anticholinergic drugs
autonomic nervous system
bacteremia
bicarbonate ion

bloat (ruminal tympany)
cathartics: osmotic, irritant
centrally or locally acting
emetics
chemoreceptor trigger zone
(CRTZ, CTZ)
chief cells
colonic
corrosive substances

dopamine receptors/antagonists
emetic
emetic center
enteric
enterochromaffin-like cells
enterotoxins
epinephrine
erosions
eructation

Animals presenting to veterinary hospitals with gastrointestinal (GI)-related problems are a daily occurrence. Clinical signs associated with GI tract injury or disease include vomiting, diarrhea, constipation, colic (abdominal pain), or bloat. Although many of these GI tract clinical signs reflect physiologic functions intended to protect the animal from harmful substances that may have been ingested, when they occur in excess, therapeutic intervention is indicated. The GI tract drugs used in veterinary medicine work by altering the normal GI tract physiology, and in so doing they help reduce the clinical signs but often produce side effects of their own. Thus, it is important the veterinary technician understand how both prescription (legend) and over-the-counter (OTC) GI tract drugs work, the mechanism by which GI tract physiology is changed, and how those changes will appear as observable clinical signs in the patient.

FUNCTION AND CONTROL OF THE GASTROINTESTINAL TRACT

Although the anatomic diversity of the GI tract among domestic species appears to be great, there are many similarities in function and control. Functionally, the monogastric (single stomach) animal has three segments of GI tract: the stomach, intestines, and cecum and colon. Functions or diseases related to the stomach are identified with the adjective gastric (e.g., gastric ulcers, gastric blood flow, gastric emptying). Those conditions related to the duodenum, jejunum, or ileum are usually referred to as enteric, and those related to the large intestine or colon are referred to as colonic.

Ruminants have a more elaborate "stomach" configuration than monogastrics. The rumen, reticulum, and omasum constitute the forestomach, and the abomasum represents the "true" stomach, similar to the monogastric stomach (Fig. 4.1). These compartments physically break down and process the ruminant's herbivorous (plant) diet by a process known as fermentative digestion. Generally, the reticulum and rumen work together to receive and mix swallowed food. Coarse materials are regurgitated from the rumen back into the mouth for further mastication before being swallowed again in a process called rumination or "chewing cud." The rumen's primary function is to serve as a large fermentation vat containing microbes (bacteria and single-celled protozoa) that enzymatically break down foodstuff into smaller, absorbable components. The complex balance among food materials, the microbes of the rumen, and the products of fermentation can be easily upset by disease, requiring therapeutic intervention. Unlike the fermentative digestion associated with rumen, the omasum and abomasum further mix the ingesta (contents of the intestinal tract), perform some enzymatic digestion, and begin the absorption of processed nutrients.

The GI tract of animals such as horses contain characteristics found both in the ruminant and the monogastric GI tract and therefore are classified as nonruminant herbivores. The nonruminant herbivores eat plants but do not have a rumen like the ruminants. Instead, they have digestive glands that secrete enzymes in a way similar to the monogastrics, and they also have microbes located in an expanded colon and cecum that perform fermentative digestion like the ruminant. The increased size and complexity of the equine colon and cecum are also factors that contribute to colic or impaction problems associated with horses.

Autonomic Nervous System Control

GI movement and secretions in all species are controlled by a balanced interaction between the nervous system, the hormones of the endocrine system, and other locally released compounds. A combination of the autonomic nervous system and local nerve reflexes within the intestinal tract wall constitute the nervous

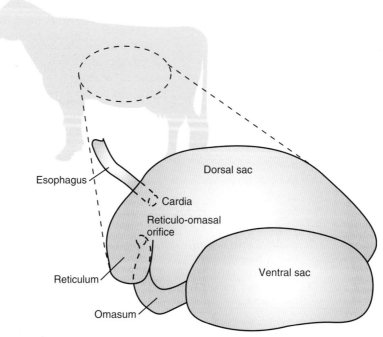

Fig. 4.1 The multiple compartments of the ruminant GI tract. (From Colville T, Bassert JA. *Clinical Anatomy & Physiology for Veterinary Technicians.* 2nd ed. St. Louis: Mosby; 2002.)

system control. The autonomic nervous system regulates bodily functions without involving conscious thought (i.e., you do not have to consciously think about digesting food for it to happen). Functionally, the autonomic nervous system has two opposing components: the parasympathetic nervous system (PSNS) and the sympathetic nervous system (SNS). At any given time both the SNS and PSNS are functioning and often exerting some control over the same organ or body system. Whichever part of the autonomic nervous system dominates at that moment determines whether the effects observed are sympathetic or parasympathetic.

The parasympathetic nervous system anatomically includes cranial nerves from the brainstem and peripheral nerves from the most caudal portion of the spinal cord. These nerves travel out from the central nervous system (CNS) and stimulate receptors in their target organs or tissues with the neurotransmitter **acetylcholine**. The vagus nerve (*vagus,* meaning "vagabond" or "wandering") is cranial nerve X (Roman numeral ten), which carries parasympathetic nerve impulses to and from a wide variety of organs in the abdominal and thoracic cavities.

Activation of the parasympathetic nervous system or using drugs that mimic the neurotransmitter acetylcholine will increase digestive secretions, improve blood flow to the GI tract, and increase gut (GI) smooth muscle tone and motility. Because the PSNS affects many other organs or tissues besides the GI tract, the same parasympathetic stimulation will also slow the heart rate, constrict the pupils, and increase secretions in the respiratory tree. The increased digestion and absorption by parasympathetic nervous system activation is what has earned the PSNS the nicknames of the "rest and restore" or the "rest and digest" system.

The sympathetic nervous system side of the autonomic nervous system balances or opposes the effects of the parasympathetic nervous system. The sympathetic nerves emerge from the spinal cord at the thoracic and lumbar segments of the spinal column and synapse with a chain of ganglia (cluster of neuron cell bodies) that run closely parallel to the spinal column first before they branch out to innervate a wide variety of organs and tissues. The neurotransmitter associated with the sympathetic nervous system effect is norepinephrine. The adrenal gland located on top of the kidney is also part of the sympathetic nervous system, and when the medulla (the inner part) is stimulated by sympathetic nerves, it releases epinephrine into the blood, which circulates throughout the body and produces more SNS effects.

As would be expected of a system that opposes or antagonizes the PSNS, the SNS or the use of drugs that mimic norepinephrine or epinephrine, decrease blood flow to the intestinal tract, decrease gastric (stomach) and enteric (small intestine) motility, and decrease secretion of digestive juices. Therefore, the net effect of the sympathetic nervous system on the GI tract is decreased digestion and absorption of nutrients.

Like the PSNS, the SNS also has other effects besides the general inhibitory effect on the GI tract. Increased activation of the SNS increases the heart rate, elevates blood pressure, dilates the pupils, opens up the respiratory airways, and redirects blood flow away from nonessential areas of the body, like the skin, to more essential organs and skeletal muscle needed for movement. These responses are part of the normal protective mechanism by which an animal can fight off prey or flee from a threatening situation. Hence the sympathetic nervous system is known as the "fight or flight" system.

In addition to the autonomic nervous system controls, there are several other hormones and locally produced compounds that regulate the GI tract. These compounds or hormones will be discussed individually with particular drugs.

EMETIC DRUGS

Emesis (vomiting) is a normal, protective mechanism designed to remove poisonous or dangerous substances that have been ingested. An emetic drug is a drug that produces vomiting needed to remove a toxic substance before it can be absorbed into the body.

The Vomiting Reflex: The Emetic Center

Like most drugs, emetics work by stimulating selected receptors, which in turn activate the physiologic mechanisms that result in the act of vomiting or emesis. Drugs that are *antiemetics* work by blocking these same receptors and in so doing reduce the stimulus that would normally produce vomiting. Therefore, the key to understanding how emetic and antiemetic drugs work requires understanding the receptors involved in this mechanism.

The vomiting center, or emetic center, is a group of special neurons located in the medullary structure of the brainstem that produces the physiologic actions associated with the period just before vomiting and during the actual act of vomiting itself (Fig. 4.2). The vomiting center coordinates the smooth muscle contraction and autonomic nervous system functions that produce the nausea, abdominal contractions, stomach contractions, and the actual act of vomiting in the species that are capable of vomiting.

In addition to the impulses the emetic center sends out to cause vomiting, the emetic center also receives input from incoming neurons that stimulate the vomiting reaction. These incoming neurons release specific neurotransmitters that are capable of binding to receptors located on the emetic center neurons, stimulating them to produce vomiting. One of the areas within the emetic center cluster that has appeared more recently in veterinary literature is the nucleus tractus solitarius (NTS). The NTS is a set of neurons that has many receptors for drugs or compounds that can stimulate vomiting and thus can also be a site of action for drugs that suppress vomiting by blocking these receptors.[1,2] Although it is important that the veterinary technician recognize the NTS when it is mentioned in veterinary literature, for purposes of simplicity in this text, we will group the receptors of the NTS with the other receptors of the emetic center and collectively refer to them as "the emetic center."

The major receptors most commonly associated with the use of emetic or antiemetic drugs in veterinary medicine include:
- Serotonin receptors (5-HT receptors)
- Acetylcholine receptors (muscarinic cholinergic receptors or M receptors)
- Histamine receptors (H_1 receptors)
- Dopamine receptors (DA receptors)
- Norepinephrine/epinephrine receptors (alpha [α] adrenergic receptors)
- Substance P receptors (NK-1 receptors)[2,3]

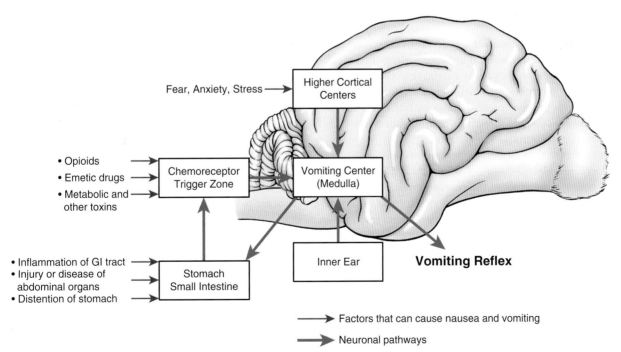

Fig. 4.2 The chemoreceptor trigger zone (CRTZ) has multiple receptors that can be stimulated by substances in the blood or the cerebral spinal fluid (CSF). Once stimulated, the CRTZ transmits signals to the vomiting center in the brainstem to initiate vomiting. The emetic center itself can be stimulated by neural input from the rest of the body through the vagus nerve, by input from the vestibular apparatus in the inner ear (motion), and from higher centers in the cerebrum (emotional responses). (Modified from Evans HE, de Lahunta A. *Guide to the Dissection of the Dog.* 8th ed. St. Louis, MO: Saunders; 2017.)

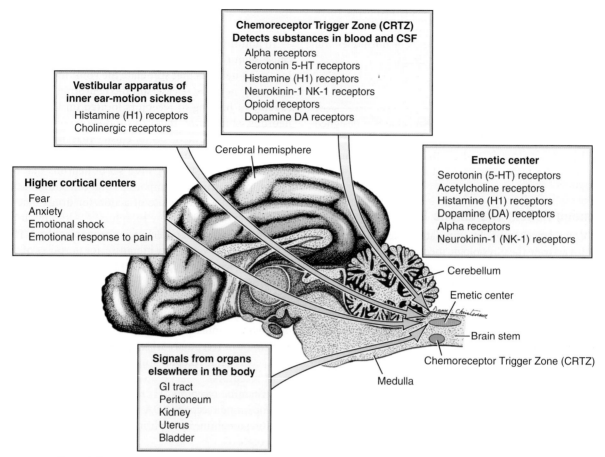

Fig. 4.3 Drugs or compounds that stimulate these major receptors in the CRTZ and emetic center produce vomiting; antiemetics block these receptors to reduce the stimulation for vomiting. (Modified from Christenson D. *Veterinary Medical Terminology.* 2nd ed. St. Louis: Saunders; 2009.)

Drugs or poisons that stimulate these emetic center receptors evoke the vomiting reflex, whereas antiemetic drugs that block these same receptors can reduce the emetic response (Fig. 4.3). Generally, these receptors on emetic center neurons can be stimulated to produce the vomiting reflex by five mechanisms:

- Drugs or chemicals bind directly to receptors on emetic center neurons and stimulate the neurons.
- Drugs or chemicals bind directly to receptors on the adjacent chemoreceptor trigger zone (CRTZ or CTZ) that, when stimulated, sends signals to the nearby emetic center.
- Nerve signals sent from distended or irritated pharynx, stomach, duodenum, small intestine, peritoneum (as in peritonitis), kidney, gallbladder, or uterus stimulate the emetic center.
- The nerves of the inner ear balance mechanism become overactive, sending signals to the emetic center (as in motion sickness).
- Higher centers of the brain or emotional centers in the brain send many signals to the emetic center as the result of emotional stimuli; intracranial trauma and subsequent swelling of the brain tissue can send signals by a similar mechanism.

The ability of an animal or a species to vomit as the result of receptor stimulation caused by any of these five general mechanisms varies depending on what type and how many receptors are located on the emetic center and CRTZ. For example, cats have a large population of alpha receptors on the emetic center that can be stimulated by epinephrine or norepinephrine, making cats more prone to vomiting caused by drugs that stimulate alpha receptors or cause a strong release of epinephrine into the blood. In contrast, dogs have fewer alpha receptors than cats but far more dopamine receptors, which means dogs vomit far more readily than cats do when given drugs that stimulate dopamine receptors (drugs like apomorphine).

Vomiting and the Chemoreceptor Trigger Zone

Adjacent to the emetic center is a specialized cluster of receptors that constantly monitor the blood and the cerebrospinal fluid for chemicals that can stimulate vomiting. This specialized cluster of receptors is called the chemoreceptor trigger zone, CRTZ, or CTZ. When the receptors of the CRTZ are stimulated, the CRTZ sends nerve signals to the emetic center, which releases neurotransmitters capable of combining with receptors on the emetic center to stimulate the act of vomiting.

Unlike the emetic center, which is protected from drugs or toxins in the blood by the blood-brain barrier, the CRTZ has a very poor blood-brain barrier and thus has greater exposure to compounds or drugs present in the cerebrospinal fluid and blood than the rest of the brain. Receptors in the CRTZ are capable of detecting many of the compounds listed for the emetic center, as well as metabolic toxins produced by diseases such as renal failure, diabetes mellitus, liver failure, or bacterial infections in the blood.

In addition to the alpha receptors, serotonin 5-HT receptors, histamine H_1 receptors, dopamine receptors, and NK-1 receptors for substance P found in the emetic center, the CRTZ also has receptors for opioids (narcotic drugs). The presence of opioid receptors on the CRTZ explains why many opioid analgesic ("painkilling") drugs at low doses produce vomiting as a side effect.

The numbers and types of receptors on the CRTZ vary among species like they did in the emetic center. The CRTZ of dogs contains more dopamine receptors and H_1 (histamine type 1) receptors than the CRTZ of cats; hence dogs are more sensitive to the effects of dopaminergic drugs or drugs that stimulate excessive release of histamine (such as with motion sickness). It also explains why antidopaminergic drugs and antihistamine drugs (like human sea sickness or motion sickness medications) work more effectively to control vomiting in the dog than in the cat.

As with the emetic center, the CRTZ of the cat is much more populated with *alpha receptors*, which explains why alpha-2 sedative agonist drugs such as xylazine (Rompun), and to a lesser extent detomidine (Dormosedan), medetomidine (Dormitor), and dexmedetomidine (Dexdomitor), produce a strong emetic effect in cats and a much lesser emetic effect in dogs.

Serotonin receptors (also called 5-hydroxytryptamine, or 5-HT_3, receptors) on the CRTZ play a significant role in vomiting, especially in patients undergoing chemotherapy for cancer treatment. Serotonin receptors are also found in the GI tract as 5-HT_3 receptors and are involved in GI tract contractions. Serotonin antagonists have been used to prevent vomiting associated with cancer chemotherapy drugs in human medicine, and in veterinary medicine serotonin antagonist drugs have been used to decrease protracted vomiting associated with cancer chemotherapy or severe viral infections of the intestinal tract. The presence of 5-HT_3 serotonin receptors in the GI tract itself may help explain why serotonin antagonists (5-HT_3 blockers) are effective in reducing vomiting from GI tract inflammation associated with diseases like parvoviral enteritis.

Motion Sickness and the Inner Ear

The vestibular apparatus in the inner ear is the organ responsible for balance. Overstimulation of motion receptors in the vestibular apparatus is a source of vomiting associated with motion sickness and inner ear infections. The eighth cranial nerve (CN VIII—vestibulocochlear nerve) carries nerve impulses from the vestibular apparatus to the CRTZ and then onto the emetic center where vomiting is stimulated. At the CRTZ, the release of histamine and acetylcholine and stimulation of H_1 receptors and cholinergic receptors are the major mechanisms by which vomiting from motion sickness occurs in the dog.[3] Drugs that block these receptors significantly reduce vomiting from inner ear hyperactivity in dogs and humans. Cats have far fewer histamine H_1 receptors in their CRTZ and emetic center; thus human antihistamine motion sickness drugs are less effective in cats than they are in dogs or humans.[3] Cats have more alpha receptors; hence alpha-2 receptor blocking drugs

like chlorpromazine are more effective in reducing motion sickness in the cat.

The drug maropitant (Cerenia) was developed and is indicated for controlling motion sickness in the dog and cat. Unlike antihistamine drugs that block specific input from the vestibular apparatus, maropitant's primary action is blocking NK-1 receptors found in the main vomiting reflex pathway in the emetic center itself.

Vomiting From Stimulation Elsewhere in the Body

Inflammation or overdistention of abdominal organs, inflammation of the peritoneum, or stimulation of the pharynx can result in vomiting. When the GI tract becomes irritated by viral or bacterial infection, a foreign body, overdistention of the lumen of the gut, or the ingestion of irritating chemicals, nerve signals are sent to the emetic center where the vomiting reflex is initiated. Additional incoming inputs from other inflamed or injured abdominal organs like the kidney, bladder, and uterus can also stimulate the CRTZ and/or the emetic center. If cancer drugs damage the intestinal tract as a side effect, GI tract serotonin is released into the blood where it can travel to the brain and stimulate 5-HT_3 receptors in the emetic center and CRTZ to produce vomiting.[3]

Although the parasympathetic nervous system and its neurotransmitter acetylcholine are most often thought of as being associated with stimulation of vomiting, nerve signals sent from the body to the CRTZ and emetic center via the sympathetic nervous system can also produce vomiting by norepinephrine stimulation of alpha receptors.

Because so many organs or systems unrelated to the GI tract can produce vomiting as a clinical sign, it is important that veterinary technicians thoroughly examine all body systems in the vomiting patient to determine whether inflammation or disease at locations other than the GI tract might be the source for the vomiting.

Emotional Vomiting

In human beings, vomiting can result from signals sent from the cerebral cortex (a higher brain center) or the limbic system (the part of the brain involved with emotion). This explains why humans under circumstances of emotional shock, such as viewing surgery for the first time or experiencing an intense emotional situation, can vomit even though there is nothing wrong with the GI tract itself. To what extent higher brain centers or the limbic system initiates vomiting in animals is uncertain, although some animals tend to vomit when stressed or excited, possibly as a result of release of sympathetic (fight or flight) neurotransmitters norepinephrine and epinephrine and subsequent stimulation of alpha receptors in the CRTZ and emetic center.

Appropriate Use of Emetic Drugs to Induce Vomiting

Emetics are most often used to intentionally induce vomiting in animals that have ingested toxic substances. However, these drugs carry with them an inherent danger that must always be considered before inducing emesis. Vomiting brings caustic, acidic stomach contents back up the esophagus to the larynx, creating the potential for aspiration of this material into the lungs and creating an aspiration pneumonia. In situations of high risk for aspiration, the veterinarian has to weigh whether the animal is more likely to die from the ingested poison or from the potential aspiration of vomitus, and then act according to his or her clinical assessment and judgment.

Vomiting should not be induced if corrosive substances such as alkali cleaning agents, acids, or oxalate products have been ingested. Corrosive substances chemically burn tissue and can extensively damage the oral and esophageal mucosa during initial ingestion and again if the corrosive is brought back up via vomiting. The esophagus is not a particularly well-protected tubular organ because it does not contain protective mucus-producing glands like the stomach. Therefore, exposure to corrosives can potentially cause deep chemical burns or even esophageal perforation. As a general rule, if burns are observed on the oral mucosa during physical examination of the mouth and there is a suspected history of having ingested an unknown substance, the ingested compound should be assumed to have corrosive properties until proven otherwise.

Emesis should not be induced in animals that have ingested volatile (easily evaporated) petroleum liquids such as gasoline, light petroleum products, and most oils. Volatile liquids such as gasoline do not stimulate the normal gag reflexes that would normally reduce the risk of aspiration into the lung, and thus these liquids can be more readily aspirated into the lungs during vomiting. If petroleum liquids are aspirated, they are highly irritating and can quickly cause potentially life-threatening pulmonary edema.

The veterinary professional should not induce emesis, or should be extremely careful during emesis induction, in an animal that is comatose, extremely depressed, unconscious, or lacking a functional gag reflex that would normally protect against accidental aspiration. If a vomiting animal needs to be heavily sedated for a diagnostic procedure or treatment, or an animal is semiconscious at the time of emesis induction, a cuffed endotracheal tube should be placed to reduce the risk of aspiration pneumonia. It is important to remember that even an inflated cuff on the endotracheal tube may not completely prevent aspiration of vomited stomach contents because the cuff is at the distal end of the endotracheal tube and does nothing to prevent vomitus from getting into the trachea proximal to the cuff or in the laryngeal area.

A side effect of animals anesthetized or sedated with barbiturates, acepromazine, or other CNS depressant drugs is that it becomes more difficult to induce emesis because the emetic center, along with the rest of the brain, is typically depressed and made less responsive by these drugs. In the event that emesis is induced in these sedated or anesthetized animals, the suppressed gag reflex makes these animals more of a risk for aspiration during the act of vomiting. If emesis is produced in a sedated or anesthetized animal, it often takes a larger dose than normal to produce the emesis. However, once the sedation or anesthetic effect wears off the patient may experience continued and protracted vomiting because of the removal of the inhibiting effect the sedatives were having on the emetic center.

Animals that are convulsing or showing preictal (preseizure) signs should not be induced to vomit. The act of vomiting can bring on seizure activity, and the uncontrolled movements increase the risk for aspirating vomitus. Some poisons like strychnine produce seizures with any significant external stimulation, and vomiting would be expected to cause strychnine seizures.

If an animal has bloat, gastric torsion, or esophageal damage, emesis should not be induced. In these conditions, the outflow tract from the stomach may be blocked, or the stomach wall may be damaged, predisposing the animal to stomach rupture with forceful vomiting. Likewise, a weakened esophagus caused by damaging chemicals could also perforate under the additional pressure of vomited materials, forcing their way upward.

Because of the anatomic arrangement between the stomach and the entrance of the esophagus into the stomach, horses are not capable of vomiting. The same is true for rabbits who, if induced to vomit, can actually damage the stomach wall because the constriction between the esophagus and stomach is so strong that it can prevent reflux of the stomach contents (the stomach would just powerfully contract without the ability to relieve the pressure). Rats and guinea pigs are likewise incapable of vomiting and also have fewer of the receptors required to actually stimulate the vomiting reflex.

Timing of administration of the emetic is also important. If the emetic is administered too late, the poison may have moved out of the stomach and beyond the proximal duodenum. At that point, vomiting will not remove the ingested poison, and the risk for aspiration would outweigh the potential benefit from emesis. Most liquid toxins pass beyond the stomach or proximal duodenum, or are absorbed into the systemic circulation, within 2 h of ingestion. Solid poisons, such as rat bait blocks and pelleted rodenticides, may still be in the stomach up to 4 h after ingestion, depending on the speed of gastric emptying.

Although the following statement should be obvious, it needs to be stated because the veterinarian or veterinary technician may want to automatically induce emesis after ingestion of a poison because it is "something" that can be done. However, as has been illustrated, there are number of circumstances where inducing emesis can be risky if not potentially life threatening. If the patient has already vomited several times on its own after ingestion of a toxic material, the body has likely removed as much toxic material by vomiting as it can, and additional emesis from an emetic drug is unlikely to produce any significant additional benefit. Before inducing emesis, it must always be asked if the risk of aspiration outweighs the benefit potential from the induced emesis, and if the animal has already vomited repeatedly the risk outweighs the potential benefit.

Centrally Acting Emetic Drugs

Emetic drugs are divided into two general categories: centrally acting emetics and **locally acting emetics**. Centrally acting emetics act by stimulating the emetic center or the CRTZ in the central nervous system and include drugs such as apomorphine and alpha-2 agonists such as xylazine. Locally acting emetics, as discussed later, act by directly stimulating the GI tract itself, which in turn sends signals to the emetic center to produce vomiting.

Ropinirole (Clevor®) is an ophthalmic drop preparation that is FDA-approved (2020) to induce vomiting in dogs weighing at least 1.8 kg (4 lb) and 4.5 months of age and older. Ropinirole induces emesis through its activity on both central and peripheral dopamine receptors, with primary activity via the D2 receptor in the chemoreceptor trigger zone. This medication, compared with other emetics discussed in this section, is preferred due to its receptor selectivity. The D2 receptor selectivity reduces the risk of unwanted side effects, such as sedation, observed with the other commonly used central acting emetics. Ropinirole causes emesis within 5–7 min in most dogs after the eye drops are applied. The total number of drops recommended to produce emesis is weight based and ranges from 1 to 3 drops, with no more than 2 drops in one eye. The same number of drops can be repeated one time if the dog has not vomited after 20 min. The most common adverse effect is protracted (uncontrolled) vomiting. Protracted vomiting should be treated with the prokinetic medication, metoclopramide.

Apomorphine is a centrally acting emetic that is an opioid drug (opium-like narcotic drug related to morphine). Apomorphine is chemically structured like dopamine and therefore relies on dopamine receptor (nonselective) stimulation in the CRTZ to produce emesis. Apomorphine does not have an FDA-approved indication to induce vomiting, so its use is always extra-label. When given intravenously (IV) or by subcutaneous (SQ) injection, apomorphine stimulates the many dopamine receptors in dogs, causing a rapid onset of emesis. Cats have fewer dopamine receptors than dogs; therefore, apomorphine is less effective as an emetic in cats and generally not recommended.

In the United States, apomorphine is available from compounding pharmacies as a tablet, capsule, or compounded into an injectable solution. Even though apomorphine is available as an oral (PO) drug, it is not consistently effective via this route for two reasons. First, apomorphine administered PO undergoes a significant first-pass effect in the liver; thus, much of the drug given PO never makes it to systemic circulation and never reaches the CRTZ.[1] Second, although apomorphine stimulates the CRTZ through its dopamine effect, as an opioid drug it also depresses the CNS overall including the emetic center in the medulla. Thus, apomorphine only induces emesis if it rapidly achieves high enough blood concentrations that it can be detected by the CRTZ receptors before the apomorphine diffuses across the blood-brain barrier and depresses the neurons of the emetic center itself. A slow rise in blood concentrations, such as would be observed with oral administration of apomorphine tablets, allows more time for apomorphine to diffuse across the blood-brain barrier and depress the emetic center before blood levels increase high enough to stimulate the CRTZ.

Although emesis is still possible within 2–10 min after oral administration of apomorphine tablets, the PO route of administration is much less reliable than other routes of administration. If the first oral dose of apomorphine fails to produce emesis, subsequent doses are not likely to be any more effective because the previous dose has already begun to depress the responsiveness of the emetic center.[4]

Intravenous or subcutaneous injection of apomorphine rapidly establishes the high drug concentrations in the blood needed to stimulate the CRTZ before emetic center depression occurs. One study suggested that the SQ route of administration was more effective than the IM route of administration.[5]

In addition to parenteral administration, apomorphine tablets can be crushed, the powder mixed with saline or water, and the suspension dropped into the dog's eye. As an alternative, the apomorphine tablet can be placed directly into the conjunctival sac of the dog's eye, where the tablet or powder dissolves quickly and is rapidly absorbed through the conjunctiva, achieving high enough blood concentrations to produce vomiting. After the desired emetic effect is achieved, any remaining residue is flushed from the eye to prevent further absorption. This method of inducing emesis is advocated (if ropinirole drops are not available) for use in drug-sniffing dogs that, in their excitement at finding a "stash," sometimes ingest the contraband they find.

Apomorphine is an opioid and depresses the CNS; therefore, it has the potential to produce respiratory depression. Apomorphine should not be given to animals that already have significant respiratory depression (e.g., breathing muscle paralysis and depression of respiratory center from poison).[1] Although apomorphine's respiratory depressant effects can be reversed with an opioid narcotic antagonist such as naloxone, the emetic effects, which are mediated by dopamine receptors, are not affected by opioid reversal agents. Prolonged vomiting from apomorphine can be reversed by dopaminergic antagonists such as phenothiazine tranquilizers (e.g., acepromazine and chlorpromazine). As previously mentioned, if an animal is tranquilized with a drug such as acepromazine, subsequent administration of apomorphine will likely not produce the desired rapid and complete vomiting because acepromazine occupies and blocks the dopaminergic receptors on which apomorphine works.

Xylazine (e.g., Rompun™ and Anased™) is another effective centrally acting emetic, and is most effective in inducing emesis in cats. This commonly available injectable sedative and anesthetic agent stimulates alpha receptors in both the CRTZ and the emetic center in cats, producing emesis in 90% of cats and 30% of dogs.[6] This emetic effect can be reversed by using alpha-2 antagonists such as yohimbine (Yobine) or atipamezole (Antisedan). The xylazine dose used to induce emesis in cats is generally lower than the dose used for sedation or preanesthesia.[1]

The newer alpha-2 agonist sedative analgesic drugs detomidine (Dormosedan™), medetomidine (Dormitor™), and dexmedetomidine (Dexdomitor™) have the ability to produce emesis in cats but are less likely to induce vomiting in dogs than xylazine.[7]

Locally Acting Emetic Drugs

Locally acting emetics typically produce their effects by locally irritating the GI tract, distending the stomach, and/or stimulating parasympathetic nerves to send signals to the emetic center in the central nervous system. The most commonly used locally acting emetic has historically been syrup of ipecac. Unfortunately, syrup of ipecac was pulled from the market in 2004 because of abuse from people with bulimia, anorexia, or compulsive eating syndromes. In addition, a study in a prominent pediatric journal indicated that use of syrup of ipecac at home did not reduce the need for subsequent emergency treatment for ingested poisons in human infants.[8] This finding was followed by a position statement from the American Association of Pediatrics recommending that parents no longer keep syrup of ipecac in the house. These factors likely led to the withdrawal of this product in the United States. Because of the widespread use of ipecac in households with children, some pet owners may still have it in their medicine cabinets, so the veterinary technician should be aware of this emetic compound.

Other locally acting emetics such as hydrogen peroxide, warm concentrated salt water solution, or a solution of powdered mustard and water produce emesis to some degree, but these emetics do not work as consistently as the centrally acting emetic drugs.

Currently **hydrogen peroxide** 3% concentration is the recommended local emetic for dogs listed on the Association for Prevention of Cruelty to Animals (ASPCA) Poison Control Center website.[9] To enhance the emesis from hydrogen peroxide, the peroxide must be "fresh" (it loses its ability to fizz after a few months) and the animal should be given a few pieces of dog food or bread to add bulk to the vomitus. Hydrogen peroxide use should be limited to 1.1–2.2 mL/kg, with a maximum of 45 mL, and no more than two doses used in a 15-min period.[9]

The use of hydrogen peroxide can irritate the stomach lining, resulting in a potentially severe *gastritis* (inflammation of the stomach). In cats, the emetic response to hydrogen peroxide is quite variable, and the risk of gastritis is reported to be more significant than it is in dogs. The subsequent froth released from the hydrogen peroxide also increases the risk for aspiration.[1]

The administration of a concentrated salt water solution may produce vomiting if it sufficiently stimulates the pharyngeal region of the throat. Placing a small amount of plain table salt directly in the pharyngeal region may also produce this effect. If a salt solution is orally administered, the animal should be given water or IV fluids to reduce the risk of salt toxicity or dehydration. Some toxicologists state that salt should not be given as an emetic because of the risk for salt toxicosis, resulting in tremors, seizures, and death by hypernatremia (increased sodium in the blood) outweighs the potential for effective emesis.[10]

Inducing vomiting by forcing a finger to the back of an animal's throat usually results in a struggle and bitten fingers, but seldom any vomiting because of the lessened sensitivity of the animal's mouth and oral pharynx to finger stimulation compared with humans.

ANTIEMETIC DRUGS

Antiemetic drugs prevent or decrease vomiting by blocking receptors in the CRTZ, blocking receptors on the emetic center, and/or blocking peripheral receptors that could send signals to the brain to produce vomiting. The veterinary professional must remember that vomiting and diarrhea are naturally protective mechanisms and that preventing vomiting with antiemetics may allow the poisonous substances to remain in the GI tract longer or may mask clinical signs used to determine the disease progression or the animal's recovery from the disease. Therefore, antiemetics should only be used when the naturally occurring vomiting reflex is considered no longer beneficial to the animal.

Phenothiazine Tranquilizers

Phenothiazine tranquilizers are considered to be broad-spectrum antiemetics because they block several types of receptors involved in the vomiting reflex. Phenothiazine tranquilizers used in veterinary medicine include the widely used veterinary tranquilizer **acepromazine** and the human drugs **chlorpromazine** (Thorazine™) and **prochlorperazine** (Compazine™). These phenothiazine tranquilizers work primarily by blocking dopamine receptors, H_1 (histamine) receptors, and to a lesser degree cholinergic (acetylcholine) muscarinic M_1 receptors in the emetic center and the CRTZ.[11]

Because the majority of the phenothiazine's antiemetic effect in dogs comes from antidopaminergic activity, and because dogs contain a greater number of dopamine receptors than cats, antidopaminergic drugs like phenothiazines generally work better in dogs than in cats. Because histamine and acetylcholine are the primary mediators of motion sickness, phenothiazine blocking of the histamine H_1 receptor and the cholinergic M_1 receptors decreases vomiting caused by motion sickness.

Although some veterinary gastroenterologists advocate the phenothiazine tranquilizer chlorpromazine for controlling vomiting associated with acute gastroenteritis (inflammation of the stomach and intestines) from canine parvovirus, better control of vomiting from cancer chemotherapy is said to come from drugs that block NK-1 (substance P) and 5-HT (serotonin) receptors.[2]

Phenothiazine drugs also have some α-adrenergic receptor antagonist activity (antialpha receptor activity) that reduce alpha receptor stimulation of vomiting. But a side effect of phenothiazine's alpha receptor blocking effect is a drop in arterial blood pressure. Whenever arterial blood pressure drops for any reason (e.g., shock, dehydration, blood loss), the sympathetic nervous system releases norepinephrine, which stimulates α_1 (alpha-1) adrenergic receptors on the smooth muscle of small peripheral blood vessels causing vasoconstriction, increasing resistance to arterial blood flow into these vessels, and causing a subsequent arterial blood pressure increase. Because phenothiazines block alpha receptors, they also block the α_1 receptor on the smooth muscle of these small blood vessels and can block the body's attempt to raise a dropping blood pressure by blocking the vasoconstriction needed to do so. For this reason, animals hypotensive (having low blood pressure) from dehydration, shock, blood loss, or any cause should have the hypotensive state corrected before phenothiazine antiemetic therapy is initiated to prevent further decreases in blood pressure. The role of α receptors in the regulation of blood pressure is discussed in greater detail in Chapter 5.

Phenothiazine drugs may produce some small degree of tranquilization at the doses usually used for antiemetic effect, and this tranquilization is one of the reasons why acepromazine is popular as a drug to prevent motion sickness associated with car travel. However, if an animal is already depressed from other causes or has already received other CNS depressant drugs, the tranquilizing effect from phenothiazines may be greater than normal at antiemetic doses.

Additional effects of acepromazine and other phenothiazine tranquilizers are discussed in Chapter 8.

⊚ MYTHS AND MISCONCEPTIONS

Acepromazine and other phenothiazines decrease the threshold for seizures in epileptic animals

False! This was a common misconception found throughout the veterinary literature (including the previous editions of this text) for a number of years based upon observations that in humans chlorpromazine was thought to increase the ease with which an epileptic human patient would go into seizures. However, subsequent studies have determined that there is no evidence in veterinary medicine that such a link occurs between veterinary patients on phenothiazines and an increase in how readily an animal experiences seizures (i.e., no evidence for a decreased seizure threshold). A 2006 retrospective study appearing in the *Journal of the American Animal Hospital Association* found no correlation between phenothiazine administration and increased seizure activity.[12] A smaller study presented at the 2004 International Veterinary Emergency and Critical Care Symposium also found no change in seizure frequency of epileptic dogs given phenothiazines.[13] However, though there is no evidence that such a link exists between phenothiazines and increased seizure activity, there is not enough evidence to REFUTE that such a link may exist. For practical purposes, contemporary thinking leans toward the conclusion that phenothiazines do NOT increase the frequency of seizure in epileptic veterinary patients.[12,13]

Antihistamine Antiemetic Drugs

Antihistamines are the main ingredient in drugs used to control motion sickness in human beings. These drugs work by blocking the H_1 receptors on the CRTZ, which decreases the ability of the histamine-mediated signals sent from the inner ear vestibular apparatus to stimulate the CRTZ. Decreased CRTZ stimulation means decreased stimulation of the emetic center and reduced vomiting. Additionally, antihistamines also block some of the acetylcholine receptors, reducing the vomiting stimulation caused by the parasympathetic nervous system stimulation.

As previously mentioned, the larger number of H_1 receptors on the dog's CRTZ than the cat's makes antihistamine antiemetic drugs more effective in the dog than the cat. Veterinarians occasionally still use **dimenhydrinate** (Dramamine™) and **diphenhydramine** (Benadryl™) to prevent motion sickness in animals even though other antimotion sickness drugs have been developed more recently. The dimenhydrinate drug is metabolized to diphenhydramine for its antihistamine activity.[3]

Antihistamines have a sedative effect on animals similar to that observed in human beings and thus may adversely affect the performance of working animals. These drugs can also decrease the wheal and flare reaction used to gauge the body's reaction to antigens during intradermal allergy testing, so antihistamines should not be used for at least 4 days before allergy testing.

Anticholinergic Antiemetic Drugs

Anticholinergic drugs block the effect of the acetylcholine neurotransmitter on acetylcholine receptors. Specifically in the CRTZ and the emetic center, this would be the muscarinic cholinergic receptor (M_1 cholinergic receptor). Although drugs that block muscarinic cholinergic receptors decrease the vomiting stimulus from parasympathetic nervous system signals, these drugs are generally not considered to be effective antiemetics in most species because vomiting can be stimulated by so many other receptors in addition to the cholinergic M_1 receptor.[1]

Because anticholinergics are not as effective antiemetics compared with other available drugs and because anticholinergic drugs have many side effects, anticholinergic drugs like scopolamine and aminopentamide (Centrine™) are no longer recommended as a first choice of antiemetic drugs for treating most causes of emesis. The veterinary product aminopentamide (Centrine™), which was used for vomiting associated with spastic colonic contractions, has been discontinued.

Scopolamine patches are still used to reduce motion sickness-induced vomiting in people by blocking the acetylcholine effect generated by overactivity of the vestibular apparatus, but they are not typically used in veterinary medicine.

Prokinetic Drugs as Antiemetics: Metoclopramide

Metoclopramide (Reglan™) is a broad-spectrum, centrally acting antiemetic that also has local antiemetic activity. Its centrally acting antiemetic effect is primarily through blocking the dopamine receptors, but at higher doses it can also block serotonin receptors on the CRTZ.[1] Because dogs have more dopamine receptors on their CRTZ than cats do, the antidopaminergic antiemetic action of metoclopramide is more effective in dogs than it is with cats. The combined antidopamine and antiserotonin antiemetic effects at higher doses contribute to metoclopramide's ability to decrease vomiting associated with some cancer chemotherapeutic agents.[3]

In addition to the centrally acting antiemetic effect, metoclopramide has a locally acting antiemetic effect in the GI tract itself. Metoclopramide is considered a prokinetic drug, meaning that it increases upper GI motility in the stomach and small intestine. The prokinetic activities of metoclopramide increase muscle tone of the lower esophagus, relax the pyloric outflow tract of the stomach, increase gastric motility in the "normal" direction without increasing secretions, and increase motility of the duodenum and jejunum. All of these increased contractions help decrease the act of vomiting by preventing gastric stasis (decreased or cessation of stomach contractions) that usually precedes the reversed peristaltic movement of vomiting.

In addition to decreasing vomiting from chemotherapeutic agents and other blood-borne vomiting stimulants, metoclopramide has been useful for intermittent vomiting of bile and mucus in otherwise healthy dogs. This syndrome is seldom problematic enough to warrant a specific trip to the veterinarian because the animal has a good appetite and feels well otherwise. However, it is annoying to the pet owner because the vomited yellow bile pigments stain fabric and carpeting. The cause of the vomiting is thought to be a reflux (reverse flow) of bile from the duodenum back into an empty stomach in animals that are not fed free choice. Bile is irritating to the stomach and produces the subsequent vomiting. Because metoclopramide enhances gastric movement in the correct direction and reduces reflux, a dose of metoclopramide given to these dogs in the evening reportedly helps correct this situation.

Metoclopramide has other CNS effects in addition to its antiemetic effect. Because it has antidopaminergic activity like phenothiazine tranquilizers, it can produce sedation and should not be used in conjunction with phenothiazine tranquilizers because of the potential added tranquilization effect. At the higher doses needed to block the serotonin receptors, some animals (especially cats) can show a seeming contradictory frenzied behavior as opposed to a more significant sedation. Likewise, some sources cite metoclopramide as being relatively contraindicated (meaning, do not use the drug unless the medical condition justifies the risk) or **absolutely contraindicated** (do not use the drug regardless of the medical condition) in animals with seizures because of an increased risk for seizure activity.[11]

Because metoclopramide relies on acetylcholine for the prokinetic gastric muscle contractions and much of its local antiemetic activity, use of anticholinergics, such as atropine or narcotic analgesics, that block acetylcholine's effect can negate the local antiemetic effect of metoclopramide.

Cisapride is another prokinetic drug similar to metoclopramide but without centrally acting dopamine-blocking antiemetic effects. It does have serotonin antagonistic effects that aid in its prokinetic function. The prokinetic activity of cisapride has been especially helpful for increasing colonic smooth muscle tone in cats with a dilated colon condition called megacolon, but has not been used successfully as an antiemetic. Cisapride is a human drug and was taken off the market in the United States in 2000 because of incidents of fatal arrhythmias in people taking the drug with certain antibiotics. It is still available for veterinarians for use in cats with megacolon and dogs with ileus through compounding pharmacies. Cardiac problems reported in human patients have not been observed in veterinary patients on cisapride.

Serotonin Antagonist Antiemetic Drugs

One of the newer classes of antiemetics to make its way from the human field to the veterinary field are the serotonin antagonists, also called the 5-HT receptor antagonists. As previously mentioned, stimulation of 5-HT receptors on the CRTZ can produce vomiting. Serotonin is also likely involved in transmitting signals from the GI tract via peripheral nerves to the emetic center to stimulate vomiting. Thus, blocking serotonin receptors and inhibiting the release of serotonin is an effective antiemetic strategy that has been used to control vomiting from cancer chemotherapy in human beings and veterinary patients.[11]

Ondansetron (Zofran™) and related 5-HT$_3$ antagonist drugs such as granisetron (Kytril™) and dolasetron (Anzemet™) have been used for dogs and cats with suspected nausea and refractory vomiting that does not respond to other drugs. In addition, these 5-HT$_3$ antagonist drugs have been used successfully to control vomiting from severe parvoviral enteritis or cancer chemotherapy in dogs and vomiting associated with pancreatitis in cats.[3]

The release of generic drug forms of ondansetron brought down the prices of 5-HT$_3$ antagonist antiemetics, making their use more cost effective for the veterinarian.

Neurokinin-1 (NK-1) Receptor Antagonist Antiemetics

In 2006, **maropitant (Cerenia™)** was released in the United States as the first of a new class of broad-spectrum veterinary antiemetic drugs called neurokinin-1 (NK-1) antagonists. Maropitant blocks substance P, a neurotransmitter peptide found in the emetic center, from combining with the neurokinin-1, or NK-1, receptor in the nucleus tractus solitarius in the emetic center. Because the emetic center's NK-1 receptors are the last step in the emetic pathway from the CRTZ, vestibular apparatus, peripheral nerve inputs, and GI tract, blocking the NK-1 receptors blocks most of these stimuli that would normally produce vomiting.[1,3,14]

This drug was used for a number of years in Europe before coming to North America. The initial United States Food and Drug Administration (FDA)-approved use for the tablet form was for prevention of acute vomiting and vomiting caused by motion sickness in dogs, and the injectable approved use was for prevention and treatment of acute vomiting. In 2012, the approved use for the injectable was extended to include treatment of acute vomiting in cats.[14] This medication is commonly used to prevent motion sickness in dogs and cats and a preanesthetic medication. Many preanesthetic protocols include maropitant to prevent vomiting from opioids, as well as to prevent postoperative vomiting.

Newer Antiemetics Are Always Coming

Because vomiting is such a common complaint in veterinary patients, new antiemetics will continue to appear. When authoritative speakers at veterinary conferences begin to suggest the use of a human drug for antiemetic purposes, it is always prudent to do additional research and identify other reliable sources to corroborate this information before using new drugs on your patients. Specifically, attempt to determine from reliable sources under what specific conditions and indications these "new" drugs should be used, what side effects are possible with their use, and what clinical research has actually been done in veterinary patients to justify the safe use of these medications in veterinary patients.

ANTIDIARRHEAL DRUGS

Antidiarrheals are drugs that change intestinal motility or reduce the secretions that contribute to diarrhea. Like vomiting, diarrhea is normally a protective mechanism that helps remove irritating or toxic substances from the intestinal tract. In many cases, mild diarrhea or loose stools are self-limiting conditions in dogs or cats. However, when diarrhea is a part of a more severe constellation of clinical signs, an antidiarrheal drug may be used to reduce the loss of bodily fluids.

Essentially, diarrhea occurs because the balance between fluid secretion from the body into the intestinal lumen and the fluid absorption from the intestinal lumen fluid into the body has been altered, resulting in more fluid being secreted into or remaining in the feces. Diarrhea takes four general forms: secretory diarrhea, exudative (increased permeability) diarrhea, motility diarrhea, and osmotic or malabsorption diarrhea. Any clinically significant case of diarrhea most likely is a combination of two more of these types.

Secretory diarrhea can be caused by bacterial enterotoxins (toxins produced by intestinal bacteria) or inflammation of the bowel, resulting in cells along the wall of the intestinal tract increasing secretion of fluids into the intestinal lumen at a rate that cannot be compensated by absorption of the fluid from the bowel. This type of diarrhea can quickly dehydrate an animal because the body is literally pumping fluid out of the body into the GI tract lumen.

Exudative diarrhea occurs when the inflammation or damage to the intestinal wall is significant enough to allow leakage of electrolytes, plasma proteins from the blood, or even blood itself into the intestinal tract. Diseases that produce ulcers or destruction of the intestinal tract lining (e.g., parvovirus diarrhea, transmissible gastroenteritis in pigs) not only result in a loss of fluid, electrolytes, protein, and blood, but they can also allow toxins from the intestinal tract to enter the body through the damaged intestinal tract wall.

Motility diarrhea results when rapid movement of the intestinal contents prevents proper digestion of food or absorption of fluids before the contents are expelled as feces. When the resulting diarrhea is composed of large volumes of liquid, this can be attributed to rapid, peristaltic movements in the small intestine and is characteristic of a "small bowel diarrhea." If the increased motility is largely confined to the large intestine or colon, the colonic contractions will produce a "large bowel diarrhea" that is characterized by small amounts of stool passed frequently and often accompanied by visible straining to defecate.

Osmotic or malabsorption diarrhea occurs whenever there are osmotic particles, such as undigested food, fiber, or laxative drugs, in the GI tract lumen that hold water by osmotic attraction and prevent the fluid from being absorbed. The increased volume of liquid feces and the liquid nature of the feces results in diarrhea. In young German shepherd dogs with exocrine pancreatic insufficiency (EPI), the pancreas is unable to produce normal amounts of digestive enzymes, resulting in food being poorly broken down into smaller molecules that can be absorbed across the GI tract wall. The undigested particles of food hold water in the lumen of the GI tract and produce a voluminous diarrhea.

Antidiarrheal drugs principally work by decreasing secretions from the GI tract wall, modifying the intestinal motility, or decreasing the underlying problem that is stimulating changes in secretion or motility (e.g., reducing inflammation or infection).

Intestinal Motility in Health and Disease

Intestinal motility involves two types of contractions: segmental contractions, which are circular contractions around a small

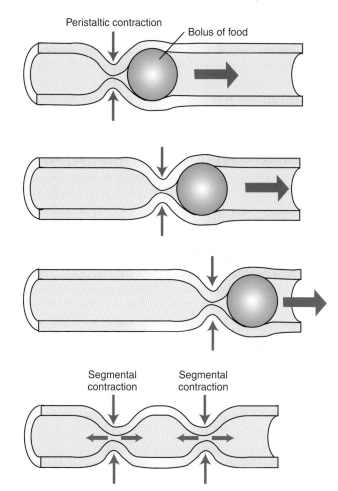

Fig. 4.4 Peristaltic contractions propel intestinal contents. (Images courtesy of Colville T, Bassert J. *Clinical Anatomy and Physiology for Veterinary Technicians.* 3rd ed. St. Louis: Elsevier; 2016.)

segment of intestine that mix the contents of the bowel, and peristaltic contractions, which move in waves to propel the food along the tract (Fig. 4.4). Increased segmental contractions constrict the size of the intestinal lumen in segments, which normally slows the passage of feces along the GI tract. Diseases that decrease segmental contractions or increase peristaltic movement result in more rapid movement of ingesta along the tract and can contribute to diarrhea.

In many small intestine diarrheal diseases, a short period of hypermotility (increased movement of bowel contents characterized by rapid peristalsis and audible gut sounds) is often followed by a longer period of hypomotility (decreased peristalsis) or atony (few or no segmental contractions, few or no audible gut sounds). When the bowel loses the smooth muscle tone for segmental contractions, the bowel loses some of the resistance that normally slows the flow of the feces. Thus, even weak peristaltic contractions can propel intestinal contents faster along the length of the intestine and result in diarrhea.

Unlike the small intestine, large bowel diarrhea from the colon is normally associated with an increased smooth muscle contraction or spasms in response to colonic or rectal inflammation and irritation. The animal is often observed to strain to defecate but produces little or no feces. In these cases, it is not the presence of fecal material that stimulates the defecation reflex but inflammation or irritation stimulating the reflex, resulting in the animal straining to defecate. This condition is called tenesmus. Owners will often mistake tenesmus as the animal being constipated and unable to pass stool when the reality is just the opposite. Well-intentioned owners may actually give their pet a laxative thinking it will help relieve the "constipation," but this only serves to make the situation worse.

Antidiarrheal Drugs That Work by Modifying Motility

Antidiarrheal drugs in general often have multiple means by which they can decrease diarrhea. Theoretically, antidiarrheal drugs should be able to decrease diarrhea by either decreasing peristaltic movements (decrease propulsion) or by increasing segmental contractions (increasing resistance to flow of feces). In fact, drugs that decrease peristalsis also tend to decrease all smooth muscle contractions, including the segmental contractions that slow the flow of feces. Thus, drugs that depress all GI motility may turn the intestine into a "garden hose" or "stovepipe" through which feces slide quickly with little resistance to flow.[3]

Narcotic (Opioid) Antidiarrheals

Opioids are drugs derived from opium, of which the prototype drug is morphine. Because these opioids can produce a state of sleepy delusion or narcosis, they are also referred to as "narcotics" (derived from the word "narcosis," meaning the state of unconsciousness or stupor). It is well known that morphine used therapeutically for pain relief can also produce constipation as a side effect in patients who are taking the drug. This same side effect is used therapeutically in OTC opioid antidiarrheal drugs such as **diphenoxylate (Lomotil™)** and **loperamide (Imodium AD™)**.

Although these antidiarrheal drugs are related chemically to potential abuse drugs such as morphine and hydrocodone, they typically do not have the ability to produce hallucinogenic effects unless taken at very high doses. Still, to discourage the potential drug abuse from ingestion of high doses of diphenoxylate, this drug also contains a small, subtherapeutic dose of atropine that, if the antidiarrheal drug is taken at very high doses, will produce dry mouth, dilated pupils, and other atropine effects that opioid abusers find uncomfortable. Because these opioid antidiarrheal drugs are not considered to pose a significant abuse potential, they are not considered to be controlled substances (not schedule drugs, drugs labeled with the capital "C" and a Roman numeral).

Loperamide and diphenoxylate decrease diarrhea by combining with mu (µ) opioid receptors, increasing the segmental contractions in the small intestine, decreasing the propulsive peristaltic movement, and simultaneously decreasing the secretory activity of cells in the GI tract wall.

Because these drugs decrease gut motility and slow the transit time of intestinal contents, they also prolong the contact time between the bowel mucosa and pathogenic bacteria, such as *Salmonella enteritidis* and enterotoxins, which could increase the damage caused by these agents. This is especially a concern in horses with bacterial enteritis. To avoid some of these detrimental effects, these compounds are often not given until it is judged that sufficient time has passed for the infectious agent or enterotoxin to have been cleared from the bowel.

Collie dogs and related breeds may have a genetic defect that produces less effective P-glycoprotein (P-gp) pump molecules as described in Chapter 3. Normally the dose of loperamide and other opioids given PO takes into account that a significant amount of the drug will not be absorbed into the brain because of the activity of the P-glycoprotein pump at the blood-brain barrier to keep drugs out of the brain. To have an effect systemically, drugs normally pumped by the P-glycoprotein have to be given at doses that overwhelm this normal protective pump and allow some of the drug to be absorbed into the body. In animals with the genetic defect that impairs the function of the P-glycoprotein, like Collies, Shelties, Australian shepherds, and related breeds, the defective P-gp results in more of the opioid antidiarrheal drug being absorbed and more of the drug being able to get to the brain because of defective P-gp pumps in the blood-brain barrier. There have been several reports of these breeds acting stuporous, sedated, or depressed when given a "normal" dose of the OTC loperamide product. If an owner should give Imodium AD™ or generic loperamide and observe sedation or signs of CNS depression, the patient should be considered a potential candidate for adverse reactions to all drugs affected by the P-gp genetic defect. This is a subtle but important clinical clue casually reported by the owner but dismissed as insignificant unless the well-educated veterinary technician recognizes its importance.

Anticholinergic Drugs as Diarrheals

Anticholinergic drugs such as atropine or scopolamine block the acetylcholine muscarinic receptor and in so doing block the parasympathetic stimulation of the intestinal motility and secretion. Although this effect might seem to reduce diarrhea, this has not been the case because the segmental contractions that would slow the transit of intestinal flow and the peristaltic contractions are decreased, resulting in the "garden hose" effect mentioned previously. In addition, anticholinergic compounds, if used in the horse, can produce a condition called ileus in which a segment of the bowel fails to contract, resulting in a functionally "dead" segment of the gut producing colic. Because anticholinergic drugs produce effects that block the parasympathetic nervous system throughout the body, they also have unwanted side effects on almost every other system in the body. Although some veterinary products have contained anticholinergic compounds in the past, today these drugs are generally regarded as ineffective.

Decreasing Diarrhea by Blocking Secretions

Increased GI tract secretions can result from stimulation by bacterial enterotoxins or by the products of inflammation itself such as prostaglandins and leukotrienes. (See Chapter 13 for further information on these inflammatory compounds.) Anything that increases the effect of acetylcholine or the activity of the parasympathetic nervous system, such as certain poisons like organophosphate insecticides, can also increase GI tract secretions. Stimulation of cells lining the GI tract can result in secretion of ions (e.g., sodium) that osmotically pull water with the ions into the lumen of the gut. This type of diarrhea can be potentially dangerous because of the risk for life-threatening dehydration, especially in younger animals.

Secretory diarrheas can become exudative (increased permeability) diarrheas when the GI inflammation also damages the tight junctions between cells lining the intestinal tract, allowing small-molecular-weight sugars, fluid, and protein molecules to be lost into the intestinal lumen. If inflammation or cellular destruction continues, the intestinal tract may become so porous that red blood cells escape into the intestinal lumen, resulting in bloody diarrhea.

Antisecretory antidiarrheal drugs used in veterinary medicine include the narcotic/opioid drugs mentioned earlier and antiinflammatory drugs that block production of inflammatory products like prostaglandins and leukotrienes. Antiinflammatory drugs used as antisecretory antidiarrheals include aspirin-like compounds (salicylates) and sulfasalazine (Azulfidine™).

Bismuth subsalicylate, the active ingredient in the OTC human antidiarrheal drug Pepto-Bismol and newer formulations of Kaopectate, breaks down in the gut to bismuth carbonate and salicylate. The bismuth coats the intestinal mucosa, protecting it from enterotoxins while producing some antibacterial activity. The major antisecretory effect, however, is probably from the salicylate, which blocks formation of inflammatory prostaglandins that would normally stimulate fluid secretion.

In addition to its antidiarrheal effect, bismuth subsalicylate has been used to treat *Helicobacter* or similar bacteria that are thought to be associated with gastric ulcers in humans and veterinary patients.[3]

Although bismuth is not well absorbed in the systemic circulation, the salicylate is absorbed very well.[15] Although salicylate absorption in cats is always a concern because of their lessened ability to metabolize the drug (see Chapter 3), the amount of salicylate absorbed systemically is typically not high enough to produce salicylate toxicity in cats if the recommended doses are not exceeded.[3] However, overzealous owners should be cautioned against using higher than normal doses of Kaopectate or Pepto-Bismol in cats, and dogs for that matter, because of the risk for salicylate toxicity if they are overdosed with these antidiarrheals.

The bismuth that remains in the bowel can make the stool appear dark and tarry, resembling melena (stools darkened by digested blood). This color change can confuse the veterinarian who might mistake its presence as an indication of gastric or small intestinal hemorrhage. Bismuth, like barium, is a radiopaque liquid that has been used as a contrast material to better show the outline of stomach and intestinal tract on radiographs. As such, the presence of bismuth in the GI tract may interfere with visualization of other abdominal organs on radiographs.

Veterinary patients commonly reject peppermint-flavored oral antidiarrheal products because of the taste. Refrigerating the liquid form reduces the peppermint flavor, which may make it easier to administer. The tablet form greatly facilitates administration of the drug.

5-HT (5-HT$_3$) serotonin antagonist drugs such as ondansetron (Zofran™) were mentioned as antiemetics and act by blocking serotonin receptors on the CRTZ and in the GI tract itself. By blocking 5-HT$_3$ receptors on the GI tract cells, serotonin antagonist drugs decrease secretion of chloride ions and water. As such, these drugs may be used as an adjunct drug (a drug used in addition to another drug) for diarrhea in addition to their antiemetic effect.[16]

Sulfasalazine (Azulfidine™) is a sulfonamide antibiotic (antimicrobial) linked chemically to a salicylate molecule called mesalamine (formerly called *5-aminosalicylic acid*). Although the antibiotic component of this combination does little to relieve intestinal inflammation or infection, the mesalamine that is cleaved from the sulfonamide antibiotic by colonic bacteria decreases prostaglandin formation and thus acts as an antiinflammatory drug in the colon. Sulfasalazine has been successfully used in the treatment of chronic bowel conditions such as ulcerative colitis, but because the cleaving of the molecule does not occur until the colon, the drug is not effective for use in treating small bowel diarrhea.

The salicylate, once cleaved from the sulfonamide antibiotic, is partially absorbed from the colon, but the rest of the salicylate remains in the colon, where it decreases production of inflammatory prostaglandins and leukotrienes.[3,17] Because the drug is a salicylate, some caution should be exercised with use in cats. However, because little of the salicylate is absorbed systemically, sulfasalazine should be safe to use in cats to treat inflammatory large bowel disease at the recommended dosages.

Because the sulfonamide antibiotic component of sulfasalazine is well absorbed, it is capable of producing side effects typically associated with sulfa antibiotics, including vomiting (if given on an empty stomach) and decreased tear production, leading to a condition called keratoconjunctivitis sicca, KCS, or dry eye. Sulfonamide antibiotic side effects are described in more detail in the antibiotic chapter (Chapter 10).

In the future, a number of other human products that contain mesalamine without the sulfonamide antibiotic are likely to find their way into veterinary use. These drugs are currently available for human use in slow-release tablet form and as enema preparations.

Adsorbents and Protectants as Antidiarrheal Agents

Adsorbents are drug molecules that cause other molecules to adhere to their outer surfaces. By adsorbing (not absorbing) toxic, irritating, or disease-causing molecules to the adsorbent drug surface, these bad compounds are less likely to be absorbed into the body or interact with GI tract cells to produce clinical signs of disease.

In contrast, protectant types of compounds are designed to cover the intestinal wall to form a physical blanket or barrier that protects the intestinal wall from contact with irritating or disease-producing compounds. Although some of these adsorbents and protectants are widely used in human medicine for control of diarrhea, their effectiveness in veterinary patients is debatable.

The bismuth in bismuth subsalicylate has adsorbent properties and may play an adsorbent and protective role in treating diarrhea. However, the antiinflammatory antisecretory effect of the subsalicylate likely contributes more to control of the diarrhea than the adsorbent or protective effect of the bismuth part of this drug. Still, bismuth has been shown to adsorb *Escherichia coli* bacterial enterotoxins, and reduce its contact with the intestinal tract wall, possibly reducing some secretory diarrhea.

The antidiarrheal products containing an adsorbent combination of kaolin and pectin were often used in people and animals. Kaolin, or more specifically **kaolinite**, is a clay-like substance thought to be able to adsorb bacteria and their enterotoxins, thereby reducing their hypersecretory effect on the ntestinal tract. However, clinical studies have shown that kaolin and pectin compounds are not very effective at adsorbing *E. coli* bacterial enterotoxins, and there is no medically based evidence to show that they reduce the duration of the diarrheal disease.[3] Hence, kaolin-pectin products for humans have been discontinued, although OTC animal products are still readily available to the public. Given their questionable effectiveness in veterinary patients, kaolin-pectin products are used far less by veterinarians to treat diarrhea.

Note that Kaopectate trade-named products stopped using kaolinite in the 1980s and switched to another clay-like product called attapulgite. In 2002, Kaopectate was then completely reformulated in the United States by removing the adsorbent clay and replacing it with bismuth subsalicylate, making the product very similar to the traditional Pepto-Bismol formulation. Thus, the same cautions regarding salicylate toxicity in Pepto-Bismol also apply to Kaopectate despite Kaopectate's name implying its ingredients are still kaolin (kaolinite) and pectin. Canada continues to produce Kaopectate with attapulgite.

Liquid barium used in contrast radiographic studies of the intestine also acts as a protectant and is likely also an adsorbent. Anecdotally veterinarians have observed that animals with chronic diarrhea may clinically improve for a while after oral administration of barium to produce intestinal radiographic contrast studies. Thus, barium likely acts similar to bismuth to reduce the effects of diarrhea.

Although not typically used as an antidiarrheal agent, **activated charcoal** adsorbs enterotoxins and many ingested poisons to its surface, preventing them from contacting the bowel wall and decreasing their ability to inflict damage or to be absorbed into the body. Although it is sometimes referred to as the "universal antidote," activated charcoal is not an antidote but merely adheres to the poison or enterotoxin, preventing it from being absorbed into the body. Because charcoal is messy to administer, it is seldom used as an adsorbent to decrease diarrhea but is formulated into veterinary and human products used to decrease absorption of ingested poisons (e.g., veterinary product Toxiban). Activated charcoal does not adsorb alcohol compounds (e.g., xylitol the artificial sweetener in candy and gum, that is toxic to dogs), metals (e.g., lead, zinc, arsenic, or iron), or petroleum products.

Because pet owners are familiar with OTC human antidiarrheal drugs and because some of these products, if used inappropriately, can potentially hurt animals, veterinary technicians need to be aware of the public's perception of these drugs so that they may knowledgeably answer questions that owners have and

help prevent these drugs from being used in ways that harm pets.

LAXATIVES, CATHARTICS, AND PURGATIVES

Laxatives, cathartics, and purgatives are used to increase the fluid content of the feces, making them softer and easing or promoting defecation. These types of drugs are used to control chronic constipation (common in some older cats), facilitate passage of trichobezoars (hairballs), evacuate the colon before radiographic procedures, and ease passage of stool after perianal surgery or in animals with severe pelvic fractures.

These drugs often have different mechanisms and degrees of aggressiveness in evacuating the bowel. Generally, laxatives are considered the gentlest of this class of drugs, whereas cathartics are more marked in their evacuating effect. Purgatives are the most potent in their actions. Although increasing the dose of some laxatives may produce a more pronounced loosening of the stool than a low dose of a cathartic, laxatives are generally used when the goal is to just soften the stool, but cathartics and purgatives are used when evacuation of the bowel is the goal.

Laxatives

Laxatives fall into two categories: **emollient** *laxatives* (lubricant oils and the so-called stool softeners) and **bulk** *laxatives* (hydrophilic colloids such as bran and plant fiber).

Emollient laxatives include lubricants such as mineral oil, cod liver oil, white petrolatum, and glycerin and are commonly used after anal surgery (e.g., after surgical removal of anal sacs or perianal fistula surgery), when passage of a firm stool may be painful.

Mineral oil (liquid petrolatum) is an emollient laxative most commonly administered by stomach tube to horses with suspected impactions. The greatest danger associated with use of this oil is accidental administration or aspiration into the lungs with subsequent aspiration pneumonia. Mineral oil has no significant taste and does not readily stimulate the swallowing reflex; therefore, the animal can fairly easily aspirate the oil if it is not given by an appropriately placed stomach tube.

Cod liver oil and **white petrolatum** are nonprescription emollients found in dog laxatives or drugs used to prevent or treat trichobezoars (hairballs) in cats (e.g., Laxatone, Katalax). These flavored semisoft tube gels are orally administered directly out of the tube or by smearing along the mouth of the cat (the cat then licks the gel and swallows it); hence there is far less risk for aspiration. Long-term use of nonabsorbable oils can decrease absorption of lipid-soluble vitamins such as A, D, E, and K.

Glycerin is most commonly used as a suppository and therefore does not carry the risk of aspiration. Glycerin suppositories facilitate stool passing through the colon or rectum of animals with severe pelvic fractures or compression of the diameter of the pelvic canal, through which the colon and rectum pass.

In addition to the lubricant oils, another group of emollient laxatives includes compounds that change the surface tension of dried fecal material, allowing water to penetrate the fecal material and soften it. **Docusate sodium succinate (DSS, Colace™)** is a stool softener that acts as a wetting agent, or surfactant. Docusate sodium succinate and related calcium and phosphate compounds may also stimulate colonic secretions, resulting in increased fluid content of feces.

Bulk laxatives osmotically pull water into the bowel lumen or retain water in the feces, softening the stool. Hydrophilic colloids or indigestible plant fiber (**bran, psyllium, methylcellulose**, Metamucil) are not digested or absorbed to any degree and therefore create an osmotic force to produce their laxative effect. Psyllium is a hydrophilic compound that has gained popularity for its purported health benefits. It is successful as a bulk laxative but increases flatulence.

Cathartics

Cathartics fall into two categories on the basis of their mechanisms: **osmotic** (saline) cathartics and **irritant** cathartics. Osmotic cathartics are more aggressive than the osmotic bulk laxatives.

Typically, osmotic or saline cathartics are hypertonic salts such as magnesium (**milk of magnesia, Epsom salts**). "Hypertonic" refers to the property that these salts are poorly absorbed and create a strong osmotic force to attract water into the bowel lumen. In addition to the direct osmotic effect, magnesium also causes release of cholecystokinin, a hormone that increases peristalsis and thus facilitates movement of the fecal material. Large doses of hypertonic salts should be avoided because they can severely dehydrate an animal.

Although osmotic cathartic salts are poorly absorbed, if they are given in large doses or if they remain in the bowel for an extended period of time, they may be absorbed in sufficient amounts to cause electrolyte imbalances within the body. For example, absorption of excessive magnesium salt can cause muscle weakness and CNS alterations. Absorption of phosphate from phosphate and sodium phosphate salt laxatives or enemas can cause hypocalcemia to the extent of producing hypocalcemic tetany. Because cats are especially susceptible to these electrolyte imbalances, phosphate laxatives and sodium phosphate enemas, including soaps with a high phosphate content, should not be used in feline patients.

Lactulose is a poorly absorbed sugar osmotic cathartic used to treat cases of chronic constipation and reduce the ammonia absorbed from the colon. It is used in a condition called *hepatic encephalopathy,* a condition in which either a poorly functioning liver or the presence of vascular shunts that bypass the liver results in elevated ammonia concentrations in the blood, disrupting/depressing normal function of the CNS and leading to death. The lactulose changes the pH of the colon, resulting in ammonia becoming more ionized, thus reducing ammonia ion absorption from the intestinal tract and helping to reduce the clinical signs associated with hepatic encephalopathy.

Irritant laxatives, including **castor oil** and **bisacodyl** (**Dulcolax™, Senokot™**), work by irritating the bowel, resulting in increased peristaltic motility and some increased secretion by glands in the intestinal tract wall. Castor oil is converted in the duodenum to ricinoleic acid, which is a highly irritating compound. Because of their stimulant activity, these compounds should not be used in animals with suspected obstructed bowel or impacted feces or those with tenesmus resulting from colonic irritation or rectal/anal surgery.

ANTACIDS AND ANTIULCER DRUGS

Physiology of Stomach Acid Secretion

The stomach contents are normally very acidic, with a pH as low as 2–3, which is sufficiently corrosive to burn a hole in tissue. Therefore, the stomach must be well equipped with safety mechanisms to contain this highly acidic liquid without damage to the stomach lining. If the balance between acid production and protective mechanisms is disrupted, the lining of the stomach can become injured and inflamed, producing gastritis (stomach inflammation) or ulceration. Understanding the way the body regulates stomach secretions and the protective function helps the veterinary technician understand the mechanisms behind the actions of antacid drugs and ulcer treatments.

The stomach is lined with gastric glands that contain hydrochloric acid-producing parietal cells (also called **oxyntic cells**), chief cells that produce an enzyme precursor called pepsinogen, and mucous cells that produce the protective mucous layer.

Hydrochloric acid is actively secreted into the stomach lumen by the oxyntic or parietal cells as separate hydrogen (H^+) and chloride (Cl^-) ions that, once secreted, combine to produce hydrochloric acid (HCl). The active transport of hydrogen ion from the oxyntic cell to the lumen of the stomach is via a "proton pump" or "H^+ pump." The proton pump uses cellular energy to actively pump the hydrogen ion against the high hydrogen ion concentration already present in the lumen of the stomach (Fig. 4.5).

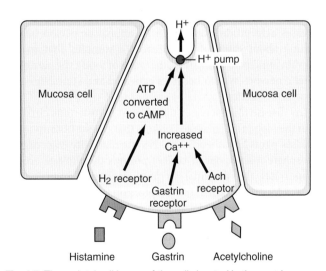

Fig. 4.5 The parietal cell is one of the cells located in the gastric mucosa lining the gastric glands, along with mucus-producing cells and chief cells that produce pepsinogen. The parietal cell actively pumps hydrogen ions (H^+) into the lumen where it combines with chloride (Cl^-) to produce hydrochloric acid (gastric acid). The parietal cell pumps hydrogen ions in response to stimulation of receptors by histamine released from the nearby enterochromaffin-like cells, gastrin produced by G cells in the stomach and proximal duodenum, and acetylcholine from the parasympathetic nervous system (PSNS).

Control of the acid production is via parietal cell stimulation from three receptors: H_2 histamine receptors, *acetylcholine receptors,* and *gastrin receptors.* Of these three receptors, stimulation of the histamine H_2 receptors has the greatest effect on acid production. Histamine is most commonly thought of in its role as one of the agents that produces the signs of inflammation (swelling, redness) after its release from basophils and mast cells. However, the histamine involved in stimulating the parietal cell's H_2 receptors is secreted by specialized cells in the stomach called enterochromaffin-like cells.

Enterochromaffin-like cells produce the histamine when stimulated by another hormone called gastrin produced by G cells located in the distal part of the stomach and proximal duodenum. G cells release gastrin hormone in response to the presence of proteins in the stomach, the stretching of the stomach with food or liquid, or as a result of increased stimulation by the parasympathetic nervous system. The function of gastrin is normally to signal relaxation of the stomach wall (so more food can be stored) and to increase stomach acid production to begin the breakdown of food in the stomach. Thus, the presence of food stimulates gastrin release, which in turn stimulates enterochromaffin-like cells to release histamine, which then locally stimulates the H_2 receptors on the parietal cells, causing stomach acid production.

As mentioned earlier, both the enterochromaffin-like cells and the parietal cells themselves have gastrin receptors, but the acid-producing effect of the parietal cell's gastrin receptor stimulation is fairly minimal compared with the effect of histamine on the H_2 receptors.

Anything that stimulates the "rest and restore" parasympathetic nervous system discussed earlier in this chapter causes release of acetylcholine at the end of parasympathetic nerves. The vagus nerve (cranial nerve X) is a parasympathetic nerve that innervates the GI tract and releases the acetylcholine that stimulates the acetylcholine receptors on parietal cells and increases acid production. When an animal or person begins to think about eating or experiences a stimulus that makes the brain anticipate eating (e.g., the smell of food), the parasympathetic nervous system becomes activated and stimulates gastric acid production.

Any disease that increases the amount of histamine circulating in the blood (e.g., mast cell tumors that release histamine) or increases parasympathetic nervous system activity (e.g., organophosphate insecticides or certain poisons that imitate acetylcholine) has the potential to produce hyperacidity in the stomach by stimulation of the receptors on the parietal cell. This is why animals diagnosed with mast cell tumors or mastocytosis often are put on H_2 blocking antacids.

When the acid contents of the stomach pass into the less protected duodenum and the pH of the duodenum drops below 4.5, another local hormone is produced by the cells in the duodenum that triggers the pancreas to secrete acid-neutralizing sodium bicarbonate into the duodenum.[18] The duodenum has far fewer protective mucus-producing glands; therefore, the sodium bicarbonate neutralization of the strong stomach acid is very important in helping to prevent duodenal ulcer formation. Anything that increases stomach acidity can also predispose the proximal duodenum to ulcer development.

Mucus Production

The acid-blocking mucus produced by the gastric glands is actually a complex of many substances that provides a gelatinous, protective coating for the stomach. *Mucins* are complex molecules produced by the mucus-producing cells in the gastric glands and are the main constituent of the **mucous** coating. In addition to the mucin, bicarbonate ions are secreted and added to the mucous coat, making it more alkaline (less acidic). By alkalinizing the mucus with sodium bicarbonate, the mucus neutralizes some of hydrochloric acid's corrosive effect before it contacts the cells of the stomach wall.

Mucus production is stimulated by prostaglandins mentioned previously with secretory diarrhea mechanisms. Locally produced prostaglandins in the stomach stimulate mucus production and inhibit acid production by parietal cells. Anything that blocks the formation of these beneficial prostaglandins, such as antiinflammatory drugs like aspirin, can predispose an animal to less mucus production, more acid production, and subsequently gastric ulcers. This explains why animals administered high or prolonged doses of antiinflammatory drugs are at risk for gastritis and ulcer formation.

! YOU NEED TO KNOW

How Mucus Is Different From Mucous

The educated veterinary technician uses the proper spelling of "mucus" vs "mucous," as well as other similar terms such as "estrus" and "estrous." Mucus and estrus, without the "o," are nouns and hence are words for things. For example, the gooey substance secreted from the nose is called *mucus*; the state of being in heat is called *estrus*. But mucous and estrous are adjectives, meaning they are words that modify a noun or tell us what type of noun it is. For example, mucous membranes describes the nature of the membrane and answers the question, "What types of membranes are they?" The estrous cycle describes a type of cycle. "What type of cycle was it? It was the estrous cycle." Thus, if a word has the "us" at the end, it describes the noun or thing, whereas a word with an "ous" at the end is an adjective that describes some characteristics of a noun.

Pepsin Production

The chief cells in the stomach produce an enzyme precursor called pepsinogen that, when secreted into the acid environment of the stomach, is activated to pepsin, an enzyme capable of digesting protein. Pepsinogen production is stimulated by acetylcholine released from increased parasympathetic nervous system activity. Thus, when the PSNS stimulates pepsinogen secretion, it also stimulates parietal cells to produce the hydrochloric acid needed to activate the pepsinogen to **pepsin**. Although the pepsin enzyme does not totally break down mucus, it can fragment the mucin molecule, making it less effective in protecting the stomach lining.

Drugs Used to Counter Gastric Acidity and Ulcer Formation

Anything that increases the stomach's acid or pepsin content to a level that overwhelms the protective mucous layer can damage the epithelial cells lining the stomach, causing inflammatory gastritis or loss of the superficial epithelial layer of cells and resulting in erosions or gastric ulcers. Gastric ulcers can be relatively shallow or superficial erosions or can be severe enough to perforate completely through the stomach wall, allowing stomach contents to leak into the surrounding peritoneal cavity.

As stated earlier, increased parasympathetic nervous system activity, excessive histamine release, or blocking beneficial prostaglandin formation all produce gastric hyperacidity and reduce mucus production, resulting in stomach cell damage. In addition to hyperacidity or decreased mucus production, anything that causes liver bile salts secreted into the duodenum to reflux back into the stomach will also damage the mucus and expose the stomach wall to injury. The accumulation of metabolic uremic toxins in diseases like renal failure can likewise disrupt the protective mechanism. In cattle, the ingestion of high concentrations of easily digestible carbohydrates (e.g., grain or very lush forage) can result in bacterial production of tremendous amounts of acid, producing rumen acidosis and severe erosions in the rumen wall. Horses can likewise suffer ulcers from a high-carbohydrate diet or from severe stress (e.g., track racing) that reduces protective prostaglandins in the equine stomach.

Regardless of the cause of the hyperacidity or ulcer formation, antacids and antiulcer drugs are used to reduce the stomach acid and enhance the mechanisms by which the stomach protects itself from its own acid. In addition, antacids are also used to decrease rumen acidosis in cattle or sheep, allowing survival of rumen microbes critical for ruminal fermentation and digestion.

Antacids decrease stomach acidity by either chemically combining with the hydrochloric acid to make a less acidic molecule or by decreasing acid production. Antacids are classified as **systemic** or **nonsystemic**, depending on whether or not they need to be absorbed systemically into the blood to produce their beneficial effect.

Nonsystemic Antacids

Nonsystemic antacids are given by mouth but are not absorbed systemically. Instead they chemically neutralize acid molecules in the stomach or rumen. Nonsystemic antacids typically come in either liquid or tablet form and are composed of calcium, magnesium, or aluminum. OTC antacids such as **Tums** and **Rolaids** are nonsystemic antacids made primarily of calcium carbonate or a combination of calcium carbonate and magnesium hydroxide. The largest group of OTC nonsystemic antacids are blends of magnesium hydroxide and aluminum hydroxide and include products such as **Mylanta™**, **Di-Gel™**, and **Maalox™**. Pure magnesium hydroxide products include **milk of magnesia**, and pure aluminum hydroxide products used in veterinary medicine include **Amphojel™**.

Side effects from nonsystemic antacids are rare because the calcium carbonate and aluminum hydroxide are not absorbed to any significant degree. Unlike calcium and aluminum products, up to 20% of the magnesium product can be absorbed. Magnesium is primarily excreted by the kidney; therefore, magnesium antacids should not be used in patients with renal disease or renal failure because of the risk of accumulating too much magnesium in the blood and disrupting the balance of electrolytes.[4]

Long-term use of calcium and aluminum antacids often cause constipation, whereas magnesium products may trigger diarrhea. Products containing both aluminum and magnesium attempt to balance these constipating and diarrheal effects.

Calcium antacids are more prone to cause gastric acid rebound syndrome than the magnesium or aluminum antacids. The calcium carbonate in these antacids triggers the release of gastrin, with a subsequent increase in hydrochloric acid production. Unfortunately, this gastrin stimulation continues after most of the calcium carbonate antacid has moved beyond the stomach into the duodenum. The result is an increased production of hydrochloric acid in the stomach without the presence of the antacid to neutralize it. Fortunately, a normal stomach can tolerate this short-lived rebound, but a stomach with gastritis or an ulcer may become more inflamed.

The pH change in the stomach lumen by antacids or the presence of calcium or magnesium in the nonsystemic antacids may interfere with absorption of other drugs from the GI tract. The alkaline pH shift in the stomach may cause some drugs (drugs that act like an acid—see Chapter 3) to shift to a more predominantly hydrophilic (ionized) form that is less able to be absorbed by passive diffusion through the stomach wall or proximal duodenum. Drugs may also combine or adhere to the calcium or magnesium in the nonsystemic antacids, causing the drug to precipitate out of solution or otherwise interfere with their absorption. For example, older tetracycline antibiotics given by mouth when calcium nonsystemic antacids are present will combine with the calcium and precipitate out of solution. Absorption of orally administered drugs like fluoroquinolone antibiotics (e.g., enrofloxacin, Baytril), the tranquilizer acepromazine, thyroid hormone supplements, and corticosteroids (antiinflammatory drugs) may also be decreased by concurrent use of nonsystemic antacids. These interactions between nonsystemic antacids and other drugs should be listed in either the package insert for the individual drugs or in the more widely used drug reference resources. In situations where such a drug is to be given to an animal also taking nonsystemic antacids, the antacid should not be administered at the same time and instead is administered no closer than 2 h before, or 3 h after, the other drug is given.

Systemic Antacids

In contrast to the local neutralizing effect of nonsystemic antacids, systemic antacids must be absorbed, circulate in the blood, and attach to receptors on the cells of the stomach to produce their effects. **H_2 blockers** are a class of systemic antacids that include **cimetidine (Tagamet), famotidine (Pepcid)**, and **nizatidine (Axid)**. H_2 antagonists or H_2 blockers work by attaching to and blocking the **H_2 histamine receptor** located on oxyntic (parietal) cells in the stomach.[17,18] H_2 blocker antacids attach to these H_2 receptors but either produce no intrinsic activity or actually decrease the basal level of acid-producing activity of the cell. Therefore, histamine released from the local enterochromaffin-like cells is blocked from reaching the H_2 receptor, preventing increased gastric acid production and reducing the basal level of acid the cells produce even when there is no H_2 receptor stimulation. These drugs are available in injectable and oral prescription forms. Cimetidine and famotidine are also available in OTC forms as Tagamet-HB™ and Pepcid-CD™, respectively.

Cimetidine (less so famotidine, and nizatidine) inhibits the hepatic enzymes responsible for metabolism and breakdown of some cardiac drugs (β-blockers, calcium channel blockers, and quinidine), the bronchodilator theophylline, and anticonvulsant drugs such as diazepam and phenytoin. Simultaneous use of cimetidine with these drugs and others results in slowed metabolism of these drugs, increases their concentrations in the body, and potentially achieves toxic drug concentrations unless the dose is reduced. Whenever using cimetidine on a patient that is also taking other drugs, it is always wise to check the drug insert or drug formulary to determine whether the other drug's metabolism would be affected by cimetidine. According to a study published in the *Journal of Veterinary Internal Medicine* in 2014 titled, Serum concentrations of gastrin after famotidine and omeprazole administration to dogs, this class of medication is only effective for about 3 days.[17] If longer acid suppression therapy is needed, it is recommended to use a proton pump inhibitor as discussed below.

Omeprazole and similar drugs in this family are described as an acid pump or proton (H+) pump inhibitors. Unlike systemic antacids that decrease acid production by blocking the stimulation of H_2, acetylcholine, or gastrin receptors, omeprazole binds to the luminal surface of the stomach's parietal cells and inhibits the pump that normally transports hydrogen ions into the stomach lumen. Fewer hydrogen ions pumped into the stomach contents means a less acidic environment.

Omeprazole is available OTC as the human product Prilosec OTC™ but is also available in an FDA-approved prescription oral paste (Gastrogard™) and an OTC version (Ulcergard™) for use in horses with gastric ulcers. Ironically, omeprazole is rapidly degraded by stomach acid so the capsules used in the human form of the drug contain enterically coated granules to prevent release of the drug until it has passed into the duodenum where it will be absorbed systemically.[3,4] Thus, if the human product it used, it must not be chewed or crushed as this could disrupt the enteric coating on the granules within the capsule and expose the drug to the degrading effects of the stomach acid. Omeprazole paste is not enterically coated but is somewhat protected by the paste medium, and the dosage is based upon a predictable loss of the drug because of exposure to gastric acid.[4]

Omeprazole is a product that has been compounded for use in small patients in veterinary medicine with varying degrees of success. If a small patient requires compounding the powder from another omeprazole preparation containing enteric-coated granules, the appropriate amount of the granules for the patient should be reinserted into another gelatin capsule to facilitate the drug dose reaching the stomach without being chewed or crushed. Omeprazole is also available in an IV formulation for patients that cannot be given oral medications. The proton pump inhibitors take about 3 days to reach therapeutic blood concentrations. To speed this up for patients with acute gastritis, clinicians will give omeprazole IV, 1 mg/kg every 12 h instead of every 24 h. This should be done for no longer than 3 days, then switch to an every 24 h dose interval.[18] The total duration of use for this medication for most patients should be no longer than 7–10 days, and should not be used as a preventative medication for any species.

There are several other members of this proton pump inhibitor family of drugs used in human and veterinary medicine (e.g., lansoprazole or Prevacid™). They can be recognized by their use as an antacid and the "-azole" suffix at the end of the drug name.

Sucralfate (Carafate) is an antiulcer drug that has been called a "gastric Band-Aid" because when exposed to stomach acid it forms a sticky paste that binds with the proteins exuding at the ulcer site. Thus, the gelatinous sucralfate selectively adheres to the ulcer site, physically protecting it from the acid, pepsin, or bile salts that could further injure the ulcer. In addition, sucralfate also stimulates local prostaglandin release, which promotes gastric protective mechanisms such as increased mucus production and improved blood flow to the ulcer site.

Sucralfate requires the presence of an acidic environment to most effectively bind to the ulcer site. Thus, theoretically, sucralfate should not be used simultaneously with antacid drugs, which would make the stomach pH more alkaline. Whether this is truly of clinical significance is still open to debate. However, avoiding the administration of sucralfate simultaneously with antacids or other drugs that alkalinize the stomach environment is likely prudent. To prevent interacting with the absorption of any medication, sucralfate should always be administered at least 30 min before any other medications or food.

Despite the need for an acidic environment to adsorb to an ulcer site, clinical investigators have compounded sucralfate to treat esophageal ulcers by crushing the tablets and mixing them with warm water to form a slurry that is administered by mouth. This formulation has only anecdotal evidence to support it efficacy for esophageal ulcers.

Misoprostol (Cytotec™) is a synthetic prostaglandin type E_1 (PgE_1) drug. Just like the naturally occurring prostaglandins, misoprostol increases mucus production, decreases acid production, and facilitates the stomach's protective mechanisms for defense and healing. It has been used to prevent ulcer formation associated with aspirin therapy in dogs and to treat ulcers associated with other nonsteroidal antiinflammatory drug (NSAID) use, but it has not been shown to be effective in decreasing ulcers caused by corticosteroid administration.[3,19] Misoprostol is relatively expensive compared with most of the other antacid and GI protective drugs and has been less widely used than the H_2 blockers or sucralfate.

Because misoprostol is a prostaglandin and because prostaglandins have so many functions throughout the body, it would be expected that misoprostol would stimulate many prostaglandin receptor sites, resulting in a wide variety of side effects. The most common side effects reflect GI stimulation and manifest themselves as diarrhea, abdominal discomfort, cramping, and colic, especially in the horse. For that reason misoprostol is generally discouraged for use in treating equine gastric ulcers.[3] Prostaglandins also increase the contractions of the uterus and can induce premature birth or abortions. Therefore, this drug should not be used to treat ulcers in animals that are pregnant. The drug, which comes in tablets, should be handled with care by pregnant humans.

DRUGS USED FOR RUMEN HEALTH

When ruminant animals become sick, one of the side effects may be rumen stasis, a condition in which the normal motility of the rumen is halted. Because normal ruminal contractions are needed for processing food, keeping the rumen microbes healthy, and balancing gas and other byproducts of rumen fermentation, rumen stasis results in poor ability to digest food, bloat from excessive gas formation, or death from bloat or rumen acidosis.

Ruminatorics: Prokinetic Drugs

Ruminatorics are prokinetic drugs that stimulate an atonic (no muscle tone) or flaccid rumen. In the past, many "barnyard" compounds have been used to "get the rumen started again." These compounds often were an integral part of a local livestock production community lore and were passed down as home remedies from generation to generation. Some of the more notable ruminatorics included mercury, strychnine, tartar, barium chloride, and various plants that contained compounds that mimicked acetylcholine.

Although some of these ruminatorics may actually have stimulated the rumen, they obviously had side effects and disadvantages and would be unacceptable today in modern livestock production. Modern ruminatoric drugs are designed to stimulate the parasympathetic nervous system and thus increase motility of the GI tract. **Neostigmine** is a ruminatoric drug that combines with the enzyme acetylcholinesterase and prevents it from breaking down the parasympathetic nervous system neurotransmitter acetylcholine. The prolonged acetylcholine effect increases the parasympathetic stimulation, resulting in increased GI stimulation, increased bronchial secretions, bronchoconstriction, decreased heart rate, miosis (constricted pupils), and urination. Other drugs that block acetylcholinesterase or mimic the neurotransmitter acetylcholine would be expected to have similar effects.

Ionophores

Ionophores are a group of antimicrobial drugs discovered in the 1950s and used in livestock to control coccidia, a common protozoa causing GI disease in poultry and cattle. The term ionophore refers to the ability of these compounds to facilitate transport of selected ions (e.g., Na^+, K^+) across a cell membrane. The transport of selected ions and the disruption of the electrolyte balance and water balance within the organism are the proposed mechanisms by which ionophores kill bacteria or protozoa like coccidia.[3]

Although very useful to control coccidiosis in poultry and livestock, the ionophore **monensin (Rumensin)** is more widely used in beef and dairy cattle to balance the rumen population of microorganisms, improve conversion of cattle feed into animal weight, and to prevent bloat. Although very safe for use in cattle and most poultry, monensin is toxic and potentially fatal to horses and should never be added to horse feed.[20]

Antibloat Medications

Antibloat medications are designed to reduce gas buildup or facilitate the removal of gas from the rumen. Normal rumen and reticulum contractions allow partially digested plant food (the cud) to be regurgitated up the esophagus into the mouth, where it is chewed and reswallowed (rumination or "chewing the cud"). This process also expels built-up carbon dioxide or methane gas from the rumen (a process called eructation), thereby reducing the risk of too much gas being trapped in the rumen and producing a condition called bloat or ruminal tympany.

Eating very lush grass or excessive clover or alfalfa can alter the rumen flora and change the surface tension of the liquid in the rumen, resulting in generation of a froth or foam in the rumen instead of a single large gas pocket, leading to an accumulation of excessive gas and bloat. Antibloat medications act either by reducing numbers of rumen microorganisms that produce the gas or by breaking up the bubbles formed in the frothy bloat. Just as home remedies were used as ruminatorics, in the past compounds such as oil of turpentine, pine oil, gasoline, creolin, and even formaldehyde have been used to kill rumen microorganisms and reduce the bloated condition. Obviously, many of these compounds carried the risk of tissue irritation, tainting of milk, and other potentially toxic side effects.

Most modern veterinary bloat medications act by decreasing the surface tension of foam in the rumen, causing the small bubbles to coalesce into much larger gas pockets that can be eructated (belched) from the rumen. Mineral oil or some vegetable oils are used to decrease the viscosity of the rumen contents, decrease the stability of the bubbles, and remove the froth. **Dioctyl sodium succinate (DSS)**, which was discussed previously as the small animal stool softener Colace, also reduces the viscosity of rumen contents, allowing the foam to dissipate. These antibloat medications are administered either by oral tube or by direct injection into the rumen through the flank with a large-bore trocar needle.

Products containing **poloxalene**, a synthetic compound that reduces the surface tension of rumen fluid and decreases froth formation, are used in conjunction with management practices as a relatively inexpensive preventative to reduce the incidence of bloat. Poloxalene is available both as a liquid drench and as large "salt lick" blocks.[21]

THE ROLE OF ANTIMICROBIALS IN GASTROINTESTINAL TRACT DISEASE

As a general rule, veterinary gastroenterologists do not recommend the use of antimicrobials (antibiotics) in the treatment of most cases of vomiting or diarrhea. In many cases, the disease is viral in nature and thus nonresponsive to antimicrobials. In other cases of bacterial origins of diarrhea (e.g., E. coli), the use of antibiotics has typically shown no clinically significant change to the course of the disease.[1,3] The use of oral antibiotics, especially those that kill Gram-positive bacteria, alters the natural flora of bacteria in the GI tract and has the potential to cause diarrhea or cramping.[1,3] In cases of Salmonella bacterial disease, antibiotics are used only if there is fever and changes in the white blood cell count that suggest bacteria may have invaded the intestinal wall and gained access to systemic circulation (bacteremia or septicemia). The use of antibiotics in less severe *Salmonella* cases may actually prolong the amount of time in which the infected animal sheds *Salmonella* into the environment, increasing the risk for spread to other animals or people.

Still, antimicrobials are commonly used to treat calf diarrhea, are used as a component of treating chronic (long-term) diarrhea or diarrhea related to bacterial overgrowth, or are used when the threat or existence of secondary spread of bacteria or their toxins to systemic circulation is likely.

Tylosin (Tylan)

Tylosin is a macrolide antibiotic belonging to the same class of antibiotics as erythromycin. Tylosin is used in cattle and swine to treat GI and respiratory infections by susceptible Gram-negative and Gram-positive bacteria, *Chlamydia,* and *Mycoplasma* organisms. Although there is an injectable form that is approved for use in dogs and cats and livestock, the oral livestock powdered formulation has been used in an extra-label manner in dogs and cats to treat bacterial overgrowth, irritable bowel disease, and colitis associated with clostridial bacteria.[3,4] The powdered form of tylosin is normally added to the livestock feed, but if added to dog or cat food the bitter taste may make small animal patients refuse their food. Tylosin can be compounded into gel capsules to improve the ability of owners to give the tylosin to the dog.

A specific tylosin-responsive chronic diarrhea syndrome has been identified in mostly middle-aged large breed dogs in which tylosin was effective in treating the diarrhea when other enteric antimicrobials and prednisone had failed.[22,23]

Most veterinarians feel that tylosin should not be used in horses because the drug may cause diarrhea potentially severe enough to cause death.[4]

Metronidazole (Flagyl)

Metronidazole is a human drug that has been used for years in veterinary medicine to treat a diarrhea-producing protozoa called *Giardia.* The trade name Flagyl is a reference to the flagellum or whip-like structure *Giardia* and other flagellate organisms use to propel themselves. Over the years of use in practice, veterinarians observed that some diarrheas not apparently caused by *Giardia* would also respond to treatment with metronidazole.[3] In addition to its antibacterial and antiprotozoal activity, it is thought that metronidazole may also decrease the intestinal inflammation by reducing bacteria (primarily anaerobic bacteria) that stimulate GI tract inflammation or by directly reducing the intestinal tract's response to the inflammatory stimuli.[3,4]

Metronidazole does have some significant side effects in some dogs at high doses or even at normal doses if the drug has been used for an extended period. These side effects include CNS signs such as weakness, head tilt, staggering, disorientation, proprioceptive deficits (inability to sense the position of the limbs), and seizures. Fortunately, these neurologic signs typically disappear a few days after metronidazole is discontinued.

Metronidazole is prohibited from use in food animals by the FDA because some studies have demonstrated potential carcinogenesis (cancer-causing properties) when used in rats and mice.

CLINICAL APPLICATION
"Brain Tumor" in a Dog

A veterinarian at a conference related a tale about an old dog that was having recurring diarrhea for a duration of several weeks. The owners had fecal samples checked repeatedly, hoping to find either some intestinal worm parasites or protozoal organisms such as *Coccidia* or *Giardia* that could be treated. The clients went to several veterinarians to try to get an answer for the continual diarrhea without much luck in getting the condition controlled. Along the way, radiographs were taken of the intestinal tract and a barium series was performed. The dog's diarrhea improved for several days after the barium series but then returned. A biopsy was done of the intestinal tract but it came back as a nonspecific diagnosis of inflammation. After several weeks of dealing with the diarrhea and not wanting to spend any more money on diagnostics, the owners tried yet another veterinarian who put the dog on metronidazole as a "shot in the dark." In 2 days, the diarrhea was remarkably better. By 4 days of metronidazole treatment the stools were firming up nicely. The owners were encouraged.

On day 8, the owners returned home from a weekend trip to find the dog wandering in a circle, staggering, and falling over. The owners feared that the dog had a brain tumor. After weeks of battling the diarrhea, this new development was too much for the owners to take. They feared their dog would never have a good quality of life again, so they took the dog to an emergency clinic where they requested euthanasia.

Unfortunately, with the history of metronidazole administration, the dog's clinical signs may have been related to the drug and not really indicative of a brain tumor. The circling behavior, the sudden onset, and the 8-day treatment with metronidazole (apparently at a significantly high dose to correct the diarrhea problem) would be consistent with central nervous system (CNS) side effects from metronidazole. Even at normal doses metronidazole has been reported to produce CNS signs in some canine patients. However, these neurologic side effects from metronidazole are reversible within a few days of the drug being stopped with no apparent long-term effects.

If the veterinarian was not aware of these neurologic side effects of metronidazole, the conclusion of a brain tumor or some acute cerebrovascular event would have been reasonable in an older dog. We will never know for sure in this case what the cause was for the neurologic event, but this case illustrates why it is important that veterinarians and veterinary technicians be aware of neurologic side effects of drugs such as metronidazole.

Erythromycin and Azithromycin

Erythromycin and azithromycin are macrolide antibiotics (antimicrobials) very similar to tylosin. It is well known for producing GI cramping as a side effect when it is used to treat bacterial infections elsewhere in the body (e.g., for bacterial pneumonia or bronchitis). At doses lower than those required to kill bacteria, erythromycin and azithromycin mimic the effects of a natural intestinal stimulatory compound called motilin and also stimulates 5-HT$_3$ (serotonin) receptors in the intestinal tract, producing increased motility. Erythromycin and azithromycin have been used in dogs and cats to stimulate gastric emptying by increasing stomach contractions or to decrease esophageal reflux of stomach acid by increasing muscle tone in the lower esophagus in dogs. In this way, erythromycin and azithromycin act as a prokinetic agents similar to metoclopramide. As mentioned, these medications are antimicrobials, so using them as a prokinetic at low, long-term dosages increases antimicrobial resistance, so should be reserved for patients not responding to other prokinetic agents (i.e., metoclopramide, cisapride).

Sulfasalazine (Azulfidine™)

Sulfasalazine (Azulfidine™), mentioned under the antidiarrheal drugs, is an antibiotic that is broken down by colonic bacteria into the sulfonamide sulfapyridine and the aspirin-like prostaglandin-blocking agent mesalamine (5-aminosalicylic acid). Sulfasalazine is typically used for its antiinflammatory effect to treat inflammatory colitis but is ineffective in treatment of small intestine inflammation because the antiinflammatory component of sulfasalazine is not released until the drug reaches the colon.

ADDITIONAL DRUGS USED TO TREAT GASTROINTESTINAL-RELATED DISEASE

Oral Electrolyte Replacements

Various liquid and powder products containing essential electrolytes (sodium, potassium, chloride) are administered orally to help replace ions lost with diarrhea or vomiting. These products are generally recommended for calves, lambs, and foals with scours (diarrhea) for which the IV administration of fluids with electrolytes would be economically or logistically impractical. They are also sometimes used in practice for dogs and cats after they are able to take fluids orally. Electrolyte replacers are most likely to be helpful when the animal has secretory diarrhea without significant dehydration and no vomiting. Absorption of electrolytes may be impaired in animals with severe intestinal damage.

Pancreatic Enzyme Supplements

Some dogs and cats may be affected by a syndrome in which the pancreas fails to produce sufficient amounts of the following digestive enzymes: lipase, which breaks down lipids; amylase, which breaks down starches; and various proteinases, which

---

GASTROINTESTINAL DRUGS

Emetics
Centrally acting emetics
  Apomorphine
  Xylazine
Locally acting emetics
  3% Hydrogen peroxide

Antiemetics
Phenothiazine tranquilizers
  Acepromazine
  Chlorpromazine (Thorazine)
  Prochlorperazine (Compazine)
Antihistamines
  Dimenhydrinate (Dramamine)
  Diphenhydramine (Benadryl)
Prokinetic drugs
  Metoclopramide (Reglan)
  Cisapride
Serotonin (5-HT) antagonists
  Ondansetron (Zofran)
Neurokinin-1 (NK-1) antagonists
  Maropitant (Cerenia)

Antidiarrheals
Narcotic (opioid) drugs
  Diphenoxylate (Lomotil)
  Loperamide (Imodium)
Bismuth subsalicylate (Pepto-Bismol, Kaopectate)
Ondansetron (Zofran)
Sulfasalazine (Azulfidine)

Adsorbents/Protectants
Bismuth
Liquid barium
Activated charcoal

Laxatives and Stool Softeners
Emollient laxatives
  Mineral oil
  Cod liver oil
  White petrolatum
  Glycerin
  Docusate sodium succinate (DSS, Colace)
Bulk laxatives
  Hydrophilic colloids (bran, psyllium, methylcellulose)

Cathartics
Osmotic (saline) cathartics
  Hypertonic salts (milk of magnesia, Epsom salts)
  Lactulose
Irritant cathartics
  Castor oil
  Bisacodyl (Dulcolax, Senokot)

Antacid/Antiulcer Drugs
Nonsystemic antacids
  Calcium carbonate (Tums, Rolaids)
  Magnesium hydroxide/aluminum hydroxide (Mylanta, Di-Gel, Maalox)
  Magnesium hydroxide (milk of magnesia)
  Aluminum hydroxide (Amphojel)
Systemic antacids or antiulcer drugs
  H_2 blockers
Cimetidine (Tagamet)
Famotidine (Pepcid)
Ranitidine (Zantac)
Nizatidine (Axid)
  Omeprazole (Prilosec OTC, Gastrogard, Ulcergard)
  Sucralfate (Carafate)
  Misoprostol (Cytotec)

Drugs Used for Rumen Health
Ruminatoric—prokinetic drugs
  Neostigmine
Ionophores
  Monensin (Rumensin)
Dioctyl sodium succinate (DSS)
Poloxalene

Antimicrobials
Tylosin (Tylan)
Metronidazole (Flagyl)
Erythromycin
Sulfasalazine (Azulfidine)

Additional Drugs Used to Treat GI Disease
Oral electrolyte replacements
Pancreatic enzyme supplements
  Pancrelipase (Viokase, Pancrezyme)
Corticosteroids

break down proteins. This condition, referred to as exocrine pancreatic insufficiency (EPI), causes a failure to properly digest food resulting in maldigestion (inadequate digestion) and subsequent malabsorption (inadequate absorption) of nutrients. The presence of these undigested nutrients creates an osmotic force that retains water in the lumen of the GI tract and may actually pull water from the body like a bulk laxative. The undigested fats will be acted upon by GI bacteria, resulting in rancid, malodorous, voluminous, pale, greasy diarrhea and subsequent weight loss.

In animals with EPI, pancreatic enzyme supplements or **pancrelipase** such as Viokase and Pancrezyme are added to the animal's food before feeding. Unfortunately, some commercially available enzyme supplements vary in their enzyme content, producing inconsistent results. Increased fat content in the diet can also reduce the enzyme supplement's effectiveness. In addition, the supplemental enzymes are denatured by the acidic environment of the stomach, rendering the lipase and proteinases (to a lesser degree) largely ineffective. Although recommendations on how best to administer these products varies, generally these enzyme products are mixed with the food at least 15–20 min before the food is offered. However, the effectiveness of lipase in breaking down fats in the food before ingestion is reduced because the enzyme depends on the proper temperature and pH to be fully active.

Because gastric acid inactivates these enzymes, it has been suggested that H_2 blockers such as cimetidine may decrease the breakdown of the enzyme supplement and make the pancreatic enzyme supplement more effective. Unfortunately, no significant improvement in fat digestion has been observed when cimetidine is used concurrently with the enzyme supplement, and the cost of the H_2 blocker may not justify its limited benefit.

Most enzyme supplements are in powder form but they are also available as tablets. The tablet form has been fairly ineffective in dogs unless crushed before administration. Enteric-coated enzyme tablets apparently have no advantage, even though the enteric coating protects the enzymes from the acidic environment of the stomach. The lack of efficacy with the enteric-coated enzymes may be related to insufficient dissolution of the coating or the relatively fast intestinal transit time in veterinary patients.

Thus, although many animals will show some resolution of the diarrhea and stabilizing of their weight, some animals with pancreatic exocrine insufficiency will continue to have subnormal digestion of fats and may not regain the weight lost since the onset of the disease.

Corticosteroids

Corticosteroid use in GI disease is controversial because the beneficial antiinflammatory effect is offset by immunosuppression (decreased immune function), increased gastric acid production, suppression of normal gastric protective and healing mechanisms, and increased risk of infection. Some chronic inflammatory bowel problems such as eosinophilic gastroenteritis may respond quite well to corticosteroids. If corticosteroids are going to be used in GI disease (or any disease), the smallest dose necessary to control clinical signs should be used, the dose should be decreased as soon as possible to minimize side effects, and the animal should be monitored closely for signs of gastric problems or other adverse systemic effects. Corticosteroids are discussed in greater detail in Chapter 13.

REFERENCES

1. Boothe DM. Gastrointestinal Pharmacology in Small Animal Clinical Pharmacology and Therapeutics. 2nd ed. Philadelphia: Saunders; 2012.
2. de la Pueta-Redondo VA, et al. Efficacy of maropitant for treatment and prevention of emesis caused by intravenous infusion of cisplatin in dogs. *Am J Vet Res.* 2007;68(1):48–56.
3. Papich MG. Drugs affecting gastrointestinal function. In: Riviere J, Papich M, eds. *Veterinary Pharmacology and Therapeutics.* Ames, Iowa: Wiley-Blackwell; 2009.
4. Plumb DC. Veterinary Drug Handbook. 7th ed. Ames, Iowa: Wiley-Blackwell; 2011.
5. Scherkl R, et al. Apomorphine-induced emesis in the dog: routes of administration, efficacy and synergism by naloxone. *J Vet Pharmacol Ther.* 1990;13(2):154–158.
6. Cullen LK. Xylazine and medetomidine in small animals. *Aust Vet J.* 1999;77(11):722–723.
7. Pfizer Animal Health. Drug Insert for Dexdomitor (Dexmedetomidine Hydrochloride); November 2012.
8. Bond GR. Home syrup of ipecac use does not reduce emergency department use or improve outcome. *Pediatrics.* 2003;112:1061–1064.
9. ASPCA. *What to Do If Your Pet Is Poisoned (Website).* www.aspca.org/pet-care/animal-poison-control/what-do-if-your-pet-poisoned. Accessed 6.13.22.
10. Casavant MJ, Fitch JA. Fatal hypernatremia from saltwater used as an emetic. *J Toxicol Clin Toxicol.* 2003;41:861–863.
11. KuKanich B. Clinical pharmacology of antiemetics in dogs and cats. In: *The Proceedings of the American Veterinary Medical Association Annual Meeting. St. Louis, MO;* July 2011.
12. Tobias KMH. A retrospective study on the use of acepromazine maleate in dogs with seizures. *J Am Anim Hosp Assoc.* 2006;42(4):283–289.
13. Garner JL, Kirby R, Rudloff E. The use of acepromazine in dogs with a history of seizures. In: *The Proceedings of the International Veterinary Emergency and Critical Care Symposium. Atlanta, Georgia;* 2004.
14. Pfizer Animal Health. Updated Drug Insert for Cerenia (Maropitant Citrate); May 2012.
15. Papich MG, Davis CA, Davis LE. Absorption of salicylate from an antidiarrheal preparation in dogs and cats. *J Am Anim Hosp Assoc.* 1987;23(2):221–226.
16. Washabau RJ. Evidence-based medicine: GI drugs in the ICU. In: *The Proceedings of the International Veterinary Emergency and Critical Care Symposium. New Orleans, LA;* 2007.
17. Parente NL, Bari Olivier N, Refsal KR, Johnson CA. Serum concentrations of gastrin after famotidine and omeprazole administration to dogs. *J Vet Intern Med.* 2014;28(5):1465–1470. https://doi.org/10.1111/jvim.12408.
18. Bersenas AM, Mathews KA, Allen DG, Conlon PD. Effects of ranitidine, famotidine, pantoprazole, and omeprazole on intragastric pH in dogs. *Am J Vet Res.* 2005;66(3):425–431.

19. Leib M. Drugs used to treat vomiting and upper GI diseases in dogs and cats. In: *The Proceedings of the Atlantic Coast Veterinary Conference. Atlantic City, NJ*; 2008.
20. Matsuoka T, et al. Review of monensin toxicosis in horses. *J Equine Vet Sci.* 1996;16(1):8–15.
21. Rasby R.J., et al. *Bloat Prevention and Treatment in Cattle, NebGuide: University of Nebraska-Lincoln Extension (Website).* http://extensionpublications.unl.edu/assets/html/g2018/build/g2018.htm. Accessed 6.13.22.
22. Westermarck E, et al. Tylosin-responsive chronic diarrhea in dogs. *J Vet Intern Med.* 2005;19(2):176–186.
23. Kilpienn S, et al. Effect of tylosin on dogs with diarrhea: a placebo-controlled, randomized, double-blinded, prospective clinical trial. *Acta Vet Scand.* 2011;53:26. http://www.actavetscand.com/content/53/1/26.

SELF-ASSESSMENT

1. Fill in the following blanks with the correct item from the Key Terms list

A. _____ This term is the adjective used to refer to items associated with the duodenum, jejunum, or ileum.

B. _____ This term is the adjective used to refer to items associated with the large intestine.

C. _____ This describes the type of digestion that occurs in the ruminant.

D. _____ This is a type of drug (not a specific drug name) that causes vomiting.

E. _____ This is the set of neurons in the brain that actually causes and coordinates the physical act of vomiting.

F. _____ This center in the brain has receptors that detect poisons, toxins, or other compounds in the blood or cerebral spinal fluid and sends signals to the structure that initiates vomiting.

G. _____ This receptor responds to the presence of substance P; blocking of this receptor reduces vomiting.

H. _____ These receptors are more prevalent in the dog's chemoreceptor trigger zone (CRTZ) than the cat's and are involved in vomiting associated with motion sickness; antimotion sickness drugs work via these receptors.

I. _____ These receptors are more prevalent in the cat CRTZ than the dog's and are involved with vomiting from common sedative drugs like xylazine.

J. _____ This is another name for 5-HT receptors.

K. _____ This is the structure in the inner ear that is responsible for balance.

L. _____ A type of drug (not a specific drug name) that produces vomiting by stimulating receptors in the CRTZ or emetic center.

M. _____ This term means "inflammation of the stomach."

N. _____ This term means the drug blocks the effects of acetylcholine and in so doing tends to block the effects of the parasympathetic nervous system (PSNS).

O. _____ This is a term applied to a type of drug to indicate that the drug increases motility in the stomach and the small intestine. Such drugs also tend to increase muscle tone of the lower esophagus, reducing reflux of stomach contents.

P. _____ This specific term means that a drug should not be used *unless the medical condition justifies the risk.*

Q. _____ This specific term means that a drug should not be used *regardless of the medical condition.*

R. _____ Type of diarrhea in which the cells along the wall of the intestinal tract pump fluid into the intestinal lumen to produce diarrhea.

S. _____ Biological poisons produced by intestinal bacteria.

T. _____ Type of diarrhea caused by leakage of electrolytes, plasma proteins, or blood through a damaged intestinal tract wall.

U. _____ Type of diarrhea associated with rapid transit of contents along the length of the bowel.

V. _____ Type of diarrhea caused by nonabsorbed osmotic particles that hold water in the gastrointestinal (GI) tract lumen or pull water from the body into the GI tract lumen.

W. _____ What "EPI" stands for in relation to GI-related disease.

X. _____ The type of intestinal contraction that mixes the contents of the bowel and provides resistance to flow of intestinal contents.

Y. _____ The type of intestinal contraction that propels food along the GI tract.

Z. _____ This term describes when an animal strains to defecate.

AA. _____ This term describes a segment of the GI tract that fails to contract.

AB. _____ This term describes stool that has a dark, tarry appearance, typically reflecting the presence of digested blood in the stool.

AC. _____ This is the compound that colonic bacteria metabolize sulfasalazine to produce an anti-inflammatory effect.

AD. _____ This is the condition called KCS that can result from the use of sulfonamide antibiotics.

AE. _____ Type of drug (not a specific drug) that works by making toxic molecules or irritating/disease-causing compounds stick to it, thus preventing their absorption.

AF. _____ Type of laxative that is a lubricant oil or stool softener.

AG. _____ Type of laxative that includes hydrophilic colloids like bran and methylcellulose from plant fiber.

AH. _____ These are the cells that produce hydrochloric acid in the stomach.

AI. _____ These are the cells in the stomach that produce the enzyme precursor pepsinogen.

AJ. _____ Stimulation of any of these three receptors found on acid-producing cells increases stomach acid production.

AK. _____ The histamine that stimulates H_2 receptors to increase acid production comes from these cells.

AL. _____ This compound normally is released from G cells and causes the stomach smooth muscles to relax; also increases gastric acid production.

AM. _____ This complex molecule forms the layer that protects the stomach lining from gastric acid.

AN. _____ This molecule is added to the mucous layer to neutralize the corrosive effect of the gastric acid that contacts the layer by making it more alkaline.

AO. _____ A family of compounds that are "local controllers" of many body systems. In the GI tract, they are generally considered to be protective of the stomach by increasing mucus production, decreasing acid production, and increasing blood supply to the stomach wall.

AP. _____ This is an enzyme that is activated by the precursor molecule secreted by the stomach cells coming into contact with the hydrochloric acid in the stomach.

AQ. _____ Type of antacid that must be absorbed into the body to be effective.

AR. _____ A type of drug (not a specific drug name) that increases the smooth muscle tone of the rumen to start it contracting again.

AS. _____ A type of drug (not a specific drug name) that facilitates the transport of selected ions across a cell's membrane.

AT. _____ This term means that bacteria or the toxins from bacteria are present in the bloodstream and usually denotes a severe medical condition.

AU. _____ Natural compound found in the intestinal tract that stimulates intestinal motility. This compound is similar in structure to the antibiotic erythromycin, which explains why erythromycin produces intestinal cramping as a side effect.

2. Fill in the following blanks with the correct drug from the Gastrointestinal Drug list. When practicing these questions, write out the answers on a separate sheet and focus on the appropriate spelling of these drug names.

   A. _____ Opioid emetic agent more effective in dogs than cats.

B. _____ Emetic agent more effective in cats than dogs. This drug is an alpha 2 agonist and is more commonly used as an injectable sedative.

C. _____ Locally acting emetic agent recommended for use if a locally acting agent is needed. Produces gastritis, especially in cats. Needs to be fresh.

D. _____ Phenothiazine antiemetic also used as a common veterinary tranquilizer.

E. _____ These two human drugs attach to and block H_1 receptors as their mechanism to decrease the effects of motion sickness.

F. _____ This prokinetic agent and antiemetic works by blocking dopamine (and probably serotonin) receptors on the CRTZ but also by increasing gastric and intestinal motility in the "normal" direction. This drug is still available as a human drug, unlike another member of this drug group that has been withdrawn from the human market and is only available by compounding.

G. _____ Serotonin antagonist antiemetic used to control vomiting from cancer chemotherapy in dogs or pancreatitis in cats that is poorly controlled by other antiemetic agents.

H. _____ Neurokinin-1 (NK-1) receptor antagonist antiemetic drug introduced in 2006 for control of motion-induced vomiting.

I. _____ These over-the-counter (OTC) opioid antidiarrhea drugs work by increasing segmental contractions and reducing intestinal secretions.

J. _____ This compound is broken down in the GI tract into a compound that coats the intestinal mucosa and another compound that is an aspirin-like antiinflammatory drug.

K. _____ This drug is an adjunct antidiarrheal drug that is also an antiemetic. It works by blocking 5-HT$_3$ receptors in the GI tract to reduce secretion of chloride ions and water.

L. _____ This drug is a sulfonamide antibiotic linked chemically to mesalamine (5-aminosalicylic acid), the latter compound being an antiinflammatory compound cleaved from the drug molecule by colonic bacteria to treat inflammatory colitis.

M. _____ This is the component of bismuth subsalicylate that is an adsorbent.

N. _____ This adsorbent is not usually used to treat diarrhea but is used to decrease absorption of ingested poisons. Is sometimes referred to as the "universal antidote."

O. _____ This emollient laxative is most commonly administered by stomach tube to horses to treat suspected impactions. A major risk of using this drug is aspiration because it has little taste.

P. _____ These two emollient laxatives are common ingredients of dog and cat laxatives used to treat hairballs.

Q. _____ This emollient laxative is used as a suppository to ease the passage of stool through the colon or rectum of animals with pelvic fractures or compression of the diameter of the pelvic canal.

R. _____ This emollient laxative is a stool softener that acts by allowing water to penetrate hard stool.

S. _____ This osmotic cathartic is also used to decrease ammonia absorption from the GI tract in patients with hepatic encephalopathy.

T. _____ These two irritant laxatives work by stimulating peristaltic activity and secretions into the bowel.

U. _____ These four drugs are H_2 antagonist antacids.

V. _____ Of the H_2 antagonist antacids, this is the one that most significantly inhibits hepatic enzymes by reducing biotransformation of other commonly used drugs and therefore requiring the veterinary technician check this drug's interaction with other drugs.

W. _____ Acid pump or proton pump inhibitor antacid.

X. _____ Antiulcer drug that forms a sticky paste that covers the ulcer.

Y. _____ Synthetic prostaglandin type E_1 drug that mimics the beneficial effects of natural GI tract prostaglandins.

Z. _____ Ruminatoric that acts by blocking acetylcholinesterase's destruction of the acetylcholine neurotransmitter.

AA. _____ Widely used ionophore in beef and dairy cattle to improve rumen health; is also used to reduce coccidiosis in livestock and poultry.

AB. _____ Stool softener also used to break up froth in frothy bloat.

AC. _____ Macrolide antibiotic used to treat both respiratory and GI tract bacterial infections in cattle and swine, as well as selected types of chronic diarrhea in the dog. Do not use it in horses.

AD. _____ Antibiotic developed initially to treat Giardia protozoa but has been found to also be effective in treating diarrhea of unknown origin in dogs and cats. Can cause neurologic side effects at higher doses or more prolonged use.

AE. _____ A macrolide antibiotic similar to tylosin that commonly causes cramping as a side effect but has also been used as a prokinetic agent to stimulate sluggish gastric emptying.

AF. _____ Pancreatic enzyme supplement for use in dogs with exocrine pancreatic insufficiency (EPI).

3. Indicate whether each effect or structure is associated with the parasympathetic (PSNS) or sympathetic nervous system (SNS):

A. _____ Emerges from the central nervous system as cranial nerves from the brainstem or peripheral nerves coming from the caudal portion of the spinal cord.

B. _____ Known as the "fight or flight" part of the autonomic nervous system.

C. _____ Vagus nerve (cranial nerve X).

D. _____ Stimulation of this part of the autonomic nervous system causes increased intestinal motility.

E. _____ Associated with norepinephrine and epinephrine effects.

F. _____ Acetylcholine is the neurotransmitter most often associated with these autonomic nervous system effects.

G. _____ Stimulation of this part of the autonomic nervous system increases GI tract secretion of digestive enzymes and acid.

H. _____ Stimulation of this part of the autonomic nervous system results in decreased perfusion of the GI tract.

4. Indicate in which of the following situations induction of vomiting would be APPROPRIATE. If the use of an emetic to induce vomiting is inappropriate, explain why.

A. A 3-month-old Labrador retriever puppy ingested a strong alkali cleaning agent 15 min ago.

B. A 2-year-old cat that otherwise appears normal ingested six of the owner's heart medication tablets 30 min ago.

C. Two hours ago, an 8-month-old golden retriever lapped up about a cup of a gasoline from a cup in which a paint brush was soaking.

D. Four hours ago, a 3-year-old Maltese mix ingested an unknown number of painkiller prescription tablets the owner had, and now the animal is semiconscious with depressed breathing and reflexes.

E. A 3-year-old "hunting dog" (German shorthair pointer mix) is presented with tonic-clonic seizures (muscles increase in tone, then begin to violently shake with rapid alternation between uncoordinated contract and relaxation). This comes after a suspected ingestion of a mole bait possibly as long as 3 h ago, but the owner is not entirely sure. Any stimulation of the patient causes an onset of seizure activity. Seizures are generating muscle heat, and the patient's body temperature is now in excess of 106°F.

F. A 4-year-old domestic shorthair cat ingested some spilled liquid cold medication 30 min ago, after which it almost immediately started vomiting and has been vomiting every 2–5 min since.

G. A 3-year-old quarter horse gelding ingested contaminated grain 30 min ago.

5. Indicate whether each statement is true or false.

A. Dogs are more sensitive to drugs that stimulate the dopamine receptor than cats.

B. Suppression of the nucleus tractus solitarius (NTS) would result in severe vomiting.

C. Drugs that stimulate the alpha receptors are more likely to cause vomiting in cats than dogs.

D. Histamine is one of the key compounds involved with the vestibular apparatus's production of motion sickness.

E. Apomorphine should be given by mouth instead of by injection because the injectable form is less effective.

F. One of the major concerns with using phenothiazine tranquilizers like acepromazine is the elevation of blood pressure in patients with heart disease.

G. One of the precautions veterinary technicians should advise owners who use the OTC drugs dimenhydrinate or diphenhydramine for motion sickness in their dogs is that the risk for increased hyperactivity and an increased heart rate is common with these drugs.

H. Substance P binds to and stimulates the NK-1 receptor, causing vomiting.

I. Exocrine pancreatic insufficiency results in a secretory or exudative diarrhea because of the increased irritation this insufficiency produces in the intestinal tract.

J. Increased segmental contractions would slow the progress of intestine lumen contents along the GI tract and increased peristaltic contractions would speed the progress.

K. Kaolin (kaolinite) and pectin are the main ingredients of the widely available human antidiarrheal drug Kaopectate.

L. Gastric acid rebound from use of local antacids is more common with aluminum antacids, like Amphojel, than it is with calcium carbonate antacids, like Tums or Rolaids.

6. Why should antihistamine drugs for motion sickness not be used before allergy skin testing?

7. With the exception of scopolamine used for motion sickness vomiting, why are anticholinergic drugs generally not considered very effective antiemetic agents?

8. In what conditions is metoclopramide relatively or absolutely contraindicated for use?

9. Why would the use of an anticholinergic drug like the scopolamine patch for motion sickness be a bad idea if the animal is also going to be treated with metoclopramide?

10. Why is it that an owner with a dog or cat exhibiting tenesmus thinks her pet is constipated? Why is she wrong?

11. How is it that an anticholinergic drug, which decreases intestinal motility and secretions, can actually increase diarrhea?

12. If anticholinergic drugs don't have any significant beneficial effect in controlling diarrhea, why is the anticholinergic drug atropine added to diphenoxylate (Lomotil) and loperamide (Imodium AD)?

13. Why should opioid antidiarrheal drugs be avoided in animals with Salmonella bacterial infections in the GI tract?

14. Why should one use drugs like diphenoxylate and loperamide with caution in collies and collie-like breeds?

15. Why should magnesium antacids like Mylanta, Di-Gel, Maalox, or milk of magnesia be avoided in patients with renal disease?

16. As a general rule, when drugs whose absorption may be impaired by antacids need to be given concurrently with antacid, how can a veterinary technician prevent the antacid from interfering with the drug's absorption?

17. Why must a veterinary patient not chew the capsule of omeprazole before swallowing it?

18. Why is metronidazole prohibited from use in food animals?

Drugs Affecting the Cardiovascular System

CHAPTER OUTLINE

OBJECTIVES

After studying this chapter, the veterinary technician should be able to:
- Describe the normal mechanism by which heart rate and force of contraction are regulated.
- Describe the normal mechanism by which the body maintains arterial blood pressure.
- Describe how these normal mechanisms are disrupted in congestive heart failure or arrhythmias.
- List the antiarrhythmic agents used in veterinary medicine and describe how they work.
- List the positive inotropic and inodilator drugs used in veterinary medicine and describe how they work.
- List the vasodilator drugs used in veterinary medicine and describe how they work.
- List the diuretics used in veterinary medicine and describe how they work.

KEY TERMS

ACE inhibitor
acetazolamide
adenosine triphosphate (ATP)
adrenergic agonists
adrenergic neurons, receptors
afterload
aldosterone
alpha-1, alpha-2 (α_1, α_2) receptors
angiotensin I and II
angiotensin-converting enzyme (ACE)
antagonist

aorta
aortic valve
arrhythmia
arteries
arterioles
atrioventricular (AV) block; first and second degree
atrioventricular (AV) node
atrioventricular (AV) valve
automaticity
baroreceptors

beta-1 (β_1) and beta-2 (β_2) receptors
beta (β) agonists, antagonists, and blockers
bradycardia/bradyarrhythmia
bundle branches
cardiomyopathy
catecholamine receptors
chlorothiazide
compensated and decompensated heart failure

conduction cells
congestive heart failure
depolarize
depolarization wave
digoxin
diuretic
dobutamine
dopamine
downregulation
ectopic focus
epinephrine
fast sodium channels
fibrillation: atrial or
    ventricular
flutter: atrial or ventricular
furosemide (Lasix)
hydrochlorothiazide
hypertension
inodilators
loop of Henle
mannitol
mitral valve

muscarinic cholinergic
    receptors
negative inotropic effect
nicotinic cholinergic
    receptors
nitroglycerin
norepinephrine
pacemaker
paroxysm
pimobendan
polarized
positive inotropic drug
preload
premature ventricular
    contractions (PVC)
PR interval
pulmonary arteries and
    veins
pulmonic valve
Purkinje fibers
P wave
QRS wave or complex

renin-angiotensin-aldosterone system
repolarization
right and left atrium
right and left ventricles
refractory period: absolute and relative
sinoatrial (SA) node
sodium-potassium-adenosine triphosphatase
    (sodium-potassium-ATPase) pump
spironolactone
supraventricular arrhythmia
supraventricular tachycardia
T wave
tachycardia/tachyarrhythmia
threshold
tolerance
tricuspid valve
upregulation
vena cava, venae cavae
venodilator
ventricular arrhythmia
ventricular tachycardia

Cardiovascular disease includes diseases that disrupt or alter the normal functioning of the heart and the blood vessels in the body. Cardiovascular disease often has a series of stages that can increasingly affect other body systems as the disease progresses. Because veterinary technicians take histories on cardiac patients, monitor cardiac patients during hospitalization, explain the effects and side effects of dispensed cardiac drugs to owners, and monitor the patient's status at home through follow-up phone calls, the well-educated veterinary technician should have a working knowledge of the normal physiology of the cardiovascular system and how cardiac drugs alter this normal physiology to achieve the therapeutic outcome. In addition, understanding how these drugs work helps the veterinary technician better understand the mechanisms by which signs of the beneficial effects or toxic side effects will appear in the patient.

This chapter presents principles of cardiac drug use. Cardiac drugs often have complex mechanisms of action and side effects affecting multiple body systems. For the sake of brevity and focus, many specifics of individual cardiac drug mechanisms and less common side effects have been excluded. Because of the complexities of these drugs and because multiple cardiac drugs may be used simultaneously, the veterinary professional should always review the package insert or published information on the specific cardiac drugs before administering them to a veterinary patient.

NORMAL CARDIAC FUNCTION

Many dynamic feedback mechanisms regulate the function of the cardiovascular system and blood pressure. This chapter contains a brief review of cardiovascular physiology and pathology as it applies to drug mechanisms. More detailed information on heart disease or regulation of the cardiovascular system can be found in veterinary cardiology, physiology, and internal medicine textbooks and resources.

Think of the Heart as Being Two Pumps

Essentially, the mammalian heart acts like a two-pump system. A fairly small pump on the right side of the heart pumps blood to the lungs and back to the heart, and a larger, stronger pump on the left pumps blood throughout the remainder of the body and back to the heart. The vessels returning blood to the right side of the heart are the venae cavae (anterior vena cava from the head, posterior vena cava from the trunk). Blood flows from the venae cavae into the right atrium, through the tricuspid, or right atrioventricular (AV) valve, and then into the right ventricle. From the right ventricle, blood is pumped through the pulmonic valve (pulmonary refers to the lungs) into the pulmonary arteries, to the lungs, and back to the heart by the pulmonary veins (Fig. 5.1).

This highly oxygenated blood in the pulmonary veins passes into the left atrium, where it is stopped from flowing into the larger and more muscular left ventricle by the mitral, or left atrioventricular (AV), valve. After passing into the left ventricle, blood is expelled from the left ventricle through the aortic valve into the large aorta that branches off into smaller vessels that carry blood to all parts of the body.

As was explained briefly with the intravenous (IV) route of drug administration, veins as a general rule carry blood toward the heart and arteries carry blood away from the heart. Drugs administered intravenously are carried by the blood toward the right side of the heart, where they mix with other blood

HEAD AND UPPER EXTREMITY

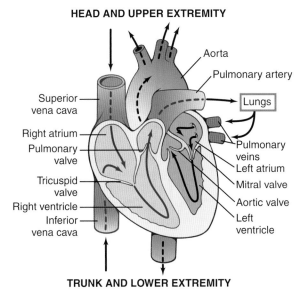

TRUNK AND LOWER EXTREMITY

Fig. 5.1 Anatomy of the heart. (From Hall J, Guyton A. *Guyton and Hall Textbook of Medical Physiology*. 12th ed. Philadelphia: Saunders; 2011.)

returning from the body, and are pumped to the lungs and back to the left side of the heart, where they then are pushed by the left ventricle to all of the tissues in the body. Thus, IV-administered drugs are diluted by the blood volume before they reach the target tissues. In contrast, drugs administered intraarterially will deliver all of the drug to the organ or tissue supplied by that artery. If given accidentally, the high concentration of drug delivered to the organ or tissue can produce a local toxicity in the tissue supplied by the artery. In special cases where a high concentration of antibiotic is intended to be delivered to a specific tissue (e.g., infected bone tissue), the intraarterial route of administration may be intentionally used by injecting the drug into a specific artery that supplies the particular targeted tissue.[1]

It is important to remember that the purpose of the valves in the heart is only to allow blood to flow in a single direction and to prevent blood from flowing backward. Valves do not pump blood but only open and close passively in response to changes in blood pressure on either side of the valve. For example, when the atria contract, the increased pressure inside the atrial chambers forces open the AV valves (mitral and tricuspid valves) and pushes blood into the relaxed ventricles. However, when the ventricles begin to contract and increase the pressure within the ventricular chambers high enough to exceed the pressure in the atria, the AV valves will slam shut, preventing blood from flowing backward into the atria. The increased pressure in the ventricles forces open the aortic and pulmonic valves, ejecting blood into the aorta and pulmonary arteries. Then the ventricles relax and the ventricular chamber pressure drops below the pressure in the aorta and pulmonary artery, and the aortic and pulmonic valves slam shut to prevent blood from flowing back into the ventricles. This sudden closing of the valves in response to the pressure change is the "lubb-dupp" sound heard when auscultating the heart.[1]

Cardiac disease related to the mechanical function of the heart occurs when either the muscular chambers of the heart fail to contract with sufficient strength; the valves fail to close or open completely; or unnatural holes connect chambers or major vessels, allowing blood to flow in abnormal directions.

❗ YOU NEED TO KNOW

What Are Preload and Afterload?

Veterinarians often talk about "preload" and "afterload" being affected by cardiac disease. As a veterinary technician, knowing what these terms mean can help understand the physical changes occurring within a patient.

Preload refers to the pressure exerted on the myocytes (muscle cells) within the walls of the ventricles by the "load" or volume of blood in the ventricles just before ventricular contraction. In other words, the force of the blood entering and stretching the ventricles during ventricular diastole (the relaxation phase between contractions) is the preload, and it correlates with the amount of blood that fills the ventricular chambers (called end diastolic volume). The greater the volume of blood pushed into the ventricles by the atria and the returning venous blood flow, the greater the preload.

Preload would decrease if blood volume were decreased by significant dehydration or blood loss because with less volume there is less "force" pushing the blood into the ventricles. Anything that decreases venous blood pressure or venous return (volume of blood returning to the heart) will result in a decreased preload.

Drugs can decrease preload by decreasing venous blood pressure through diuresis (decreased blood volume as the result of water loss through the kidneys) or vasodilation. In contrast, IV fluids can increase preload by increasing the overall volume of blood returning to the heart and hence the pressure by which blood is pushed into the ventricles.

If preload increases too much, the increased pressure within the ventricles during the relaxation phase (diastole) will cause pressure to increase "upstream" in the incoming venous return system (large veins carrying blood back to the heart from the body). When pressure within the venous system increases, it eventually also increases pressure within capillaries that feed into the veins. Remember that capillaries are "leaky" and have fenestrations that allow small molecules like water to readily leave the capillary. When pressure builds up in the capillaries, water is pushed out into the tissues and edema, ascites (fluid in the abdomen), or pulmonary edema occurs. Thus, an increased preload can result in signs of edema or fluid accumulation in body tissues.

Afterload refers to the tension or pressure the ventricles must create to eject blood out of the ventricles and into the aorta and pulmonary arteries. If the animal has a disease that makes it harder (takes more ventricular contraction pressure or effort) to eject the blood from the ventricles, the animal has a greater afterload. Diseases like systemic hypertension (increased blood pressure within systemic arteries) create a greater afterload on the left ventricle because the increased blood pressure already in the aorta and the rest of the arterial system "pushes back" against any blood trying to be ejected from the left ventricle and added to the arteries.

An aortic stenosis (narrowing of the opening around the aortic valve) creates an increased afterload because the stricture creates resistance against which the ventricles must push harder to eject blood into the aorta.

In contrast to the aortic stenosis, a mitral valve insufficiency (damage to the valve between the left atrium and left ventricle) creates a decreased afterload on the left ventricle because in addition to the blood ejected in the normal direction into the aorta, some of the blood from the left ventricle flows backward into the left atrium through the defective mitral valve. Because there are more paths for the blood to flow from the ventricle, it is easier to eject more of the blood from the left ventricle and the afterload is decreased.

Drugs like arteriole vasodilators decrease afterload by opening up the small arterioles, decreasing the resistance of blood flowing through these arterioles, and making it easier (requiring less pressure or force of contraction) for the left ventricle to eject blood into the aorta. Less effort means less afterload.

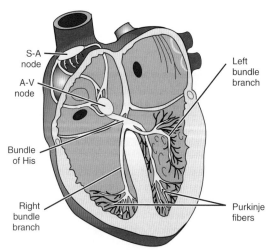

Fig. 5.2 Anatomy of the conduction system. (Modified from Tilley LP. *Essentials of Canine and Feline Electrocardiography: Interpretation and Treatment.* 4th ed. St. Louis: Saunders; 2008.)

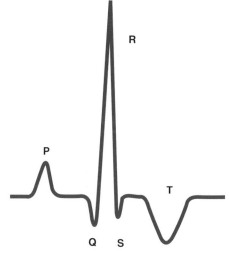

Fig. 5.3 Basic components of the electrocardiogram (ECG): P wave, QRS wave, and T wave.

Electrical Conduction Through the Heart

The coordinated mechanical contraction of the heart is totally dependent on the proper electrical conduction of the depolarization wave, or "firing" of cells through the heart (Fig. 5.2). All of the cardiac muscle cells are linked to each other such that if a stimulus is applied to one part of the heart, theoretically the entire heart could contract at once. However, this would result in very inefficient pumping of blood (think of squeezing a tube of toothpaste along its entire length all at once). Because such simultaneous or uncoordinated contraction would result in ineffective pumping of blood, the electrical activity and the depolarization wave must produce a specific sequence of coordinated muscle contractions to eject the blood most effectively.

There are two general types of cardiac muscle cells that make up the heart: the contractile muscle cells that actually pump the blood and modified muscle cells called conduction cells that initiate and conduct the depolarization wave along a specific conduction pathway so that the muscle cells contract in the proper order. The conduction cells in each segment of the specialized conduction pathway possess automaticity, which is the ability to depolarize (fire) spontaneously and independently without any external stimulation to do so. If one of these specialized cardiac muscle cells were to be removed from the heart and placed in a special physiologic solution to keep it alive, the cell would spontaneously depolarize at a rate determined by that cell's physical and biochemical makeup.

A group of specialized conduction cells in the right atrium (Fig. 5.2) depolarizes more rapidly than any other cells in the heart. By doing so, these cells set the pace of depolarization of the heart and subsequent contraction that is felt as a pulse rate. This group of cells is called the sinoatrial (SA) node and is often referred to as the heart's pacemaker. Cells in the SA node depolarize about 15 times per minute in the adult horse and around 350 times per minute in the rat: larger species generally have slower rates than smaller ones.[2,3]

Because the cardiac muscle fibers are connected to each other, SA node depolarization sends a wave of depolarization

outward in all directions through the right atrium and left atrium. As the wave of depolarization passes from one cardiac muscle cell to another, each cell contracts. This wave passes so quickly that both atria contract almost simultaneously, pushing blood through the AV valves into the ventricles. On the electrocardiogram (ECG) strip, this atrial depolarization (and subsequent contraction of atrial muscle cells) appears as a small bump or deflection called the P wave. The wave components of the ECG shown in Fig. 5.3 proceed in alphabetical order, from P through T, as the strip is viewed from left to right.

The wave of depolarization spreads around the atria but is prevented from entering the ventricles by a cellular barrier that acts like an electric insulator. In normal animals, the depolarization wave can only reach the ventricles through a specialized cluster of conducting cells called the atrioventricular (AV) node. The atrial wave of depolarization enters the atrial side of the AV node and is delayed there for a fraction of a second before entering the ventricles. This short delay allows the atria to complete their contraction and physically move the blood from the atria into the ventricles before the ventricles are stimulated to contract. Without this slight delay in the AV node, the atria and ventricles would contract at the same time and blood would not be pumped efficiently. On the ECG, this period of conduction delay in the AV node shows up as a flat line after the P wave and is referred to as the PR interval or the P-QRS interval in reference to the atrial P wave and the large QRS wave or QRS complex that represents ventricular depolarization.

After the depolarization wave passes through the AV node, it travels rapidly in the interventricular septum (wall between the right and left ventricles) along a specialized conduction cell pathway that splits into right and left parallel tracts known as the bundle branches. The bundle branches rapidly conduct the electrical impulse to the Purkinje fibers located at the apex of the heart (the conical end or "bottom of the heart"). The depolarization wave finally emerges from the Purkinje fibers at the apex and spreads rapidly throughout the ventricular muscle cells, causing them to contract from the apex toward the heart valves, pushing blood through the pulmonic and aortic valves and out to the lungs and body.

Depolarization (and contraction) of the ventricles is seen on the ECG as a large three-part wave called the *QRS complex*. The QRS complex is composed of a very small Q wave, a much larger R wave, and a small S wave, all clumped together. After the ventricles contract, the ventricular muscle cells relax and repolarize (reset) to prepare electrically for the next depolarization wave. This period of ventricular repolarization appears as the T wave on the ECG strip.

An ECG pattern shows the way electrical impulses travel through the heart. Any deviation from the normal pattern of cardiac depolarization or repolarization is referred to as an arrhythmia and can appear as abnormal P waves, bizarre QRS complexes, or skewed T waves. It is important to remember that the ECG is not used to diagnose mechanical abnormalities of the heart (such as poorly functioning valves or weak cardiac muscle); it is only useful in identifying electrical abnormalities in the conduction pathway or in detecting an increase in overall mass of the heart as reflected by the longer period of time it takes for the enlarged atria and ventricles to completely depolarize (seen as enlarged or wide P waves or QRS complexes).[4]

What Are Depolarization and Repolarization?

When a cardiac cell or specialized conducting cell "fires," it is said to depolarize. When a cell resets itself in preparation to fire again, it is called repolarization. What actually happens in depolarization and repolarization is a small set of charged ions (sodium ($[Na^+]$), potassium ($[K^+]$), and calcium ($[Ca^{2+}]$)) exchange places across the cardiac cell membrane, changing the relative charge on either side of the cell membrane. This change in cellular charge causes the cardiac muscle cells to contract but also stimulates adjacent cells to depolarize, setting off a rolling wave of depolarization that extends from cell to cell and eventually causes the entire heart to contract. Because many cardiac drugs affect depolarization or repolarization, either as an intended effect or as a side effect, the veterinary technician should have a basic understanding of the processes that take place within cardiac cells during depolarization and repolarization.

The cycle of depolarization and repolarization may be compared with the mechanics of a mousetrap. A mousetrap is set by moving the spring-loaded wire loop into place. After the trap is tripped by the mouse and snaps shut, it cannot snap (i.e., fire) again until it is reset. In its *resting state*, a cardiac cell is much like the mousetrap: ready to snap when triggered to do so. When the cardiac cell is stimulated, it fires or depolarizes and, like the tripped (i.e., depolarized) mousetrap, the cardiac cell cannot depolarize again until it repolarizes (i.e., resets). Repolarization of the cardiac cell would be like resetting the mousetrap to fire again.

Depolarization and repolarization of cardiac cells, skeletal muscle cells, and neurons primarily involve movement of sodium (Na^+) and potassium (K^+) ions across the cell membrane (Fig. 5.4A–C). In its resting state, the cell is polarized, meaning that it has two distinct "poles," or segregated areas, of electrical charge on either side of the cell membrane. In resting cells, the polarization occurs between sodium ions, which are found in high concentrations outside the cell membrane, and potassium ions, which are found in high concentrations inside the cell membrane (Fig. 5.4A). At resting state, some sodium ions (Na^+) may still leak into the cell, and some potassium ions (K^+) leak out of the cell. Thus, to keep sodium ions at high concentrations outside the cell and potassium concentrations high inside the cell, the cell continually expends energy to pump stray Na^+ ions back out of the cell while simultaneously pumping stray K^+ ions back into the cell. The pump that maintains the separation of sodium and potassium is a specialized

! YOU NEED TO KNOW

It Is Not Just Table Salt

Sodium and chloride together are table salt. Potassium is often used in food as a "salt substitute." However, when it comes to normal functions in the body, the distribution and concentrations of sodium, chloride, and potassium are tightly regulated. These three ions constitute the largest numbers of ions in the body, and any disruption of their location or numbers causes significant malfunction of nerves and muscles. The body expends a tremendous amount of energy to pump these ions or *electrolytes* so that there are significant ion concentration differences on either side of the cell membranes.

The highest concentrations of sodium and chloride ions are mostly located *outside* of cells, and the highest concentrations of potassium ions are mostly located *inside* cells. Sodium (Na^+) is positively charged and chloride (Cl^-) is negatively charged. Because opposite charges attract each other, where sodium goes chloride wants to follow. Potassium (K^+) is also a positively charged ion. This unequal distribution of positive and negative ions on either side of a cell membrane is what allows nerves and muscles to "fire" when stimulated. Anything that alters ion concentrations or the body's ability to keep these ions in unequal distribution across a cell membrane damages the function of nerves and muscles.

For example, in kidney disease or damage potassium ions accumulate outside of the cell in the tissue fluid to higher than normal concentrations (potassium is usually concentrated inside the cell). When this happens the normal flow of sodium and potassium ions during depolarization and repolarization is disrupted, and muscles or nerves are unable to contract or fire. The same thing happens if too much potassium is administered in IV fluids. Indeed, such high accumulation of potassium in the blood or tissue fluids can stop the heart and cause death. This is why potassium is sometimes given IV as part of a euthanasia protocol.

If too much chloride (normally an extracellular ion) enters a nerve cell, the nerve cell will become more negative than normal and will not be able to fire when stimulated to do so. When this occurs in the brain, the neurons fail to depolarize and the brain is unable to function.

A lowered concentration of sodium in the blood or tissue fluids (sodium is normally found in high concentrations outside of the cell) will also disrupt nerves or muscles from firing also by disrupting the normal flow of ions during depolarization or repolarization.

Thus, tight regulation of sodium, potassium, and chloride ions is necessary for the life and normal function of the animal. As a veterinary technician, it is important to never take administration of these ions or electrolytes in IV fluids lightly because a miscalculation or an accidental administration of chloride, potassium, or sodium could result in serious harm or death of a patient.

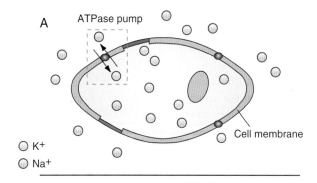

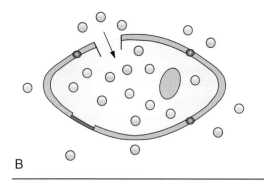

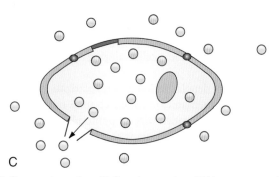

Fig. 5.4 Changes in sodium (Na$^+$) and potassium (K$^+$) ion concentration during depolarization and repolarization. (A) In the resting state, the Na$^+$/K$^+$ ATPase pump keeps K$^+$ concentrations high inside the cell while keeping Na$^+$ inside the cell low by pumping Na$^+$ out of the cell. (B) During depolarization, the fast Na$^+$ channels open, allowing Na$^+$ to rapidly move into the cell driven by its concentration gradient. (C) During repolarization, the Na$^+$ channels close, the K$^+$ channels open, and K$^+$ moves out of the cell. When the potassium channels close, the Na$^+$/K$^+$ ATPase pump returns the potassium back inside the cell and moves the sodium inside the cell back out to reset the cell to be depolarized again.

protein located within the cell membrane called the sodium-potassium-adenosine triphosphatase (sodium-potassium-ATPase) pump. The enzyme *ATPase* creates the energy needed for the pump's active transport of sodium and potassium by breaking down adenosine triphosphate (ATP), which is the cell's stored energy molecule.

The cardiac cell remains in this p"lari'ed resting state until the appropriate stimulus occurs. This stimulus is either the depolarization of adjoining cardiac cells or a change in electrical charge within the cardiac cell itself. When the stimulus occurs, the fast sodium (Na$^+$) channels snap open, allowing Na$^+$ to rapidly flood into the cell. The Na$^+$ is pushed inside by the concentration gradient of high sodium outside the cell to low sodium inside and also by the negatively charged intracellular proteins that attract

the positively charged sodium ions (Fig. 5.4B). This rapid sodium influx is called depolarization because the two ion populations are no longer kept separated or polarized across the cellular membrane. Depolarization of skeletal muscle cells and neurons is essentially the same process as described for cardiac cells.

As the positively charged Na$^+$ ions flood into the cell during depolarization, the net charge inside the cardiac cell becomes more positive (phase 0 in Fig. 5.5). When the charge within the cell becomes positive enough, the fast Na$^+$ channels close and the K$^+$ channels open (Fig. 5.4C). With the potassium channels open, the concentration gradient of K$^+$ (high inside the membrane, low outside) and the increasingly positive charge within the cell caused by the influx of positive sodium ions drives the K$^+$ out of the cell, taking with them their positive charges and causing the charge inside of the cardiac cell to become more negative again. This movement of K$^+$ out of the cell is called repolarization because the ion populations are once again separated and the cell is polarized again.

When neurons or skeletal muscle fibers repolarize, the potassium outflow causes repolarization to occur very rapidly, much as described in the previous paragraph. However, when cardiac muscle cells start to repolarize (phase 1 in Fig. 5.5) they have a plateau phase that occurs as the potassium starts to flow out during initial repolarization. During this plateau phase (phase 2 in Fig. 5.5), Ca^{2+} and some Na$^+$ ions continue to move into the cell through so-called slow channels, thus maintaining the positive charge inside the cell despite the K$^+$ beginning to flow out. Once these slow Ca^{2+} and Na$^+$ channels close, repolarization continues rapidly from the continued potassium outflow (phase 3 in Fig. 5.5) until the baseline charge is achieved and the cell enters the resting state again (phase 4 in Fig. 5.5). The cardiac muscle cell remains in phase 4 until stimulated to depolarize again.

Note how at the completion of K$^+$ efflux of repolarization, the Na$^+$ and K$^+$ ions are located on the "wrong" sides of the cellular membrane, having passed through their respective channels during depolarization and repolarization. At this point, the sodium-potassium pump quickly reestablishes the correct location of Na$^+$ and K$^+$ by pumping the Na$^+$ out of the cell and pumping the K$^+$ into the cell. Once the sodium and potassium ions are relocated, the cell is ready to depolarize once again (Fig. 5.5).

Conduction Cells Depolarize Differently From Cardiac Muscle Cells

The specialized cells of the heart's electrical cardiac conduction system (SA node, AV node, bundle branches, Purkinje cells) depolarize and repolarize with sodium and potassium in the same way as cardiac muscle cells, except that the conduction cells do not have a plateau phase, and their phase 4 is slightly different.

Note how the part of the line in phase 4 of the cardiac muscle cell (Fig. 5.5) remains flat and the charge inside the cell remains the same until the cell is stimulated to depolarize again. However, unlike the cardiac muscle cell, the phase 4 in the conduction cell moves gradually upward immediately after completion of repolarization. This increased intracellular positive charge during phase 4 is because of the inherent "leakiness" of the conducting cell membrane which, in turn, allows sodium (Na$^+$) and some calcium (Ca^{2+}) ions to slowly and continuously move into the cell.

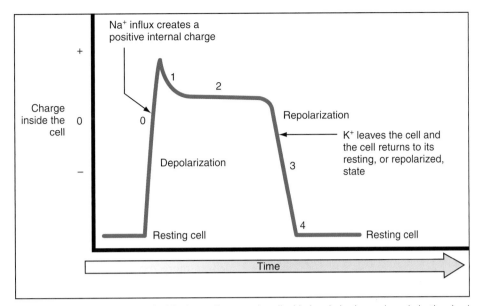

Fig. 5.5 Phases of charge changes inside the cardiac muscle cell with depolarization and repolarization. In phase 0, the sodium fast channels have opened, allowing positive sodium ions to rush into the cell and making it more positive inside. Shortly after this sodium influx the sodium channels close and potassium channels open. The positive potassium leaving the cell starts to cause the change to inside the cell to become less positive in phase 1. However, in phase 2 the opening of other sodium slow channels and calcium channels causes a further influx of positively charged ions that offsets the loss of the potassium, creating a plateau at phase 2 of the depolarization/repolarization curve. When the slow sodium and calcium channels shut, the continued outward movement of positive potassium ions now takes the charge inside the cell to the negatively charged baseline in phase 3. The potassium channels close at the beginning of phase 4, and the sodium-potassium-ATPase pump redistributes the sodium ions from phase 0 back outside the cell while moving the potassium ions from phase 1, 2, and 3 back into the cell. Because there is no net change in charge inside the cell at this point, the line in phase 4 remains flat until the next stimulus opens the fast sodium channels to begin phase 0 again.

Once the phase 4 slope attains a certain level of positive charge (called the threshold), the conducting cell depolarizes (fires), opening sodium and calcium channels and allowing the ions to flow in producing the characteristic phase 0 positive charge upswing associated with depolarization. Like with the cardiac muscle cells, conduction cell repolarization is caused by the potassium moving out of the cell, returning the cell charge back toward baseline. However, as soon as the "resting state" charge has been reestablished in the conducting cell at the end of phase 3, the charge inside the conducting cell again begins creeping upward. This continued cycle of leaking and depolarization without any external stimulus explains why these cells exhibit automaticity and can spontaneously fire on their own. The rate at which the conducting cell leaks sodium and calcium in phase 4 determines the inherent rate at which the conducting cell depolarizes spontaneously. The faster the leak, the quicker the cell depolarizes again.

Because the SA node has the "leakiest" conducting cells, the SA nodal cells reach the threshold more quickly than the rest of the cells in the conducting system and therefore set the rate or pace at which the heart contacts. Because the SA node sets this pace, it is called the pacemaker of the heart. If a cell elsewhere in the heart becomes injured or damaged by disease and becomes leakier than the cells in the SA node, this cell can acquire a more rapid automaticity and begin to fire on its own at a rate faster than the SA node, making this cell an abnormal pacemaker that produces irregular heartbeats or abnormal rhythms called arrhythmias. This topic will be discussed further with the antiarrhythmic drugs.

The Refractory Period

After a cardiac cell has depolarized, it cannot depolarize again until it has completed the repolarization phase of the cycle. The time in the depolarization/repolarization cycle when the cardiac cell cannot again depolarize is called the refractory period. The refractory period is divided into the **absolute refractory period** and the **relative refractory period**. A cardiac cell (or nerve) is absolutely refractory to depolarization stimulus during phase 0 of the cycle because no matter how strongly the cell is stimulated again to depolarize, it cannot open the sodium channels that are already open. Thus, no amount of stimulus can cause another depolarization and the cell is considered absolutely refractory to such stimulus.

As the sodium channels close and the cell begins to repolarize in phases 2 and 3, a sufficiently strong stimulus may be able to cause the sodium channels to open again and elicit a weak depolarization response. The cell is said to be relatively refractory to stimulus at this point because only a stronger than normal stimulus can evoke a depolarization response. As the cycle continues into phase 3, the cell becomes less refractory to depolarization stimuli and can produce a stronger depolarization response if given a sufficiently strong stimulus.

The refractory period is essential to prevent a wave of depolarization from traveling continuously from one end of the heart to the other and back again in a continuous and uncontrolled series of depolarization waves. For example, when the SA node depolarizes and sends a wave of depolarization around the atria, the wave is stopped when it encounters already depolarized cells that are in the refractory period of the cycle. If the refractory period of cells in the atria were shortened for some reason and the cells were capable of depolarizing again when the depolarization wave returned, the wave would continue on and the coordinated contraction of the heart would quickly turn into a continuous series of rapid, uncoordinated contractions. Such uncoordinated muscle contractions are called flutter or fibrillation of the atria or ventricles.

ROLE OF THE AUTONOMIC NERVOUS SYSTEM IN CARDIOVASCULAR FUNCTION

As mentioned in Chapter 4, regarding the gastrointestinal (GI) tract function, the autonomic nervous system is composed of the sympathetic and parasympathetic branches and automatically regulates many organ and system functions at an unconscious level (Fig. 5.6).

◎ MYTHS AND MISCONCEPTIONS

The Term "Vasoconstriction" Makes It Sound Like All of the Blood Vessels Are Squeezing Down and Constricting

False! When vasoconstriction occurs, it does not squeeze the entire circulatory system but only a very small part of it. Large blood vessels like the aorta or the arteries are too thick-walled to be compressed significantly by the smooth muscle in their walls. Thus, vasoconstriction only occurs at the arterioles (small arteries), which are very small blood vessels located between the arteries and the single-cell-wall-thick capillaries. The thin wall of these precapillary arterioles only contains one or two layers of smooth muscle that can squeeze the vessel when stimulated by drugs, natural catecholamines (epinephrine and norepinephrine), or other hormones that regulate blood pressure.

When precapillary arterioles constrict all over the body, the resistance to blood flow is increased, making it harder for the heart to push blood through these constricted arterioles. Because the heart continues to pump blood into the aorta and arterial system, this increased resistance at the end of the arterial system causes the blood to "back up" in the arteries, resulting in increased arterial blood pressure. When these same smooth muscles in the arterioles relax, the arterioles dilate and blood flows more readily through them, dropping the arterial blood pressure. Thus, vasoconstriction and vasodilation of precapillary arterioles are two of the most important mechanisms in regulating blood pressure.

When the veterinary technician measures the *capillary refill time* (CRT) by pressing on an animal's gums and counting how long it takes for the color to return to the pressed area, she is measuring both the resistance to blood flow back into the capillaries (presence or absence of vasoconstriction) and the arterial pressure that is pushing the blood from the arteries into the arterioles and capillaries. Vasoconstriction from epinephrine, norepinephrine, or other vasoconstrictive substances in the body would prolong the CRT (it would take longer for the capillary to refill with blood), whereas vasodilation would result in a shorter CRT. Animals with any condition that drops arterial blood pressure (e.g., hemorrhage, dehydration, shock) will display a prolonged CRT because the arterial blood pressure driving the blood into the capillaries is reduced; in addition, the body is causing profound vasoconstriction (and hence increasing resistance to flow) in an attempt to raise the arterial blood pressure. The combination of these two factors explains why animals that are in shock from being hit by a car, are profoundly dehydrated from profuse diarrhea, or have lost blood because of acute hemorrhage will have a prolonged CRT.

The Sympathetic Nervous System Control of the Cardiovascular System

In the cardiovascular system, the sympathetic nervous system (the "fight or flight" response system) increases the rate and force of contraction of the heart, elevates blood pressure, causes constriction of small peripheral arterioles (small artery blood vessels), decreases perfusion of nonessential organs and tissues, dilates arterioles in the skeletal muscle to increase blood flow, decreases activity of the GI tract, dilates the bronchioles, and dilates the pupil size.

All these functions improve the body's ability to survive a "fight or flight" crisis. Bronchodilation allows more oxygen to reach the alveoli of the lungs and oxygenate the blood. The increased heart rate and force of contraction plus the dilation of the arterioles in the skeletal muscle deliver more oxygenated blood to the skeletal muscles so they can function to fight or flee. Because there is a limited volume of blood, the blood supply must be directed away from the skin, GI tract, and the kidney by vasoconstriction and sent to the vasodilated skeletal muscle blood vessels instead. The combination of peripheral arteriole vasoconstriction and increased heart rate causes increased arterial blood pressure, much in the same way that blowing through one end of a rubber tube and squeezing off the other end would cause an increase in pressure within the tube. The increased arterial blood pressure helps assure fight or flight tissues are receiving adequate oxygenated blood supply during the crisis. These emergency responses occur very rapidly and are normally intended only for short-term changes needed to remove or defend the animal from danger. Persistent sympathetic response can be damaging to the body over time.

The sympathetic nervous system response is the result of two neurotransmitter hormones: epinephrine (old name: adrenaline) released from the adrenal medulla (the center of the adrenal gland) and norepinephrine released from adrenergic neurons (adrenergic: referring to adrenaline). Norepinephrine, **epinephrine**, and similarly structured molecules like dopamine are collectively called *catecholamines*. These catecholamines bind to **adrenergic receptors**, which are also called catecholamine receptors. The combination of the catecholamines with the adrenergic receptors found on tissues and organs produces the physiologic changes observed as the fight or flight response.

Any drugs that have intrinsic activity on these receptors can mimic the effects of epinephrine and norepinephrine and are called adrenergic agonists. They may also be called *sympathomimetic drugs* because their actions mimic the catecholamine sympathetic nervous system effects. In contrast, drugs that are able to bind to these receptors but have no intrinsic activity are called *adrenergic antagonists* because they block catecholamine molecules from combining with the receptors and, in so doing, block the sympathetic effect.

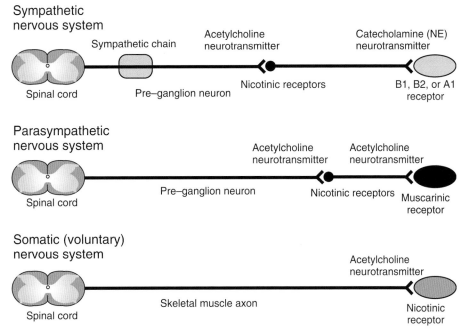

Sympathetic nervous system

Sympathetic chain

Acetylcholine neurotransmitter

Catecholamine (NE) neurotransmitter

Spinal cord   Pre–ganglion neuron

Nicotinic receptors

B1, B2, or A1 receptor

Parasympathetic nervous system

Acetylcholine neurotransmitter

Acetylcholine neurotransmitter

Spinal cord   Pre–ganglion neuron

Nicotinic receptors   Muscarinic receptor

Somatic (voluntary) nervous system

Acetylcholine neurotransmitter

Spinal cord   Skeletal muscle axon

Nicotinic receptor

Fig. 5.6 Distribution of muscarinic cholinergic receptors for acetylcholine, nicotinic cholinergic receptors for acetylcholine, and catecholamine adrenergic receptors (alpha-1, beta-1, and beta-2 receptors) for epinephrine and norepinephrine.

! YOU NEED TO KNOW

The Receptors by Which the Autonomic System Works

Because many drugs work by modifying the autonomic nervous system by either blocking or stimulating the sympathetic or parasympathetic receptors, it is essential the veterinary technician remember what these receptors do when stimulated.

Alpha-1 (α_1) adrenergic	Stimulation causes vasoconstriction of precapillary arterioles in skin, abdominal organs including the GI tract, and kidney
	Stimulation causes dilation of pupil (mydriasis)
Alpha-2 (α_2) adrenergic	Stimulation causes inhibition of release of further norepinephrine from nerve terminal
Beta-1 (β_1) adrenergic	Stimulation causes increased heart rate and force of contraction (think "Beta for beat")

Parasympathetic Nervous System (Rest and Restore, Rest and Digest)

Beta-2 (β_2) adrenergic	Stimulation causes increased bronchiole diameter (bronchodilation) by relaxing smooth muscle (think "Beta-2 for bronchioles")
	Stimulation causes dilation of blood vessels in skeletal muscle (for fleeing or fighting)
Cholinergic (muscarinic)	Stimulation causes increased secretion, motility of the gastrointestinal tract
	Stimulation slows heart rate—but has no effect on force of contraction
	Stimulation causes urination
	Stimulation causes bronchoconstriction
Cholinergic (nicotinic)	Stimulation causes voluntary skeletal muscle contraction (at neuromuscular junction between nerve and skeletal muscle)

The natural catecholamines epinephrine and norepinephrine, along with other adrenergic agonist drugs, can bind to several types of adrenergic receptors, each of which produces a different effect in the body. Although there are many different types of adrenergic receptors, the four adrenergic receptors having the greatest role in adrenergic drug actions are α-1 (α_1), α-2 (α_2), **beta-1 (β_1)**, and beta-2 (β_2) adrenergic receptors.

β_1-Receptors are located primarily in the heart. When stimulated, they increase the heart rate, the strength of contraction by the cardiac muscle, and the speed through which the depolarization wave passes through the heart's conduction system. Stimulation of β_1-adrenergic receptors by norepinephrine or adrenergic agonist drugs is responsible for the racing heart (tachycardia) experienced during exercise, fear, or excitement. An easy way to remember that β_1-receptors are responsible for this is to think of the β as standing for "beat" or to remember that the letters for "beta" can be rearranged into "beat."

β_2-Receptors are found on the smooth muscle cells surrounding arterioles that supply the heart muscle and skeletal muscles and surrounding the terminal bronchioles (smallest bronchioles) in the airway of the lungs. When stimulated, β_2-adrenergic receptors cause smooth muscle surrounding blood vessels or bronchioles to relax, causing dilation. Therefore, β_2-receptor stimulation causes vasodilation of blood vessels in the skeletal muscle and heart and bronchodilation of airways in the lungs.

α_1-Receptors cause smooth muscle surrounding the small arteriole blood vessels in the skin, kidney, and intestinal tract to contract (vasoconstriction), decreasing blood flow to these tissues. Thus, in fight or flight situations, the α_1-vasoconstriction shunts blood away from the skin, kidney, and digestive tract and toward the heart and skeletal muscles (β_2-effect) so that the pounding heart and rapidly moving skeletal muscles (fleeing or fighting) can receive more oxygenated blood.

Note that this arteriole vasoconstriction occurs only with the smallest vessels on the arterial side of the vasculature where they regulate blood flow into the capillaries by vasoconstriction or vasodilation. The larger arterial vessels themselves do not constrict. Thus, α_1-receptor vasoconstriction reduces the flow of blood from the arterioles into the capillaries and can prolong the *capillary refill time* measured by pressing on the gums of the patient and observing how quickly the color returns to the pressed area, reflecting the speed with which capillaries refill with blood.

Although α_2-*receptors* are adrenergic receptors with which norepinephrine can combine, they are located on the ends of adrenergic neurons where they help regulate the release of norepinephrine. This alpha-2 function is not directly related to cardiovascular function but helps prevent excessive release of norepinephrine from the adrenergic neurons. Because this function can be used to sedate an animal, α_2-receptors are discussed in greater detail with anesthetic and sedative agents in Chapter 8.

Autonomic drugs can be selective or nonselective for particular receptors or may produce specific or nonspecific effects. For example, older bronchodilator drugs are fairly *nonselective* and will combine with β_2-receptors to produce bronchodilation but may also combine with β_1-receptors and cause tachycardia as a side effect. These drugs are said to act in a *nonspecific* manner because the drug effects include both bronchodilation (β_2-stimulating effect) and an increased heart rate (β_1-stimulating effect). Newer bronchodilators are more *selective* because they combine only with β_2-receptors, and they are also more *specific* in their effect because they produce only bronchodilation with little or no increased heart rate. When given the choice, veterinarians prefer to use autonomic drugs that are more selective (fewer receptor types combined with) and more specific (fewer types of effects) so these powerful drugs produce the maximal beneficial effect with the fewest side effects.

Although α_1-, α_2-, β_1-, and β_2-receptors are all stimulated by sympathetic catecholamine neurotransmitters and adrenergic agonist drugs, they are not necessarily stimulated equally. For example, epinephrine has a very strong α_1-effect (strong vasoconstriction of peripheral arteriole blood vessels) but a weaker β_2-effect (weaker vasodilation of cardiac and skeletal muscle arterioles and bronchodilation). The ability to cause arteriole vasoconstriction and subsequent increase in arterial blood pressure means that epinephrine is sometimes used to increase arterial blood pressure in patients that are hypotensive (i.e., have low blood pressure).

The Parasympathetic Nervous System Control of the Cardiovascular System

The parasympathetic nervous system (the "rest and restore" system) antagonizes or works against many of the effects of the sympathetic nervous system. Increased parasympathetic system activity or the use of drugs that combine with cholinergic receptors and mimic the actions of acetylcholine slows the heart rate (opposite of the β_1-adrenergic effect), increases blood flow to the intestinal tract and kidney (opposite of the α_1-adrenergic effect), and decreases the diameter of the bronchioles (opposite of the β_2-adrenergic effect). The parasympathetic nervous system has little effect on peripheral superficial arteriole blood vessels and thus does not antagonize the arteriole vasoconstriction of skin vessels caused by the sympathetic nervous system. In addition to these effects, the parasympathetic nervous system dilates the blood vessels in the GI tract, increases GI activity and secretions, and causes pupillary constriction.

As described in Chapter 4 and as shown in Fig. 5.6, neurons of the parasympathetic nervous system produce their effect through secretion of acetylcholine and stimulation of *cholinergic receptors.* Drugs that mimic the effect of acetylcholine are called *parasympathomimetic drugs* because they mimic the effects of that part of the autonomic nervous system.

Just as there are different types of adrenergic receptors in the sympathetic nervous system, there are also different types of cholinergic receptors in the parasympathetic system called muscarinic cholinergic receptors and nicotinic cholinergic receptors. Muscarinic receptors are typically found in tissues and organs that produce the observed physiologic changes associated with the parasympathetic nervous system effects. Thus, drugs that stimulate muscarinic cholinergic receptors tend to increase GI stimulation, slow the heart rate, and cause the pupil to constrict.

As shown in Fig. 5.6, the nicotinic cholinergic receptors are found in both the parasympathetic and sympathetic nervous system pathways; therefore, stimulation of these specific receptors by nicotine-like drugs (e.g., tobacco) often shows a mixture of both sympathetic and parasympathetic effects. With stimulation of nicotinic receptors, the sympathetic signs tend to dominate over the parasympathetic signs; thus, patients will tend to show tachycardia instead of bradycardia, pupillary dilation instead of constriction, and increased arterial blood pressure.

Unlike the muscarinic cholinergic receptors, nicotinic cholinergic receptors are also found on skeletal muscles, where they receive nerve signals to produce the conscious movements of the body via the acetylcholine released by voluntary motor nervous system nerves. When drugs or poisons stimulate these same skeletal muscle nicotinic receptors, they may produce visible muscle tremors or shaking. However, as these nicotinic receptors are increasingly stimulated, they get to a point where they depolarize but then fail to repolarize. As described in the mechanism of depolarization and repolarization, a receptor that has been depolarized cannot depolarize again until it is repolarized, much like a snapped mousetrap cannot snap again until it has been reset. Because the overstimulated nicotinic receptor becomes unable to respond to further acetylcholine signals sent by the voluntary motor nerves, the skeletal muscle cell is unable to be stimulated to contract and the affected muscle appears to become paralyzed. Animals with toxicity from drugs or poisons (e.g., insecticides) that stimulate the nicotinic cholinergic receptor thus show tremors and shaking at low-dose toxicity followed by weakness and paralysis at high-dose toxicity.

The Autonomic Tug-of-War

The parasympathetic and sympathetic nervous systems are always producing, often simultaneously, some effect on the body or even the same organ or tissues. Whichever of the two parts of the autonomic system produces the stronger effect at any particular moment determines whether the body shows sympathetic or parasympathetic physiologic signs.

Parasympathetic nervous system signs can appear if either the parasympathetic nervous system or cholinergic receptors are being strongly stimulated or if the sympathetic nervous system activity or the adrenergic receptors are being blocked. Adrenergic receptor antagonist drugs (e.g., β_1-blockers) decrease sympathetic nervous system effects, allowing parasympathetic nervous system effects to dominate and producing a slowed heart rate. Conversely, drugs that are cholinergic antagonists and block the parasympathetic nervous system effect (e.g., atropine) would allow the sympathetic nervous system signs to dominate, producing an elevated heart rate, dilated bronchioles, and dilated pupils. This concept of the continuous balance between the two parts of the autonomic nervous system helps explain the mechanism by which almost any autonomic drug or poison produces its outward clinical signs.

ANTIARRHYTHMIC DRUGS

An arrhythmia is any abnormal pattern of electrical activity in the heart. Arrhythmias can result in a faster than normal heart rate (tachycardia, tachyarrhythmias) or slow the heart rate (bradycardia, bradyarrhythmias). Arrhythmias can result from cardiac cells firing rapidly or out of sequence or conduction cells failing to depolarize at all when they are stimulated. Because there are different causes of arrhythmias, there are multiple types of *antiarrhythmic drugs* used to control arrhythmias.

As previously discussed, the waves of depolarization that cause the coordinated contraction of the heart follow a specific sequence, starting in the SA node and ending with contraction of the ventricular muscle cells. If another area of the myocardium (heart muscle) or the conduction cell system begins to depolarize out of sequence or more to depolarize at a rate that is faster than the SA node, the normal electrical pattern of P-QRS-T waves is disrupted. The abnormal site of initial depolarization is called an ectopic focus and often results from a damaged myocardial cell or conducting cell with membranes that leak Na^+ into the cell more rapidly than normal, producing the spontaneous depolarization.

An ECG detects arrhythmias caused by ectopic foci or other abnormalities. If the ectopic focus is located in the ventricles, it will generate a single, large, bizarre wave on the ECG in place of the normal QRS complex of ventricular depolarization. Because this bizarre-looking wave occurs before the ventricles have the opportunity to contract from the normal conduction pathway, the wave pattern seen on the ECG is called a premature ventricular contraction (PVC) (Fig. 5.7). Single, intermittent PVCs on the ECG do not significantly affect the heart's overall ability to pump blood and sometimes occur in healthy animals under general anesthesia or in humans who have had too much coffee or other stimulants.

Although most PVCs occur as isolated waveforms, multiple PVCs can also occur one after the other in a short series of waves called a paroxysm. A longer series of PVCs is referred to as *ventricular flutter*. If the conduction disturbance is severe and the depolarization wave so totally disrupted so as to not even be recognizable on the ECG, this means that the ventricles are simply quivering and unable to produce any resemblance of a coordinated contraction to eject blood. This is a rapidly fatal condition called *ventricular fibrillation*. Fibrillation and flutter can also occur in the atria, resulting in *atrial flutter* or *atrial fibrillation*. Atrial fibrillation, atrial flutter, and ventricular flutter are examples of *tachyarrhythmias* because they are associated with a faster (but uncoordinated) ventricular contraction rate. Ventricular fibrillation could also be considered a tachyarrhythmia, but the ventricular contraction is so uncoordinated from the fibrillation that no discernible ventricular contraction rate can be identified.

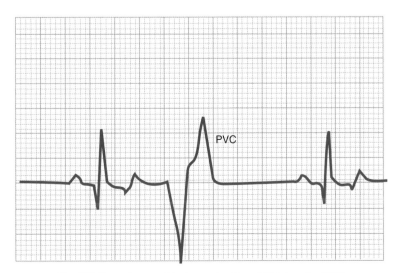

Fig. 5.7 Premature ventricular contractions (PVCs) on the ECG.

Classify the Arrhythmia to Understand Which Drug to Use

Before the veterinary professional can choose the appropriate drug to control arrhythmias, the arrhythmia has to be classified according to its effect and the location of the arrhythmia's source. One method to classify arrhythmias is to divide them into two general groups: fast arrhythmias vs slow arrhythmias. A fast abnormal rhythm is called a tachyarrhythmia and can result in a fast ventricular heart rate, or tachycardia, whereas a slow abnormal rhythm is called a bradyarrhythmia and can produce a slower than normal heart rate, or bradycardia.

Arrhythmias are then further subdivided into *supraventricular arrhythmias* or *ventricular arrhythmias* according to location of the ectopic foci or lesion that is causing the arrhythmia. A supraventricular arrhythmia indicates that the source of the arrhythmia is "above" (supra-) the ventricles and thus originates in the atria, SA node, or AV node. A ventricular arrhythmia indicates that the problem originates somewhere within the ventricles or the conduction pathways in the ventricles.

The terms for speed and location of the arrhythmia are then combined to describe the arrhythmia. For example, atrial fibrillation results in a rapid heart rate (tachycardia) caused by a problem in the atria (supraventricular origin) and would therefore be classified as a *supraventricular* tachyarrhythmia or supraventricular tachycardia. Conversely a problem with the SA node resulting in slower than normal rhythm and irregularity would be a supraventricular bradyarrhythmia or supraventricular bradycardia. An abnormal cell in the ventricles rapidly depolarizing and causing a rapid heartbeat would be classified as a ventricular tachycardia or ventricular tachyarrhythmia.

Once the type of arrhythmia has been determined, an effective antiarrhythmic drug is used to reestablish a normal conduction sequence, or *sinus rhythm* (normal rhythm controlled by the SA node). The characteristics of the antiarrhythmic drug determine whether it will work in the atria or ventricles and whether the drug is capable of correcting bradycardia or tachycardia.

Antiarrhythmic Drugs That Inhibit Sodium Influx: The Sodium Channel Blockers

Antiarrhythmic drugs are classified as belonging to Class I, II, III, or IV based on their mechanisms of action. Thus, the veterinary technician may hear the veterinarian refer to a drug as a "Class I" or "Class II" antiarrhythmic drug. In this chapter, we will refer to these classes primarily by their descriptive names, such as "β-blockers," "sodium channel blockers," or "calcium channel blockers."

Lidocaine, quinidine, and procainamide are Class I sodium channel blocker antiarrhythmics that work primarily by decreasing the rate of Na^+ movement into the cell through the sodium fast channels mentioned previously (see Fig. 5.5). Without normal Na^+ influx at depolarization, the steep phase 0 is retarded, resulting in a longer depolarization phase, a longer time spent in the refractory period (which stabilizes the cell by decreasing the risk for firing again too soon), and decreased spontaneous depolarization of ectopic foci.

Lidocaine (also called "lignocaine" in Australia) is one of the major drugs of choice for controlling PVCs and ventricular arrhythmias in canine cardiac patients, animals under anesthesia, or where the heart has experienced trauma. Although lidocaine works well in controlling ventricular ectopic foci and PVCs, it has little efficacy against atrial ectopic foci, atrial fibrillation, or atrial flutter.

Lidocaine blocks the sodium fast channels, reducing sodium influx; however, it also slows the rate at which the phase 4 automaticity occurs in ectopic foci cells, reducing their ability to spontaneously depolarize. The drug concentrations needed to achieve this suppression of the ectopic foci do not affect the automaticity of the SA node (the heart rate does not slow), and the automaticity of the AV node, bundle branches, and Purkinje fibers are minimally affected.[5] Thus, lidocaine works well to selectively decrease the firing of ectopic focus cells without significantly depressing the function of the normal conduction system.

Lidocaine, if given orally, has extensive biotransformation by the liver before the drug can reach systemic circulation (first-pass effect) and produces GI irritation. Therefore, lidocaine is used to treat ventricular arrhythmias only as an IV-administered drug. And because the drug is metabolized so quickly, lidocaine needs to be given as a constant rate infusion (CRI) or as multiple slow bolus doses to maintain sufficient blood concentrations to work.

Cats appear to be more sensitive to the side effects of lidocaine than other species and therefore require lower doses than what is used in dogs (about one tenth of the dog dose).[5] The cat heart's conduction cells seem to be more susceptible to depression by lidocaine than the dog's, and use of lidocaine can result in decreased depolarization of the AV node, a condition called first- or second-degree AV block. Because reports of adverse reactions in cats from lidocaine do exist, lidocaine must be used cautiously in cats.[6] However, some sources go further than this and state that because of the cat's reduced ability to metabolize lidocaine, lidocaine should not be used in cats as an antiarrhythmic drug at all, especially if the cat is ill or under anesthesia.[7]

Low-dose lidocaine toxicosis signs include sedation, ataxia, and drowsiness. As the dose of toxicity increases, the sedation and ataxia are replaced by excitement and seizures. The seemingly opposite clinical signs (central nervous system [CNS] depression followed by CNS excitation) are likely because lower dose lidocaine toxicity inhibits excitatory neurons, but higher dose toxicity inhibits the inhibitory neurons, allowing the remaining excitatory neurons to depolarize more readily and producing CNS excitation (seizures, tremors). Because lidocaine is so rapidly metabolized by the liver, seizure activity from lidocaine toxicity stops soon after lidocaine administration is halted and seldom requires additional treatment.

Veterinary technicians must realize that lidocaine is also used as a local anesthetic. However, the local anesthetic version of lidocaine also contains epinephrine. The epinephrine is added to the local anesthetic to cause local vasoconstriction at the injection site, thus decreasing tissue perfusion, slowing the absorption of the injected lidocaine, and prolonging the activity of the local anesthetic where it was injected. If the lidocaine with epinephrine is mistakenly given IV to treat an animal with an arrhythmia, the epinephrine will stimulate the heart, possibly making it more electrically unstable and potentially worsening the arrhythmias. Because most veterinary hospitals stock both forms of lidocaine (with and without epinephrine), the bottles of the different forms should be clearly marked with colored tape or other distinctive marking so the wrong type is not picked up by accident during an arrhythmic emergency.

In addition to its use as a local anesthetic in both small and large animals, lidocaine without epinephrine is also used IV in some anesthesia/analgesia protocols.

Mexiletine is an orally administered drug in the same class as lidocaine and can be used for long-term control of lidocaine-responsive arrhythmias. Because lidocaine can only be given by the IV route of administration and because its rapid metabolism requires constant dosing, it is unsuitable for dispensing to clients for long-term control of PVCs or other ventricular arrhythmias. Mexiletine, in contrast to lidocaine, has minimal first-pass effect and longer half-life and is very well absorbed from the GI tract when given orally (PO). Mexiletine may still produce some GI and CNS side effects similar to lidocaine, but at normal therapeutic doses these effects are minimal. Mexiletine is currently available as a generic drug from veterinary drug distributors and is also available as a compounded drug from compounding pharmacies.

Procainamide and quinidine are Class I sodium channel blocking drugs belonging to the same general class as lidocaine; however, they differ from lidocaine in their ability to control both ventricular ectopic foci and atrial flutter/fibrillation. Quinidine and procainamide decrease the velocity of phase 0 depolarization like lidocaine does and lengthen the phase 4 return to depolarization threshold, extending the refractory period. The extended refractory period controls atrial fibrillation and atrial flutter by preventing perpetuation of multiple atrial depolarization waves caused by constant restimulation and depolarization of atrial cells that have just completed the depolarization-repolarization cycle.

Neither procainamide nor quinidine is readily available to veterinarians because their use for human medical purposes has sharply declined and therefore manufacture has likewise decreased. Note that quinidine is used in human medicine not only for control of arrhythmias but also to treat malaria. Although injectable procainamide is still sometimes used in small animal medicine, quinidine is no longer used in small animal medicine but continues to be used to control atrial fibrillation or atrial flutter in horses.[8]

When quinidine is used to treat atrial tachyarrhythmias in horses, it would normally be expected that the ventricular rate (as monitored by the pulse) would decrease and become more regular as the number of uncoordinated atrial fibrillation depolarization waves reaching the AV node decreases. However, when quinidine is used to control these supraventricular tachycardia arrhythmias, the veterinary technician may initially detect the pulse becoming more rhythmic but remaining faster than normal or even accelerating slightly. This is because one of the side effects of quinidine is to block the slowing effect that

acetylcholine would normally have on the AV node, allowing more rapid depolarization wave conduction from the atria to the ventricles and resulting in a faster ventricular rate. This acetylcholine blocking effect is called the "antivagal" or vagolytic effect in reference to the vagus nerve that is the source of the acetylcholine that normally slows conduction through the AV node. Procainamide does not have this vagolytic effect.

β-Blocker Antiarrhythmic Drugs

β **(beta)-Antagonists or β (beta)-blockers,** also referred to as Class II antiarrhythmics, are recognized by the "-olol" ending on the drug names (e.g., propranolol, atenolol, esmolol, metoprolol, and carvedilol). As the name implies, these antiarrhythmic drugs work by blocking the β_1-sympathetic nervous system receptors on the heart. Although stimulation of β_1-receptors by catecholamines normally increases the cardiac output by increasing the heart rate (action on the SA and AV node) and force of contraction (effect on the cardiac muscle), the increased stimulation of the heart also makes the heart more electrically unstable, which can allow ectopic foci and arrhythmias to appear. Thus, blocking the β_1-receptors blocks the sympathetic nervous system stimulation of the heart, helping reduce the generation of ectopic foci and arrhythmias.

Because β-blockers block the sympathetic nervous system, they allow the parasympathetic nervous system effects to dominate through acetylcholine action on muscarinic cholinergic receptors on the heart's conduction system, slowing both the heart rate (SA node effect) and the rate that depolarization waves pass through the AV node. As was mentioned previously, this parasympathetic dominance on the AV node when β-blocker drugs are used slows the conduction of the depolarization wave through the AV node, producing first- or second-degree atrioventricular (AV) block. First-degree AV block appears on the ECG as a prolongation of the PR interval between the P wave (atrial depolarization) and the large R wave of the QRS complex. If conduction through the AV node is delayed long enough by parasympathetic stimulation of the AV node, the depolarization wave may fade out in the AV node and not reach the ventricles. This phenomenon appears on the ECG as a P wave (atria depolarizing) without a corresponding QRS complex (ventricles depolarizing) and is referred to as second-degree AV block. The veterinary technician might detect the second-degree AV block on auscultation or pulse palpation as an intermittent missed beat.

Because the AV block is from parasympathetic stimulation of cholinergic receptors, the resulting AV block or bradycardia can itself be reversed using cholinergic receptor-blocking drugs such as atropine. As a general rule, when attempting to reverse bradycardia or early AV block associated with the use of β_1-blocker antiarrhythmics, better results are obtained by either decreasing the β-blocker dose or using an anticholinergic drug rather than attempting to overcome the β-block by using a β_1-stimulating drug to increase sympathetic dominance over the parasympathetic effect.

Note that there are no cholinergic receptors on the cardiac muscle itself, so any decreased force of cardiac muscle contraction from β-blocker antiarrhythmic drugs comes from the lack of sympathetic stimulation via the β_1-receptors, not from stimulation of, or dominance by, the parasympathetic nervous system.

Animals that have been receiving a β_1-blocking antiarrhythmic drug for some time may appear to become resistant to the effects of the β-blocker drug (tolerance) as evidenced by a return of an accelerated heart rate or the appearance of previously well-controlled arrhythmias. This tolerance is not caused by induction of drug metabolism by the liver as observed with opioid or barbiturate drugs but results from upregulation of the β_1-adrenergic receptors by the cell.[6]

Upregulation occurs after β_1-adrenergic receptors have been blocked by β-blocker drugs for a long period of time. The β-blocker effect decreases sympathetic stimulation from normal amounts of epinephrine and norepinephrine, and this causes the cell to begin to produce more β_1-receptors on the cell surface to give the cell more opportunity to respond to the catecholamines. By creating more receptors available for catecholamines to stimulate, the antiarrhythmic β-blocker drug is unable to block all of the normal catecholamines produced by the body, the cell again becomes sensitive and able to respond to the effects of normally released epinephrine and norepinephrine, the heart rate increases, and the arrhythmias return.[6,9]

If the dose of the β-blocker drug is increased to compensate for the increased number of β_1-receptors generated by the cell, the cell will further upregulate and respond by producing still more β_1 receptors. Eventually the cell's upregulation process and increased dose of β_1-blocking drugs will hit a balance point where the cell is no longer producing as many new receptors and further drug tolerance appears to decrease. However, at this balance point the cell surface is now loaded with many β_1-receptors, potentially making these cells very sensitive to the presence of catecholamine compounds (e.g., epinephrine, norepinephrine).[9]

Should the owner suddenly stop the β-blocker drug and the β-blocker drug molecules cease to block the β_1-receptors, the normal release of epinephrine or norepinephrine from excitement or fear (e.g., the dog chasing its ball or a trip to the veterinarian) can result in a much greater sympathetic stimulation of the cells than normal, resulting in tachycardia (SA and AV node effect) or severe arrhythmias (overstimulation of cardiac cells). This phenomenon has been documented in humans and is assumed to likely occur in veterinary patients. Thus, if a patient has been on β-blocker antiarrhythmic drugs for several days or weeks and the drug needs to be discontinued, the drug should be withdrawn gradually over several days to several weeks to allow the body to downregulate the β_1-receptors (remove the extraneous receptors) to a normal level.[6]

Propranolol is the old prototype β_1-antagonist drug. It is referred to as a *nonselective* antagonist of beta receptors because it combines with both β_1- and β_2-receptors. Propranolol blocks β_1-receptors on the SA node and AV node, depressing the automaticity of the SA node and slowing conduction of the depolarization wave through the AV node. This decreases the heart rate and prevents the heart from speeding up and working harder in response to stress, fear, excitement, or other fight or flight responses. Propranolol is also used to decrease the rapid heart rate associated with feline hyperthyroidism (increased thyroid hormone production).

In addition to slowing the conducting system, propranolol decreases the automaticity of ventricular ectopic foci, effectively controlling arrhythmias made worse by sympathetic nervous system stimulation.

The nonspecific antagonist effect of propranolol means this drug also has the capacity to block stimulation of β_2-adrenergic receptors that dilate skeletal muscle vasculature and cause bronchodilation. When the sympathetic nervous system's dilating effect on the terminal bronchioles is blocked by a nonspecific/nonselective β-blocker drug like propranolol, the parasympathetic nervous system dominates, allowing bronchoconstriction, especially in animals with prior bronchoconstrictive disease.[6,9]

The newer β-blocker antiarrhythmic drugs are more selective for β_1-receptors, thus significantly reducing, but not totally eliminating, the β_2-antagonist side effects on the bronchioles, especially at higher drug doses. These newer drugs include **atenolol** (also used to treat hypertension and feline cardiomyopathy), **esmolol** (a very short-acting β-blocker drug used to test if an arrhythmia is responsive to β-blockers), **metoprolol** (which is also used to help control signs of cardiomyopathy in cats), and other "-olol" drugs like **carvedilol**.[6,9]

Because all β-blockers decrease sympathetic stimulation, they have the potential to cause the heart to contract with less force.[9,10] In healthy animals, this is of little consequence. However, in those animals with congestive heart failure (weakening of the heart muscle), the sympathetic nervous system "boost" to the cardiac output may be the only thing keeping the animal from going into uncompensated congestive heart failure and death. When an animal has congestive heart failure, the decreased cardiac output causes a decreased arterial blood pressure. This drop in blood pressure is detected by receptors in the arterial vasculature and causes increased sympathetic nervous system activity in an attempt to increase the cardiac output and return arterial pressure to near normal. Under these conditions the use of a β-blocker antiarrhythmic drug would have a negative inotropic effect (cause a decreased force of contraction), which could cause the congestive heart failure to worsen and the animal to progress into full heart failure. For this reason, β-blockers must be used with caution or not at all in animals with myocardial failure in which sympathetic nervous system activity may be keeping the patient alive.

This trade-off between the antiarrhythmic effect and the negative inotropic effect of β-blocker drugs makes it very difficult to treat a patient for both congestive heart failure and a ventricular arrhythmia that would normally require a β-blocker. The use of the β-blocker antiarrhythmic would increase the odds of the patient dying from congestive heart failure, and the use of a drug to stimulate the heart to beat with greater force would likely also increase the risk for more severe arrhythmias. Thus, the veterinarian faced with this dilemma often has to decide which condition, the failing heart or the arrhythmia, is more life-threatening and to treat that condition knowing that the treatment will adversely affect the other condition.

Because β-blockers slow SA node rate and conduction through the AV node, they should not be used in animals that already have slowed conduction associated with disease involving the heart's conduction system or administration of other drugs that produce slowed conduction as a side effect.

Other Antiarrhythmic Drugs

Sotalol and **amiodarone** are two antiarrhythmic drugs belonging to the Class III antiarrhythmics. As such they do not work by affecting sodium channels but by inhibiting potassium channels, making them slower to open and thus prolonging the repolarization period and extending the refractory period. As the "-olol" part of the "sotalol" name suggests, this drug also has some β-blocking effects at lower doses. Although various uses are mentioned in veterinary literature, experience overall with this group of drugs is still less than that found with the Class I sodium channel blockers or Class II β-blockers. These drugs may be used alone or with other antiarrhythmic drugs to control selected types of arrhythmias such as those found in boxer dogs with ventricular cardiomyopathy (disease of the ventricle muscle).[7] Because these drugs can have serious side effects under some conditions (e.g., partial AV block, SA node disease, bronchoconstrictive disease) and because new and different arrhythmias may, ironically, suddenly appear with the slow heart rate caused by these drugs, these drugs are most often used only when other antiarrhythmic drugs have not been successful.

Calcium channel blocker antiarrhythmics are Class IV antiarrhythmic drugs that block the slow calcium channels in conduction system cells, especially the SA node and AV node, resulting in a prolonged phase 4 upslope to threshold and reduced spontaneous depolarization (the drug decreases automaticity). Calcium channel blockers also prolong the plateau phase of the cardiac muscle cell depolarization and as such prolong the refractory period, making it harder for the cell to repolarize and be stimulated to depolarize again. Thus, calcium channel blockers like **verapamil** and **diltiazem** have been used successfully to treat supraventricular tachycardia, atrial fibrillation, and atrial flutter. Unfortunately, blocking the calcium channels can also decrease the strength of heart muscle contraction and reduce cardiac output. Therefore, calcium channel blockers should be used with caution or not at all in animals with congestive heart failure because of their negative inotropic effect.

Although the calcium channel blocker diltiazem was used in cats in the past to reduce the effects of feline hypertrophic cardiomyopathy, use of diltiazem has decreased over recent years primarily because of inconsistent beneficial clinical outcomes when the drug is used for this purpose.[6] It is still used with other drugs, like digoxin, to decrease the ventricular contraction rate in animals with atrial fibrillation.[7,11]

Digoxin is an old drug used previously as a positive inotropic agent (a drug that increases the force of contraction). But it is one of digoxin's side effects that make it useful for controlling the effects of atrial fibrillation or flutter.[7] When animals have atrial fibrillation, the ventricular contraction rate accelerates because of the bombardment of impulses from the atria on the AV node, subsequently increasing the number of depolarization waves reaching the ventricles. The increased parasympathetic side effect that digoxin normally has on the SA node and AV node slows the pacemaker rate and delays conduction of impulses through the AV node (first-degree AV block). Giving digoxin to a patient with ventricular tachycardia caused by atrial fibrillation causes the impulses passing through the AV node to slow, decreasing the number of depolarization waves that reach the ventricles, slowing the ventricular rate, and allowing more effective filling of the ventricles between ventricular contractions.[6,11]

POSITIVE INOTROPIC DRUGS AND INODILATORS

Positive inotropic drugs (positive inotropes) increase the strength of contraction of a weakened heart. More recently drugs have been used in human and veterinary medicine that have both a positive inotropic effect and a vasodilation effect. These drugs are called inodilators. The positive inotropic effect will be discussed in this section and the vasodilatory effect discussed in the next section.

Most positive inotropic agents work by directly or indirectly making more calcium available to the contractile proteins within the muscle cell or by increasing the affinity between calcium and contractile proteins that shorten the muscle cell. By increasing the calcium available for the contractile proteins, each muscle fiber contracts with greater force.

Catecholamines

Catecholamines (*norepinephrine, epinephrine,* and *dopamine*) are the body's natural positive inotropic agents and are used by the sympathetic nervous system to increase the force of cardiac contraction and speed of depolarization wave conduction, subsequently increasing the cardiac output of blood. Adrenergic drugs of the natural catecholamines (e.g., the drug form of epinephrine) or other adrenergic drugs like dobutamine produce a similar positive inotropic effect by stimulating β$_1$-receptors in the cardiac muscle and the conducting system cells.[12]

Catecholamines increase the force of contraction through the β$_1$-receptors by causing a greater release of calcium from intracellular storage sites within the cardiac muscle cell. This intracellular calcium combines with the contractile elements (filaments) of the muscle cell, allowing the overlapping sliding filaments to bind to each other and move past each other in a ratchet-type fashion, resulting in a shortening of the cardiac cell (muscle cell contraction). By increasing the amount of calcium released from storage to combine with the contractile filaments, the resulting muscle contraction is stronger, producing the positive inotropic effect.

Although adrenergic drugs are strong positive inotropes, they only improve cardiac contractility for a relatively short period of time because of downregulation of β$_1$-receptors. Downregulation means that the cells remove some of the β$_1$-receptors from the cell surface (downregulation), which reduces the number of receptors available to bind with adrenergic drugs or catecholamines, reducing the cell's ability to respond to the adrenergic drug stimulation and decreases the positive inotropic effect. Thus, catecholamines are not used for any long-term positive inotropic treatment because of downregulation of the receptors.

Pimobendan

Pimobendan ("pee-moh-BEN-dan") is an inodilator drug approved for veterinary use in 2007 (Vetmedin™). Being an *inodilator* drug means that pimobendan acts as both a vasodilator and a positive inotropic drug. It is used to treat congestive heart failure, primarily in dogs with mitral valve disease or when the heart chambers dilate because of thin and weakened ventricular muscle walls (dilated cardiomyopathy).[13,14] According to a 2011 consensus panel of the American College of Veterinary Internal Medicine, pimobendan has largely supplanted the use of the older traditional positive inotropic drug digoxin for use in congestive heart failure related to mitral valve disease.[14]

Unlike catecholamines, pimobendan does not increase release of calcium from storage sites inside the cell but instead increases the calcium binding with the contractile elements, resulting in a more effective contraction of the cardiac muscle cell. This mechanism of increased binding ability is an advantage because the increased release of calcium within the cardiac cell seen with older positive inotropic drugs like the catecholamine dobutamine or digoxin is thought to have a role in reducing long-term survivability of the patients on these drugs.[15]

The mechanism by which pimobendan causes vasodilation involves inhibition of an enzyme and is a different mechanism than its positive inotropic mechanism. The vasodilator effect of pimobendan will be discussed with the vasodilators later in this chapter.

Pimobendan is contraindicated in circumstances where the increased force of contraction of the heart muscle would be harmful to the animal. For example, hypertrophic cardiomyopathy (different from dilated cardiomyopathy, mentioned earlier) is a condition in cats where parts of the ventricular muscle wall of the heart become very thickened. The abnormal thickening constricts the outflow tract from the left ventricle into the aorta. During ventricular contraction, this reduced opening in the outflow tract can narrow even further, obstructing the flow from the left ventricle to an even greater degree. Thus, stimulating greater force of contraction may actually produce greater obstruction of blood outflow from the left ventricle. Although pimobendan should not be used in hypertrophic cardiomyopathy in cats, it has been used to treat congestive heart failure in that species.[7]

According to the EPIC study, published in 2016, pimobendan should be used in canine patients with Myxomatous Mitral Valve Disease (MMVD) and echocardiographic and radiographic evidence of cardiomegaly before clinical signs are present. Prior to this study, pimobendan was not given to these patients prior to the development of clinical signs. This study demonstrated no significant adverse events and prolonged the preclinical period by an average of 15 months.[14,16,17]

Digoxin

Digoxin has historically been the most commonly used long-term positive inotrope. With the emergence of pimobendan and more tactical use of vasodilator drugs to control congestive heart failure, digoxin use has decreased in veterinary medicine. Still, it does have a place in controlling cardiac disease.

Digoxin exerts its positive inotropic effect primarily by causing more calcium to be released from intracellular storage sites, making more calcium available for the contractile elements, and therefore enhancing the strength of contraction. Digoxin increases intracellular calcium secondarily to decreasing the action of the cell's *sodium-potassium-ATPase pump*. As previously discussed, the sodium-potassium-ATPase pump normally pumps Na^+ out and K^+ into the cell to maintain the cell's polarized "resting" state. When this pump is inhibited by digoxin, Na^+ is not pumped out as effectively and begins to accumulate within the cardiac cell. This relatively small increase in intracellular Na^+ displaces calcium from its storage site in the cardiac cell, making more calcium available to contractile elements and resulting in an increased force of contraction.[12] Unfortunately, the increased Na^+ inside the cardiac muscle cell also makes the cell more electrically unstable, increasing the risk of spontaneous depolarization and ectopic foci. Therefore, one of the side effects of digoxin therapy can be the appearance of arrhythmias associated with ectopic foci.

Digoxin is a cardiac glycoside and is a poison found in nature. Specifically, digoxin was originally derived from digitalis compounds naturally found in the foxglove plant. Because digoxin is a biologic toxin, the dosages that achieve therapeutic concentrations are very close to the dosages and concentrations that produce toxic side effects. The relatively high risk for toxic side effects for digoxin and pimobendan's fewer side effects constitute the major reason digoxin is not used as much today as a positive inotrope.

Early signs of digoxin toxicity reflect the drug's ability to directly stimulate the chemoreceptor trigger zone involved with the vomiting reflex (see Chapter 4). The first signs of digoxin toxicosis noticed by an owner or veterinary technician would include anorexia, vomiting, and diarrhea. Owners of animals receiving digoxin should be instructed to contact the veterinarian immediately if these early signs of toxicity occur.

Cardiac signs of digoxin toxicity typically occur at higher concentrations than the GI effects. As concentrations of digoxin accumulate, the parasympathetic effect of digoxin on the SA node slows the heart rate, and the effect on the AV node increases the PR interval on the ECG, producing first-degree AV block. As toxicity increases and causes greater suppression of the AV node, the PR interval lengthens until occasional waves of depolarization traveling through the AV node fade out and do not reach the ventricles, resulting in a P wave without a QRS complex (second-degree AV block). Third-degree, or complete, AV block is characterized by no waves of depolarization getting through the AV node and the ventricles beating at a rate that is independent of the atria. *Third-degree AV block* is usually associated with severe myocardial disease rather than AV-blocking drugs such as digoxin. Because the SA and AV node effects of digoxin are mostly through enhancement of the parasympathetic effect on the nodes, most of the AV block and SA bradycardia can be reversed using cholinergic receptor antagonists like atropine.

Because digoxin is primarily excreted by the kidneys, animals with impaired kidney function (e.g., older animals with early renal failure) must receive lower digoxin doses to avoid accumulating toxic concentrations. Some clinicians prefer to calculate doses for cats, small dogs, and very large dogs based on the surface area of the animal (milligrams of drug per square meter of surface area) on the premise that these specific animals tend to be overdosed or underdosed if their dose is calculated by body weight (in milligrams per kilogram). Many texts or drug formularies contain tables for converting weight, in kilograms, to square meters (m^2) of surface area.

VASODILATOR DRUGS

Vasodilator drugs increase the diameter of blood vessels and are very important in treating congestive heart failure, especially when used in conjunction with positive inotropic drugs like pimobendan and diuretics like furosemide. Vasodilators are often classified as pure arterial vasodilators, pure venodilators (dilate veins), or mixed vasodilators that balance dilation of both the arterial and the venous system. Realistically all vasodilator drugs have activity on both the arterial and venous sides of the circulatory system, but if a particular drug's action is predominantly one side or the other, it is often referred to as an arterial vasodilator or a venodilator.

Arterial vasodilators used in veterinary medicine include amlodipine and hydralazine, and the key venous dilator is nitroglycerin. Nitroprusside and the angiotensin-converting enzyme (ACE) inhibitors (enalapril and others) constitute the bulk of the mixed vasodilators used in veterinary medicine. To understand why vasodilators are so effective, it is important to understand why vasoconstriction is so detrimental to a failing heart.

Vasoconstriction is one of the normal protective mechanisms by which the autonomic nervous system regulates arterial blood pressure. As discussed previously, when arterial blood pressure drops, there is increased sympathetic nervous system activity, which increases the heart rate (β_1-effect) and also causes peripheral arteriole vasoconstriction (α_1-effect). Inhibition of the sympathetic nervous system and/or stimulation of the parasympathetic nervous system decreases arterial blood pressure by reducing vasoconstriction and slowing the heart rate. Although both sympathetic effects contribute to elevating arterial blood pressure, the α_1-vasoconstriction increases arterial blood pressure to a greater degree than the β_1-increased heart rate.

How Does Vasoconstriction Come About in Heart Disease?

Congestive heart failure means that the heart muscle is too weak to eject sufficient blood to maintain normal tissue functions. The decreased cardiac output from the weakened heart results in a decreased arterial blood pressure. When arterial blood pressure decreases, special pressure receptors called baroreceptors located in the walls of large arterial blood vessels (primarily the carotid artery and aortic arch) detect the change. Under normal blood pressure, these same baroreceptors send a constant low-level inhibitory signal to the brain to inhibit activation of the sympathetic nervous system. However, when arterial blood pressure decreases, the baroreceptors stop sending the inhibitory signal, allowing the sympathetic nervous system to become activated. The activated sympathetic nervous system

releases epinephrine and norepinephrine, which stimulate β_1- and α_1-receptors and produce the increased arterial blood pressure described previously.

The body responds to the decreased cardiac output and lowered arterial blood pressure in congestive heart failure patients by activating the sympathetic nervous system and causing peripheral vasoconstriction and increased stimulation of the heart. The effect of these sympathetic nervous system changes on cardiac output and arterial blood pressure is similar to forcefully blowing into a rubber tube (β_1-effect on heart rate and force) while pinching off the far end of the tube (vasoconstriction at the peripheral arterioles). When pinched, the rubber tube will inflate, reflecting an increased pressure within the tube (the arterial system). Notice how pinching the rubber tube has a greater effect on the degree of inflation of the tube than blowing harder into the tube. This parallels what was said earlier about α_1 vasoconstriction effects having a greater effect on arterial blood pressure than the β_1-effects.

Unfortunately, the vasoconstriction that is needed to elevate the arterial blood pressure in the congestive heart failure patient also increases resistance to arterial blood flow through the arterioles and into the capillaries beyond. This increased resistance requires the weakened, damaged heart to work harder to eject blood against this vascular resistance, and if unable to effectively do so, the cardiac output to the peripheral tissues may decrease even further (Fig. 5.8). To get an idea of how changing the diameter of the blood vessels affects the force needed to push blood through them, think about how much harder it is to suck a milkshake through a small-diameter straw vs a large-diameter straw. Therefore, one of the major roles of vasodilator drugs is to open the constricted arterioles, decreasing resistance to blood flow and making it easier for the weakened heart to pump blood through these vessels.

If the combination of increased cardiac output from the sympathetic nervous system stimulation (β_1-receptor effect)

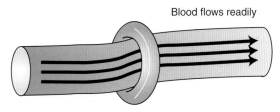

Blood flows readily

Precapillary sphincter (relaxed)

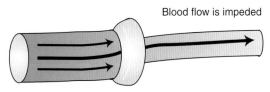

Blood flow is impeded

Precapillary sphincter (constricted)

Fig. 5.8 Vasoconstriction of precapillary arterioles. Vasoconstriction increases the resistance to blood flow from the arterioles into the capillary and increases arterial blood pressure.

increases the perfusion of the tissue sufficiently to meet the body's need for circulating blood, the animal with congestive heart failure will survive for the moment. A patient whose body has successfully initiated this autonomic compensatory response to the weakened heart and falling arterial blood pressure is referred to as being in a state of compensated heart failure. However, if the vasoconstriction used to increase arterial blood pressure creates too much blood flow resistance, the heart will not be able to pump sufficient blood to the tissues even with the β_1 stimulatory boost and the patient becomes **decompensated** and quickly spirals into full cardiac failure and death.

The Kidney's Role in Heart Disease: The Renin-Angiotensin System

When the sympathetic nervous system catecholamines cause vasoconstriction of peripheral arterioles by α_1-stimulation, they also cause vasoconstriction of the arterial blood supply to the renal tubules. This constriction reduces the amount of blood flowing into the glomerulus where ions, water, some drugs, and other small molecules are filtered into the kidney tubules. With the decreased blood flow (decreased renal perfusion), the blood pressure that forces water and other molecules out of the glomerulus is reduced and urine formation slows. When specialized cells in the renal tubules detect decreased blood flow, they release a compound called *renin* into the blood (Fig. 5.9). Renin converts angiotensinogen, a compound produced by the liver, to angiotensin I, which is then quickly converted by the angiotensin-converting enzyme (ACE) to **angiotensin II**.

Angiotensin II is one of the body's most potent vasoconstrictors; therefore, the release of angiotensin II because of poor blood flow to the kidneys is designed to increase the arterial blood pressure and theoretically restore renal blood flow and urine formation. However, as a side effect of the marked vasoconstriction to increase arterial blood pressure, angiotensin II also increases the workload on the heart by creating increased blood flow resistance through the peripheral constricted arterioles.

Angiotensin II also increases the heart workload by increasing the volume of circulating blood. Angiotensin II stimulates release of the hormone aldosterone from the adrenal cortex. Aldosterone increases sodium (Na^+) reabsorption from the urine and pulls it back into the blood, causing a greater retention of Na^+ in the body. The increased sodium in the blood osmotically attracts and holds water in the blood, causing an increased blood volume. Although the increased fluid volume of the blood helps restore or maintain arterial blood pressure, it also creates a larger volume of blood that the heart must pump, thereby increasing the workload on a failing heart.

Vasoconstriction's Role in Systemic Hypertension

Hypertension (increased blood pressure) is most commonly associated with hyperthyroid cats and chronic renal disease. Other systemic diseases, such as diabetes mellitus (a lack of insulin production) and tumors that overproduce aldosterone (the hormone that increases sodium retention and increases blood volume) can also produce systemic hypertension. The hypertension caused by these diseases typically results from a

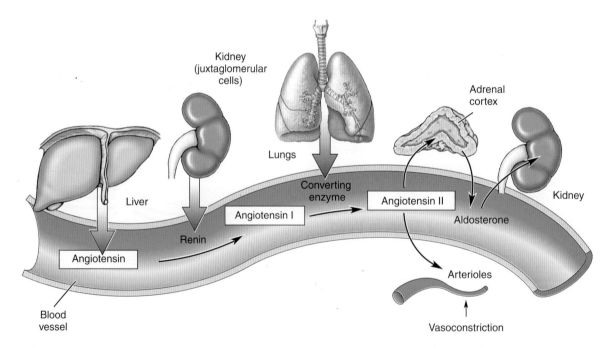

Fig. 5.9 Renin-angiotensin cascade. The cascade is started by anything that decreases arterial blood pressure (blood loss, dehydration, shock, etc.). The decreased arterial blood pressure reduces blood flow to the kidney and decreases urine filtration. The kidney senses this change and releases renin into the blood. Renin converts the precursor molecule angiotensinogen into angiotensin I. Angiotensin I, as it passes through the lungs, is acted upon by angiotensin-converting enzyme (ACE) and becomes the potent vasoconstrictor angiotensin II. Angiotensin II stimulates the adrenal gland to produce aldosterone, which causes increased reabsorption and retention of sodium drugs and water in the blood, the cardvolume. The combination of vasoconstriction of precapillary arterioles and increased blood volume raises the arterial blood pressure back to normal. (From Herlihy B. *The Human Body in Health and Illness.* 4th ed. St. Louis: Saunders; 2011.)

combination of increased cardiac output (increased heart rate, increased volume of blood, or both) and vasoconstriction. The result of uncontrolled systemic hypertension can be retinal detachment, retinal bleeding, hyphema (bleeding into the interior chambers of the eye), or cerebrovascular accident (stroke). Note that strokes are fairly rare in veterinary patients but they do occur. Treatment for hypertension is targeted toward correcting any underlying problem (hyperthyroidism, renal disease) and then using low-sodium diets, diuretics (to remove excess fluid from the blood), β-blockers (to reduce heart rate and cardiac output), and vasodilator drugs.

Principles of Safe Vasodilator Drug Use

Most vasodilators reverse vasoconstriction by blocking the α_1-receptor or the renin-angiotensin system (also called the renin-angiotensin-aldosterone system), reducing production of angiotensin II and aldosterone.

When vasodilators are used for the first time in a patient, the patient may experience hypotension (blood pressure below normal) that would cause clinical signs of ataxia (weakness), syncope (fainting), or lethargy. These signs may be most evident when the animal rises after being recumbent for some time. In response to this transient hypotension, the baroreceptors stop sending the inhibitory signal to the sympathetic nervous system as described earlier, and activation of the sympathetic nervous system quickly corrects the arterial blood pressure.

However, if animals are being treated simultaneously with vasodilators and β-blocker antiarrhythmic drugs, the expected rebound in arterial blood pressure from vasodilator-induced hypotension may not be observed because the β-blocker drugs prevent sympathetic stimulation of the heart rate and force of contraction. Thus, animals already on β-blocker antiarrhythmic drugs that are then placed on vasodilators should be closely monitored for signs of excessive hypotension when the vasodilator drug is given. Animals on diuretics (drugs that increase water loss and reduce blood volume) are also more likely to have an excessive initial hypotensive effect from the vasodilation.

To avoid a clinically significant hypotensive effect, vasodilators are usually started at small initial doses that are slowly increased until early signs of hypotension appear or an adequate beneficial clinical response is attained. If significant hypotension develops during initial dosing, the drug is discontinued for 12 h and then resumed in slightly smaller doses. Mild hypotensive signs, such as lethargy, observed at the start of vasodilator therapy often disappear after a few days of vasodilator drug treatment as the body adapts to the effect of the drug.

Unfortunately, the body's ability to adapt to vasodilator drugs can be a problem for long-term control over excessive vasoconstriction. Because each vasodilator drug typically affects only one of the vasoconstrictive mechanisms in the body (e.g., α_1-stimulation or angiotensin II vasoconstriction) the other remaining vasoconstrictive mechanisms are intact and are likely to respond to any hypotension caused by the vasodilator drug. Therefore, after a few weeks or months, these other vasoconstrictive mechanisms may compensate for the vasodilator drug effect, resulting in a return of vasoconstriction, increased workload on the heart, and a subsequent increase or return of heart failure signs in the congestive heart failure patient.

Arterial Vasodilators: Amlodipine and Hydralazine

Arterial vasodilation directly reduces the resistance the heart must overcome to successfully eject the blood from the ventricles. As such, it reduces the amount of blood left in the ventricles after ejection, which reduces the backup of blood in the atria and vessels returning blood to the heart. The reduced backup and lowered pressure in the venous system decreases the pressure in the capillaries, which in turn reduces the force pushing water into the tissues, ultimately decreasing edema formation. Thus, arterial vasodilation can reduce systemic hypertension, improve ventricular blood ejection despite defective AV valves, reduce tissue edema, and ease the workload on a weakened or dilated heart (e.g., dilated cardiomyopathy).

! YOU NEED TO KNOW

What Causes Ascites and Pulmonary Edema?

Ascites is the accumulation of fluid within the abdominal cavity, and pulmonary edema is the accumulation of fluid within the tissue of the lungs. Both can result from cardiac disease, and understanding why they occur can help the veterinary technician better understand the reasons for the treatment their patient is receiving.

Ascites and pulmonary edema both occur whenever the forces pushing water (fluid) out of the capillaries are greater than the forces pulling water from the tissue or retaining water in the capillaries. In the case of ascites and pulmonary edema associated with heart disease, the force of pressure pushing water out through the small capillary fenestrations is called *hydrostatic pressure* and occurs as the result of blood backing up in the capillaries such as occurs in conditions like congestive heart failure. In congestive heart failure, the heart muscle is weak or damaged and is not able to effectively push blood forward into the aorta and/or pulmonary artery. This results in incomplete ejection of the blood from the ventricles, more blood remaining in the ventricular chamber after ejection is completed, and an increased pressure of blood in the ventricles as they relax. This increased pressure in the ventricles as they relax is referred to as an increase in preload (see You Need to Know box: "What Are Preload and Afterload").

The increased pressure in the ventricles pushes back against the blood incoming from the atria and the venous system, causing a pressure increase in those structures. When this pressure continues to build "backward" to the capillaries, the increased capillary pressure forces water out through the capillary fenestrations into the tissues. The net result is that water "oozes" into the tissue and edema is formed.

When the left side of the heart fails, this increase in left ventricular preload pressure causes an increase in pressure in the left atrium, the vena cava bringing blood into the left atrium, and eventually the capillaries that feed into those veins. Because the capillaries feeding blood into the veins that return blood to the left side of the heart are located throughout the body (everywhere except the lungs), edema can appear in the body tissues and spaces including the peritoneal (abdominal) cavity. Fluid in the abdomen appears on physical examination as a distended abdomen that feel fluid filled when pushed or compressed. This fluid is called ascites.

When the right side of the heart fails, the increase in right ventricular pressure builds backward into the pulmonary veins and capillaries, producing pulmonary edema in the lung tissue. Pulmonary edema may interfere with proper oxygenation, causing the patient to have poor exercise tolerance (gets tired easily), generalized weakness, rapid breathing, and a thoracic radiograph that shows increased radiodensity (more white) throughout the lung field.

Thus, ascites and pulmonary edema occur from the same general mechanism, but the location of the edema (body or lungs) reflects whether the heart is failing on the right or left side.

Amlodipine is an arterial vasodilator used in dogs and cats for hypertension but is primarily used in cats with hypertension secondary to chronic kidney disease, hyperthyroidism, or diabetes mellitus. Amlodipine is classified as a calcium channel blocker, and, as discussed with calcium channel blocker antiarrhythmic drugs, it works by reducing the calcium entering the vasculature smooth muscle cells through the cell's calcium channels, decreasing the calcium available for muscle contraction. The end result is less contraction and more relaxation of the smooth muscles dilating the small arterioles. Although other calcium channel blockers may be used to control arrhythmias or reduce the progression of hypertrophic cardiomyopathy (thickened heart muscle walls), amlodipine is not generally used to assist treatment of cardiac disease.

Hydralazine is an arterial vasodilator that directly causes arteriolar smooth muscle to relax. The mechanism by which smooth muscle relaxation occurs with hydralazine is not yet completely understood but is thought to reflect either some inhibition of calcium movement into smooth muscle cells or a reduced calcium availability to the muscle filaments. Hydralazine is still used to relieve some signs of congestive heart failure caused by severe mitral valve insufficiency (valve damage) by reducing arterial blood pressure and allowing more blood to flow from the left ventricle outward through the aorta instead of regurgitating back through the left AV valve into the left atrium. Hydralazine is sometimes used when other mixed vasodilators like ACE inhibitor drugs fail to adequately control clinical signs of heart failure on their own.

One of the major drawbacks of hydralazine and amlodipine vs the mixed vasodilators is the potential for stimulating the renin-angiotensin system because of decreased arterial blood pressure. Stimulating the renin-angiotensin system can result in additional vasoconstriction from the angiotensin II and retention of sodium and water in the blood from the increased release of aldosterone. Both of these effects can increase the arterial blood pressure and increase the workload on the heart despite the vasodilating effects of these two drugs.

Venous Vasodilator: Nitroglycerin

Nitroglycerin primarily relaxes the blood vessels on the venous side of the circulation, resulting in blood "pooling" in the expanding venous blood vessels, which reduces the volume of blood in the arterial side of circulation and decreases arterial blood pressure. By dilating primarily veins in the systemic circulation, blood volume shifts from the pulmonary circulation (pulmonary artery to lungs to pulmonary vein) to the systemic circulation, decreasing the pulmonary blood volume and subsequently decreasing pulmonary blood pressure. The decreased pressure within pulmonary capillaries reduces the force with which water is forced from the capillaries into the tissues and reduces pulmonary edema formation. Thus, nitroglycerin is used to treat pulmonary edema secondary to heart failure.

In addition to venodilation, nitroglycerin dilates the heart's coronary arterioles and improves blood flow to the myocardium by relaxing the vascular smooth muscles. People with angina pectoris (chest pain) caused by spasms of the coronary arteries take nitroglycerin by putting a tablet under the tongue to speed absorption of the drug and relieve the arteriole spasms.

Nitroglycerin has a significant first-pass effect that negates the use of the drug via the PO route of administration. The use of the tablets placed under the tongue delivers the drug directly into systemic circulation and bypasses the liver and its first-pass effect. As would be suggested by this use, nitroglycerin also readily crosses the skin and is absorbed from topical application sites.

Because the drug is also metabolized very quickly and has a half-life measured in minutes, the drug is typically administered as a topically applied cream or a transdermal patch that is capable of providing a more continuous supply of the drug.[6] When nitroglycerin cream is used, it is applied every 8–12 h to the hairless inner aspect of the pinna of the ear, axilla under the arm, or groin. In animals that already have low blood pressure, reflex vasoconstriction of peripheral arterioles, and less perfusion of the skin or mucous membranes, the nitroglycerin should be applied to the axilla or groin instead of the inner surface of the pinna of the ear. The degree of hypotension and reduced perfusion of skin or mucous membranes can be estimated by the degree of prolonged capillary refill time, fast heart rate, or arterial blood pressure measurements.

When the nitroglycerin patch is used, it provides drug for 24 h and can be cut into smaller pieces to adjust the dose for smaller patients. The site of nitroglycerin application by the patch should be changed with each dose.

Because the drug can be absorbed through the skin, including the animal owner's skin, clients should be instructed to always wear gloves when applying nitroglycerin. Children and others should be instructed not to pet the animal where the cream or patch has been applied.

Although this compound is the same chemical used in explosives, danger of explosion does not exist because the drug has been diluted with several other compounds (mainly dextrose, lactose, and propylene glycol).

Mixed Vasodilators: Nitroprusside and Angiotensin-Converting Enzyme Inhibitors (ACE Inhibitors)

Mixed or "balanced" vasodilators theoretically combine the benefits of arterial vasodilation (lowered arterial blood pressure, ease of ventricular ejection of blood) and venodilation (lowered pulmonary circulation blood pressure, decreased edema formation).

Nitroprusside is a potent mixed vasodilator that is typically used as a short-term drug to help stabilize dogs or cats with severe dyspnea (difficulty breathing) caused by pulmonary edema secondary to heart failure. The drug works very quickly and therefore is typically given as an IV infusion as needed. Nitroprusside works by creating nitric oxide (NO), which in turn inhibits the smooth muscle fiber coupling mechanism that causes muscle contraction, resulting in relaxation of the muscle and vasodilation. This mechanism is the same mechanism by which sildenafil (Viagra) and tadalafil (Cialis) work.

Nitroprusside requires special handling. It must be given IV and should not be allowed to escape into the tissues surrounding the IV catheter. It is sensitive to light and must be shielded from any light. It has to be diluted to be given to veterinary patients, and any drug left over should be discarded. Because it is such a powerful vasodilator, it must not be used in patients that are already hypotensive and its administration must be carefully monitored and titrated.

ACE inhibitors are mixed or "balanced" vasodilators that relax the smooth muscles of both arterioles and veins, and so are useful in treating animals with cardiac disease that involves either the right or left ventricle (or both), such as in severe cardiac valve disease or cardiomyopathy. ACE inhibitors used in veterinary medicine include **enalapril** (Enacard), **captopril**, **benazepril**, and **lisinopril.** Other ACE-inhibiting human drugs are sometimes used in veterinary medicine and can be recognized by the "-pril" at the end of the nonproprietary (generic) name.

ACE inhibitors produce vasodilation by blocking or inhibiting the angiotensin-converting enzyme (ACE), which prevents formation of angiotensin II (the potent vasoconstrictor) and aldosterone (the hormone that increases blood volume by causing sodium retention). Many veterinary cardiologists believe that stimulation of the renin-angiotensin system during congestive heart failure and the subsequent production of angiotensin II has a detrimental effect on the heart that goes beyond the increased workload caused by the vasoconstriction and increased blood volume effects.[7] Consistent with this idea, ACE inhibitor drugs that would disrupt formation of angiotensin II have been shown to significantly improve the quality of life and increase length of survival in dogs with heart failure.[18] Therefore, ACE inhibitors have become an essential component of many therapeutic regimens for treating heart failure.

Although ACE inhibitors have a marked beneficial effect in animals with congestive heart failure, normal animals show little response to these drugs because normal animals have not activated the renin-angiotensin system; hence no ACE is present to inhibit.

Vasodilators, like ACE inhibitors, can be used in animals with heart failure caused by poorly functioning or damaged atrioventricular heart valves (the mitral valve on the left side and the tricuspid valve on the right). When the ventricles contract the incompetent valves allow blood from the ventricles to flow backward into the atria instead of being effectively ejected into the aorta and pulmonary artery. This decreases the amount of blood being delivered to the tissues and results in the clinical signs of heart failure. As described for hydralazine, vasodilation of the arterial side of the vascular system decreases arterial blood pressure, reduces the resistance to ejection of blood from the ventricles into the aorta and pulmonary artery, and allows more of the ventricular ejection to flow in the "normal" direction. So even though the valve remains damaged or incompetent, blood flow from the ventricles to the rest of the body in the normal direction is improved. Clinical studies of ACE inhibitor drugs have shown some improved survivability and delay of full heart failure in dogs already showing clinical signs of mitral valve disease at the time of treatment.[18]

ACE inhibitors must be used with caution in animals with preexisting kidney disease because the initial drop in arterial blood pressure from the drug's vasodilation can significantly decrease the blood flow to the kidney, further reducing its ability to filter the blood. In animals presented with acute heart failure and evidence of poor kidney function (e.g., increased blood urea nitrogen [BUN] and creatinine as a result of reduced glomerular filtration), ACE inhibitors should not be used until the low arterial blood pressure from the congestive heart failure is stabilized with other drugs or treatments. As the blood pressure is brought up, the ACE inhibitor can be used to relieve the vasoconstriction and ease the workload on the failing heart while simultaneously maintaining sufficient blood pressure to keep the kidneys filtering blood.

Hyperkalemia (high concentrations of K^+ in the blood) may occur if ACE inhibitors are used simultaneously with potassium-sparing diuretics or K^+ supplements. Hyperkalemia results from ACE inhibitors blocking the angiotensin II stimulation of aldosterone production. Aldosterone normally causes Na^+ and water reabsorption from the urine back into the body at the expense of K^+ excretion into the urine. Therefore, if aldosterone production is blocked by ACE inhibitors, normal K^+ excretion is decreased and potassium can accumulate in systemic circulation and the body tissues.

For the same reason that ACE inhibitors should not be used in animals with high potassium levels, ACE inhibitors should be used with caution in animals with low sodium levels in the blood and body (*hyponatremia*). Aldosterone normally enhances Na^+ reabsorption from the urine back into the body and systemic circulation, and because ACE inhibitors block aldosterone formation and its Na^+ reabsorption, ACE inhibitors should not be used in patients with hyponatremia.

As with other vasodilators, the initial doses of ACE inhibitors should start small and then be progressively increased to the most effective dose.

DIURETICS

Diuretics increase urine formation and promote water loss (diuresis). They are used for a variety of purposes that usually involve reducing inappropriate accumulation of tissue fluid (e.g., pulmonary edema, cerebral edema), reducing blood volume and arterial blood pressure, and decreasing the workload on a failing heart in congestive heart failure.

Often one side of the heart will fail before the other. For example, the left side tends to fail in congestive heart failure, but the right side could fail because of canine heartworm disease. Tissue edema occurs because the side of the heart that is not failing continues to eject blood into circulation in the normal amount. Because the systemic circulation is a closed loop, the volume of blood pushed out from one side of the heart has to eventually be handled with equal efficiency by the other side of the heart. Unfortunately, if one side of the heart is failing, the blood returning to that failing side is not pumped through as quickly as it is being pumped out by the "normal" side. Hence blood returning to the failing side tends to "back up" into the atria and veins, bringing the blood to the failing ventricle. The increased buildup of blood, or congestion, increases pressure in the veins returning blood to the failing side, and eventually the pressure increases in the capillaries that flow into those veins. The increased pressure in those capillaries causes water to be pushed from the capillaries into the tissues, producing edema.

In the case of left-sided heart failure, the failing left side causes increased blood pressure to build up in the left atrium pulmonary veins and the pulmonary capillaries. The increased pressure in the pulmonary capillaries produces pulmonary edema at the pulmonary capillary beds. Likewise, in the case of right-sided heart failure, the failing right side causes increased blood pressure to build up in the right atrium, the venae cavae that are returning blood from the whole body and capillaries everywhere in the body except in the pulmonary system. Thus, in right-sided heart failure, the edema produced in veterinary patients typically appears as fluid accumulation in the abdomen (ascites). Because humans stand upright, some increase in fluid appears in the abdomen, but a great deal of tissue swelling occurs in the lower extremities of the legs due to the effect of gravity and congestion. Diuretics are used to reduce the blood volume, reduce the pressure within the compromised part of circulation, and reduce the production of tissue edema. See the You Need to Know box "What Causes Ascites and Pulmonary Edema?" for further explanation.

All diuretics act by roughly the same basic mechanism. Diuretics either prevent reabsorption of Na^+ or K^+ from the renal tubules or they enhance their secretion into the tubules. The net increase in Na^+ or K^+ in the renal tubules creates an osmotic force that draws water into, or retains water within, the renal tubules, removing water from the body as urine. Diuretics should be used cautiously in any animal with hypovolemia (low blood volume) or hypotension (low blood pressure) because diuretics will further reduce both blood fluid volume and blood pressure.

Loop Diuretics: Furosemide

Loop diuretics such as furosemide (Lasix) are the most commonly used diuretics in veterinary medicine. The term *loop* refers to the kidney's loop of Henle, which is the location within the renal tubule where these drugs produce diuresis (Fig. 5.10). When loop diuretics inhibit the reabsorption of sodium from the urine at the thick ascending segment of the loop of Henle, Na^+ is retained in the forming urine, which osmotically retains water in the urine and results in water loss via urine.

Loop diuretics do not result in sodium loss from the body, even though they primarily work by preventing reclamation of sodium from the renal tubules. Because sodium is so important to the body, the distal convoluted tubule (downstream from the loop of Henle) has an active transport mechanism by which sodium is reabsorbed and potassium is excreted in exchange for the sodium. Because the number of solutes (ions) in the urine remains approximately the same and exerts the same degree of osmotic pressure to draw water into the urine and retain it, the diuretic effect continues despite the removal of sodium from

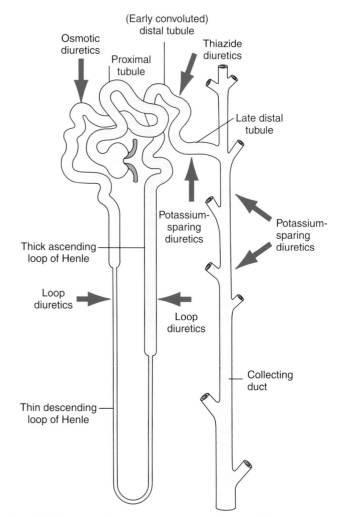

Fig. 5.10 Anatomy of the nephron and site of action of diuretics.

the forming urine. Prolonged use of loop diuretics, which would result in continual potassium loss, may result in hypokalemia (low blood potassium) if the animal's diet is not supplemented with additional potassium.

Loop diuretic drugs are not normally filtered into the urine at the glomerulus but require active transport (secretion) into the forming urine in the lumen of the proximal convoluted tubule where they flow downstream to reach their sites of action within the loop of Henle. Although furosemide can increase diuresis in early stages of renal damage or disease, in more advanced stages of renal failure the proximal convoluted tubule itself is damaged and cannot actively transport and deliver furosemide from the blood into the renal tubule, significantly decreasing furosemide's effectiveness.[19]

Furosemide is sometimes used to help control exercise-induced pulmonary hemorrhage (EIPH) in horses. However, its use remains controversial. The theoretical benefit of furosemide is through its blood volume reduction, the subsequent reduced pulmonary vascular pressure, and ultimately the reduced spontaneous hemorrhage in lungs of horses engaged in athletic activity.[19] Because furosemide use in race-horses is regulated, legal doses or use of furosemide can vary from state to state or even from track to track.

Furosemide and other loop diuretics have been implicated in ototoxicity (toxicity associated with hearing or the inner ear). Ion imbalances, especially with use of large IV doses of furosemide in cats, are believed to change the electrolyte balance in the inner ear, resulting in a loss of hearing. The risk of ototoxicosis is increased if other ototoxic compounds, such as aminoglycoside antibiotics (e.g., gentamicin, amikacin), are used concurrently with the loop diuretic. Unless permanent damage is done to the cochlea or other parts of the hearing apparatus, hearing apparently returns after diuretic use is discontinued.

Thiazide Diuretics: Chlorothiazide and Hydrochlorothiazide

Thiazide diuretics such as chlorothiazide, hydrochlorothiazide, and other thiazide-like diuretics are not often used by themselves in veterinary medicine for cardiac problems because of the greater effectiveness of furosemide. After administration, thiazides are secreted into the forming urine by the proximal convoluted tubule, pass by the loop of Henle without causing any effect, and then flow downstream to the initial (early) segment of the distal convoluted tubule (Fig. 5.10), where they act to decrease resorption of sodium and chloride. As with loop diuretics, the increased sodium in the urine is exchanged for potassium as it moves through the rest of the distal convoluted tubule. Thus, thiazide diuretics can also cause a loss of K^+, resulting in hypokalemia.

Thiazides are less potent than loop diuretics because of their site of action in the distal convoluted tubule. Normally 90% of the urine sodium is resorbed back into the body in the loop of Henle, such that the urine arriving in the distal convoluted tubule contains significantly less sodium. Blocking reabsorption of Na^+ at the distal convoluted tubule only slightly increases the osmotic force within the urine, meaning that less osmotic force is available to retain water within the tubule; hence thiazides have less diuretic effect than furosemide. With long-term use of thiazides, the body seems to adjust to the thiazide-induced Na^+ loss, resulting in a further reduction of the diuretic effect.

Thiazides may be used in the early stages of congestive heart failure because they produce moderate diuresis without significantly altering the overall body balance of electrolytes. More commonly they are used in conjunction with furosemide when the kidneys become less responsive to furosemide alone.

Potassium-Sparing Diuretics: Spironolactone

Spironolactone is a diuretic that is a competitive antagonist of aldosterone, the hormone that normally causes sodium reabsorption from the distal renal tubules and collection ducts. In animals with congestive heart failure, the overall weakened ejection of blood from the heart into systemic circulation decreases arterial blood pressure, stimulating the renin-angiotensin system and release of aldosterone to increase blood volume by body sodium retention (Fig. 5.10). By blocking aldosterone's effect on the distal convoluted tubule, less sodium is reabsorbed from the renal tubule back into the body, more Na^+ remains in the lumen of the renal tubules, and water is osmotically held in the tubule, preventing its reabsorption and increasing diuresis.

Unlike the previously mentioned diuretics, spironolactone actually increases sodium ion excretion and retains potassium in the body instead. Because they do not excrete potassium, drugs like spironolactone are called **potassium-sparing diuretics**. These drugs are not as effective as loop diuretics for the reasons described for the thiazide diuretics (90% of sodium is reabsorbed before the distal convoluted tubule). Still, spironolactone can be useful for animals with excessive fluid retention from congestive heart failure that is unresponsive to furosemide or thiazide alone or in situations in which hypokalemia is a concern.

Osmotic Diuretics

Although not used for diuresis associated with cardiac problems, mannitol and other osmotic diuretics have their roles in veterinary medicine. Mannitol is a carbohydrate (sugar), and, unlike the other diuretics that work by inhibiting renal tubular resorption of Na^+ or K^+, mannitol retains water in the renal tubules by its physical presence within the lumen of the renal tubule. This sugar is freely filtered from the blood (glomerular capillaries) into the Bowman's capsule but is poorly reabsorbed from the renal tubule. Its presence provides a solute that osmotically retains water in the renal tubular lumen, resulting in increased urine production and diuresis. Mannitol is primarily used to reduce cerebral edema associated with head trauma, reduce some of the damage to the kidneys when they are first injured by a poison or drug, and increase excretion of renally eliminated toxins.[19]

Carbonic Anhydrase Inhibitors

Carbonic anhydrase inhibitors such as acetazolamide are not often used as systemic diuretics in veterinary medicine but may be used to decrease production of aqueous humor in the eye and reduce intraocular pressure in animals with glaucoma. Because of its relatively weak diuretic effect and the ready availability of more effective diuretics, acetazolamide is not used to treat cardiac problems in veterinary patients. Veterinary ophthalmology texts will contain more information on the use of this diuretic in the treatment of glaucoma.

OTHER DRUGS USED IN TREATING CARDIOVASCULAR DISEASE

Aspirin

Aspirin (acetylsalicylic acid) inhibits platelet formation of prostaglandins and thromboxanes. Thromboxanes are released by traumatized tissue and make platelets sticky so that they will adhere to each other at small breaks in blood vessels to form a platelet plug that stops the bleeding. Reduction of platelet thromboxanes reduces aggregation (clumping) of platelets, among other actions, and therefore reduces the chances for spontaneous platelet plug formation and subsequent larger fibrin clot (thrombus) formation. In cats, aspirin can reduce the risk for spontaneous platelet adhesion and thrombus formation associated with hypertrophic or congestive cardiomyopathy. If clots are spontaneously formed in a diseased heart, they may break off (form emboli) and pass into the vasculature only to lodge and occlude smaller blood vessels. In some cats, the site for this occlusion occurs at the branches of the femoral arteries where they split to supply blood to the rear legs. The clots can lodge here and expand until they almost totally obstruct blood flow to the rear legs and tail. The use of aspirin reduces this risk. However, aspirin must be used cautiously in cats because they do not metabolize the drug as readily as other species do. Aspirin is relatively safe to use in cats if the drug is given with a 48-h dose interval to allow sufficient time for the cat to metabolize and eliminate the drug. Daily use of low-dose aspirin in human beings is advocated to decrease the risk of stroke or myocardial infarction by reducing the chance for spontaneous clot formation in the coronary arteries or vessels in the brain. Aspirin is discussed in greater detail in Chapter 13.

Clopidogrel (Plavix™)

Clopidogrel is an antithrombotic (antiplatelet) medication that is commonly used in both dogs and cats, and occasionally in horses. Recent studies have demonstrated that clopidogrel is a more effective and has less side effects as an antithrombotic agent than aspirin.[20] The reason for this is due to its unique mechanism of action compared with Aspirin. Clopidogrel inhibits platelet aggregation through inhibition of cyclooxygenase with thromboxane A_2 production. It is also an irreversible antagonist of the platelet adenosine diphosphate $(ADP)_{2Y12}$ receptor that inhibits primary and secondary platelet aggregation and inhibiting the ADP induced conformational change of the glycoprotein IIb/IIIa receptor complex.

Clopidogrel is used to prevent blood clots in patients with diseases such as immune mediated hemolytic anemia or feline cardiomyopathy. According to the most recent (2019) consensus on the rational use of antithrombotics in veterinary critical care guidelines, clopidogrel is preferred over aspirin; however, it is more expensive, so may be cost prohibitive in some cases.

Antiplatelet therapy does not always need to be discontinued before an invasive procedure. The veterinarian must evaluate the risk of bleeding compared with the risk of a thromboembolic event if the antiplatelet medication is discontinued prior to the procedure.

Rivaroxaban

Rivaroxaban is a novel oral anticoagulation medication that is not commonly used in veterinary medicine due to its high cost; however, it has demonstrated efficacy in preventing clots in high-risk cats and dogs as monotherapy and when combined with clopidogrel or aspirin. Rivaroxaban inhibits clot formation via irreversible inhibition of activated clotting factor X (FXa) and prothombinase activity. This medication does not have a reversal agent; therefore, if the patient is hemorrhaging, the patient will require a whole blood or plasma transfusion to stop the bleeding.[20,21]

Sedatives and Tranquilizers

If an animal has severe pulmonary edema secondary to advanced congestive heart failure, it may experience aerophagia, a condition in which the animal is gasping for breath. Sedatives and tranquilizers may be used to calm the anxious animal, thereby allowing the heart to slow, reduce the heart muscle's oxygen consumption, and improve the heart muscle's effectiveness.

The combination of fear-induced sympathetic nervous system–stimulated tachycardia combined with the insufficient oxygenation of the stimulated heart because of the pulmonary edema can result in death from arrhythmias. Sometimes merely calming the animal reduces the heart rate and reduces the risk of fatal arrhythmias. However, the beneficial effects of tranquilization need to be weighed against any possible adverse side effects of sedative drugs related to lowered blood pressure or decreased heart function.

CARDIAC DRUGS

Antiarrhythmic Drugs	Vasodilator Drugs
Sodium influx inhibitors	Arterial vasodilators
Lidocaine (Lignocaine)	Amlodipine
Mexiletine	Hydralazine
Procainamide	Venous vasodilator
Quinidine	Nitroglycerine
β-Blockers ("-olol" drugs)	Mixed vasodilators
Propranolol	Nitroprusside
Atenolol	ACE inhibitors ("-pril" drugs)
Esmolol	Enalapril
Metoprolol	Captopril
Carvedilol	Benazepril
Other antiarrhythmic drugs	Lisinopril
Sotalol	
Amiodarone	**Diuretics**
Calcium channel blockers	Loop diuretics
Diltiazem	Furosemide (Lasix)
Verapamil	Thiazide diuretics
Digoxin	Chlorothiazide
	Hydrochlorothiazide
Positive Inotropic Drugs and Inodilators	Potassium-sparing diuretics
	Spironolactone
Catecholamines	Osmotic diuretics
Norepinephrine/epinephrine	Mannitol
Dopamine	Carbonic anhydrase inhibitors
Dobutamine	Acetazolamide
Pimobendan	
Digoxin	**Other Drugs**
	Aspirin
	Clopidogrel
	Rivaroxaban
	Sedatives, tranquilizers

REFERENCES

1. Guyton AC, Hall JE. Textbook of Medical Physiology. 13th ed. Philadelphia: Saunders; 2016.
2. Azar T, Sharp J, Lawson D. Heart rates of male and female Sprague-Dawley and spontaneously hypertensive rats housed singly or in groups. *J Am Assoc Lab Anim Sci.* 2011;50(2):175–184.
3. Kahn CM, ed. *The Merck Veterinary Manual.* 9th ed. Whitehouse Station: Merck and Company; 2005.
4. Tilley L, Burtnick N. ECG for the Small Animal Practitioner. Jackson: Teton NewMedia; 2009.
5. Plumb's Formulary Online: https://academic-plumbs-com. ezproxy.lib.purdue.edu/drug-monograph/Ehf1HkfFUePROD? source=search&search. Accessed 06.14.22.

6. Miller WM, Adams HR. Antiarrhythmic agents. In: Riviere J, Papich M, eds. *Veterinary Pharmacology and Therapeutics.* Ames, Iowa: Wiley-Blackwell; 2009.

7. DeFrancesco T. Basic review of cardiac drugs for the ER and ICU. In: *Proceedings of the International Veterinary Emergency and Critical Care Symposium, San Diego, California, September 7–11;* 2013.

8. Van Loon G. Treatment of common arrhythmias (equine). In: *Proceedings of the American College of Veterinary Internal Medicine Forum, Seattle, Washington, June 12–15;* 2013.

9. Ware W. Drugs acting on the cardiovascular system. In: Hsu WH, ed. *Handbook of Veterinary Pharmacology.* 2nd ed. Seoul: Shinilbooks Company; 2013:277–320.

10. Boothe DM. Therapy of Cardiovascular Disease in Small Animal Clinical Pharmacology and Therapeutics. Philadelphia: Saunders; 2012.

11. Sleeper MM. Management of canine atrial fibrillation. In: *Proceedings of the American Veterinary Medical Association Annual Meeting, St. Louis, Missouri, July 16–19;* 2011.

12. Miller WM, Adams HR. Digitalis, positive inotropics, and vasodilators. In: Riviere J, Papich M, eds. *Veterinary Pharmacology and Therapeutics.* Ames, Iowa: Wiley-Blackwell; 2009.

13. Gordon SG, Miller MW, Saunders AB. Pimobendan in heart failure therapy—a silver bullet? *J Am Anim Hosp Assoc.* 2006;42(2):90–93.

14. Bowles D, Fry D. Pimobendan and its use in treating canine congestive heart failure. *Compend Contin Educ Vet.* 2011;33(11): E1–E6.

15. Cote E. Positive inotropes: digoxin, pimobendan, and others. In: *Proceedings of the 2008 World Veterinary Congress, Vancouver, British Columbia, Canada, July 27–31;* 2008.

16. Boswood A, Häggström J, Gordon SG, et al. Effect of pimobendan in dogs with preclinical myxomatous mitral valve disease and cardiomegaly: the EPIC study—a randomized clinical trial. *J Vet Intern Med.* 2016;30(6):1765–1779. https://doi.org/10.1111/jvim.14586.

17. Conversy B, Blais MC, Dunn M, Gara-Boivin C, Del Castillo JRE. Anticoagulant activity of oral rivaroxaban in healthy dogs. *Vet J.* 2017;223:5–11. https://doi.org/10.1016/j.tvjl.2017.03.006. Erratum in: Vet J. 2020;263:105522.

18. Atkins C, Bonagura J, Ettinger S, et al. Guidelines for the diagnosis and treatment of canine chronic valvular heart disease. *J Vet Intern Med.* 2009;23:1142–1150.

19. Kochevar DT. Diuretics. In: Riviere J, Papich M, eds. *Veterinary Pharmacology and Therapeutics.* Ames, Iowa: Wiley-Blackwell; 2009.

20. Hogan DF, Fox PR, Jacob K, et al. Secondary prevention of cardiogenic arterial thromboembolism in the CAT: the double-blind, randomized, positive-controlled feline arterial thromboembolism; clopidogrel vs. aspirin trial (FAT CAT). *J Vet Cardiol.* 2015;17(Suppl. 1):S306–S317. https://doi.org/10.1016/j.jvc.2015.10.004.

21. Goggs R, Bacek L, Bianco D, Koenigshof A, Li RHL. Consensus on the Rational Use of Antithrombotics in Veterinary Critical Care (CURATIVE): domain 2-defining rational therapeutic usage. *J Vet Emerg Crit Care (San Antonio).* 2019;29(1):49–59. https://doi.org/10.1111/vec.12791.

FURTHER READING

Atkins CE, Keene BW, Brown WA, et al. Results of the veterinary enalapril trial to prove reduction in onset of heart failure in dogs chronically treated with enalapril alone for compensated, naturally occurring mitral valve insufficiency. *J Am Vet Med Assoc.* 2007;231 (7):1061–1069.

Chetboul V, Lefebvre HP, Sampedrano CC, et al. Comparative adverse cardiac effects of pimobendan and benazepril monotherapy in dogs with mild degenerative mitral valve disease: a prospective, controlled, blinded and randomized study. *J Vet Intern Med.* 2007;21 (4):742–753.

SELF-ASSESSMENT

1. Fill in the following blanks with the correct item from the Key Terms list.

    A. _____ This term describes the pressure exerted on the ventricle wall by the "load" or volume of blood in the ventricles just before ventricular contraction.

    B. _____ This term describes the special cardiac cells that quickly pass along a depolarization wave throughout the heart, resulting in a coordinated contraction.

    C. _____ This is the property that describes the ability of certain heart cells to depolarize spontaneously on their own.

    D. _____ This is the pacemaker of the heart.

    E. _____ This term is the part of the ECG that represents atrial depolarization.

    F. _____ This is the specialized structure through which depolarization waves in the atria must pass to get to the ventricles; it delays the depolarization wave as it passes.

    G. _____ That part of the ECG that represents movement of the depolarization wave through the AV node.

    H. _____ This is the part of the ECG that represents ventricular depolarization.

    I. _____ This is the part of the ECG that represents ventricular repolarization.

    J. _____ When a cardiac cell is in the resting, polarized state, this ion is mostly concentrated on the inside of the cell.

    K. _____ This ion rushes into the cardiac cell to initiate depolarization.

    L. _____ This is the specialized pump that maintains concentrations of sodium and potassium in their respective locations during the polarized resting state.

    M. _____ The influx of what ion produces the plateau phase of cardiac muscle cell depolarization?

N. _____ This is any abnormal or irregular heart rhythm.

O. _____ These are the two catecholamines released by the sympathetic nervous system that produce its effects.

P. _____ Stimulation of this receptor increases heart rate.

Q. _____ Stimulation of this receptor slows heart rate.

R. _____ Stimulation of this receptor causes bronchodilation.

S. _____ Stimulation of this receptor causes increased GI activity.

T. _____ Stimulation of this receptor causes peripheral vasoconstriction.

U. _____ This term means a fast heart rate.

V. _____ This is a site of depolarization in the heart that is other than on the normal conduction pathway sequence (SA node, AV node).

W. _____ Large, bizarre-looking wave on the ECG caused by some cell in the ventricles depolarizing on its own out of sequence and disrupting normal ventricular depolarization.

X. _____ Abnormality seen on ECG as a prolongation of the PR interval, representing decreased conduction of the depolarization wave through the atrioventricular (AV) node.

Y. _____ At the end of a drug name, this often indicates the drug is a β-blocker (β_1 antagonist) antiarrhythmic drug.

Z. _____ This is the process by which cardiac cells become less sensitive to the effects of β-blocker antiarrhythmics; the process involves increasing the number of β_1 receptors on the cardiac cell surface, making it more sensitive to catecholamines like norepinephrine.

AA. _____ These detect changes in arterial blood pressure.

AB. _____ This system helps regulate arterial blood pressure, water, and electrolytes through its action on the kidneys and peripheral blood vessels.

AC. _____ The body's most potent vasoconstrictor, converted to its active form by ACE.

AD. _____ The hormone that regulates sodium reabsorption from the urine.

AE. _____ The term applied to drugs that selectively dilate veins.

AF. _____ This is the type of cardiac drug recognizable by the "-pril" at the end.

AG. _____ What "ACE" stands for.

AH. _____ This is the term applied to drugs that cause increased production of urine.

2. Fill in the following blanks with the correct drug from the Cardiovascular Drug list. When practicing these questions, write out the answers on a separate sheet, focusing also on the appropriate spelling of these drug names.

A. _____ Antiarrhythmic drug that acts by blocking the sodium channels; the drug of choice for control of ventricular ectopic foci, but not effective against atrial ectopic foci; must be given IV; not effective PO because of GI irritation and first-pass effect.

B. _____ Orally administered sodium channel blocker antiarrhythmic that is used to treat ventricular arrhythmias; minimal first-pass effect; typically available as a compounded drug.

C. _____ Nonspecific prototype β_1 antagonist antiarrhythmic drug.

D. _____ Name at least three other β-blocker antiarrhythmics that are more specific for β_1-receptors than the nonspecific prototype β-blocker.

E. _____ Name two calcium channel blocker antiarrhythmics.

F. _____ Drug used as an antiarrhythmic only to slow conduction through the AV node (produces first- or second-degree AV block), reducing the ventricular contraction rate in animals with atrial fibrillation; does not reduce atrial fibrillation itself.

G. _____ Positive inotropic drug used only for short periods of time because of the downregulation effect.

H. _____ Inodilator.

I. _____ Old positive inotropic drug; increases amount of calcium available inside the cell by a chain reaction that starts with poisoning the sodium-potassium-ATPase pump.

J. _____ Calcium channel blocker arterial vasodilator used in cats for hypertension caused by renal disease, hyperthyroidism, or diabetes mellitus.

K. _____ Direct arterial vasodilator used to relieve signs of congestive heart failure caused by mitral valve disease or used when ACE inhibitors fail to adequately control clinical signs of heart failure on their own.

L. _____ Venous vasodilator applied as a cream.

M. _____ Mixed (balanced) vasodilator quite commonly used to treat dogs exhibiting clinical signs of cardiac disease; works by inhibition of ACE.

N. _____ Loop diuretic.

O. _____ Diuretic that works on the distal convoluted tubule to block sodium reabsorption; not as strong a diuretic as loop diuretics.

P. _____ Potassium-sparing diuretic.

Q. _____ Used to reduce spontaneous clot formation, such as in cats with hypertrophic cardiomyopathy.

3. Describe the blood flow through the heart, starting with the anterior vena cava and ending with the aorta. Include all the chambers of the heart, the valves between each chamber, and the major blood vessels carrying blood to and from the atria and ventricles.

4. If the veterinarian were to thread a catheter into the heart by way of the jugular vein into the anterior vena cava and then into the heart, what would be the first chamber of the heart the catheter would enter? What if the catheter were threaded up the femoral artery to the dorsal aorta and into the aorta itself?

5. What is the difference between the absolute and relative refractory periods in the depolarization cycle of the heart cells?

6. Describe the path of a depolarization wave from the SA node to the ventricles. What physiologic purpose does the delay at the AV node serve?

7. What characteristic of the SA node makes it the pacemaker of the normal heart?

8. Which part of the autonomic nervous system causes the heart to speed up and which causes it to slow down?

9. What is the difference between what an adrenergic receptor does vs a cholinergic receptor?

10. Name the effect sympathetic and parasympathetic stimulation would have on the following: heart rate, heart force of contraction, GI tract activity, size of bronchioles, size of the arterioles, and pupil size.

11. Why is it preferred to use a selective adrenergic drug as opposed to a less selective one?

12. What is the difference between fibrillation and flutter? Which is worse: atrial fibrillation or ventricular fibrillation? Are these arrhythmias or are they bradyarrhythmias or tachyarrhythmias?

13. Classify the following arrhythmias according to heart rate (tachycardia or bradycardia) and the location of the problem (supraventricular or ventricular):

    A. Arrhythmia in a dog with ventricular contraction rate of 200 beats/min caused by atrial fibrillation.

    B. Arrhythmia in a dog with a ventricular contraction rate of 40 beats/min caused by inability of the SA node to depolarize at its normal rate.

    C. Arrhythmia in a dog with a series of PVCs that increases the heart rate to 150 beats/min for approximately 30 s.

14. What is the difference between first-degree and second-degree AV block?

15. Why should β-blocker antiarrhythmics not be used in animals with significant congestive heart failure?

16. Mrs. Jones's dog has been on a β-blocker to control a ventricular tachyarrhythmia. It was started 2 weeks ago, and the heart rate decreased as expected, along with the tachyarrhythmias. However, on the recheck today the heart rate has crept upward toward its pretreatment heart rate, and the ECG shows signs of intermittent tachyarrhythmias. Can you explain why the drug appears to be failing 2 weeks after starting it? Should the dog be taken off the drug immediately?

17. Why does digoxin toxicosis start out as exhibiting GI signs instead of cardiac signs?

18. Why is peripheral arteriole vasoconstriction a bad thing in a weak heart if the vasoconstriction keeps arterial blood pressure up in the normal range?

19. How does aldosterone increase arterial blood pressure? Why is this bad for a congestive heart failure patient?

20. Mrs. Jones's 14-year-old poodle has just been put on a vasodilator. About what precautions should veterinary technicians tell clients like Mrs. Jones when their pets first start on vasodilator drugs? Why is it that veterinarians have to be careful when using a vasodilator on a patient at the same time as a β-blocker antiarrhythmic drug?

21. Why do vasodilator drugs often lose their effect after a period of time?

22. Why must ACE inhibitors be used with caution in animals with preexisting kidney disease or elevated levels of potassium in the body (often accompanies renal failure) or if an animal is on potassium supplementation?

23. Why does enalapril cause vasodilation in animals with heart failure but have little effect in normal animals?

24. If the veterinarian prescribes nitroglycerin cream for use on a canine patient, what precautions should owners take to protect themselves when treating their animal with the topical nitroglycerin product?

25. How do diuretics reduce edema formation?

26. Why is furosemide more effective at producing diuresis than chlorothiazide?

27. How is it that spironolactone causes less loss of potassium than furosemide or thiazide diuretics?

28. For what is acetazolamide diuretic used?

29. Mannitol is kept on the shelf for use as a diuretic. Why is mannitol not used in congestive heart failure to cause diuresis, as are the other diuretics such as furosemide, chlorothiazide, and spironolactone?

30. You overhear the veterinarian telling the owner of a cat with cardiomyopathy to administer aspirin. However, you remember that aspirin must be used with caution in cats. Is the doctor wrong to recommend aspirin for this cat?

31. Why might sedatives or tranquilizers be used in patients in a crisis with congestive heart failure?

32. Indicate whether each statement is true or false.

    A. Parasympathomimetic drugs would be expected to decrease the heart rate.

    B. An adrenergic antagonist drug would be expected to increase the heart rate.

    C. Vasoconstriction of the peripheral arterioles would be expected to cause an immediate decrease in arterial blood pressure.

    D. The most oxygenated blood in the body can be found in the pulmonary arteries.

    E. First- or second-degree AV blocks are more likely to occur with increased activation of the parasympathetic nervous system than activation of the sympathetic.

    F. Sodium moves out of the cell during depolarization.

    G. Dogs are more sensitive to the effects of lidocaine than cats.

    H. A drug that imitates the effects of acetylcholine would slow the heart rate.

    I. A drug that blocks α_1-receptors would cause a drop in arterial blood pressure.

J. Lidocaine formulated as a local anesthetic for subcutaneous use is okay to use IV for control of ventricular arrhythmias.

K. The initial dose of quinidine sometimes causes an increased heart rate in animals experiencing atrial fibrillation or flutter.

L. Upregulation occurs with β-blocker drugs, and downregulation occurs with β-agonist drugs.

M. Digoxin toxicity is more likely to cause bradycardia than tachycardia.

N. A negative inotropic effect means that the drug slows the heart rate.

O. Increased inotropic effect comes from the increased release of sodium or the increased availability of sodium to combine with the muscle contractile filaments.

P. The advantage of β-blocker drugs over other antiarrhythmics is that if problems arise after several weeks of therapy, the drug can be safely stopped immediately.

Q. Pimobendan would be safe to use in cats with congestive heart failure but should NOT be used in cats with hypertrophic cardiomyopathy.

R. ACE converts angiotensinogen to renin.

S. Stimulating baroreceptors (by stretching) results in activation of the sympathetic nervous system.

T. Furosemide is considered to be a stronger diuretic than the thiazide diuretics.

U. Mannitol is a vasodilator.

V. Aspirin can be safely used in cats.

Drugs Affecting the Respiratory System

OBJECTIVES

After studying this chapter, the veterinary technician should be able to:

- Describe the mechanisms by which the respiratory system protects itself and how these mechanisms can be altered by disease.
- Explain the mechanisms by which antitussives work.
- Describe how mucolytics, expectorants, and decongestants work to relieve signs of respiratory disease, how they alter physiology to produce their effects, and whether they serve any significant purpose in veterinary medicine.
- Describe the types of bronchodilators and how they produce their beneficial effects.
- Explain how corticosteroids and antihistamines are useful in respiratory disease and how they differ from each other in their mechanisms.
- Describe the role of diuretics and oxygen in the treatment of respiratory disease.

KEY TERMS

aerosolization
aerosol therapy
alpha-1 (α_1) receptor
antitussive drugs
beta-1 (β_1) receptor
beta-2 (β_2) receptor
bronchoconstriction
centrally acting antitussive
cor pulmonale
cyclic adenosine monophosphate (cAMP)

decongestants
dyspnea
expectorants
histamine type 1 (H_1) receptors
inspissated
locally acting antitussive
metered-dose inhaler (MDI)
mucociliary apparatus
mucolytic

nebulization
opioid
phosphodiesterase
productive/nonproductive cough
recurrent airway obstruction (RAO)
serotonin
tachypnea

THE RESPIRATORY SYSTEM'S PROTECTIVE MECHANISMS

The body is quite effective at protecting the respiratory tract from injury or infection by either preventing foreign substances from reaching the alveoli or expelling offensive substances from the respiratory tract. The upper respiratory tract decreases the ability of materials or offensive substances to enter the respiratory tree by causing sneezing or excessive mucous secretions to expel or dilute the offending substances. If a substance makes it past the nose, any stimulation of the laryngeal area, trachea, or bronchial tree elicits a coughing response that can range from a deep, subtle cough to a retching gag. The vocal folds of the larynx can slam shut with a spasm if they are irritated or mechanically stimulated (e.g., laryngospasm when trying to place an endotracheal tube).[1]

In the trachea and larger bronchioles, a sheet of sticky mucus traps particles. The mucus is then swept upward by microscopic, hairlike cilia that line the respiratory tract so that the mucus and trapped materials are coughed up and expelled. This combination of mucus and cilia constitutes the mucociliary apparatus.[2] Because this apparatus moves mucus and trapped materials up the bronchi and trachea, it is sometimes referred to as the mucociliary escalator. As the airways divide into smaller and smaller branches, they lose the benefit of the mucociliary apparatus because the presence of the mucus would likely obstruct very small openings.

At the level of the terminal bronchioles—the smallest bronchial airways that connect with the alveoli—the last line of defense is ring of smooth muscle that surrounds the small terminal bronchioles and can narrow or close off the airway (bronchoconstriction), preventing foreign materials from entering and damaging the alveoli. Finally, if foreign particles or bacteria do make it to the alveoli, macrophages (i.e., phagocytic cells) can engulf them.[1]

When these protective mechanisms work effectively, potential pathogens (i.e., disease-causing organisms) and noxious gasses are prevented from entering the body. But under certain conditions these protective mechanisms become overstimulated or act when they are not needed for protection. Under these circumstances the protective mechanism is now contributing to the signs of clinical disease itself.

For example, a dry cough that continues for months may lead to deterioration of the cartilage rings in the trachea, resulting in partial tracheal collapse or vascular changes in the lungs that can lead to heart problems (a condition called cor pulmonale).[1] Another example would be asthma, in which an overabundance of bronchoconstrictive activity would deprive the animal of the ability to bring oxygen into the alveoli.

Just like in the gastrointestinal (GI) tract or cardiovascular physiology illustrated in the previous chapters, the veterinarian must intervene to attenuate or reduce the body's overzealous protective reaction to prevent further tissue damage or death. Whenever respiratory drugs are used to treat a cough, nasal secretions, or sneezing, the benefit of the treatment must be weighed against the effect it has in depressing the body's natural protective mechanisms.

ANTITUSSIVES

Antitussive drugs block the cough reflex. The cough reflex is coordinated by the cough center, which is a cluster of neurons located next to the respiratory centers in the medullary area of the brainstem. The presence of irritation or stimulation of cough receptors in the larynx, trachea, bronchi, or bronchioles sends impulses to the brainstem, where the cough reflex causes contraction of the appropriate respiratory muscles to produce a sharp, forceful expiration (i.e., cough).

The nature of the cough is determined to some degree by the location of the cough receptors that are stimulated and whether mucus is brought up with the cough.[3] When the larynx or pharynx is stimulated by irritation or pressure from food or other materials, receptors send impulses to the brainstem by way of the vagus nerve, resulting in a sudden gagging, violent, retching type of coughing. Stimulation of these receptors can also produce a reflex constriction of the small terminal bronchioles (i.e., bronchoconstriction). This choking cough is observed when food is accidentally inhaled or anything irritates the pharynx.

Receptors located lower in the trachea and those located in the bronchi respond to mechanical and chemical irritation or the release of histamine by producing a deep, forceful cough mediated by the cough center. Tachypnea (i.e., rapid breathing) and reflex bronchoconstriction may also accompany this type of stimulation. This deeper type of cough is associated with bronchitis, inhalation of irritating gases, allergic bronchoconstriction, or pressure of the bronchi from an enlarged heart.[3]

Coughs can also be classified as productive or nonproductive according to the amount of mucus associated with the cough. A productive cough produces mucus, whereas a nonproductive cough is dry and hacking, with no significant mucus brought up. A nonproductive cough may occur in the early stages of infection or inflammation when the mucous glands lining the respiratory tree have not yet significantly increased production of mucus. A nonproductive cough may become productive as the disease progresses. A nonproductive cough may also be associated with chronic conditions such as chronic bronchitis, in which the mucus produced becomes inspissated (i.e., dry) and sticky and thus accumulates in the bronchi instead of being effectively coughed up. A nonproductive cough may also occur in an animal that is significantly dehydrated, preventing the mucous glands from producing sufficient liquid secretions.

Antitussive drugs suppress the coughing mechanism that the body uses to remove mucus, cellular debris, exudates, and other products that accumulate within the bronchi as a result of infection or inflammation. Therefore, veterinarians should use antitussives cautiously or avoid large doses in animals with a very productive cough or a nonproductive cough in which the mucus is very sticky and not easily moved by the mucociliary apparatus (e.g., chronic bronchitis). Some sources state that antitussives are contraindicated for use in very productive coughs.[1] In such situations, the mucociliary apparatus may not be able to adequately clear the respiratory tree debris by itself, and the body may be relying on the cough itself to prevent obstruction of the airways or accumulation of excessive mucus and debris.

Antitussives are sometimes described as centrally acting or locally acting. A centrally acting antitussive, such as the codeine or hydrocodone found in cough syrups, reduces coughing by suppressing the cough center neurons in the brainstem. In contrast, a locally acting antitussive, such as a cough lozenge, reduces coughing by directly soothing the irritated respiratory mucosa that is initiating the cough. Centrally acting antitussives are the only type used in veterinary medicine because veterinary patients are unwilling to hold lozenges in their mouth long enough to be effective.

Antitussives are commonly used to treat animals with dry, nonproductive coughs generated by inflammation in the trachea (i.e., tracheitis) or both trachea and bronchi (i.e., tracheobronchitis). Although these inflammatory diseases are often mild by themselves, they may keep the pet and the owner awake at night and often delay resolution of the underlying cause of the cough because the cough itself promotes further irritation to the already inflamed airway.

One of the most common uses of antitussives is for treatment of uncomplicated tracheobronchitis in dogs, commonly called "kennel cough." The retching type of cough associated with kennel cough is often punctuated by gagging and produces a small amount of mucus that the owner interprets as vomitus. The harsh coughing irritates the trachea, which stimulates more coughing, which further irritates the airway. This pattern can continue for weeks after the inciting agent has been removed or successfully treated unless the cough itself is treated. Cases of untreated tracheobronchitis can result in chronic bronchitis, secondary bacterial bronchitis or pneumonia, cardiac problems (e.g., cor pulmonale), or eventual weakening of the cartilaginous tracheal rings and subsequent tracheal collapse. In this situation, the protective mechanism of the body is doing more harm than good and needs to be suppressed.

Butorphanol

Butorphanol (Torbutrol) is a centrally acting opioid cough suppressant that is the only FDA-approved veterinary antitussive. Because it is an opioid drug (meaning *opium-like*), it is considered a narcotic drug with potential for abuse and is therefore classified as a class C-IV controlled substance. Butorphanol is also commonly used as an analgesic (pain-killing) drug. All opioid drugs suppress the respiratory center and cough by stimulating opioid receptors in the medulla of the brainstem. This suppression of the respiratory center is commonly observed when opioids are used as part of an anesthetic or analgesic protocol for surgical patients, and it is this same suppression that constitutes the antitussive mechanism for opioid cough medications.[4] Interestingly, butorphanol's cough suppressant effect can be reversed by the opioid antagonist drug naloxone. This lends support to the idea that opioid receptor stimulation produces the antitussive effects of opioid-based drugs.[2]

Because butorphanol is commonly used as an analgesic sedative in anesthetic protocols, it would be expected that larger antitussive doses of butorphanol could produce some degree of sedation. Butorphanol is available in both injectable and tablet forms, but different doses for antitussive activity are required for the different routes of administration. Orally administered butorphanol has a low overall bioavailability because of a significant first-pass effect. A smaller percentage of the orally administered drug is absorbed compared with the equivalent injectable dose, and hence the oral dose of butorphanol is about 10 times higher than the equivalent injectable dose.[2]

Hydrocodone

Hydrocodone (Hycodan) is an orally administered potent mu (mu [μ]-opioid receptor agonist that is synthesized from codeine but considered to be more potent than codeine.[5] It is

a human drug (all veterinary use is extra-label) and is listed as a CII controlled substance for most cough preparations.

As would be expected, sedation can be noted with the use of this drug. Additionally, long-term administration of this drug can result in constipation because opioids slow GI motility and decrease intestinal secretions (see Chapter 4).

Because hydrocodone has been a target for diversion (i.e., stealing drugs for purposes of selling them illegally for abuse purposes) this drug is not as widely available as it has been in the past. In the United States, hydrocodone commercial preparations are commonly mixed with a low dose of an atropine compound designed to discourage abuse of the drug by causing an uncomfortable dry mouth. In Canada, hydrocodone can be found without the atropine.[2] Veterinary technicians should take notice of any client who makes repeated requests for strong opioid antitussive prescriptions or drug refills to relieve a pet's cough and should date and document such requests in the patient's record and report it to the veterinarian.

Codeine

Codeine is a relatively weak μ-opioid receptor agonist antitussive and is found in a variety of oral cough and cold preparations.[4] All prescription products containing codeine have either a C-II (pure codeine) or C-III (e.g., acetaminophen plus codeine) rating. Products with lower concentrations of codeine may be incorporated with other drugs to treat the symptoms of cold and flu (e.g., acetaminophen, antihistamines, decongestants, expectorants) and may be obtained through a pharmacist with or without a prescription, depending on the state or provincial law.[1,2] The sedative and constipation effects of codeine are similar to those of hydrocodone.[2]

Because orally administered codeine is poorly and inconsistently absorbed in the dog, its use is more common in humans than it is for canine coughs. Codeine plus acetaminophen combinations would be contraindicated for use in cats because of the toxic effect of acetaminophen in cats.

Dextromethorphan

Unlike the opioids from which it is chemically derived, dextromethorphan is an antitussive that is considered a nonnarcotic because it does not combine with either the μ- or kappa (κ)-opioid receptor to produce its antitussive effect.[2] Because it is not a narcotic, it is not a controlled substance and therefore is a common ingredient in over-the-counter (OTC) nonprescription cough, flu, and cold preparations. Although dextromethorphan has demonstrated antitussive activity in humans, its use in dogs is questionable because of its relatively poor absorption when given orally and little documentation of its effectiveness.[2]

Dextromethorphan is not recommended for use to control coughing in dogs or cats. However, veterinary technicians should be aware of this drug because owners may attempt to medicate pets for colds or cough at home by using human cold products containing dextromethorphan. Although dextromethorphan in OTC products is fairly harmless to animals by itself, most cold or flu preparations contain many other ingredients like acetaminophen or decongestants that potentially could have more serious side effects.

⚠ YOU NEED TO KNOW

Reverse Sneezing

Reverse sneezing is condition in dogs that is typically reported by clients as the pet being "unable to catch its breath" or "making a weird gagging, snorting sound." On closer inspection of history, the owners will report that it is not a cough nor is it a real sneeze. The animal typically does not seem to be bothered by it excessively, and often the owner is more upset by it than the pet.

Reverse sneezing can be caused by any irritation in the nasal cavity ranging from an allergic response to inhaled antigens to nasal polyps and tumors. Though most cases are benign allergic reactions to environmental stimuli, a diagnosis, or at least a rule-out, of other more serious conditions requires doing an endoscopic examination of the reach of the nasal cavity.

Because most of these reverse sneeze situations are the result of an allergic reaction, they can be controlled or reduced by the use of antihistamines or, in more advanced cases, corticosteroids.

Padrid P. Diagnosis and treatment of upper airway disorders. In *Proceedings of the 2013 American Board of Veterinary Practitioners*, Phoenix, Arizona, 2013.

MUCOLYTICS, EXPECTORANTS, AND DECONGESTANTS

As mentioned at the beginning of this chapter, glands and mucus-producing cells line the respiratory tree, where they produce the sticky mucous layer that traps particles that enter the lower respiratory tree. Columnar epithelial cells with cilia also line the respiratory tree from the larger bronchioles to the laryngeal area where the cilia sweep mucus and particulate matter up the respiratory tree to the oropharynx, where they are coughed up and swallowed or expectorated (spit out) (Fig. 6.1).

In respiratory diseases or physiologic changes, the protective mechanism of the mucociliary apparatus can be overwhelmed or significantly impaired. For example, in severely dehydrated animals, the mucous membranes become dry and the mucus layer becomes very sticky, preventing the cilia from moving the mucus up and out of the respiratory tree. Therefore, dehydrated animals often exhibit a nonproductive cough because they are unable to remove much of the dried, inspissated mucus. However, after the patient is rehydrated the mucus regains its normal fluid consistency and the cough may become quite productive. Thus, the veterinary professional should ideally correct

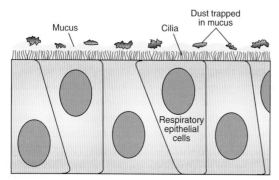

Fig. 6.1 The mucociliary apparatus traps dust particles and other debris in a blanket of mucus.

for systemic dehydration before deciding whether to give a drug that modifies or increases the activity of the mucociliary apparatus.

Mucolytics

Mucolytic agents, as the name implies, are designed to break up, or lyse, mucus and reduce its viscosity so the cilia can more readily move it out of the respiratory tract. For example, when there is an infection or inflammation occurring on the surface of the cells lining the respiratory tree (because that is the side inhaled bacteria or irritants would come from), inflammatory cells move into the affected area to combat the infectious agent or to help clean up the cellular debris. During this process, these inflammatory cells die and lyse, releasing their contents. When the cells die in the mucus, the sulfhydryl groups located on the deoxyribonucleic acid (DNA) in the dead and lysed inflammatory cells react with protein in mucus to create disulfide bonds (S—S), causing the mucus to become more viscous (thicker) and sticky. When this happens, the cilia cannot adequately move the viscous mucus and the mucociliary apparatus becomes less effective. By breaking apart the bonds that make mucus sticky, mucolytic drugs can improve the mucociliary apparatus function again.

Acetylcysteine (Mucomyst) is a mucolytic agent that decreases the viscosity of mucus by breaking apart the disulfide bonds that were contributed to the mucus by DNA strands and that contribute significantly to the viscosity of the mucus. When acetylcysteine is used as a mucolytic, it can be administered by mouth or by nebulization, which is the inhalation of a fine mist containing the drug. Although nebulization can deliver drug to the surface of the bronchi and bronchioles in humans, it is less effective for veterinary patients because the animals resist inhaling the mist deeply. Acetylcysteine is also used as the orally or intravenously administered antidote for acetaminophen (Tylenol) toxicosis in cats by helping convert the toxic acetaminophen metabolite to a nontoxic metabolite and preventing acetaminophen's conversion of hemoglobin to nonfunctional methemoglobin.

Sometimes owners create a mucolytic effect in a pet by placing the animal in a steamy bathroom or using a humidifier in a closed space. Although this practice increases the fluidity of secretions in the upper respiratory tract, it does not significantly increase the fluidity of the mucus in the lower airways because the comparatively large steam droplets precipitate in the trachea and are not inhaled deeply enough to penetrate the lower airways.[1]

When oxygen is administered to animals with respiratory problems or other disease, the very dry nature of the gas can dehydrate the mucociliary apparatus and decrease its efficiency. Therefore, if a patient has significant respiratory disease or is going to be on oxygen long term, moisture may be added to the oxygen by bubbling it through a container of water.

Expectorants

Expectorants also improve the effectiveness of the mucociliary apparatus by increasing the fluidity of mucus in the respiratory tract. As opposed to mucolytics, which reduce the viscosity of mucus by chemically altering it, expectorants increase the fluidity of mucus by generating watery secretions by respiratory tract cells. To expectorate means "to spit"; therefore, expectorants increase the amount of fluid moved up from the lower respiratory tract to a point where it can be coughed up or spit out.

Although expectorants are commonly included in human OTC cold preparations, they are of questionable benefit in veterinary patients. A more effective expectorant-like effect can be achieved by maintaining proper systemic hydration of the patient and increasing the humidity of inspired air. The benefits of expectorants must also be weighed against the increased volume of fluid that would have to be removed from the respiratory tree by the mucociliary apparatus.

Guaifenesin (glyceryl guaiacolate) and **saline expectorants** such as ammonium chloride, potassium iodide, and sodium citrate are given by mouth and increase watery secretions in the respiratory tree. These drugs slightly irritate the gastric mucosa, stimulating the parasympathetic nervous system to create respiratory secretions. This link between GI tract stimulation of the parasympathetic nervous system and bronchiole secretions can be demonstrated in people who eat a large meal when they have a cold. Within 5–15 min after eating, the person will begin to cough from the expectorant action caused by increased parasympathetic stimulation associated with increased GI tract function.

When animals accidentally ingest cold medications with these expectorants, they often vomit because of the irritant action of these medications on the gastric mucosa. Guaifenesin, sometimes referred to as "GG" for glyceryl guaiacolate, is also administered intravenously to produce muscle relaxation in equine anesthesia protocols.

In contrast to expectorants that act by irritating the gastric mucosa, the **volatile oil** expectorants such as terpin hydrate, eucalyptus oil, and pine oil directly stimulate watery respiratory secretions when their vapors are inhaled or when the absorbed volatile oil is excreted by the respiratory tract.

Decongestants

Many OTC human cold preparations also contain decongestants such as pseudoephedrine and phenylephrine for relief of nasal congestion. Decongestants reduce congestion (i.e., vascular engorgement) of swollen nasal tissues by stimulating the sympathetic nervous system's alpha-1 (α_1) receptors on the smooth muscle of blood vessels in the skin and mucous membranes. When stimulated, α_1 receptors cause vasoconstriction in the swollen mucous membranes of the nasal passages, which decreases the flow of blood through capillaries, reduces the amount of fluid leaking out into the tissues, and thereby decreases tissue edema and secretions by mucous glands.

Because the molecules in decongestants are not specific for α_1 receptors, most have some beta-1 (β_1)-receptor activity and therefore increase the heart rate as a side effect. In most animals, this does not cause significant problems; however, if the animal has cardiovascular disease, the additional oxygen demand by the β_1-stimulated myocardial cells could result in arrhythmia.

Because the decongestant ingredient pseudoephedrine closely resembles methamphetamine in its chemical structure, cold medications containing this decongestant have provided the raw material for the creation of methamphetamine in meth labs. For this reason, the ability to purchase cold medications with pseudoephedrine is regulated either by prescription or having to purchase the product from the pharmacist ("behind-the-counter" drug). The other decongestant phenylephrine is not a precursor for methamphetamine production and hence is not regulated like pseudoephedrine, but it is also considered to be a less effective decongestant than pseudoephedrine.[2]

Decongestants are typically not used in veterinary medicine. However, because pet owners sometimes treat their animals with their own OTC human cold and flu medications, veterinary professionals must understand the dangers involved with use of these products and be able to explain to pet owners the reasons these preparations should not be used in pets.

BRONCHODILATORS

What Causes Bronchoconstriction or Asthma?

Bronchoconstriction is the contraction of smooth muscles surrounding the small terminal bronchioles deep within the respiratory tree. Bronchoconstriction in veterinary patients is considered to be a complex effect caused by a variety of different cellular mechanisms or by alteration of the balance between sympathetic and parasympathetic nervous system control over the bronchioles.

The parasympathetic nervous system effect is slightly more dominant than the sympathetic nervous system on the bronchioles during normal, healthy conditions. The effect of the release of acetylcholine and stimulation of the bronchiolar smooth muscle muscarinic receptors creates a constant, slight degree of bronchoconstriction. The sympathetic nervous system antagonizes this primary effect by causing bronchodilation via norepinephrine stimulation of β_2 receptors.

Thus, drugs or poisons that mimic acetylcholine or stimulate the muscarinic cholinergic receptor produce bronchoconstriction and dyspnea (i.e., difficult breathing). Also, any drugs or poisons that inhibit *acetylcholinesterase*, the enzyme that normally breaks down acetylcholine and terminates its activity, would allow acetylcholine to have a greater effect on the bronchiolar smooth muscle and cause bronchoconstriction. This latter mechanism is what causes dyspnea related to organophosphate insecticide toxicity.

β-Blocker antiarrhythmic drugs (see Chapter 5) could block the β_2 receptors as a side effect of their antiarrhythmic action. This blocks the sympathetic effect and allows the parasympathetic influence to dominate, producing greater bronchoconstriction. The reason β-blocker antiarrhythmics are contraindicated for use in cats that also have feline asthma is that, as the drugs block the arrhythmias, they also block the vasodilating effect of the sympathetic nervous system and worsen the degree of bronchoconstriction from the asthma. In contrast, β_2-agonist drugs would produce bronchodilation, which explains why many asthma rescue inhalers used to reverse the effects of an asthmatic attack are β_2-agonist drugs (Fig. 6.2).

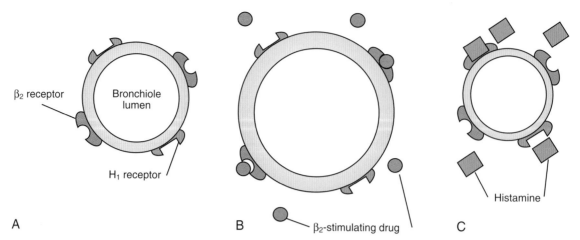

Fig. 6.2 Bronchoconstriction mechanisms. Effects of β₂- and H₁-receptor stimulation on bronchiolar smooth muscle. (A) Smooth muscle layer surrounds the bronchiole. (B) Smooth muscle relaxation and bronchiole dilation are caused by a predominance of a β₂-stimulating drug. (C) Smooth muscle contraction and bronchiole constriction are caused by a predominance of histamine.

In addition to the autonomic effects, there are a variety of local effects on the bronchioles mediated through release of different inflammatory compounds. The compound that is thought to be the principal cause of bronchoconstriction from allergies and inflammation is histamine. Histamine is released by mast cells located in the respiratory tract to varying degrees depending on the species. Though histamine stimulates several types of histamine receptors, the major one causing bronchoconstriction is the histamine type 1 (H_1) receptor located on bronchiolar smooth muscle cells.

Because histamine causes bronchoconstriction, inflammation, and edema typically found in asthma, it was thought to be the major cause of asthma bronchoconstriction. However, the lack of therapeutic response to selective H_1-receptor antagonist drugs suggested that other mediators must play an important role.[1] We now know that other inflammatory mediators released by inflammatory cells including serotonin, prostaglandins, and leukotrienes (discussed in Chapter 13) all play a role in bronchoconstriction and airway inflammation, although the importance of the role of each inflammatory mediator may vary by species. For example, serotonin probably does not play a key role in canine or human asthma, but when present in cats, serotonin produces a profound bronchoconstriction and likely plays a major role in feline asthma syndromes. One of the additional effects of β₂-receptor stimulation is the stabilization of mast cells decreasing the release of histamine and other mediators of inflammation.

Beta-Adrenergic Agonist Bronchodilators

Because beta-2 (β₂)-receptor stimulation is involved in bronchodilation and stabilization of mast cells, β-agonist drugs are often used as bronchodilators. Older β-agonist bronchodilators like epinephrine and isoproterenol were nonselective β agonists and thus stimulated β₁ receptors and the β₂ receptors, increasing the heart rate and force of contraction as a side effect when these drugs were used. Such cardiac stimulation in a healthy animal would have little consequence; however, in a patient experiencing asthma and consequently having a difficult time breathing or getting enough oxygen, an increased heart rate without sufficient oxygen could lead to arrhythmias or poor cardiac function. However, epinephrine is still used for the emergency treatment of life-threatening bronchoconstriction.[2]

The more recent generations of bronchodilator drugs—**terbutaline, albuterol,** and metaproterenol—are more selective β₂ agonists and have fewer, but still some, β₁ side effects. Unlike epinephrine, these drugs last longer and are incorporated into metered-dose inhalers (MDIs) "rescue inhalers" or "puffers," tablets, oral syrups, and injections. The oral forms of these drugs require higher doses than the parenteral forms because of the extensive first-pass effect for the oral drugs.

In addition to treating bronchoconstriction or asthma-like syndromes in small animals, terbutaline and albuterol are both used to treat an asthma syndrome in horses called equine recurrent airway obstruction (RAO) and formerly called chronic obstructive pulmonary disease (COPD). Though the terbutaline is used as the injectable form, an aerosol form of terbutaline and albuterol can be administered to horses with a pressurized MDI and a special adapter that fits over the horse's nose.

Like the β₁ agonists used as positive inotropic agents discussed in Chapter 5, the β₂-agonist drugs can begin to lose their effectiveness as a result of frequent stimulation of the receptor and subsequent downregulation of receptors. Over time, the removal of available receptors by the bronchiolar smooth muscle cells makes the cell become less responsive to the drug. Therefore, to prevent the progressive loss of function caused by downregulation, the β₂ bronchodilators should be used only intermittently for acute asthma attacks (hence the term *rescue inhaler*).

Methylxanthine Bronchodilators

The methylxanthine compounds include bronchodilators such as **theophylline** and **aminophylline,** as well as the nervous system stimulants caffeine and theobromine (the active ingredient in chocolate toxicity). Although theophylline was used in humans for many years as a bronchodilator, the side effects and the development of newer bronchodilating drugs have diminished its use. However, theophylline continues to be used in veterinary medicine, particularly in dogs.[1,2]

The mechanism by which methylxanthine produces bronchodilation remains debatable. Two different mechanisms have been reported in previous editions of this text, reflecting the predominant theories prevalent at the time of those publication dates. Therefore, although there is likely more than one mechanism by which methylxanthines cause bronchodilation, it appears that the science seems to favor acceptance of the phosphodiesterase inhibition mechanism. When the β_2 receptor is stimulated by β agonists, like albuterol and terbutaline, the cell produces a compound called cyclic adenosine monophosphate (cAMP), which in turn causes relaxation of the bronchiolar smooth muscles. When cAMP is destroyed by the cellular enzyme phosphodiesterase, the bronchodilating effect ceases. It is thought that the major mechanism by which methylxanthine drugs cause bronchodilation is by inhibiting the action of phosphodiesterase, thus prolonging the bronchodilating effect of cAMP.[2] Other possible mechanisms involve blocking of adenosine receptors or direct interference with the calcium mobilization required for the contractile elements of muscle to connect, thus forcing the bronchiolar smooth muscles to remain in a relaxed state.[1]

Aminophylline is essentially 80% theophylline plus 20% ethylenediamine salt to make the drug better tolerated by the GI tract when given orally. Although aminophylline is still available and dosages exist for its use in veterinary medicine, theophylline is the methylxanthine bronchodilator used most often because of refinements in the sustained-release theophylline formulations now available, which are capable of establishing longer therapeutic concentrations in dogs.

Theophylline has been used to treat recurrent airway obstruction (RAO) in horses. However, theophylline has a narrow therapeutic index in horses, meaning that the dose that causes the beneficial effect is close to the dose that produces toxic side effects. Toxic side effects can include gastritis (with oral administration) and nervous system stimulation or agitation. In addition, this drug is classified as a Class III drug in the Association of Racing Commissioners International, Inc. Uniform Classification Guidelines for Foreign Substances, and administration in a race horse may alter the eligibility of that horse to run on some tracks. For further information on this topic, use "UCGFS" in any Internet search engine or browser.

Finally, aminophylline and theophylline can interact with a wide variety of drugs. Theophylline is metabolized by the liver and therefore can increase or decrease the metabolism of other drugs, including phenobarbital, the antacid cimetidine, and the antibiotics clindamycin, erythromycin, and lincomycin. Some of these drugs, if used concurrently with theophylline, will decrease the metabolism of theophylline, slowing its elimination and potentially allowing the drug to accumulate to potentially toxic concentrations. Therefore, before methylxanthines are used in an animal that is already on other medications, the

veterinary professional should review the package insert or a reliable source to determine whether a significant drug interaction exists.

OTHER DRUGS USED TO TREAT RESPIRATORY PROBLEMS

Antimicrobials

Antimicrobials are drugs used to combat infections by a variety of microorganisms, including bacteria, fungi, and protozoa. They are discussed in greater detail in Chapter 10. The philosophy of using antimicrobials differs between small animal medicine, food animal medicine, and equine medicine.

For food animals, antimicrobials are frequently used to treat respiratory disease because bacteria typically play an important role in respiratory infections in cattle, sheep, swine, and other food animals. Often the choice of antimicrobials for herd control of respiratory disease is selected based on empiric decisions. That is to say, the choice of antimicrobial drug is based on an estimation of which bacteria is most likely causing the current disease based on the clinical signs, the progression of the disease, the age of the animals affected, the time of the year, and any prior history of disease diagnosed on that particular farm or livestock operation. Because livestock production is a business, the use of antimicrobials is an expense not likely to be recovered when the animals are sent to market or their food products (milk, eggs) sold. For that reason the antimicrobial will be selected without extensive diagnostic tests and used only until any significant disease clinical signs are controlled.

In equine medicine, there may be more diagnostics performed before choosing an antimicrobial, but antimicrobials may not be used if the primary cause of the respiratory disease is suspected to be viral in origin or resulting from a noninfectious inflammatory disease. Investment by the animal owner into more diagnostics and longer duration of antimicrobial treatment is more likely than it would be in a livestock operation.

In small animal medicine, ideally the presence of a bacterial infection and the antibiotic susceptibility of the involved bacteria should be established before antimicrobials are used in respiratory disease. Many respiratory infections in small animal medicine are caused by viruses or allergens (i.e., allergy-producing substances), against which antimicrobials are completely ineffective. Additionally, the repeated use of antimicrobials under such conditions does little to help the animal, creates a false sense of security ("we're doing something"), and creates opportunities for bacteria present to develop resistance to the antimicrobial.

Bacterial specimens can be obtained by a transtracheal wash, bronchoscopic wash, or other sampling techniques. Even if the specimens obtained are not submitted for culture identification and antimicrobial sensitivity testing, the sample can be stained to determine the general type of bacteria involved (e.g., Gram negative vs Gram positive; bacilli vs cocci). Based on the shape and Gram stain of the bacteria, an empiric selection of an antimicrobial can be made.

Although part of successful treatment of infectious respiratory disease depends on selection of the appropriate antimicrobial, the other critical element is duration of therapy. Many animal owners stop giving the animal an antimicrobial after just a few days when clinical signs begin to subside and the animal feels better. Unfortunately, the improvement in clinical signs does not mean the infectious organism has been eliminated. If the owners fail to give the drug for the entire prescribed duration or do not give the drug as prescribed, resistant bacteria may survive the treatment and go on to reemerge as the predominant infectious bacteria in a new infection of the respiratory tract. When the new infection is treated with the same antimicrobial, the drug may be ineffective against the bacterial infection. Thus, animals with respiratory infections should be treated with antimicrobials for at least 7–10 days, with some treatments for long-duration diseases such as chronic bronchitis lasting 4–6 weeks.

The other challenge with antimicrobial use for respiratory infections is being able to deliver the drug to the bacteria's location. When bacteria are breathed in, they first land on and propagate on the surface of the cells lining the airways. Bacteria in this location are essentially outside the body, making it hard for an orally or parenterally administered antimicrobial absorbed antimicrobial and absorbed into systemic circulation to reach this surface. Many otherwise effective antimicrobials may not be effective when administered systemically because they do not reach the lumen infection site (i.e., the surface of the cell facing the airway) in concentrations sufficient to inhibit or kill the bacteria. Certain antimicrobials, however, are incorporated into the respiratory secretions and thus delivered to the luminal surface where the bacteria reside. Other drugs reach this location by being incorporated into inflammatory cells that migrate to the site of the infection and deliver antimicrobial drug directly to the bacteria.

An additional option is to deliver the drug by nebulization. Nebulization (also called aerosolization or aerosol therapy) was mentioned previously as a delivery method for the mucolytic drug acetylcysteine and β-agonist rescue inhalers for asthma and is the process of administering a drug as a fine mist that the animal inhales into the airways. When properly performed this technique would deposit the drug directly onto the surface of the bronchiolar epithelium. However, a significant disadvantage of nebulization in veterinary patients compared with human patients is that the dog, cat, or horse will not breathe deeply to inhale the mist. Thus, the nebulized mist tends to precipitate on the surfaces of the upper respiratory tract and not achieve significant concentrations in the lower respiratory tract.[6]

Animals frequently fight having a mask placed over the face or nostrils, making nebulization a struggle. If an animal is already hypoxic from respiratory disease and airway compromise, it may be at risk for potentially fatal cardiac arrhythmias if it struggles with the nebulizing mask. Sedation may be needed in animals that fight the mask, but sedation itself is not without risk to the compromised patient.

The use of nebulizing chambers reduces some of the animal's anxiety with having a mask placed over its nose; however, the same problem with precipitation of the mist still exists. Nebulization can be carried out with an endotracheal tube; however, this requires anesthesia or heavy sedation, with its inherent risks of depressing the respiratory centers or decreasing cardiovascular function.

Poor-quality nebulizers result in relatively large droplets of moisture being inhaled, which strike the wall of the upper respiratory tree and then are swallowed, sneezed, or coughed out. Even fine-mist nebulizers lose a significant amount of mist in the trachea and upper parts of the main bronchi because the animal resists taking deep breaths.

Another potential problem with aerosol therapy is the risk of reflex bronchoconstriction in response to introduction of the mist into the respiratory tree. Thus, a bronchodilator may be needed before nebulization is performed if the aerosolized drug is irritating.

One of the advances in aerosol therapy in human medicine that has moved over to veterinary medicine is the previously described MDI. The drug is packaged in a pressurized container with a propellant and is released in a measured amount with each depression of the trigger or plunger. The resultant mist is then inhaled, theoretically delivering a set amount or dose.[7] Specialized masks with spacers to dilute the mist with air before it is inhaled have been developed to accommodate MDIs in an attempt to use this technology to treat canine, feline, and equine respiratory diseases. Despite the challenges to using this method of drug delivery, nebulization in its various forms remains a tool used by veterinarians to treat selected respiratory conditions.

Corticosteroids

Corticosteroid use in the treatment of respiratory disease remains controversial, with some veterinarians strongly recommending its use and others warning against its use because of corticosteroids' immunosuppressing effect.

Generally, corticosteroids, or specifically glucocorticoids, are indicated in those situations in which the inflammation itself is potentially more life threatening than a temporary suppression of the immune response. For example, smoke inhalation triggers an acute inflammatory response that, if not held in check to some degree, can cause accumulation of fluid in and around the alveoli, causing pulmonary edema and interfering with the ability of oxygen to pass from the alveolus into the blood. If the degree of swelling and inflammation is suppressed by corticosteroids, the animal would have a greater chance of surviving.

Corticosteroids also stabilize the histamine-containing mast cells, thus decreasing their release of potent inflammatory mediators that cause swelling and edema of the bronchiolar tissues. Corticosteroids also help stabilize the integrity of the capillaries, reducing fluid loss from the capillary into the tissues. Both effects decrease the clinical signs associated with inflammation. Allergic responses, aspiration of chemicals, inhalation of caustic fumes, and eosinophilic bronchitis all initially respond well to corticosteroids.

Corticosteroids have long been used as supplements for human treatment of asthma because they are believed to improve the activity of methylxanthine and β-agonist bronchodilators. They are used less often today because of the side effects of many corticosteroids (see Chapter 13). Cats with feline asthma syndrome appear to respond well to corticosteroid treatment. Horses with recurrent airway obstruction may be treated with aerosolized corticosteroids as part of their treatment.[2]

Considerable debate exists about whether corticosteroids should be used in the treatment of chronic bronchitis or respiratory conditions involving a significant infectious component. Some veterinary internal medicine specialists who treat animals with chronic respiratory disease believe that corticosteroids are essential to maintain function of the respiratory tree; others are less adamant about the beneficial role of corticosteroids. Large doses of corticosteroids are known to impair the immune system response to infection and have the potential to delay healing. Corticosteroids also reduce cell-mediated immunity, which is the body's primary defense against fungal infections; therefore, the use of corticosteroids could result in a significant worsening of fungal infections in the lungs.

Because many positives and negatives exist regarding glucocorticoid use in respiratory disease, the veterinary professional must carefully weigh the benefits and risks of corticosteroids before using them in a critically ill patient or one that could potentially become critical.

Antihistamines

As previously discussed, histamine causes constriction of the bronchioles and is involved in the inflammatory response of the respiratory tract, but it has also been shown that blocking H_1 receptors by itself does little to alleviate clinical signs of respiratory disease. Therefore, antihistamines are usually much less effective in treating respiratory problems of small animals than they are in human beings.

In horses, histamine release is involved in recurrent airway obstruction disease and other bronchial problems related to dust and particulate matter like "stable cough." Horses predisposed to respiratory problems from dust or airborne allergens may be kept on antihistamine continuously during the worst times of the year. However, more serious respiratory disease treatment has shifted away from antihistamines and more toward the judicious use of corticosteroids by parenteral and aerosol routes of administration.

In contrast to corticosteroids, which can reverse or stabilize much of the damage caused by inflammation or allergic insult, antihistamines only prevent inflammation if they reach the H_1 receptors on bronchial or vascular smooth muscles in large quantities before the arrival of histamines released from mast cells. If histamine gets to the H_1 cell receptors first, antihistamine drugs do little to reverse the histamine effects. Theoretically, then, antihistamines should either be used prophylactically before the histamine is released or when exposure to the allergic substance and histamine release is continuous. This explains why antihistamine granules may be fed to horses that are continuously exposed to dust or molds in the barn environment.

Diuretics

Diuretics are used to remove accumulated fluid from the lungs, such as in animals with edema from pneumonia or congestive heart failure. As explained in Chapter 5, diuretics promote loss of body water through decreased reabsorption of water by the kidneys. The decreased water content in the blood increases the osmotic force within the capillaries that attracts water from body tissues into the bloodstream. Through this mechanism, the fluid of ascites or pulmonary edema is slowly moved out of the tissues, into the blood and then out of the body through the kidneys. The use of diuretics can be thought of as therapeutic tissue dehydration. A disadvantage of using diuretics to treat animals with respiratory disease is that they tend to dry the respiratory secretions, rendering the mucociliary apparatus less effective. This side effect must be measured against the potential benefits.

Oxygen

Oxygen administration with an oxygen cage or a mask is indicated in animals that are transiently hypoxic. For an animal, the stress of having the oxygen mask applied or being placed in an oxygen cage can sometimes precipitate collapse. Some cats and dogs tolerate a small-diameter tube that is hooked to an oxygen source, placed into the nasal passages, and glued or taped to the hair of the head to hold it in place. Some veterinary professionals create a portable oxygen cage by placing an Elizabethan collar on the animal, partially covering the large end of the funnel with plastic wrap, and running an oxygen line to the inside of the collar. To allow heat to escape, the opening of the Elizabethan collar funnel head should never be totally covered with plastic wrap. It is important to remember that oxygen gas is very dry so it should be humidified to prevent severe drying of the mucous membranes and mucociliary apparatus.

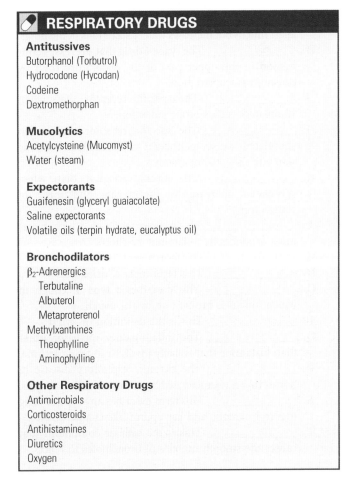

RESPIRATORY DRUGS

Antitussives
Butorphanol (Torbutrol)
Hydrocodone (Hycodan)
Codeine
Dextromethorphan

Mucolytics
Acetylcysteine (Mucomyst)
Water (steam)

Expectorants
Guaifenesin (glyceryl guaiacolate)
Saline expectorants
Volatile oils (terpin hydrate, eucalyptus oil)

Bronchodilators
β_2-Adrenergics
   Terbutaline
   Albuterol
   Metaproterenol
Methylxanthines
   Theophylline
   Aminophylline

Other Respiratory Drugs
Antimicrobials
Corticosteroids
Antihistamines
Diuretics
Oxygen

REFERENCES

1. Boothe DM. Drugs affecting the respiratory system. In: Boothe DM, ed. *Small Animal Clinical Pharmacology and Therapeutics.* Philadelphia: Saunders; 2012.
2. Papich MG. Drugs that affect the respiratory system. In: Riviere J, Papich M, eds. *Veterinary Pharmacology and Therapeutics.* Ames, Iowa: Wiley-Blackwell; 2009.
3. Carey SA. Localization of respiratory disease. In: *Proceedings of the 65th Convention of the Canadian Veterinary Medical Association.* Canada: Victoria, British Columbia; 2013.
4. Accessed online: https://academic-plumbs-com.ezproxy.lib.purdue.edu/drug-monograph/Ehf1HkfFUePROD?source=search&search Accessed on 06.14.2022.
5. Karch SB. *Pharmacokinetics and Pharmacodynamics of Abused Drugs.* Boca Raton, Florida: CRC Press; 2008.
6. Schulman RL, Crochik SS, Kneur SK, et al. Investigation of pulmonary deposition of a nebulized radiopharmaceutical agent. *Am J Vet Res.* 2004;65(6):806–809.
7. Dowling PM. Using metered dose inhalers in veterinary patients. In: *Proceedings of the Western Veterinary Conference*, Las Vegas, Nevada; 2004.

SELF-ASSESSMENT

1. Fill in the following blanks with the correct item from the Key Terms list.

   A. _____ This term means the administration a drug by a mist that is inhaled.

   B. _____ This is the mechanism that traps inhaled particles in a mucous layer and moves it up and out of the respiratory tree.

   C. _____ This term describes pulmonary disease that causes cardiac disease.

   D. _____ This is the term that describes the narrowing of the terminal bronchioles.

   E. _____ The type of drug that suppresses cough.

   F. _____ The type of drug that chemically breaks apart mucus.

   G. _____ The type of drug that does not break apart mucus but increases watery secretions in the lungs.

   H. _____ The type of drug that decreases congestion in the upper part of the respiratory tract by causing vasoconstriction.

   I. _____ The specific receptor that, when stimulated, causes bronchodilation.

   J. _____ The specific receptor that, when stimulated, causes peripheral vasoconstriction in the skin and mucous membranes.

   K. _____ The specific receptor that, when stimulated, increase the heart rate and force of contraction.

   L. _____ The receptor through which histamine produces its inflammatory effects.

   M. _____ This term means "difficult breathing."

   N. _____ This term means "dried out."

   O. _____ This describes a type of cough in which mucus is brought up by the cough.

   P. _____ This is the definition of "MDI."

   Q. _____ The inflammatory mediator other than histamine that is likely involved in feline asthma.

   R. _____ The chronic respiratory disease in horses that is characterized by asthmalike clinical signs.

   S. _____ This term describes any type of drug that is a narcotic and has opium-like characteristics.

   T. _____ This is the cellular compound that causes the smooth muscles of bronchioles to relax.

   U. _____ This is the enzyme that degrades cAMP.

2. Fill in the following blanks with the correct drug from the Respiratory Drug list. When practicing these questions, write out the answers on a separate sheet; focus also on the appropriate spelling of these drug names.

   A. _____ Expectorant; works by irritating the gastric lining.

   B. _____ Centrally acting opioid antitussive; the only Food and Drug Administration (FDA)-approved veterinary product for cough.

   C. _____ Same drug group as caffeine and theobromine (in chocolate); a bronchodilator that contains 80% active ingredient and 20% salt.

   D. _____ Used in patients in which the inflammatory process is life threatening; not to be used with respiratory fungal disease; stabilizes cellular membranes more than antihistamines.

   E. _____ Mucolytic that breaks apart sulfhydryl bonds (S—S).

   F. _____ Prophylactic antiinflammatory that decreases inflammatory response only if it is at the site of inflammation before the inflammation starts.

   G. _____ Potent narcotic antitussive; human product; C-II or C-III controlled substance.

   H. _____ Type of drug used to decrease pulmonary edema.

   I. _____ Common antitussive ingredient in over-the-counter (OTC) cold preparations; not a controlled substance; not very effective in veterinary patients.

   J. _____ Also used as an intravenously (IV) administered muscle relaxant for equine patients.

   K. _____ Also used as an antidote in cats with acetaminophen toxicosis.

   L. _____ Active ingredient of aminophylline.

   M. _____ Used to dilate bronchioles by directly stimulating β_2 receptors.

   N. _____ Human prescription opioid antitussive that is widely used in human medicine, often in conjunction with other cold or flu medications; a strongly abused opioid; not used much in veterinary medicine.

   O. _____ Bronchodilator that works by inhibiting phosphodiesterase.

3. Indicate whether the following statements are true or false.
   A. Inflammation and migration of inflammatory cells (e.g., neutrophils) into the mucus cause the mucus to become stickier or more viscous.
   B. Rapid breathing is called dyspnea.
   C. Inspissated mucus means that the mucus is dried out.
   D. Use of a diuretic drug would decrease the efficiency of the mucociliary apparatus.
   E. Dextromethorphan is more effective than butorphanol as an antitussive.
   F. In dehydrated animals the cough is usually nonproductive.
   G. A common side effect of most direct bronchodilators is decreased heart rate.
   H. If an animal is in distress from bronchoconstriction, antihistamine drugs should be used to dilate the bronchioles.
   I. Decongestants primarily work by causing vasoconstriction in the nasal mucosa.
   J. Prescribing dextromethorphan antitussive requires a controlled substance license or permit.
   K. Nebulization describes the process by which macrophages move into the alveoli and clean up debris that made it down that far.
   L. Stimulation of the larynx produces a more forceful and gagging cough than bronchiolar irritation.
   M. Theophylline is the methylxanthine active ingredient, and aminophylline is composed of theophylline plus a salt.
   N. Stimulation of the parasympathetic nervous system in the bronchioles causes bronchoconstriction.
   O. Centrally acting cough suppressants work better than locally acting ones in veterinary patients.
   P. Overdose of the opioid narcotic antitussives causes respiratory depression.
   Q. Drugs that stimulate acetylcholine receptors in the respiratory tree cause bronchodilation.
   R. Stimulation of H_1 receptors on the bronchioles produces an effect opposite of what stimulation of β_2 receptors would do to the bronchioles.
   S. Butorphanol and hydrocodone are Controlled Substances.
4. Stimulation of which branch of the autonomic nervous system produces bronchodilation?
5. What effect do methylxanthines have on the central nervous system (CNS) activity?
6. Which neurotransmitter is associated with the effects of the parasympathetic nervous system?
7. What substance is released by mast cells and causes inflammation and bronchoconstriction?
8. What role does cyclic adenosine monophosphate (cAMP) play in regulation of the diameter of the terminal bronchioles?
9. Different levels of the respiratory tree prevent foreign particles (e.g., food, dust, and molds) from reaching the deepest levels of the respiratory system. What are the normal mechanisms by which the larynx protects the respiratory tract? How do they differ from the reactions of the bronchi and trachea? What about the protective mechanisms at the level of the terminal bronchioles and alveoli?
10. A dehydrated animal with a high temperature and a nonproductive cough is admitted to the clinic. The veterinarian wants to correct the dehydration and determine whether the character of the cough changes before using antitussives. Why does he or she do this?
11. A veterinary pharmaceutical sales representative is offering a special price on locally acting antitussives for your veterinary patients. Should you make such a purchase?
12. Why is inspissated mucus a bad thing as far as the respiratory tract protecting itself? How do expectorants and mucolytics help correct this? What is the difference in mechanism between expectorants and mucolytics?
13. What effect would an owner likely see if a cat lapped up several milliliters of the owner's spilled liquid decongestant?
14. What effect would stimulation of β_2 receptors have on cAMP and the respiratory tree? What effect would β-blocking antiarrhythmic drugs have on these?
15. Why are terbutaline and albuterol used more commonly for bronchodilation than epinephrine, even though they have similar mechanisms of action?
16. What are the differences among aminophylline, theophylline, and methylxanthine?
17. Why should the owner not stop antibiotics for a respiratory disease as soon as the pet seems back to normal?
18. What is the rationalization for using nebulization in animals with respiratory disease? What is the challenge with nebulizing an animal compared with nebulizing a human being? What techniques have been used to increase the effectiveness of nebulization?
19. Of what benefits are corticosteroids in respiratory disease? Why are they not used all the time?
20. What role might diuretics play in respiratory-related disease? Why do they decrease the effectiveness of some of the other respiratory-protective mechanisms?
21. Oxygen administration can be beneficial to hypoxic animals. Why does oxygen therapy often reduce an animal's ability to remove inflammatory products, cellular debris, or excess mucus from the respiratory tract?

Drugs Affecting the Endocrine System

OBJECTIVES

After studying this chapter, the veterinary technician should be able to:

- Apply concepts of negative feedback and general endocrine control to all endocrine systems.
- Describe how thyroid function is controlled, how thyroid disease alters the physiology of the animal, and how drugs can restore physiologic balance to this hormonal system.
- Describe the mechanism of action and key side effects of drugs used to treat thyroid disease.
- Describe how insulin is produced, what insulin does, and what clinical signs result from insufficient insulin or ineffective insulin action.

- Describe the types of insulin and other drugs used to control insulin-dependent or non–insulin-independent diabetes mellitus, and what additional concepts need to be considered when using insulin products.
- Describe the mechanism by which the normal estrous cycle occurs, what hormonal changes maintain pregnancy, and which hormones inhibit the release of other hormones to maintain a balanced estrous cycle.
- Describe the drug interventions used for common reproductive system problems and how the drugs work to correct them.
- Describe the precautions and potential threat to humans handling these drugs.

KEY TERMS

aplastic anemia
anestrus
basal metabolic rate
beta cells
carcinogenic
Controlled Internal Drug Release (CIDR)
corpus luteum (CL)
cortisol
diethylstilbestrol (DES)
dystocia
endogenous
equine chorionic gonadotropin
estrogen
estrous/estrus
euthyroid
exogenous
foal heat

follicle-stimulating hormone (FSH)
follicular phase
goiter
gonadotropin-releasing hormone (GnRH)
gonadorelins
gonadotropins
human chorionic gonadotropin
hyperthyroidism
hypoglycemic agents
hypothyroidism
inhibin
insulin-dependent diabetes mellitus (IDDM)
luteal phase
luteinizing hormone (LH)
metritis

myometrium
negative feedback regulatory mechanism
non–insulin-dependent diabetes mellitus (NIDDM)
oocytes
oxytocin
parturition
primary hypothyroidism
progestagen
progestational hormone
progesterone
progestin
prostaglandins
protamine
pyometra
recombinant human insulin
seasonal anestrus

secondary hypothyroidism
sulfonylurea compound
tertiary hypothyroidism
tetraiodothyronine
thyrotropin-releasing hormone
  (TRH)

thyroid-stimulating hormone
  (TSH)
thyroidectomy
thyrotoxicosis
thyroxine (T₄)
timed artificial insemination
  (timed AI)

triiodothyronine (T₃)
type 1 diabetes
type 2 diabetes
U-40 and U-100 insulin

The endocrine system is composed of the thyroid gland, ovaries, testicles, pancreas, adrenal glands, and other glands that produce hormones that, in conjunction with the nervous system, control most functions in the body. To function properly, the amount of hormone produced must be precisely balanced with the need of the body. Unfortunately, this balance is easily upset by diseases or drugs that alter the amount of hormone produced or change the ability of the hormone to produce its intended effect. Correcting hormonal imbalances requires understanding what the natural hormone does, how it is controlled, and how any hormonal therapy is going to alter the physiology back toward normal. Because veterinary technicians are often involved with client education and patient monitoring for animals receiving different hormonal therapies, a solid understanding of basic hormone functions and hormonal therapy mechanisms is needed.

THE NEGATIVE FEEDBACK SYSTEM

All endocrine systems are regulated by a feedback mechanism in much the same way that a thermostat and furnace regulate the temperature inside the house. When a house gets cold, the thermostat detects the lowered temperature and signals the furnace to produce heat until the desired temperature level is achieved, at which point the thermostat sends a signal that turns off further heat production by the furnace. This signal from the thermostat to the furnace to stop heat production when sufficient heat has been generated is an example of a simple negative feedback regulatory mechanism. Understanding the negative feedback mechanism is the key to understanding how a hormone level (i.e., the warmer temperature generated by the heat from the furnace) controls the function of endocrine glands (i.e., the furnace generating the heat).

As shown in Fig. 7.1, endocrine gland A produces its hormone until concentrations of the hormone reach a certain level, at which point the cells in the endocrine gland detect this and shut off further hormone production (i.e., the negative feedback mechanism). As long as hormone levels are high enough, the negative feedback signal keeps the endocrine gland turned off because no further hormone needs to be generated. However, when the body metabolizes the circulating hormone and active hormone concentrations drop below the critical concentration, the negative feedback signal stops and endocrine gland A begins to secrete hormone again.

Although this simple negative feedback loop mechanism is used to regulate many body system functions, many other endocrine

glands are regulated by a slightly more complex feedback that involves a chain or sequence of glands and hormones. As shown in Fig. 7.2, endocrine gland A produces a hormone that does not stimulate the target organ or tissue but instead stimulates endocrine gland B to produce its hormone. Endocrine gland B produces the hormone that the body actually needs to regulate a system. Endocrine gland A would be like the thermostat sending an electrical current that turns on the furnace (endocrine gland B) to produce the heat that the house actually needs. Notice in Fig. 7.2 that the

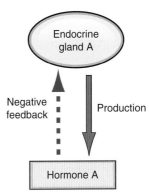

Fig. 7.1 Basic feedback mechanism for regulation of endocrine glands.

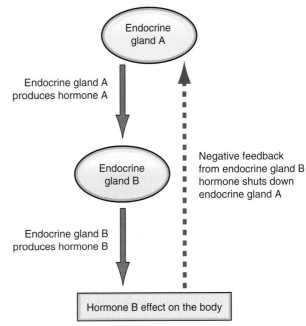

Fig. 7.2 Regulation of endocrine glands when more than one gland is involved.

hormone produced by endocrine gland B also provides the negative feedback that inhibits endocrine gland A's hormone production just like the heat produced by the furnace turns off the thermostat's signal to the furnace. Thus, the same concepts of the simple negative feedback mechanism also pertain to this two-gland sequence of hormone production.

If an exogenous (i.e., a compound that originates outside the body) drug is chemically similar to an endogenous, or naturally occurring, hormone, the drug can produce similar physiologic effects and exert the same negative feedback as the natural hormone. For example, if a drug that did the same thing as endocrine gland B's hormone was injected into the patient, the drug would produce the same bodily effect as gland B's hormone, and it would also inhibit endocrine gland A. Again referring to the furnace analogy, this action would be similar to bringing in a secondary heating source (e.g., sunshine, a kerosene heater) to bring the temperature of the house up. With the house temperature up, the thermostat does not turn the furnace on; as far as the thermostat is concerned, there is enough heat in the house regardless of where the heat came from.

Conversely, if the drug injected into the patient imitated endocrine gland A's hormone, the drug would stimulate endocrine gland B, resulting in increased production of endocrine gland B's hormone, much like sending an electrical signal from somewhere other than the thermostat to turn on the furnace.

Thus, it is important to remember that any exogenous hormone or hormone-like drug can easily upset the hormonal balance and produce unintended effects. This chapter discusses thyroid, pancreatic, and reproductive hormones because these endocrine systems are the targets for most endocrine-related drugs used in veterinary medicine. Corticosteroids are also hormone-like drugs that emulate natural endocrine hormones, but they are discussed with other antiinflammatory drugs in Chapter 13.

THYROID DISEASE AND DRUG THERAPIES

Normal Thyroid Control

Hormones of the thyroid gland enter almost all cells in the body, where they combine with receptors in the nucleus to turn on functions that regulate the cell's metabolic functions. Because of this, the thyroid is said to regulate the cell's basal metabolic rate, which is the overall rate at which cellular functions occur.

The control of thyroid hormone production is a sequential mechanism involving the hypothalamus and pituitary glands in the brain, and the thyroid gland itself in the neck (Fig. 7.3). Normally, low concentrations of thyroid hormone in the blood cause the hypothalamus to release a stimulating hormone called thyrotropin-releasing hormone (TRH), whose function is to stimulate the pituitary gland to release thyroid-stimulating hormone (TSH) into the blood. The pituitary TSH circulating in the blood stimulates the follicular cells of the thyroid gland to absorb iodine and incorporate it into tyrosine molecules to produce two functional thyroid hormones: triiodothyronine (T_3) and tetraiodothyronine, or thyroxine (T_4). The numbers 3 and 4 refer to the number of iodines attached to the thyroid hormone molecule: T_4 has four iodines and T_3 has three.

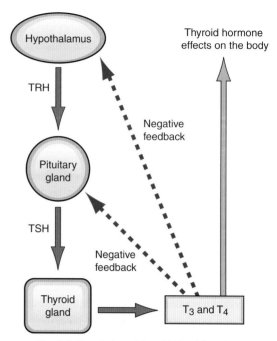

Fig. 7.3 Regulation of thyroid gland function.

The T_4 and T_3 molecules are then released by the thyroid gland into circulation, enter cells of the body, and combine with receptors in the nucleus as previously described. T_3 is considered to be the hormone that produces the physiologic effect of thyroid hormones even though T_3 is produced in smaller quantities than T_4. The larger amount of T_4 serves as a storage pool for the more active T_3 because the majority of tissues derives most of their needed T_3 by enzymatically removing one iodine from T_4 and converting it to T_3.[1] Both T_3 and T_4, to varying degrees, play some role in providing the negative feedback to the hypothalamus and pituitary to decrease release of TRH and TSH when sufficient thyroid hormone has been produced.[2] In addition, TSH by itself may also produce negative feedback to inhibit further TRH release (the so-called short feedback loop).[3]

Thyroid Disease

Different species develop different problems with their thyroid glands. For example, dogs are prone to develop hypothyroidism (low production of thyroid hormone), whereas cats are prone to develop hyperthyroidism (an excessive production of thyroid hormone). Reports of hypothyroidism also exist in horses and cattle, but apparently these species are either less affected by hypothyroidism than are dogs or the condition is not recognized or treated to the same extent as in dogs.

Many endocrine diseases, including those of the thyroid, classify the location of the cause of the disease as primary, secondary, or tertiary. The primary form of an endocrine disease means that the source of the problem for the disease resides in the organ itself that produces the final hormone. For example, primary hypothyroidism is a disease of the thyroid gland itself that results in lower T_3 and T_4 hormones. The secondary form of an endocrine disease means that the end organ is normal, but the location of the problem is in the organ that directly regulates the end endocrine gland. For example, secondary hypothyroidism means that the thyroid gland itself functions normally, but the low quantities of T_3 and T_4 hormones result from the pituitary gland being unable to produce TSH for some reason. Without the stimulation of TSH, the thyroid gland does not produce thyroid hormones, and hypothyroidism results.

In tertiary hypothyroidism, the thyroid gland is again normal, but unlike in secondary hypothyroidism, the pituitary is also normal. In tertiary hypothyroidism, the problem is located two steps away in the hypothalamus. Without hypothalamic TRH to stimulate the pituitary gland, no TSH will be released to stimulate the thyroid gland and no T_3 and T_4 hormones will be produced, resulting in hypothyroidism.

Although clinical signs in primary, secondary, and tertiary hypothyroidism can all be explained by low levels of T_3 and T_4, and all are treated with T_3 and T_4 supplementation, the prognosis for full recovery from secondary and tertiary hypothyroidism is poorer because any disease that affects the pituitary or hypothalamus is likely to affect multiple endocrine systems and body functions.[2]

Goiter is another hypothyroid condition that results not from a damaged thyroid gland, but from a lack of iodine needed to manufacture T_3 or T_4 hormones. In goiter, the thyroid gland becomes very large, which would seem to be counterintuitive when the animal has low levels of thyroid hormone circulating in the body. However, if the concept of negative feedback is applied, it makes sense. Without the iodine the thyroid cannot produce T_3 or T_4 hormones, the thyroid hormone levels drop very low, negative feedback on the hypothalamus and the pituitary is removed, and both glands release large amounts of TRH and TSH to stimulate increased thyroid hormone production. Unfortunately, without iodine, no amount of stimulation of the thyroid gland will increase thyroid hormone production. But with the continual TSH stimulation of the thyroid tissue, the thyroid gland itself hypertrophies (increases in size), producing the increasingly larger and larger goiter.[3]

Goiter is easily treated by feeding the patient iodinated foods and is now considered a rare disease because of the wide availability of commercially prepared, well-balanced animal feeds. Still goiter is occasionally seen in range cattle that feed off plants on sandy soil, which typically have low amounts of natural iodine, or calves nursing from cows that have low amounts iodine in their diets.

Regardless of the cause of hypothyroidism, the clinical signs reflect an overall decreased metabolic rate and slowed cellular metabolism. Signs of hypothyroidism include lethargy, weight gain despite normal consumption of food, heat-seeking behavior (e.g., dogs will huddle over warm air duct vents), bradycardia, decreased function of the estrous cycle, decreased growth in young animals, hair loss (alopecia), and dry and scaly skin (altered dermal metabolism).[1–3] Many of these signs are only evident when hypothyroidism has been chronic or has progressed to a fairly advanced stage. Early stages of hypothyroidism may have few signs or only subtle clinical signs.

Because thyroid hormone is so important to normal development of the fetal neural and skeletal systems, young born from hypothyroid mothers can have serious clinical signs.[3] Foals of hypothyroid mares may have contracted tendons, poor development of respiratory epithelium, and appear lethargic ("dull") and uncoordinated.

Drugs Used to Treat Hypothyroidism

The most common treatment for hypothyroidism is the use of thyroid drugs as hormone supplements. Drugs used to treat hypothyroidism include thyroid extracts, synthetic T_4 (**levothyroxine**), and synthetic T_3 (**liothyronine**). Thyroid extracts, sometimes called desiccated thyroid extract, are no longer commonly used to treat hypothyroid veterinary patients, but some products are still available through health food outlets labeled as "raw thyroid." Thyroid extracts are most commonly made from bovine or porcine thyroid glands acquired from slaughterhouses, and as such, the actual amount of T_3 or T_4 can vary considerably among batches.[2] Therefore, it is strongly recommended to use synthetic thyroid hormone to treat hypothyroidism.

The synthetic T_4 product levothyroxine is the drug of choice for treatment of hypothyroidism.[2,3] T_4 therapy has several advantages over synthetic T_3; the most important is that T_4 allows each tissue to individually convert T_4 to T_3 to meet its specific metabolic need. For example, the central nervous system (CNS) has a high metabolic rate and therefore has an increased requirement for thyroid hormone.[2] With levothyroxine therapy, both T_3 and T_4 levels will return to normal, whereas with synthetic T_3 therapy, T_4 levels remain low.[3] Levothyroxine may also more closely imitate the negative feedback mechanism on the pituitary because T_4 levels seem more closely inversely correlated with TSH levels (as T_4 goes up, TSH goes down due to negative feedback on the pituitary) than T_3. Finally, levothyroxine has a longer half-life than liothyronine, meaning it can be dosed less frequently, enhancing client compliance with life-long hormone supplementation. Synthetic T_3 is still used in those patients who do not respond successfully to conventional T_4 supplementation therapy.

Additional Clinical Considerations of Hypothyroid Therapy

When starting levothyroxine therapy for hypothyroidism, many endocrinologists and internal medicine specialists recommend using a well-known brand name or a reliable generic synthetic T_4 drug because these products may achieve more consistent systemic concentrations of T_4 than other brands of thyroxine.[2,3] Regardless of what brand is ultimately selected, the product used should not be arbitrarily changed to another brand just because of availability or price because subtle differences in the manufacture of the drug can alter the amount of drug absorbed.

Sometimes levothyroxine therapy is started on a canine patient without performing the diagnostic tests to confirm hypothyroidism because the client does not want to or is unable to spend the money for the necessary tests. Because supplementation of thyroid hormone is the therapy for suspected hypothyroidism, this means an animal with a normal thyroid that shows clinical signs similar to hypothyroidism would be receiving a treatment that would potentially elevate T_3 and T_4 levels above the normal range. Fortunately, levothyroxine has a relatively wide therapeutic (safety) index in the dog, meaning higher than normal thyroid hormone concentrations can be safely tolerated. Human physicians or nurses may be alarmed by the possibility of their pet having a "thyroxine overdose" because human beings with even a relatively small thyroxine overdose may have thyroid storms, or thyrotoxicosis, causing hyperthyroidism signs, such as tachycardia, agitation, nervousness, and polyuria.[2] An animal receiving such a therapeutic trial to "diagnose" hypothyroidism generally would have to be on the levothyroxine for at least 4 weeks before significant improvement in outward clinical signs (skin, weight, hair coat) can be observed. Even then, the outward changes might be marginal or caused by other conditions unrelated to the therapy, making a definitive diagnosis of hypothyroidism difficult using just the therapeutic trial of supplemental drug. Thus, in the long run it is usually worth the client's investment to get a definitive diagnosis early on by running the needed laboratory tests for thyroid function.

⚠ YOU NEED TO KNOW

Acute Overdose of Levothyroxine in a Dog

A 6-year-old male Keeshond was presented after being observed ingesting 850 of 0.2-mg levothyroxine sodium tablets. The owner initiated vomiting with hydrogen peroxide at home. Some of the dissolved tablets may have come up with the vomitus. At the time of admission, 3–9 h after ingestion, the dog showed no significant clinical abnormalities. The rectal temperature was 102.4°F, and the heart rate was 92 beats/min.

The National Animal Poison Control Center at the University of Illinois recommended treatment with activated charcoal (adsorbent) and diluted magnesium sulfate (saline cathartic). Blood was taken to determine T_4 concentration. The owner declined hospitalization.

The dog was reexamined and blood taken for T_3 and T_4 concentrations on days 3, 6, 9, 15, and 36 after ingestion. The initial T_4 concentration was 4900 nmol/L (normal range, 5.3 to 26.7 nmol/L). Although the concentrations of T_4 decreased significantly in the first 6 days (day 6 was less than 100 nmol/L), the concentrations did not return to normal until day 36. T_3 concentration at day 3 was 5.3 nmol/L (normal range, 0.4–1.4 nmol/L) but had returned to normal by day 6. The heart rate increased to 136 beats/min on day 3 and then to 156 beats/min on day 6. The owner reported no observable behavior changes.

Although problems with long-term overdose of thyroid supplements are cited in both the human and veterinary literature, seldom do acute overdoses of thyroid supplements produce severe degrees of tachycardia, hyperactivity, tachypnea (rapid breathing), abnormal pupillary light responses, or diarrhea. The veterinarian speculated that because only the nonprotein-bound (unbound) form of levothyroxine is physiologically active and also because of the very large capacity of protein binding of T_4 in the dog, perhaps not as much T_4 was physiologically available as the very high concentration would suggest.

What should be learned from this situation: A wide therapeutic index appears to exist for thyroid medications. Thus, when veterinarians try a therapeutic trial of thyroid supplementation in animals suspected of being hypothyroid, the risk of producing thyroid toxicosis is small. T_3 toxicosis would potentially be more of a risk for clinical toxicosis because of the direct cellular effect this hormone has. In human beings, overdose with T_3 typically produces signs sooner but of a shorter duration than T_4 toxicosis. Regardless of whether T_3 or T_4 toxicosis is the diagnosis, the animals at most risk for a fatal toxicosis would be elderly dogs that have concurrent heart disease.

As would be expected from a hormone that has effects on so many body systems, the thyroid supplementation therapy itself is going to significantly alter the animal's physiology as the patient is returned to a normal thyroid (euthyroid) state. For example, hypothyroid animals typically have insulin receptors that become less receptive to insulin's action to move glucose from the blood into the body's cells. Thus, animals with diabetes and hypothyroidism may have higher levels of blood glucose because the insulin used to control the diabetes is less effective on the insulin receptors. Once levothyroxine therapy is instituted, the receptors become more responsive to insulin therapy and the same dose of insulin may cause blood glucose levels to plummet, causing a hypoglycemic crisis. Thus, diabetic animals being placed on levothyroxine for hypothyroidism treatment should have their blood glucose closely monitored and their insulin doses decreased appropriately as the body adjusts to the euthyroid state.

As mentioned previously, liothyronine, or synthetic T_3, may be used if levothyroxine therapy fails to produce adequate blood concentrations of thyroid hormone or a satisfactory clinical response. Liothyronine is generally absorbed more effectively than levothyroxine because synthetic T_4 more readily combines with intestinal contents, trapping the drug in the gastrointestinal (GI) tract lumen. Normally T_3 has a bioavailability of 0.95, so 95% of T_3 is absorbed from the GI tract, compared with only 40%–80% absorption of T_4.[4] However, because there are other reasons for an inadequate T_4 concentration or less than desirable improvement in clinical signs after starting levothyroxine therapy, a consultation with a veterinary endocrinologist or internal medicine specialist is recommended before switching to synthetic T_3 therapy.

A few human products are available that contain both liothyronine and levothyroxine. The 4:1 ratio of T_3 to T_4 in these products is designed to meet the needs of human beings with hypothyroidism. But dogs require a different ratio, and if dogs are given the human combination product with this 4:1 ratio, the dog would receive excessive concentrations of T_3. In addition, T_3 and T_4 are metabolized at different rates in the dog (hence the different half-lives for each hormone), meaning that the dose interval for the T_4 fraction of the drug would be different from that required to maintain T_3 concentrations.[3] Because levothyroxine therapy achieves the therapeutic goals by itself and at a lesser cost than the combined human T_3/T_4 products, there is little use for this product in veterinary medicine.

Drugs Used to Treat Hyperthyroidism

Although dogs, horses, and cattle experience hypothyroidism, hyperthyroidism is more often diagnosed in middle-aged to elderly cats. Hyperthyroidism (thyrotoxicosis) is caused by a functional, hormone-secreting tumor of the thyroid gland and characterized as an increase in circulating concentrations of T_3 and T_4 thyroid hormones.

Feline hyperthyroidism is a disease that was not "discovered" until the early 1980s, at which point practitioners began to recognize and identify cases on a frequent basis. This has led to a great deal of speculation as to what changes in the environment or other factors lead to this disease emerging during that time. Since that time, owner and veterinary awareness of the disease has made measurement of serum thyroxine concentrations a routine part of the older cat's physical examination and wellness workup.

In contrast to hypothyroidism, hyperthyroidism is manifested by increased physical activity, diarrhea from increased GI motility, weight loss despite a voracious appetite, tachycardia (with heart rates exceeding 240 beats/min), heat intolerance (they get overheated more easily), polyuria (increased urination), and polydipsia (increased water intake). Owners of hyperthyroid cats often do not present their pets to a veterinary hospital until later in the disease because early signs of increased activity, alertness, good appetite, and loss of excessive body fat are viewed as signs of a very healthy middle-aged to elderly cat. Clients often complain that the old cat is acting more like a kitten with its aggressive, playful activity and appetite. In addition to these clinical signs, the thyroid mass itself can usually be palpated on the ventral aspect of the trachea near the top few cartilaginous rings.[3] Because of the prevalence of this condition, veterinary technicians should include palpation of the ventral neck in their routine physical examination of every cat.

There are four treatment modalities used to treat hyperthyroidism. The thyroid tumor can be removed and the disease cured by either surgical removal of the thyroid tumor (**thyroidectomy**) or the injection of radioactive iodine (^{131}I) to destroy the tumorous thyroid tissue. Control of hyperthyroidism signs, but not cure of the disease, can be achieved using medications that block thyroid hormone production or diets that restrict the amount of iodine needed to create thyroid hormones. Each of the four therapies has advantages and disadvantages, and the choice of which therapy to use is made based on client preferences (e.g., giving daily medication or restricting diet), financial consideration, what the cat can tolerate (e.g., anesthesia for surgery), and the availability of a skilled surgeon or special facility capable of handling radiation therapy. The nonsurgical treatments for hyperthyroidism will be discussed in this text.

Methimazole (Tapazole) is an orally administered antithyroid drug has been used to control hyperthyroidism in cats by blocking the thyroid tumor's ability to use iodine to produce T_3 and T_4. The drug is inexpensive and relatively safe and is tolerated by old cats. As an alternative to orally administered tablets, methimazole has also been compounded into a topically applied gel that is absorbed through the skin.[3]

Because methimazole only prevents hormone formation but does not destroy existing T_3 and T_4 molecules, signs of hyperthyroidism do not abate until previously released thyroid hormones have been metabolized. Cessation of methimazole treatment results in recurrence of hyperthyroid signs because methimazole is not toxic to the tumor itself and the mechanism for producing thyroid hormones is not permanently disabled by the drug. Cats with hyperthyroidism must take this drug for the rest of their lives to control the hyperthyroid signs.

Side effects occur in approximately 10%–25% of cats treated with methimazole.[5] The most common side effects are vomiting, lethargy, and anorexia; however, these signs may resolve after a few weeks of methimazole treatment or with a decrease in the administered dose.[5] Mild changes in the complete blood count (CBC) are common and include eosinophilia (increased eosinophils), lymphocytosis (increased lymphocytes), and leukopenia (decreased overall white cell count).[3] Typically, the drug does not need to be stopped with these mild hematologic changes. More severe reactions requiring medical intervention and possible discontinuation of the drug occur in 3%–9% of the cats and include liver problems, bleeding, and more severe changes in white blood cell or platelet counts.[3]

Some veterinarians choose to use methimazole in hyperthyroid cats for a few weeks to reduce the hyperthyroid signs, stabilize the heart, and make the cat a better surgical risk for thyroidectomy. A short trial of methimazole may also be used, especially in older cats, to bring the cat into a euthyroid state so the renal function of the cat can be assessed. Hyperthyroidism typically increases arterial blood pressure and therefore also increases pressure within the renal glomerulus, which filters drugs, small molecules, and wastes out of the blood into the urine. When a cat is returned to the euthyroid state, the reduced blood pressure may decrease glomerular filtration below normal levels, revealing a kidney that is in partial renal failure. Therefore, before a cat is returned to a normal euthyroid state by surgery or radioactive iodine, methimazole therapy may be tried to see how well the kidneys function in the euthyroid state.

Carbimazole is another antithyroid drug available in Australia and Europe that is metabolized to methimazole for its active drug state.

Radioactive iodine (^{131}I) is used if the patient is a poor surgical candidate or the owner is reluctant or unable to give oral medication on a daily basis for the rest of the cat's life. Because ^{131}I is easily administered subcutaneously (SQ) or intravenously (IV) and is 95% effective in destroying the tumorous part of the thyroid gland that produces hyperthyroidism, for some veterinarians with access to an appropriate facility, it is the treatment of choice.[3]

Because iodine is a normal component of thyroid hormone, the radioactive iodine is actively taken up and concentrated within the thyroid tumor cells, causing them to receive a lethal dose of beta particle radiation. The beta particle radiation only penetrates 1–2 mm into tissue, which means the ^{131}I destroys thyroid tumor cells while sparing the normal thyroid tissue and surrounding tissue like the parathyroid glands.

Why does normal thyroid tissue not take up ^{131}I and avoids irradiation and destruction like the thyroid tumor cells? Because the thyroid tumorous tissue produces high levels of T_3 and T_4, the negative feedback loop depresses release of TRH and TSH, removing stimulation on any of the nontumorous thyroid tissue. Although the tumorous thyroid tissue continues to function regardless of any TSH stimulation, the normal tissue atrophies without the effect of TSH. Thus, at the time of ^{131}I administration, the atrophied normal thyroid tissue does not take up any significant amount of radioactive iodine and is spared from its lethal cellular effects.

Although the killing activity of ^{131}I is because of beta particle radiation, ^{131}I also emits gamma radiation, which is far more penetrating than beta particle radiation. Thus, cats treated with ^{131}I are considered a potential source of hazardous radiation.

Cats treated with ^{131}I must be isolated from other animals and their urine and feces collected and disposed of as hazardous radiation waste. Thus, special facilities conforming with state and federal law are required to administer ^{131}I. Personnel treating the cats must wear protective clothing and gloves, wear radiation detection devices, and receive training in radiation safety procedures. Cats treated with ^{131}I are monitored for gamma radiation and, depending on local regulations, are required to be hospitalized in the special facility from 3 days to 3 weeks.[3] Some clients choose not to elect this treatment because of the cost of housing the cat in such an approved facility. Fortunately, with a proliferation of facilities designed to accommodate use of radiation treatment, these specialized hospitals are far more conveniently located than they were a few years ago.

Iodine-limited diets have been developed to "starve" the thyroid tumor of the iodine needed to produce high levels of T_3 and T_4. Once normal thyroid cells have converted to tumorous cells, they continue to live and function without TSH stimulation or a supply of iodine. Thus, iodine-limited diets would decrease thyroid hormone production but would not adversely affect the underlying tumorous tissue itself.[3]

Although this diet may be used in the short term or long term for cats that are not good surgical candidates or whose owner elects not to have radioactive iodine treatment, there are drawbacks to using these diets. Cats must be strictly confined to this diet without additional treats or food that may contain iodine. If the diet is unpalatable to the cat, the cat may not be able to be maintained on the diet. Cats with other medical conditions that require specialized diets may not be able to use the iodine-limited diet. In multiple-cat households, the other cats need to be monitored to insure the cat needing the diet eats the iodine-limited diet food and it is not eaten by other cats.

As of this writing in 2015, experience with long-term effects of iodine-deficient diets in cats is unknown. There is some concern that thyroid adenomas (the most common type of thyroid tumor found in earlier stages of feline hyperthyroidism) could over time convert to thyroid carcinoma, a more aggressive type of tumor, if not removed.[3] Thus, treatments like methimazole and iodine-limited diets, which do not destroy or remove the tumor but only control the levels of thyroid hormone, could allow for the adenoma to convert over to a thyroid carcinoma at some point. Cats on long-term therapy with iodine-limited diets or methimazole should have their thyroid glands palpated regularly and the size recorded in the medical record to document any increased size that would potentially indicate a carcinoma.

Additional Clinical Considerations of Hyperthyroid Therapy

In hyperthyroidism, the elevated levels of thyroid hormones produced by the thyroid tumor increase the number of β_1 receptors on cardiac cells, making the heart more sensitive to sympathetic stimulation. Thus, normal sympathetic stimulation produces tachycardia, with heart rates in the cat often exceeding 240 beats/min. β_1 antagonists (see Chapter 5) such as **propranolol** or **atenolol** decrease the effect of sympathetic stimulation by preventing the normal sympathetic neurotransmitter molecules of epinephrine and norepinephrine from combining with the β_1 receptors. Consequently, the heartbeat slows to a more normal rate, allows more efficient filling of the ventricles, and has less myocardial oxygen demand. The drawback to using propranolol is that it is a nonselective β-blocker and will also block β_2 receptors in the bronchioles, causing bronchoconstriction in cats with reactive airway disease (asthma).[3] Atenolol is more selective for β_1 and has a longer duration of action than propranolol. Both β-blockers are started at low doses and increased until the desired effect is achieved. Although β-blockers can help a little with hypertension from hyperthyroidism, significant hyperthyroidism requires more aggressive drugs like the calcium channel blocker **amlodipine** to reduce the risk of sustained hypertension damage to organs and tissue like the retina.

ENDOCRINE PANCREATIC DRUGS

The pancreas plays a role in both endocrine (hormone) and exocrine (digestive enzyme) functions in the body. Insulin, glucagon, and somatostatin are the hormones normally produced by the pancreas. Of the three, insulin is the only pancreatic hormone that is used for therapeutic purposes with any regularity.

The major effect of insulin is to move glucose from the blood into tissue cells. Insulin also causes the liver to store glucose as glycogen and facilitates deposition of fat in adipose tissue. The net effect of insulin is to decrease blood glucose concentrations by enhancing distribution of glucose to body tissues. Lack of insulin results in diabetes mellitus, a disease characterized by high blood glucose levels (hyperglycemia), and the presence of glucose in the urine (glucosuria).

The most common cause of diabetes mellitus in veterinary patients is destruction or lack of function of the pancreatic beta cells, which produce insulin. This type of diabetes is characterized by decreased insulin and is referred to as type 1, or insulin-dependent diabetes mellitus (IDDM). Although type 1 diabetes is related to the number of functional pancreatic beta cells, type 2 diabetes, or non–insulin-dependent diabetes mellitus (NIDDM), results from a decreased effectiveness of insulin even though the pancreatic beta cells are potentially capable of producing adequate insulin. A decreased number of insulin receptors on tissue cells, decreased sensitivity of insulin receptors present, or a decreased sensitivity of the pancreatic beta cells to hyperglycemia can all result in hyperglycemia classified as type 2 diabetes or NIDDM.[6]

Diabetes mellitus is very different in the cat than the dog. Cats exhibit type 2 diabetes mellitus or NIDDM, and dogs exhibit type 1 or IDDM. The cat response to insulin is quite variable, with some cats being very sensitive to the insulin effects and others very resistant to the insulin effects. Cats may go into spontaneous diabetic remission during the course of treatment, but dogs rarely achieve remission of disease and have to be treated for the rest of their lives. Cats are very susceptible to signs of diabetes mellitus being produced, in part, by other diseases like hyperadrenocorticism (Cushing's disease). The duration of most insulin drugs in cats is shorter than the duration of the same insulin drug in dogs. Thus, treatment of diabetes mellitus in cats requires a very different approach than treatment in dogs.

Unfortunately, the administration of insulin by injection fails to mimic the body's normal production of insulin in response to elevated blood glucose concentrations. Therefore, insulin administration must be scheduled and regulated in conjunction with the animal's diet and exercise 24 h a day, 7 days a week, 365 days of the year. Treatment of a diabetic patient requires a strong commitment from the pet owner.

Owners are often initially hesitant about giving injections to their animal and ask if they can give an oral medication. Because insulin is a protein, it would be destroyed (denatured) by the stomach's gastric acid and therefore cannot be given orally. Even if the insulin molecule was not denatured by the gastric acid, the insulin molecule is too large to be absorbed through the bowel mucosa. The technician's role in educating the client to properly administer the insulin and in explaining the dietary and lifestyle changes and the need for blood or urine glucose testing is very important in helping the client understand what is required to regulate the diabetic patient.

Types of Insulins

Various types of insulins are available, but the availability of certain insulins is in a constant state of flux. What is presented is an overview and guidelines of the types of insulins. Insulins are classified by their duration of activity (short-, intermediate-, and long-acting) and according to the species from which the insulin is derived (pork or genetically engineered human-type insulin).

Insulin derived from purified pork was the main type available to both the human and veterinary markets for many years. Differences in insulin structure between species are thought to have contributed to the development of insulin antibodies, which can lead to erratic control of blood glucose levels. Fortunately pork insulin is antigenically similar to canine insulin and is still one of the insulins of choice, currently available as **porcine insulin zinc suspension** (trade name Vetsulin).

The genetically engineered human **insulin glargine** and **insulin detemir** are called recombinant human insulin because they are created by bringing together (recombining) genetic material from different sources and producing DNA sequences that are capable of producing these insulins that would not be otherwise produced by biological organisms. Human recombinant insulins are not as close in structure to canine insulin as is pork insulin but are close enough to prevent significant antibody production. Insulin glargine has been used for many years in cats, but experience with detemir insulin in veterinary medicine is far less.[6]

As previously stated and as shown in Table 7.1, insulins are also classified by the duration of effect they have in the body. The duration of activity of insulin relates to the differences in absorption based on what the insulin is combined with and the solubility of the resulting insulin crystals. For example, **neutral protamine Hagedorn insulin (NPH)** and **protamine zinc insulin (PZI)** are formed by mixing insulin, zinc, and a fish protein called protamine. The combination is allowed to precipitate into crystals that are poorly soluble (slow to dissolve) and

that release the insulin slowly when injected SQ. The difference in absorption speed between NPH and PZI is the result of the different protamine and zinc ratios. The lente family of insulins derives its duration from higher concentrations of zinc (no protamine) and the size of the crystals.

The short-acting insulin is **regular (crystalline) insulin**; the intermediate-acting insulins include **NPH** and **porcine insulin zinc suspension**; and the long-acting insulin is **PZI**. The human analogs mentioned—insulin glargine and insulin detemir—are both considered long-acting insulins. Recently, combination insulins incorporating two types of insulins have been marketed as an attempt to provide more consistent peaks of insulin activity with one injectable product.

Initial stabilization of the new canine diabetic patient can be done either starting with the intermediate-duration insulins (recombinant human, NPH, and porcine insulin zinc suspension), or, if the animal has a very high blood glucose and ketoacidosis, regular or crystalline insulin is used initially to bring the blood glucose down to a safe level at which point the intermediate insulins can be used.[6] In the cat, regular insulin is used to stabilize the cat that is severely hyperglycemic or exhibiting diabetic ketoacidosis signs from poor control of the diabetic condition. NPH insulin does not last as long in the cat as it does in the dog and so is not a convenient choice for long-term diabetes control in the cat. The longer acting human recombinant PZI insulin is commonly used to control diabetes in the cat. Human recombinant PZI insulin is not used very often in the dog because of its longer duration that makes twice daily dosing too often and once daily dosing not often enough to control blood glucose levels. Insulin glargine and insulin detemir have been used to some degree in the dog, but degree of control is more difficult to predict in some dogs than porcine insulin zinc suspension or NPH.

Insulin Syringes and Additional Considerations in Using Insulin

Insulin is administered in syringes that are marked differently from a typical 3-cc or 6-mL syringe. Unlike most drugs, which are measured in milligrams, insulin is measured in units. The bottles of insulin are listed as U-40 or U-100, meaning the bottle contains 40 or 100 insulin units per milliliter. Likewise, the insulin syringes are calibrated for the different unit concentration bottles, meaning that U-40 syringes are to be used only with U-40 bottles of insulin and U-100 syringes are to be used only with U-100 insulin bottles. The special insulin syringes help a client accurately measure the amount of insulin to give because the markings on the syringe are calibrated in units based on the unit rating of the insulin and matching syringe. Thus, instead of the client having to calculate a dose in milliliters, he or she simply withdraws the required number of units from the appropriate insulin bottle. It is important that the client understand the difference in U-40 vs U-100 insulin because some brands of insulin come in both concentrations, and using the wrong syringe with a bottle can result in a serious hypoglycemic crisis or the insulin dose being totally ineffective.

Most of the insulins are suspensions, meaning that the insulin is not dissolved in the liquid but must be resuspended before

TABLE 7.1	Comparison of Types of Insulin Used for Dogs and Cats				
Insulin Type	Route of Administration	Species Source	Duration of Effect (Dog)	Duration of Effect (Cat)
Regular crystalline	IV infusion	Recombinant human	Based on infusion	Based on infusion
	IM	Recombinant human	4–6 h	4–6 h
	SQ	Recombinant human	6–8 h	6–8 h
NPH	SQ	Recombinant human	6–12 h	6–10 h
Porcine zinc insulin	SQ	Porcine (Pig)	10–24 h*	8–24 h*
PZI	SQ	Recombinant human	10–16 h	10–14 h

IV, Intravenous; *IM*, intramuscular; *SQ*, subcutaneous; *NPH*, neutral protamine Hagedorn; *PZI*, protamine zinc insulin.
*Information from Vetsulin product label.
Adapted from Feldman EC, Nelson RW. *Canine and Feline Endocrinology*. Philadelphia: Saunders; 2015:223.

each withdrawal of insulin from the bottle. Historically resuspension of the insulin crystals was recommended to be done only by gently rolling the bottle between the palms of the hands instead of vigorously shaking the bottle for fear of physically breaking the insulin molecule and inactivating the drug. However, more recent information provided by the manufacturer of the porcine insulin zinc suspension (Vetsulin) specifically states that shaking does not adversely affect insulin activity and more uniformly resuspends the drug throughout the liquid medium than rolling.[6] Note that the pharmaceutical companies that produce NPH and PZI insulin have not followed these changes recommended by the manufacturer of porcine zinc suspension and still recommend rolling to resuspend the insulin.

Suspensions need to be stored at the proper temperatures to avoid extremes of hot or cold, which could alter the crystalline structure of the insulin or denature the insulin, resulting in alteration of absorption of the drug or inactivation of the insulin itself. The proper storage and mixing of insulin should provide full activity of the insulin up to and beyond the shelf life date on the bottle. If there is any question about possible contamination of the insulin or the patient begins to show signs of loss of control over the diabetic condition, replacement of the insulin bottle should be considered.

Because insulin doses are timed to have their maximal effect near the time when blood glucose concentrations are peaking after consumption of a meal, reliable patterns of absorption are important for the intermediate- and long-acting insulins. With the exception of regular insulin that can be administered IV, intramuscularly (IM), and SQ, the rest of the insulins are administered SQ, typically in the neck or lumbar area (although some authors may advocate other areas).

For the insulin to be absorbed consistently from dose to dose, the pet owner must administer the drug in areas that have consistent perfusion. If the client injects too deeply and administers the insulin intramuscularly, the drug is likely to be absorbed more quickly than if it were injected SQ, and the peak effect of the insulin may therefore occur before the anticipated rise in blood glucose from eating a meal. At the other extreme, insulin injected into a poorly perfused fat pad may remain at that site for hours beyond what it would if injected SQ. Thus, proper depth and consistent location of insulin injection are essential for regulation of the diabetic patient by its owner.

Many veterinary diabetic patients can benefit from diets that are lower in absorbable sugars or that reduce the amount of sugars available to be absorbed. However, regardless of what diet is prescribed for the diabetic, consistent administration of the diet and exclusion of "treats" (unless incorporated into the regular diet regimen) is essential for preventing an inadvertent hypoglycemic crisis or poorly controlling the diabetic condition, resulting in hyperglycemia and the metabolic derangement called *diabetic ketoacidosis*. It is also recommended, especially in cats, to reduce obesity and maintain exercise; suggestions include using walks for dogs, toys for cats, or other interactions that stimulate activity and play.

Other Drugs to Control Diabetes and Drugs to Avoid

The use of other drugs in diabetic patients can alter insulin requirements and may necessitate changing the insulin dosage. For example, corticosteroids (glucocorticoids) such as prednisone and dexamethasone mobilize glycogen stores, elevate blood glucose levels, and interfere with insulin receptors, all of which can produce significant hyperglycemia in a diabetic animal. Other drugs that elevate blood glucose levels include thiazide diuretics, phenothiazine tranquilizers (such as acepromazine), progesterone, and catecholamines such as epinephrine.

Clients often ask about use of alternative medications or human oral hypoglycemic agents (drugs that lower blood glucose) for their pets as an alternative to daily injections of insulin. They know of relatives or friends who are type 2 diabetics who are well controlled with these oral drugs and do not require insulin injections.

Preliminary experiences with most of the human products have not been encouraging in veterinary medicine; however, the FDA recently (12/6/2022) approved an oral glycemic control medication for cats. The medication is Bexacat™ (bexagliflozin tablets). This medication is a sodium-glucose cotransporter 2 inhibitor causing the glucose to be excreted into the urine. This is achieved by reducing reabsorption of filtered glucose in the kidneys resulting in increased urinary glucose excretion.[7] This medication has shown promising glucose control in otherwise healthy cats. These patients need to be monitored closely for urinary tract infections, dehydration, diarrhea or loose stool, anorexia and lethargy in addition to appropriate blood glucose monitoring. As a veterinary technician, you will play a key role in educating owners on how to monitor their cats on this medication. Another hypoglycemic drug for which the most experience has been gained is the sulfonylurea compound called

glipizide. Sulfonylurea compounds combine with the β cells in the pancreas and stimulate release of additional insulin. Drugs like glipizide do not work if the beta cells have been exhausted, destroyed, or are otherwise incapable of producing sufficient insulin regardless of the degree of stimulation.[1,8] This medication is used in an extra label use for cats and has demonstrated poor efficacy in glycemic control for our feline patients.

Because a relatively high incidence of type 2 diabetes or NIDDM is believed to occur in cats and almost never occurs in dogs, glipizide has been tried in cats for over 15 years. It has been suggested that glipizide may accelerate beta cell loss, rendering the glipizide ineffective and making the diabetic condition worse. The major authors of many of these studies have concluded that, because of glipizide's potential side effect, the lack of medical advantage of glipizide over insulin therapy, and less client compliance with daily oral administration of glipizide tablets for the life of the cat vs insulin injections, the use of insulin in cats is recommended over the use of any sulfonylurea medications.[8]

DRUGS AFFECTING REPRODUCTION

Hormone drugs, either natural or synthetic, are used in food animals and horses to synchronize estrous cycles, terminate pregnancies, and induce ovulation. In dogs and cats, these drugs are used primarily to prevent pregnancy or alter the state of the uterus. Because the degree of response to reproductive hormone therapy varies among species, the dosage regimen or therapeutic protocol in one species should not be assumed to produce the same effect in another species. The information provided in this section provides the veterinary technician with an understanding of the way the drugs are used as "tools" to manipulate reproductive functions. The information will not include specific drug regimens used to manipulate the functions, as these vary widely and change frequently based on emerging research or field experience with these protocols. Further information on theriogenology (the study of reproduction) in cattle and horses can be found in food animal or equine internal medicine resources.

Hormonal Control of the Estrous Cycle

Although there are species variations in how the estrous cycle is controlled, there are some general principles that extend across all the major domestic animal species. More detailed descriptions can be found in reproductive physiology or theriogenology resources for each individual species.

In female animals, hormone therapies often block or enhance the effect of the endogenous reproductive hormones by either mimicking the effect of the natural hormone or by triggering the normal negative feedback mechanisms the body uses to control hormone production. But doing this successfully to modify the activity of the estrous cycle is tricky because the hormones controlling the cycle and producing the bodily effects vary depending on which part of the cycle the animal is in. Hence, reproductive hormone drugs can be effective or ineffective, indicated or contraindicated, at different stages of the estrous cycle (proestrus, estrus, metestrus/diestrus, and anestrus).

The estrous cycle is sometimes described as having two phases: the follicular phase, in which hormones produced by the ovarian follicle exert predominant control and prepare the animal to become inseminated, and the luteal phase, in which hormones of the corpus luteum (CL) on the ovary predominate, focusing on sustaining a fertilized egg. The follicular phase includes proestrus, when follicles are developing, and estrus, when the female animal is receptive to mating and ovulates. The luteal phase usually includes metestrus or diestrus, in which the follicle turns into a CL to prepare for and sustain a pregnancy. Anestrus is the period of time in which little or no cycling activity is occurring and hormone levels in general are very low. Anestrus occurs during the winter months in animals whose reproductive systems are tied to the length of day (seasonal breeders). An important note: **estrus** is a noun referring to the state of being in heat. *Estrous* is an adjective, as indicated by *-ous,* and is used to describe the noun "cycle."

The proper progression of this rather complex cycle is a coordinated and integrated activity between the hypothalamus in the brain, the pituitary gland located just below the hypothalamus, and the gonads (the ovaries in the female). Early in the follicular phase the hypothalamus responds to neural input, the presence of estrogen, or the absence of progesterone to release gonadotropin-releasing hormone (GnRH) from the hypothalamus. The GnRH travels a short distance to the anterior pituitary gland and releases follicle-stimulating hormone (FSH), which in turn stimulates the ovary (female gonads) to produce follicles containing egg cells, or oocytes (Fig. 7.4).

Under the influence of FSH the follicular tissue also begins to produce estrogens. The behavioral and physical changes associated with estrus ("heat") are largely related to changes in

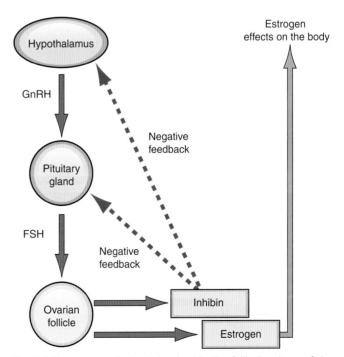

Fig. 7.4 Hormones and glands involved in the follicular phase of the estrous cycle.

estrogen levels. Estrogen production usually peaks near the time of estrus, although considerable variation exists among species.

A second hormone, inhibin, is also produced by the developing follicular tissue and serves as a negative feedback mechanism to decrease release of GnRH and FSH. By decreasing the release of FSH, inhibin allows only the most developed follicle to continue maturation until it can release an ovum. Thus, inhibin helps prevent development of multiple mature follicles that could potentially each release a viable egg and therefore decreases the potential for multiple births in animals that normally have only one or two offspring per birth.

The follicular phase terminates with GnRH signals from the hypothalamus that causes release of a surge of luteinizing hormone (LH) from the pituitary gland. The LH surge lyses the mature ovarian follicles, releases the ova, and transforms the ruptured follicle into a CL, ushering in the luteal phase.

Progesterone produced by the CL is the principal hormone in charge of the luteal phase (Fig. 7.5). Progesterone causes the lining of the uterus to thicken and secrete a nutrient-rich fluid in preparation for implantation of the ovum or ova. In addition, progesterone keeps the uterine smooth muscles (myometrium) in a quiescent, noncontractile state and activates negative feedback on the hypothalamus to inhibit further release of GnRH, which shuts down release of pituitary FSH and LH. If the animal becomes pregnant, progesterone continues to create an environment in the uterus that is conducive to fetal development. Hence, progesterone is considered to be the "hormone of pregnancy."

The CL only lasts for a short period of time (a few days to a few weeks depending on species) after which, if the animal is not pregnant, it degenerates, causing a drop in progesterone production and subsequently reduced progesterone concentrations. This decrease in progesterone removes the inhibition on

hypothalamic GnRH production and allows GnRH once again to stimulate pituitary FSH and LH release, resulting in initiation of a new estrous cycle.

Hormonal Changes During Pregnancy and Parturition

If, after ovulation, the animal becomes pregnant, adequate levels of progesterone must be produced by the CL and the placenta to maintain the pregnancy. At the end of pregnancy, the fetus initiates parturition (the birth process) by producing pituitary adrenocorticotropic hormone (ACTH), which stimulates production of cortisol (a natural corticosteroid) from the adrenal glands of both the fetus and the pregnant female animal. In response to the elevated cortisol levels, the uterus begins to produce estrogens and prostaglandins, both of which make the myometrium more prone to contraction and produce physical changes in the cervix and birth canal that favor passage of the newborn.

The prostaglandins produced by the uterus lyse (destroy) the CL, terminating its production of progesterone and removing the "calming" effect on the myometrium. Estrogen and prostaglandins both make the uterus more prone to contraction, and additionally they increase the number of oxytocin receptors on the myometrial cells, making these smooth muscle cells more sensitive to the powerful contracting effect of oxytocin. Stimulation of the cervix or vagina, such as from entry of the fetus into the birth canal, or stimulation of the nipples in a nursing animal causes the pituitary gland to release oxytocin, which produces the forceful uterine contractions associated with labor and postpartum contractions and the contraction of smooth muscles around milk glands causing release of milk (milk letdown).

Types of Reproductive Drugs

Gonadotropin-releasing hormone drugs (GnRH analogs) or gonadorelins have a similar, but not identical, structure when compared with endogenous GnRH and stimulate release of LH and FSH. Unfortunately, these analogs cannot exactly mimic the natural GnRH because endogenous GnRH is normally released in pulses from the hypothalamus that signal whether FSH or LH is to be released by the pituitary gland.

Gonadorelins are approved for short-term use in beef and dairy cattle to lyse persistent ovarian follicles or follicular cysts through stimulation of LH release. In addition, these drugs have also found a purpose in timed artificial insemination (timed AI) protocols, where the use of drugs in a specific, timed order brings the entire group of cattle into estrus at the same time, regardless of where they were in their estrous cycle, thus eliminating the time-consuming and labor-intensive work of identifying where individual cows are in their cycles. Additional information on timed AI protocols is readily available on the web and can be found by searching for protocol names such as "Ovsynch," "Co-Synch," or "Select Synch." Trade names for gonadorelins include products like Cystorelin, Factrel, Fertagyl, and OvaCyst. These drugs are modified so as to preferentially release LH more than FSH; however, both hormones are typically released to some degree.

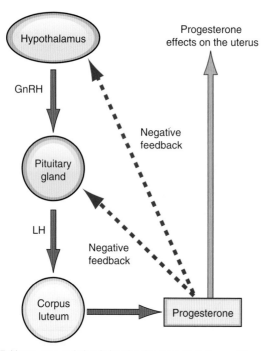

Fig. 7.5 Hormones and glands involved in the luteal phase of the estrous cycle.

Gonadotropins are not the same as gonadorelins but are drugs that are FSH- and LH-like, as opposed to causing the release of FSH or LH like gonadorelins do. The word fragment *-tropin* means "an affinity for"; therefore, the pituitary gonadotropins FSH and LH have an affinity for, and produce their effects on, the gonads (ovaries, testes).

Although we think of gonadotropins as being released from the pituitary in response to GnRH stimulation, gonadotropins can be produced by other tissues in the body, and those substances can be harvested for use as drug gonadotropins. Human chorionic gonadotropin is a hormone produced by the human placenta and has LH-like effects with few or no FSH effects. Certain fetal cells in the horse produce equine chorionic gonadotropin, also known historically as pregnant mare serum gonadotropin, which has FSH and LH effects. These drugs are sometimes used in food animals to induce superovulation (release of ova from multiple follicles). Chorionic gonadotropins have also been used to stimulate testicular descent in cryptorchid males with undescended testicles.

With the success of the more modern GnRH analog gonadorelins to stimulate endogenous LH or FSH, drug gonadotropins are used less frequently in veterinary medicine today.

Progestins, progestagens (also spelled progestogens), and progestational hormones are terms used to describe drugs that have similar chemical structures and effects as the natural hormone progesterone. **Progestins** refers to the group of progesterone-like hormones, and the term **progestational hormones** is synonymous with progestins. A **progestagen** refers to a synthesized drug that mimics progestins.

Remember that progesterone has a negative feedback effect on the release of hypothalamic GnRH and pituitary FSH and LH—as such, progestins are used during the follicular phase to inhibit FSH release and slow development of the follicles. When used in this manner, progestins can prevent an animal from coming into estrus. Drugs like the orally administered drench **altrenogest** (Regu-Mate is a trade name) are used to regulate the onset of heat for more effective breeding or to delay the onset of estrus when the mare may be competing in an event or stallions are around.

In the luteal phase of the estrous cycle, progestins can be used to prolong diestrus beyond the time when the CL production of progesterone has naturally regressed. By controlling how long the progestin is given and when it is stopped, the veterinarian can imitate the end of diestrus, initiate a new estrous cycle, and control when estrus occurs for optimal management of breeding.

Altrenogest is not approved for use in cattle, but there is a feed additive called **melengestrol acetate**, or **MGA**, that can do the same thing. MGA is an FDA-approved progestagen that is added to the cattle feed to suppress the estrous cycle or prolong diestrus in groups of feedlot heifers to facilitate the heifers all coming into heat at the same time and managing artificial insemination.

As an alternative to using MGA to prolong diestrus in cattle, a Controlled Internal Drug Release (CIDR) apparatus can be used in cattle to provide a continuous supply of progesterone for several days. The CIDRs are FDA approved for use in cattle, are long, slender silicone rubber implants containing progesterone, and are inserted vaginally for several days (varying with whatever breeding protocol or purpose it is being used), after which the implant is removed to imitate the lysis of the CL and the end of diestrus.

The veterinary professional should be aware of certain precautions when using progestins in general. Progesterone causes the endometrium (uterine lining) to produce nutrient-rich secretions ("uterine milk") that favor implantation of ova after fertilization. These progesterone-induced changes also provide an environment conducive for bacterial growth in the uterus. Thus, the use of progestins or progestagens at higher than normal levels or for extended periods predisposes the uterus to infection, metritis (inflammation of the uterus), or pyometra (a uterine infection with pus). If the cervix is relaxed, the purulent material (pus) produced within the uterus can escape and be evident on the vulva as a purulent discharge, a condition called open-cervix pyometra. If the cervix is closed, the pus may accumulate within the uterus, creating a life-threatening condition called closed-cervix pyometra.[9] For this reason, the use of progestins is contraindicated in any animal that might have inflammation or infection of the uterus.

Progesterone and other progestins have an antagonistic effect on insulin receptors and interfere with insulin's ability to dock with its receptor on cells, reducing insulin's ability to move glucose from the blood into cells. This effect of progestins helps explain the hyperglycemia and a temporary diabetic-like syndrome (gestational diabetes) that is frequently seen in pregnant women and female animals in other species. Because of its insulin antagonism, progestational compounds should not be used in diabetic animals.

Progestin drugs can be well absorbed across the skin of those who handle these drugs. Thus, latex gloves should always be worn when handling a progesterone CIDR and care should be taken not to spill oral progesterone drug on the skin of the person administering the drug. Oil-based progesterone products may penetrate some cheaper, more porous gloves, so good quality latex gloves should always be used, and if there is any suspicion of a tear or puncture, the gloves should be replaced.

The label for Regu-Mate (altrenogest) states that pregnant women, or those who suspect they are pregnant, should not handle the product because of the risk of prolonging the pregnancy beyond its natural end. This caution is especially important for women working with these drugs on a regular basis where potential repeated exposures could provide a near-constant exogenous supply of progesterone when it is not needed. In the event of accidental exposure, the recommendation is to immediately wash the drug off the skin with water and soap.

Most of these conditions relate directly to the progestin effects. However, most progestational drugs also have some estrogen effect, and therefore some warnings, such as avoiding the drug if the administrator is using estrogen contraceptives or has an estrogen-dependent neoplasia, relate to a secondary estrogen-enhancing effect of the drug.

It is important that the veterinary technician not only be aware of the effects of these progestin drugs for their own health and safety but that they also help protect veterinary staff, clients/owners, or other nonveterinary personnel who are likely to be unaware of the potential dangers from exposure to these drugs.

Estrogen drugs have historically been used for a variety of reproductive and nonreproductive functions. However, with refinement of medical treatments, the availability of newer drugs, and banning of some estrogen products from any use in food animals, the legitimate estrogen uses in veterinary medicine are far more limited.

Estrogen products still used include **estradiol** tablets and **estriol** (trade name Incurin) tablets that are primarily used in spayed female dogs to treat urinary incontinence, usually in conjunction with another drug that tightens the internal urinary outflow sphincter. Diethylstilbestrol (DES) is another estrogen compound that several years ago was used extensively in food animals as a growth-promoting, or anabolic, steroid. However, after DES was found to have significant carcinogenic (cancer-producing) potential in human beings, the drug was banned from use in food animals. DES is still available in an oral form from compounding pharmacies, but because of the newer compounds like estriol approved for treating dogs with urinary incontinence, DES is seldom used.

Estrogens in general are prone to some potentially serious side effects that every veterinary technician must know. Estrogens can predispose the uterus to infection and pyometra by increasing the number of progesterone receptors on uterine cells, making the uterus more sensitive to progesterone and increasing the progesterone effect, including the conditions that predispose the uterus to infection.

Estrogens also can suppress the blood cell production by the bone marrow, resulting in a condition called aplastic anemia. Estrogen-induced aplastic anemia usually appears 2–8 weeks after estrogen administration and is manifested as low platelet counts (thrombocytopenia), pinpoint hemorrhages in the skin or mucous membranes (caused by low platelet levels), evidence of bruising, leukopenia (low white blood cell count), and severe anemia. Aplastic anemia may slowly resolve after discontinuation of estrogen therapy; however, the anemia can continue to progress, resulting in death of the animal.

Prostaglandins, along with GnRH and progestins, play a major role in synchronizing estrous cycles. By lysing the CL, prostaglandins terminate the major source of progesterone during the luteal phase, causing progesterone levels to drop, terminating diestrus, and initiating a new estrous cycle.

Synthetic prostaglandin drugs, most of which are analogs or derivations of prostaglandin $F_{2\alpha}$, are used to lyse an active CL in an animal in the diestrus period of the luteal phase or to cause contractions of the uterus. Prostaglandins are marketed under a variety of trade names. Most can be recognized by the stem -*prost* in the chemical or generic name. Common prostaglandin drugs include **dinoprost tromethamine** (Lutalyse, ProstaMate, In-Sync) and **cloprostenol** (Estrumate).

Prostaglandins can only function in the luteal phase when an active CL is present to lyse. If prostaglandins are administered during the follicular phase when no CL is present, no clinical effect related to progesterone levels will be observed. Timed AI protocols, which do not assess the animal's stage of the estrous cycle but rely on the drugs to bring the animal back into estrus regardless of the current estrous stage it is in, often repeat the injection of prostaglandin to catch cattle that were in the follicular phase at the time of the first prostaglandin injection.

Significant species differences exist in the susceptibility of the CL to prostaglandin lysis, with horses and cattle significantly more sensitive to lysis than dogs or cats. Also, a younger CL is more resistant to lysis than a more mature CL.

Prostaglandins have a direct and indirect effect on the uterus. By decreasing progesterone through CL lysis, prostaglandins remove the hormone responsible for the quiescent state of the myometrium (uterine muscle), making the uterus more prone to contractions with time as progesterone levels decrease. Prostaglandins also have a more immediate effect by directly stimulating the myometrium to contract.

Endogenous prostaglandins affect many body systems, and exogenous-administered prostaglandins similarly cause a wide variety of side effects. The most common side effects include unintended abortion in pregnant animals because of CL lysis; bronchoconstriction in animals with respiratory disease (such as horses with heaves); vomiting (in dogs and cats); colic and sweating (in horses); and, in larger doses, CNS effects such as anxiety, hyperpnea (rapid breathing), and pupillary dilation.

Technicians who handle prostaglandins should be aware that these drugs are easily absorbed through the skin and can easily produce CL lysis and bronchoconstriction in people, as well as in animals. Technicians should take precautions such as wearing good quality latex gloves when handling these drugs. Women of childbearing age and those with asthma should completely avoid handling these drugs at any time.

Within the past few years a rumor has been reported in newspapers in several states that teenage girls were stealing or obtaining prostaglandin to terminate unwanted pregnancies. As a result of several inquiries about this topic in 2009, the American Veterinary Medical Association warned its members to more tightly control prostaglandin products within their practice. Regardless of whether these stories are true or urban legend, they raise a concern about making sure that prostaglandin drugs are handled safely, stored safely, and do not fall into the hands of untrained individuals, where use could result in a tragic outcome.

Specific Uses for Reproductive Drugs

By knowing how the individual drugs affect the reproductive tract, the veterinary technician should be able to understand how the drugs act as tools to manipulate breeding, the estrous cycle, or pregnancy. These specific uses will be summarized later on.

Drugs Used to Control Estrous Cycling

Livestock breeders use estrus synchronization in female animals so that artificial insemination can be planned in advance and a number of animals can be inseminated at the same time. By synchronizing heat and insemination dates, all offspring are born at approximately the same time, which facilitates management of parturition and better neonatal care.

Injecting cows with prostaglandins during diestrus results in CL lysis, which subsequently causes progesterone concentrations to fall and the animal to return to estrus within 2–5 days of prostaglandin administration. Prostaglandins are used similarly in mares but with more variable results because, among other reasons, the equine CL is less sensitive to the lysing effects of prostaglandins for up to 5 days after ovulation and the transformation of the follicle into the CL.

Prostaglandins are not used in this manner in small animals because synchronizing groups of animals for breeding is not common, and the CL of cats and dogs tends to be resistant to the effects of exogenous prostaglandin for most of the luteal phase.

Using progestins to prolong the diestrus phase beyond the natural length determined by the CL and then stopping the drug when needed to imitate the lysis of the CL and terminate diestrus is another way to synchronize estrus in a herd of livestock. In mares, progesterone drugs are used in a similar way, although some equine breeding regimens are now including estrogen with the progestin to suppress follicular development and provide a more predictable return to estrus.

Gonadorelins have been used on cows or mares with persistent ovarian follicles or cysts that are resistant to the normal regression that should occur at the end of estrus. Because of the persistent follicle, the animals remain in a prolonged estrus (nymphomania) and often exhibit aggressive behavior. Gonadorelins and the subsequent surge of LH are usually successful in lysing the follicle, terminating the prolonged estrus, and allowing the animal to continue on into metestrus/diestrus.

Drugs Used in Foal Heat

Mares that come into heat soon after foaling generally have a significantly lower conception rate than mares that come into heat at a later time. It used to be that breeding managers would attempt to delay this foal heat to increase the chances of conception at a later breeding by using progesterone to inhibit release of FSH and LH by negative feedback. However, this did not seem to significantly increase the conception rate.

A second technique was to shorten the diestrus phase of the first cycle by using prostaglandins to lyse the CL and initiate a new cycle (short cycling). This has met with variable success also. Because successful reproduction in the mare is influenced by multiple factors related to hormones, nutrition, and the state of the uterus and the environment, it is often difficult to implement a protocol that is predictably successful in improving conception during foal heat.

Drugs Used to Treat Anestrus

As the days grow shorter in autumn and the photoperiod decreases, the reproductive hormones in mares begin to decrease to minimal amounts, causing most mares to stop cycling and enter a period of seasonal anestrus.[10] Because

equine breed registries encourage the birth of foals as soon as possible after January 1, breeders often ask veterinarians to help mares conceive during the spring, when the animals are in transition from seasonal anestrus to full reproductive capacity. During this period of transitional estrus, several follicles may grow and regress, causing periods of estrus that are frequently long and during which the exact time of ovulation is unknown.

A variety of techniques using drugs have been tried, but no one drug method seems to consistently work. Administration of progesterone or a progestin drug for 10–14 days to mimic diestrus and then halted to mimic CL lysis seems to work on mares near the end of the transitional anestrous period or when multiple large follicles are already on the ovaries.

GnRH analog drugs have been used to stimulate release of FSH and LH in an attempt to promote follicular development. Another technique has been to use **dopamine antagonist** drugs, which promote the release of prolactin from the pituitary. Prolactin injections have been shown to increase follicular activity in anestrus mares. However, endocrine neurons from the hypothalamus normally release dopamine that suppresses prolactin release from the pituitary. By using dopamine antagonist drugs to block dopamine receptors, the prolactin-suppressing effect of dopamine is blocked and prolactin is released from the pituitary in greater amounts, facilitating follicular development.

Although each of these techniques has had some measure of success, the results are quite variable, and what works in one animal may not work in another. Thus, proposed solutions to this particular reproductive problem will continue to evolve.

Drugs Used to Maintain Pregnancy

Because progesterone is the normal hormone that maintains pregnancy, progestagens and progesterone have been advocated for use in maintaining pregnancy in mares prone to abortion. These drugs may help if the reason for pregnancy failure is related to low progesterone levels because of a poorly functioning CL. Altrenogest has been used with varying success in mares to prevent premature parturition. Because altrenogest is slightly different from progesterone, it does not produce negative feedback on endogenous progesterone production and thus can be given as an oral progesterone supplement. Unfortunately, because abortion and premature parturition have multiple causes, the success of progestin therapy in maintaining pregnancy varies considerably.

Drugs Used to Prevent Pregnancy

Pregnancy can be prevented by suppressing the estrous cycle or preventing implantation of the fertilized ova in the uterine wall. **Megestrol acetate** is an orally administered progestin used for contraception in female dogs and cats. The drug is similar to progesterone and is thought to suppress release of GnRH and subsequent release of FSH and LH, causing cessation of cycling.[9] Because megestrol is a progestin, it causes endometrial changes such as thickened, increased secretions consistent with progesterone stimulation. Use of megestrol increases the risk of cystic hyperplasia of the endometrium, endometritis, or pyometra, although the risk of pyometra appears to be fairly low.

Prolonged use of megestrol can result in mammary hyperplasia (proliferation of mammary tissue). For these reasons, megestrol acetate is contraindicated in animals with any disease of the reproductive organs, mammary tumors, or mammary growth. Megestrol is contraindicated in pregnant females because the drug can have a masculinizing effect on female fetuses and can delay parturition. As with progesterone and other progestins, megestrol has an antagonistic effect on insulin, reduces insulin's ability to move glucose from blood into cells, and can create a hyperglycemia in diabetic animals, requiring an increased insulin dose.

The adrenal gland in cats is apparently sensitive to the suppressive effects of megestrol acetate. Plasma cortisol levels in cats treated with megestrol can drop well below normal, producing a syndrome resembling hypoadrenocorticism. Most cats treated with megestrol do not show severe signs with this effect; however, administration of prednisone or other corticosteroids should be considered if such cats are to have surgery, be hospitalized, or be subjected to other stress. Low-dose megestrol treatment has been suggested for control of feral cat populations.[9]

Mibolerone is another contraceptive previously commercially available for controlling the onset of estrus in female dogs. Mibolerone is an androgen hormone similar to testosterone and interrupts estrous cycling by inhibiting LH release. Follicles develop to a point but do not lyse and consequently do not release their ova. Because this drug is a testosterone analog and therefore an anabolic steroid subject to human abuse for athletes and others who might abuse steroids, it is only available on a case-by-case basis from compounding pharmacies and carries a controlled substance designation.[11]

Drugs Used to Terminate Pregnancy

Several drugs are used to induce abortion or initiate parturition. These drugs are used in animals carrying a dead fetus, mares carrying twins, or heifers that have been bred too young to safely deliver a live calf. Prostaglandins are the most commonly used drugs for termination of pregnancy. Prostaglandin administration causes CL lysis, resulting in a decrease in progesterone levels and subsequent fetal death.

The effectiveness of **prostaglandin $F_{2\alpha}$** and its analogs varies among species because of the resistance of some CLs to prostaglandin and the placenta's role in providing some progesterone necessary to maintain pregnancy. In cows, the CL continues to produce progesterone for the entire pregnancy; however, the placenta can produce sufficient progesterone to maintain pregnancy without the CL after the fourth or fifth month. Therefore, prostaglandins are only effective in cows if given before the fourth month of pregnancy.

In dogs, the CL is relatively resistant to the lytic effects of prostaglandins during the first 2–4 weeks of pregnancy. Canine CL sensitivity to prostaglandin increases after this time. Although prostaglandins are quite effective in terminating pregnancy, they often cause side effects such as panting, salivation, respiratory distress, GI stimulation (vomiting and diarrhea), tachycardia, and increased urination. If side effects occur, they last approximately 20 min.

Dinoprost tromethamine is the prostaglandin $F_{2\alpha}$ analog approved for termination of pregnancy in mares. As in dogs, side effects include increased respiratory and heart rates, sweating, transient fever, and some abdominal discomfort. These signs usually disappear approximately 1 h after administration.

Dopamine agonists are a group of compounds that, as the name implies, bind with and stimulate dopamine receptors, unlike the previously mentioned dopamine antagonists that block dopamine receptors. Dopamine normally inhibits release of pituitary prolactin, a hormone that helps maintain an active CL. If a dopamine agonist drug is used, prolactin is inhibited and the CL may degenerate, resulting in a decline of progesterone necessary for maintaining pregnancy and terminating the pregnancy. **Bromocriptine** is a drug that has been advocated in the past to terminate pregnancies and treat pseudopregnancy in dogs. Because of the high incidence of vomiting and other side effects, it has not been widely used.

Corticosteroids may induce abortion or premature parturition in mares or cows by mimicking the elevated levels of cortisol that occur at the beginning of normal parturition. In dogs, corticosteroids such as dexamethasone have been reported to cause intrauterine death and fetal resorption if given after 30 days of gestation (pregnancy) and premature parturition if given during the last 3 weeks of gestation. If corticosteroids are used to intentionally terminate the pregnancy, their efficacy is unpredictable. Using corticosteroids to initiate parturition and terminate the pregnancy in cows is associated with a fairly high incidence of retained placenta.

Because prostaglandins are usually much more effective at terminating pregnancy, corticosteroids are not often used for intentionally inducing parturition or abortion. However, the inadvertent administration of a significant dose of a corticosteroid in a pregnant animal for a problem unrelated to pregnancy, such as joint inflammation or immune-mediated disease, can induce unintended abortion.

Other Uses of Reproductive Drugs

Oxytocin is an endogenous hormone released from the pituitary gland that causes contraction of the *myometrium* (muscles of the uterus). Just before parturition the increased concentrations of prostaglandins and estrogens cause increased numbers of oxytocin receptors to appear on the smooth muscle cells of the uterus, making these cells more sensitive to the effects of oxytocin. When the entrance of the fetus into the birth canal stimulates oxytocin release, the uterus contracts to expel the newborn. Exogenous oxytocin is most commonly used to increase uterine contractions in animals with dystocia (difficult labor) related to a weakened or fatigued uterus. Calcium gluconate is sometimes given in conjunction with oxytocin to facilitate uterine contraction in dystocia.

Veterinarians may also give an oxytocin injection to increase expulsion of placental materials after birth and to decrease uterine hemorrhage. Controversy exists regarding whether this is of any significant benefit. Administration of oxytocin causes both contraction of mammary smooth muscles and milk letdown and therefore may also result in dripping of milk from the teats after administration for uterine contraction.

ENDOCRINE DRUGS

Drugs Used to Treat Hypothyroidism
Levothyroxine
Liothyronine

Drugs Used to Treat Hyperthyroidism
Methimazole (Tapazole)
Radioactive iodine (^{131}I)
Iodine-limited diets
Propranolol/atenolol
Amlodipine

Endocrine Pancreatic Drugs
Regular crystalline insulin
NPH (neutral protamine Hagedorn) insulin
Porcine insulin zinc suspension
PZI (protamine zinc insulin)
Insulin glargine
Insulin detemir
Glipizide (sulfonylurea compound)

Reproductive Drugs
GnRH (gonadotropin-releasing hormone) analogs/gonadorelins

Gonadotropins
Equine chorionic gonadotropin
Human chorionic gonadotropin
Progestins, progestagens, progestational hormones
Altrenogest (Regu-Mate)
Melengestrol acetate (MGA)
Estrogen
Estradiol
Estriol
Prostaglandin $F_{2\alpha}$ analogs
Dinoprost tromethamine
Cloprostenol
Dopamine antagonists
Megestrol acetate
Mibolerone
Dopamine agonists
Bromocriptine
Corticosteroids
Oxytocin

REFERENCES

1. Behrend EN, Civco TD, Boothe DM. Drug therapy for endocrinopathies. In: Boothe DM, ed. *Small Animal Clinical Pharmacology and Therapeutics*. Philadelphia: Saunders; 2012.
2. Ferguson DC. Thyroid hormones and antithyroid drugs. In: Riviere J, Papich M, eds. *Veterinary Pharmacology and Therapeutics*. Ames, Iowa: Wiley-Blackwell; 2009.
3. Scott-Moncrieff JC. Hypothyroidism. In: Feldman EC, Nelson RW, et al., eds. *Canine and Feline Endocrinology*. 4th ed. Philadelphia: Saunders; 2015.
4. Accessed online: https://academic-plumbs-com.ezproxy.lib.purdue.edu/drug-monograph/Ehf1HkfFUePROD?source=search&search. Accessed 06.14.2022.
5. Peterson ME, et al. Methimazole treatment of 262 cats with hyperthyroidism. *J Vet Intern Med*. 1988;2(3):150–157.
6. Nelson RW. Canine diabetes mellitus. In: Feldman EC, Nelson RW, et al., eds. *Canine and Feline Endocrinology*. 4th ed. Philadelphia: Saunders; 2015.
7. Accessed online: https://animaldrugsatfda.fda.gov/adafda/app/search/public/document/downloadFoi/13222#:~:text=Bexacat%E2%84%A2%20(bexagliflozin%20tablets)%20is,regardless%20of%20blood%20glucose%20level. Accessed 03.03.2023.
8. Reusch CE. Feline diabetes mellitus. In: Feldman EC, Nelson RW, et al., eds. *Canine and Feline Endocrinology*. 4th ed. Philadelphia: Saunders; 2015.
9. Doodipla SD, Gadsby JE. Hormones affecting reproduction. In: Riviere J, Papich M, eds. *Veterinary Pharmacology and Therapeutics*. Ames, Iowa: Wiley-Blackwell; 2009.
10. Oberhaus EL, Paccamonti D. Review of management of anestrus and transitional mares. In: *Proceedings of the American Association of Equine Practitioners Annual Convention, Nashville, Tennessee, December 7-11*; 2013.
11. Greer ML. Canine Reproduction and Neonatology. Philadelphia: CRC Press; 2014.

SELF-ASSESSMENT

1. Fill in the following blanks with the correct item from the Key Terms list.
   A. _____ This term means the mechanism by which a hormone inhibits its own production or generation.
   B. _____ The hypothalamic hormone that stimulates the pituitary gland to release the hormone that directly stimulates the thyroid gland.
   C. _____ The pituitary hormone that directly stimulates the thyroid gland.
   D. _____ The thyroid hormone that is the more biologically active hormone.
   E. _____ The thyroid hormone that acts as a reserve of biologically active hormone and is converted by the tissues into the biologically active hormone to meet the specific tissue need.
   F. _____ The state of having lower than normal thyroid hormones.
   G. _____ The state of having higher than normal thyroid hormones.
   H. _____ The type of hypothyroidism caused by damage or disease of the thyroid gland itself.
   I. _____ The type of hypothyroidism caused by damage or disease of the hypothalamus.

J. _____ The type of hypothyroidism caused by damage or disease of the pituitary gland.

K. _____ An enlargement of the thyroid gland caused by lack of iodine in the diet.

L. _____ Term (adjective) that describes the reproductive cycle (spell it correctly!).

M. _____ What T_3 stands for.

N. _____ What T_4 stands for.

O. _____ This term means "normal thyroid" state.

P. _____ This is the term that describes the surgical removal of the thyroid gland.

Q. _____ Type of diabetes mellitus that does not require treatment with insulin.

R. _____ Type of diabetes mellitus that does require insulin treatment.

S. _____ What does IDDM stand for?

T. _____ What does NIDDM stand for?

U. _____ This term describes the production of insulin drug by combining DNA in a way that produces an insulin molecule not normally produced by biological organisms.

V. _____ Fish protein added to insulin to slow absorption of the drug.

W. _____ Designation on an insulin syringe that means 40 units of insulin are found in every 1 mL of insulin product.

X. _____ What does PZI stand for?

Y. _____ These are human drugs, usually given as oral medications, that decrease the blood sugar.

Z. _____ The drug group to which glipizide belongs to.

AA. _____ The part of the estrous cycle phase dominated by the follicle.

AB. _____ The part of the estrous cycle phase dominated by the CL.

AC. _____ The hypothalamic hormone that causes release of FSH and LH.

AD. _____ What does FSH stand for?

AE. _____ What does LH stand for?

AF. _____ This is a term meaning "egg cells."

AG. _____ The term for "heat"; the period of receptivity to mating (spell it correctly!).

AH. _____ The hormone produced by the developing follicle cells that prevents too many egg follicles from maturing in those species that normally only produce one or two young at a time.

AI. _____ The hormone of pregnancy.

AJ. _____ The hormone produced by the CL.

AK. _____ What does CL stand for?

AL. _____ The term for the smooth muscle layers of the uterus.

AM. _____ The hormone in the fetus that initiates parturition.

AN. _____ The hormone that is elevated in the fetus and mother by ACTH during early stages of parturition.

AO. _____ The hormone that destroys the CL at time of parturition.

AP. _____ The types of receptors that proliferate on the uterus just before parturition because of elevated levels of estrogen and prostaglandin.

AQ. _____ The hormone released from the pituitary gland when the fetus moves into the birth canal and stimulates the cervix.

AR. _____ The hormone responsible for most of the strong labor contractions.

AS. _____ The hormone responsible for milk letdown.

AT. _____ This term describes a drug that is a synthesized analog of GnRH.

AU. _____ This describes a breeding program in which cattle are not checked individually for signs of heat but are given a series of drugs designed to bring all the cows back into heat about the same time regardless of where they were in their estrous cycle.

AV. _____ The term that describes drugs that have an affinity for the ovaries and testes.

AW. _____ This term describes drugs that have effects like FSH and LH.

AX. _____ The drug derived from human placenta that has LH-like effects.

AY. _____ The drug derived from horse placenta that has FSH and LH effects.

AZ. _____ The term that describes a group of progesterone-like hormones.

BA. _____ The term that describes a synthesized drug that mimics progesterone.

BB. _____ What does CIDR stand for?

BC. _____ The term that describes inflammation of the uterus.

BD. _____ The term that describes a pus-filled, infected uterus.

BE. _____ The term that means "cancer causing."

BF. _____ The term that describes damage to the bone marrow resulting in an inability to generate any blood cells by the marrow.

BG. _____ The first estrus after a mare gives birth.

BH. _____ The term that describes a period of time related to shortened length of daylight in which the estrous cycle stops cycling.

BI. _____ This term means "difficult labor."

2. Fill in the following blanks with the correct drug from the Endocrine Drug list. When practicing these questions, write out the answers on a separate sheet, focusing also on the appropriate spelling of these drug names.

A. _____ The drug of choice for correcting canine hypothyroidism.

B. _____ Synthetic thyroid hormone only used to treat hypothyroidism if the drug of choice does not adequately correct the hypothyroidism.

C. _____ Oral medication given to hyperthyroid patients that works by preventing available dietary iodine from being incorporated into thyroid hormone.

D. _____ Only drug treatment that actually eliminates thyroid tumor.

E. _____ Drug used to slow the heart rate in hyperthyroid patients by blocking β_1-receptor sites on the heart.

F. _____ Drug of choice for controlling hypertension caused by hyperthyroidism.

G. _____ Only type of insulin that can be given intravenously (IV).

H. _____ Two types of insulins made from recombinant human DNA.

I. _____ Three types of intermediate-duration insulins.

J. _____ Long-acting insulin.

K. _____ Insulin used to initially control diabetic patients with very high blood glucose and diabetic ketoacidosis.

L. _____ Sulfonylurea compound; hypoglycemic agent.

M. _____ Types of drugs used to lyse ovarian follicles or follicular cysts.

N. _____ A progestagen given orally by drench.

O. _____ Types of drugs used to prolong diestrus; stopping the drug imitates CL lysis.

P. _____ Oral feed additive that is a progestagen.

Q. _____ Drug used to treat urinary incontinence in spayed female dogs.

R. _____ Used to lyse the CL and bring an animal back into proestrus.

S. _____ Two synthetic prostaglandin drugs commonly used in veterinary medicine.

T. _____ Type of drug that can cause abortion in humans.

U. _____ Type of drug used to "short cycle" mares after foaling so as to bypass a foal heat and have another estrus that is more likely to result in conceiving if bred.

V. _____ Type of drug used to delay the onset of foal heat by suppression of follicle-stimulating hormone (FSH) and luteinizing hormone (LH) release.

W. _____ Type of drug given for 10–14 days to a transitional anestrus mare to make the body think it is in diestrus; the drug is then withdrawn to hopefully stimulate a new estrous cycle.

X. _____ Type of drug given to increase FSH and LH release so as to start an estrous cycle in a transitional anestrus mare.

Y. _____ Type of drug that promotes release of prolactin, which should increase follicular activity in transitional anestrus mares.

Z. _____ Progestagen used to maintain pregnancy in mares with low natural progesterone.

AA. _____ Orally administered progestin used as a female canine and feline contraceptive by suppressing progression of the estrous cycle by inhibiting GnRH release and release of FSH and LH.

AB. _____ Androgen hormone similar to testosterone used as a contraceptive for suppressing the onset of estrus in female dogs.

AC. _____ Drug that causes suppression of prolactin release, degeneration of the CL, and termination of pregnancy or pseudopregnancy.

AD. _____ Type of drug that is used for anti-inflammatory effects but can also initiate the parturition process in near-term cows or mares, resulting in premature birth.

AE. _____ Drug used to stimulate contraction of the uterus during parturition.

3. An endocrine gland A secretes hormone A, which causes gland B to produce hormone B. Hormone B produces the needed effect on other body tissues. What effect will high levels of hormone B likely have on gland A and hormone A?

4. If an animal has primary hypothyroidism, would you expect the serum T_3/T_4 level to be increased or decreased? What about serum TSH and TRH levels? What would the levels of T_3/T_4, TSH, and TRH be if the hypothyroidism was secondary or tertiary? What about if the animal had goiter caused by iodine deficiency?

5. Indicate which of the following clinical signs are most often associated with hypothyroidism and which are associated with hyperthyroidism.

Hypo	Hyper	
Hypo	Hyper	Bradycardia
Hypo	Hyper	Intolerance of warm environments
Hypo	Hyper	Increased activity, alertness
Hypo	Hyper	Dry, scaly skin
Hypo	Hyper	Increased size of thyroid gland or part of thyroid gland
Hypo	Hyper	Heat-seeking behavior
Hypo	Hyper	Weight gain despite normal food consumption
Hypo	Hyper	Polyuria, polydipsia
Hypo	Hyper	Loss of weight despite normal or increased appetite
Hypo	Hyper	Tachycardia

6. Why is it that liothyronine or the human combination T_3/T_4 products are not used in veterinary medicine that much?

7. What drugs are used to reduce elevated thyroid hormones in cats with hyperthyroidism? Which of these treatments cures and which controls the hyperthyroidism?

8. What effect would successfully treating hypothyroidism in a dog that was also a diabetic have on the insulin required to keep the diabetic condition under control?

9. Why is it that cats with hyperthyroidism often are not presented to a veterinary hospital for complaints related to the disease until months after the first clinical signs appear?

10. What does methimazole do to suppress production of thyroid hormones in a thyroid tumor?
11. What chronic organ disease might be "covered up" in a cat that has hyperthyroidism and the clinical signs not become apparent until after the hyperthyroidism has been corrected?
12. What is carbimazole?
13. Why does radioactive iodine not destroy all of the thyroid tissue instead of just the thyroid tumor?
14. What causes tachycardia in hyperthyroid cats? How do drugs like propranolol and atenolol counteract tachycardia?
15. In which species does non–insulin-dependent diabetes mellitus (NIDDM) more frequently occur? Is NIDDM (type 2 diabetes) treated the same way as insulin-dependent diabetes mellitus (IDDM)? Why or why not? How do these two diseases differ physiologically?
16. What is the concern about pork or human insulin not being identical to canine insulin?
17. What in insulin determines whether it is short acting, intermediate acting, or long acting?
18. Why are special syringes used for insulin administration? What does the designation "U-40" on an insulin bottle or syringe mean?
19. What is the "controversy" about the way insulin is resuspended before withdrawal from the bottle with a syringe? What types of insulins get which type of resuspension method?
20. Why should the owner not switch around injection sites on a daily basis?
21. In what species have oral hypoglycemics been used? Under what conditions might this therapy work? Why can insulin not be given by mouth instead? Why are oral hypoglycemics not used in dogs?
22. How is it that progesterone can prevent an animal from coming into heat?
23. In what estrous cycle phase can prostaglandins work? How do prostaglandins initiate a new estrous cycle? Why will they not work in the follicular phase?
24. How does the body keep humans or horses from having litters of young each time they are pregnant?
25. What starts the parturition process? How does this affect the uterus? Where does oxytocin come in? Could oxytocin be as effective in producing uterine contractions if given as a drug earlier in the pregnancy?
26. What does it mean when it is said that oxytocin causes milk letdown? What is happening?
27. Why is timed artificial insemination (timed AI) considered to be a labor-saving technique in breeding operations?
28. How is it that gonadotropins are able to lyse mature follicles on the ovary? How is this different from a gonadorelin?
29. What effect would human chorionic gonadotropin have on the follicular phase of an animal? What effect would it have on the luteal phase? How about equine chorionic gonadotropin?

30. Why is altrenogest used to maintain pregnancy? In what physiologically abnormal conditions would altrenogest be most effective?
31. How does melengestrol acetate (MGA) suppress the estrous cycle?
32. What is a controlled internal drug release (CIDR)? How is it used to regulate the estrous cycle in cows?
33. What are the concerns related to uterine health when using high doses or long-term doses of progesterone in the intact female animal?
34. What precautions should a human take when administering progesterone as a drench or as a CIDR? What potentially could happen to the human?
35. What are estrogen products used for in the dog these days? Why is the estrogen DES not used anymore in food animals even though it was so useful in the past?
36. What is the concern about misuse of veterinary prostaglandins by individuals outside of the veterinary profession? What is the health risk to veterinary technicians who handle prostaglandins? What can technicians do to prevent this risk?
37. What drugs are used to treat nymphomania, and how do they work to fix this problem?
38. How would a dopamine antagonist drug stimulate a transitional anestrous mare to come into heat? What is the role of prolactin?
39. What are the two pregnancy preventive medications for dogs? Why is one a controlled substance?
40. How can dopamine agonists cause premature parturition or terminate pregnancy?
41. If Mrs. Jones gives her near-term pregnant mare an injection of a glucocorticoid (corticosteroid) drug to relieve the swelling her mare has in one of her hocks, how might this result in the mare dropping the foal prematurely?
42. Indicate whether each statement is true or false.
    A. Hyperthyroidism occurs more frequently in dogs than cats.
    B. Thyrotoxicosis from excessive thyroid hormones is typically more severe in the dog than it is in humans.
    C. Radioactive iodine is given orally.
    D. Iodine-limited diets need only be given for a short period of time to hyperthyroid patients because the iodine deficiency starves the thyroid tumor, causing the cells to die.
    E. NPH, protamine zinc insulin (PZI), and porcine insulin zinc suspension insulin are all given subcutaneously (SQ).
    F. Estrogen compounds can cause a proliferation of increased red blood cells and white blood cells from the bone marrow.

Drugs Affecting the Nervous System: Analgesics, Tranquilizers, Sedatives, and Anesthetics

CHAPTER OUTLINE

OBJECTIVES

After studying this chapter, the veterinary technician should be able to:

- Differentiate between the roles analgesics, tranquilizers, sedatives, and anesthetics play in controlling pain or for producing a balanced anesthetic regimen.
- Describe the steps in the pain pathway and how drugs can modify the transmission of pain in the pathway from nociceptor to brain.
- Explain how opioid analgesics work and what effects the three opioid receptors play in producing analgesia or side effects.
- Describe the opioid agonist and antagonist drugs commonly used in veterinary medicine and be able to differentiate the drugs based upon their key characteristics.
- Explain the difference between a tranquilizer and a sedative and list the common drugs used in veterinary medicine that fit into these categories.

- Describe the important adverse effects or contraindications for use of key analgesics, sedatives, and tranquilizers in veterinary medicine.
- Explain the cardiovascular effects of alpha-2 (α_2) agonist drugs and the physiologic mechanisms for the associated clinical signs.
- Describe the mechanism of action, key effects, and significant side effects or precautions to be taken with propofol and dissociative anesthetics.
- Describe the three major gas anesthetics used in veterinary medicine and the key characteristics that differentiate them from each other.
- Describe what central nervous system (CNS) stimulants are used in veterinary medicine and for what specific purposes they are used.

KEY TERMS

agonist
alpha-2 (α_2) receptor
analgesic
anesthesia/anesthetic
apnea
apneustic breathing
  pattern
antagonist
anxiolytic
baroreceptors
bradycardic
bradypnea
catalepsy

ceiling effect
compound A
diffusion hypoxia
dissociative anesthetic
dopamine receptor
dysphoria
efficacy
euphoria
GABA$_A$ receptor
gamma (γ)-aminobutyric acid
  (GABA)
general anesthesia
hyperalgesia

hyperthermia
hyperesthesia
idiosyncratic reaction
local anesthesia
minimum alveolar concentration
  (MAC)
mixed agonists and antagonists
modulation (of pain)
N-methyl-D-aspartate (NMDA)
  receptor
narcosis
narcotics
neuroleptanalgesics

neurosteroid/neuroactive steroid
nociceptor
opiates
opioid receptors (μ, κ, δ)
opioids
partial agonists and antagonists

phenothiazines
potency
redistribution
sedative
somatic pain

tachycardic/tachycardia
transduction
tranquilizer
visceral pain
wind-up (pain)

Numerous drugs used in veterinary medicine alter the function of the nervous system. The categories of these drugs include analgesics, tranquilizers, sedatives, anesthetics, anticonvulsants, and stimulants. Veterinary anesthesiology texts provide a more thorough description of specific anesthetic regimens and their application to different species. This chapter provides an overview of the anesthetic, tranquilizing, sedating, and analgesic drugs; their mechanisms of action; and problems encountered when using these drugs.

ANALGESICS

Analgesics are drugs that reduce the perception of pain without significant loss of other sensations.

The Pain Pathway

Because of continued research on pain and its expression in veterinary patients, we have a better understanding of the causes of pain perception, the pain pathway from site of injury to the brain, and why the perception of pain changes with time (Fig. 8.1).

Essentially, pain can be thought of as having four steps. Step one is the stimulus of sensory nerve endings to the painful stimulus, whether it be an incision made by a surgeon, a burn, excessive pressure, chemical irritation, or inflammation from trauma or disease. This process of translating a physical stimulus into excitation or depolarization of the pain receptor (the nociceptor) is called transduction. The pain pathway can be blocked at this starting point by local anesthetic drugs, which prevent depolarization of nociceptors and hence block the transduction.

Step two is the transmission of the depolarization wave from the stimulated receptor to a sensory nerve that carries the nerve impulse to the spinal cord. This peripheral sensory nerve step can be blocked by injecting local anesthetic drugs near the sensory nerve, blocking any depolarization waves coming from the nociceptor. Nerve blocking is commonly done in cattle surgery where the cow is required to stand during surgery but needs to have large sections of the skin and underlying tissue anesthetized. By blocking a sensory nerve bundle comprised of dozens or hundreds of individual sensory nerves, each carrying sensory

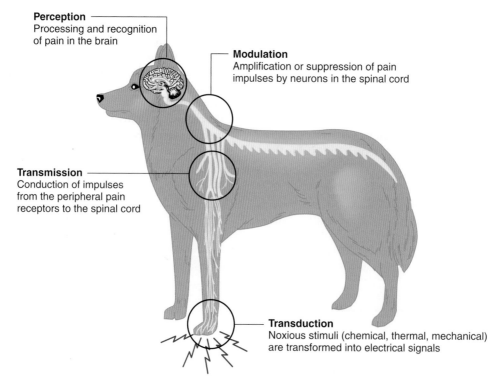

Fig. 8.1 The Pain Pathway. A painful stimulus is converted into a depolarization wave by the pain receptor (transduction) sent along the sensory nerve to the spinal cord (transmission), where it may be modified in intensity (modulation) before ascending the spinal cord and reaching the conscious areas of the brain (perception). (From Thomas J. *Anesthesia and Analgesia for Veterinary Technicians*, 5th ed. St. Louis: Mosby; 2017.)

impulses from nociceptors over a wide area of the skin, a single local anesthesia injection point located closer to the spinal cord than the surgery site can anesthetize a much wider area and is far easier to do than attempting to block each individual nociceptor in the skin.

Step three is the transmission of this sensory depolarization wave up the spinal cord and toward the brain. The depolarization wave can be modified (depressed or sometimes enhanced) in the spinal cord or lower brain by other neurotransmitters, naturally occurring painkilling compounds (e.g., natural opioids such as enkephalins or endorphins), or other nerve pathways that dampen the sensory signal. This third step of the pain pathway is called modulation and explains why the sensation of pain during the first few minutes of the injury is different from that felt hours later. Modulation decreases the pain perception at the brain level by decreasing the number of pain signals that actually reach the brain, despite the nociceptor's continual transmission of the pain sensation. Many painkillers or analgesics work by increasing the degree of inhibition or dampening of pain signals traveling along the spinal cord, thus decreasing the number that actually reaches the brain and consciousness.

The fourth step in pain perception is the actual perception of the pain impulse at the conscious level. Only when the impulse reaches the higher areas of the brain does the animal become aware of the pain. An example of this is seen when human beings experience a traumatic event that emotionally overwhelms an individual to such a degree that he or she is unaware (does not perceive) of a severe physical injury because perception of the pain signal is blocked by the emotional turmoil in the brain itself. In this case, the pain is being successfully transmitted to the brain, but the brain is unable to process this perception at a conscious level because of so many other competing sensory signals and the emotional state. General anesthesia produces unconsciousness, which in turn prevents conscious perception of pain. However, pain transmission in the unconscious patient still occurs at all levels below the brain.

As mentioned earlier, pain perception changes over time, as anyone who has had an injury knows. The pain may progress from the initial acute, focal pain to a more diffuse, throbbing pain that seems to emanate from a wider area around the trauma. This change in perception has a physiologic explanation. When a tissue is traumatized, the resulting inflammatory process is carried out by the arachidonic acid pathway (see Chapter 13), producing all of the inflammatory compounds that increase the ease with which the pain receptors in and around the site of inflammation can depolarize. In other words, the inflammation makes pain receptors in the adjacent areas much more sensitive and responsive to any potentially painful stimulation (e.g., touch, pressure), a condition called hyperalgesia. A similar term, hyperesthesia, is an increased sensitivity to any sensation, not just painful stimuli. By decreasing the inflammation process shortly after the trauma or injury, the increased sensitivity of receptors to stimuli can be reduced or avoided.

In addition to this local hyperalgesia caused by inflammatory mediator compounds, the spinal cord also becomes more effective at transmitting pain impulses up to the brain. Initially some of the pain impulses passing up the spinal cord are dampened, reducing pain perception at the brain level, but over time (hours) this dampening effect is significantly reduced and pain is more effectively transmitted up the spinal cord to the brain, increasing pain perception. This process of increasing success in transmitting pain up the spinal cord is sometimes referred to as wind-up.[1]

It is important to note that the process of wind-up occurs whether or not the patient is unconscious. Thus, even though an anesthetized patient may be unconscious during a surgical procedure and unable to perceive the pain at a conscious level, the spinal cord may be modulating its pain transmitting ability by wind-up, resulting in the patients having a higher level of pain perception when it wakes up from the general anesthesia. If analgesic or antiinflammatory drugs are used to prevent or reduce spinal cord wind-up, pain perception can be more effectively controlled for an animal in postoperative recovery.

Opioid Receptors and Their Actions

Typically the most potent analgesics used in veterinary medicine are the opioids. Opiates are drugs derived as extracts from poppy seeds, whereas opioids are chemically synthesized, opiate-like drugs. All opioids bind specifically to opioid receptors to produce their analgesic effect.

Opioids are often called narcotics because of the narcosis, or stuporous state, that they produce, from which the animal is not easily aroused. Opioids are incorporated into a preanesthetic or general anesthetic protocol to specifically reduce the need for general anesthetic agents (which cause unconsciousness). They are also commonly used alone for animals with existing pain or before starting painful surgeries or procedures to reduce wind-up.

Neuroleptanalgesics are opioid drugs combined with a tranquilizer or *sedative* (e.g., butorphanol opioid with a diazepam tranquilizer). The intent of these combination drugs is to use the tranquilizer effects to decrease some of the adverse effects of the opioids. When using these types of drugs, the veterinary technician needs to be aware of the side effects of both drugs used in the neuroleptanalgesic combination.

As stated earlier, opioids act by binding to opioid receptors in the central nervous system (both brain and spinal cord, including the chemoreceptor trigger zone [CRTZ]), gastrointestinal (GI) tract, urinary tract, and smooth muscle. Three major types of opioid receptors are recognized in mammals: *mu* (μ) *receptors, kappa* (κ) *receptors,* and *delta* (δ) *receptors.* A fourth receptor, the sigma (σ) receptor, is sometimes described in veterinary literature, but its role in veterinary patients is still debated. Hence opioid drug mechanisms described in veterinary patients typically cite the three main receptors, with most emphasis placed on the μ- and κ-opioid receptor activities.

Species and even individual animals will vary in their responses to opioid drugs, reinforcing Rule #2 presented in Chapter 1: "All doses are guesses." Some of the variable response can be attributed to differences in metabolism, but much of the variability appears to be caused by slight modifications of the opioid receptors themselves. μ Receptors are thought to have various subtypes or subtle changes in their molecular arrangement that alters the ability of opioid drugs to combine with the receptor. This may help explain why some animal species or individual animals are more prone to hallucinations or bad effects (dysphoria) from opioids, but other animals seem to be more resistant to the dysphoric effects of opioids.[2] Knowing that such variability exists, the recommended dose for an opioid drug is typically considered to be just the starting point for identifying how much drug an individual patient will actually need to control its pain.

Opioid drugs vary in their ability to combine with each of the three opioid receptor types (their affinity for the receptor) and the degree of intrinsic activity they will stimulate once they have bound to the receptor. The degree of intrinsic activity is reflected by whether the opioid is considered to be an agonist, a **partial agonist**, or an antagonist (see Chapter 3). Thus, most opioids are described by the type of receptor to which they attach (mu, kappa, or delta) and whether the drug exerts a noticeable effect (agonist), a partial effect (partial agonist), or no effect (an antagonist).

As described in Chapter 3, a **partial agonist** opioid drug has some intrinsic activity but can reverse some of the stronger effect of a full opioid agonist when it replaces the full agonist molecules at the opioid receptor site. In this situation, the strong analgesia and strong respiratory depression caused by the full μ-opioid agonist drug is replaced by the weaker analgesia and lessened respiratory depression of the partial opioid agonist drug. The weaker drug is therefore a **partial antagonist** to the stronger drug because the weaker drug did not completely reverse the analgesic or respiratory depressant effect of the full agonist because the partial antagonist has some intrinsic agonist activity of its own. Thus, such "weaker" opioid drugs are sometimes referred to as partial agonist/partial antagonist drugs.

Opioids are also often classified as mixed agonists/antagonists, meaning that the drug combines with multiple types of opioid receptors. Thus, one drug might stimulate a μ receptor (i.e., be a μ agonist) but at the same time also stimulate a κ receptor (i.e., be a κ agonist). Such a drug would be a mixed agonist. A drug that is an antagonist on more than one opioid receptor would be a mixed antagonist. Some opioid drugs are combinations of both in that, like the drug butorphanol, the drug molecule combines with and stimulates a κ receptor (i.e., is a κ agonist) but at the same time combines with the μ receptor and produces little or no effect (i.e., is a μ antagonist). Butorphanol would then be called a mixed agonist/antagonist.

It does not take much reading about opioid drugs in veterinary medicine to see that the research on opioid mechanisms in veterinary patients is still emerging. Many of the original concepts of opioid mechanisms in veterinary patients were extrapolated from mechanisms in human medicine. As time and clinical studies have revealed, some of these extrapolations did not accurately reflect what appeared to occur in veterinary patients. Thus, information on veterinary use of opioids today often does not align exactly with information found in older sources. Despite the continued revision of our understanding of opioid drug effects in all of our domestic animal species, there are still key principles of how opioids work that the well-educated veterinary technician should understand so as to accurately monitor and anticipate problems with opioid drugs before they occur.

μ Receptors are found on nerves associated with the pain pathways throughout the brain and spinal cord; it is the μ-agonist effect that is primarily responsible for the profound analgesic effect observed with opioid drugs. Most full μ-receptor agonists also stimulate κ receptors and, in so doing, have an enhanced analgesic effect.

Full μ agonists include drugs like morphine, hydromorphone, oxymorphone, and fentanyl; partial μ agonists like buprenorphine produce a more moderate amount of analgesia suitable for controlling mild pain. Butorphanol is considered to be somewhere between a partial μ agonist and a μ antagonist, but it still produces analgesia because it produces a moderate analgesic effect from being a κ-receptor agonist. Naloxone is a μ antagonist with no other opioid effects, making naloxone a reversal agent for the opioid analgesic drugs.

The μ-mediated analgesia occurs primarily by decreasing the release of excitatory neurotransmitters (e.g., acetylcholine, dopamine, serotonin) and dampening excitation of the postsynaptic sites where these neurotransmitters would normally act. The net effect is that the pain signals sent as depolarization waves or release of neurotransmitter are blocked or significantly depressed.[3]

In addition to the analgesia and narcotic sedation, μ-receptor stimulation of respiratory center neurons depresses the respiratory center function; for that reason, it reduces the respiratory reflexes that produce cough. Several opioids mentioned in Chapter 6 are very effective antitussive (cough) medications. Strong μ stimulation produces the respiratory depression that is characteristic of most strong opioid drugs. In most cases opioid respiratory depression will have little clinical impact and require no therapeutic intervention in a healthy, conscious animal. However, in an anesthetized animal or an animal whose respiratory function has already been depressed by disease or other drugs, there may be clinically significant respiratory depression from the opioids, and closer monitoring of respiratory function and oxygenation is prudent. Although this concern over respiratory depression has been widely disseminated in the veterinary literature, part of the original concern over respiratory depression in veterinary patients came from human medicine, where fatal opioid respiratory depression has been reported. However, experience and evaluation of opioids in veterinary medicine have revealed that even high-risk veterinary patients rarely have fatal opioid respiratory depression unless the animal is not being monitored properly or serious underlying neurologic disease is present.[2]

Additional effects attributed to μ receptors include decreased GI secretions and movement (useful in treating diarrhea with opioid antidiarrheal drugs); euphoria (i.e., pleasant hallucinatory effect); and pupillary miosis (i.e., constriction) or mydriasis (i.e., dilation), which is species dependent. Bradycardia occurs by opioid stimulation of μ-receptor centers in the brain that send parasympathetic signals down the vagus nerve to the heart to slow the heart rate. However, in healthy animals, the bradycardia does not result in a significant decrease in cardiac output (the actual amount of blood pumped per minute) because the force of contraction and stroke volume (amount pumped per beat) compensates to some degree.[3,4]

κ-Receptor stimulation produces a milder degree of analgesia than the μ-receptor response and contributes to sedation without as much respiratory depression or bradycardia as seen with μ-receptor stimulation.[4] As mentioned previously, most full μ-receptor agonist analgesics also are κ-receptor agonists, and this κ-receptor analgesia adds to the μ–analgesic effect to produce a strong analgesic action. Conversely, full κ-agonist drugs are often μ antagonists, and this partially explains why they are much weaker analgesic drugs. Butorphanol is a κ-agonist drug that also has μ-partial agonist or μ-antagonist effects.

κ-Receptor stimulation in conjunction with the μ-receptor agonist effect produces the sedation seen with opioid administration. Additionally, κ-agonist drugs also have the antidiarrheal effect and the effects on the pupils previously described with the μ-agonist drugs.

δ-Receptors are also thought to provide some spinal cord analgesia and perhaps to modulate μ receptors.[1,4] There are no specific δ-receptor drugs used in veterinary medicine.

Opioid Analgesic Drugs

Commonly used opioid drugs in veterinary medicine are classified by their agonist/antagonist activity (Table 8.1). Many of the drugs are mixed in their degree of agonist and antagonist activity.

Morphine is the prototypical opioid drug against whose potency all other opioids tend to be measured. For example, hydromorphone is said to have five times the analgesic potency of morphine. Increased potency means that it takes a lower dose of the hydromorphone to produce the same level of effect as a higher dose of morphine. Potency does not tell the maximum effect of the opioid; the maximum effect is expressed as effect or efficacy.

Morphine primarily stimulates μ-receptors and has some activity with κ-receptors at higher doses. Therefore, morphine is an effective drug for visceral (i.e., organ-related) **pain** and somatic (i.e., superficial tissues and skin) **pain**. However, the efficacy (i.e., maximum analgesic effect) of morphine may not be sufficient by itself to provide adequate analgesia from pain associated with surgical procedures if the drug is used alone. The opioids in general are better at blocking pain sent by the smaller, so-called unmyelinated C-fiber nociceptor nerves, which are associated with dull aching pain, than they are at blocking the larger, myelinated alpha nerves, which quickly transmit sharp,

discretely located pain, as might be experienced during a surgical incision. Thus, morphine and the other opioids must be combined with other analgesics or anesthetics to provide adequate blocking for surgical pain.

Morphine is also used as an epidural drug (i.e., drug injected into the space surrounding the spinal cord) to provide regional analgesia for painful procedures involving the hind limbs, pelvis, perineal area (i.e., under the tail), or posterior abdomen.

Dogs injected intramuscularly (IM) or subcutaneously (SQ) with morphine at low doses often salivate and vomit. In contrast, the same dogs injected with a larger morphine dose or given morphine intravenously (IV) do not vomit or vomit only for a short period of time before stopping. Opioid-induced vomiting occurs when morphine stimulates dopamine receptors on the chemoreceptor trigger zone (CRTZ—see Chapter 4), which in turn triggers the emetic center to produce the act of vomiting. The CRTZ is quick to respond to low doses of opioids in the blood because, unlike the emetic center, the CRTZ is not protected by the blood–brain barrier and is readily accessible from the blood. However, when these same opioids are given IV or another opioid is given that is especially quick to penetrate the blood–brain barrier, the opioid stimulates more rapidly penetrates the blood–brain barrier, accesses the emetic center μ- or κ-opioid receptors, and depresses the activity of the emetic center, which stops the vomiting reflex. The slower rise of blood concentrations associated with IM or SQ injection means that the drug will initially stimulate the CRTZ dopamine receptors before the opioid can cross the blood–brain barrier, enter the brain, and suppress the emetic center through stimulation of μ or κ receptors. Thus, any circumstance in which the opioid drug reaches the CRTZ before it suppresses the emetic center activity will result in vomiting.

Interestingly, most studies of vomiting from opioids have been done in pain-free, healthy animals. But it has been observed and reported in the veterinary literature that animals actually experiencing pain vomit far less and are less likely to experience dysphoria when given opioids than animals that are pain free. Thus, a healthy animal given opioids before surgery is more likely to vomit than if given the same opioid dose after surgery when the animal is showing signs of pain.[2,5]

Morphine stimulates the cells of the nucleus of cranial nerve III (oculomotor nerve) in the brain, resulting in signals being sent to the pupil that cause it to constrict. In dogs, rabbits, and rats, the presence of morphine results in pupillary constriction (miosis).[2] However, in cats and horses, morphine administration results in pupillary dilation by a mechanism not well understood. Because the pupil diameter can be affected by other drugs or release of catecholamines from fear or stress, the pupil size can vary with opioid use and does not correlate well with the degree of analgesia.

One of the side effects of morphine seen less with other opioids is the release of histamine after intravenous injection. Among its other effects, histamine causes vasodilation and a drop in arterial blood pressure. In healthy animals, this histamine release from IV morphine at therapeutic doses usually

TABLE 8.1 Agonist/Antagonist Activity of Commonly Used Opioid Drugs in Veterinary Medicine

Full agonists	Morphine (μ agonist, κ agonist at higher doses)
	Fentanyl (μ agonist)
	Hydromorphone (μ agonist)
	Oxymorphone (μ agonist)
	Methadone (μ agonist)
	Meperidine (μ agonist)
Partial agonists	Butorphanol (μ partial agonist to antagonist, κ agonist),
	Buprenorphine (μ partial agonist, κ antagonist)
Full antagonists	Naloxone (μ antagonist, κ antagonist, δ antagonist)

produces no clinically significant decrease in arterial blood pressure. However, the histamine-mediated arterial hypotension is more profound when morphine is given with drugs that depress the cardiac output (e.g., some anesthetic agents) or decrease the ability of the vasculature to maintain vasoconstriction (e.g., phenothiazine tranquilizers like acepromazine or alpha-2 (α_2) sedative analgesics like xylazine). Still, some authors state that the histamine effect is fairly negligible and that any observed hypotension is the effect of the other drugs more than the histamine release.[2]

The effect of morphine on the release of histamine-containing mast cell tumors has not been investigated in veterinary medicine; therefore in patients with this tumor, the use of morphine should be via SQ or IM injection (not IV), or another opioid should be used.[2]

Previously it was stated in veterinary literature that morphine or other full agonist opioids were not to be given in head trauma cases because any decreased respiratory function from the opioids could elevate carbon dioxide levels in the brain, causing vasodilation and potentially increasing blood flow and edema or hemorrhage in the brain. This phenomenon is well documented in human medicine. However, the general thinking in veterinary medicine is that the amount of respiratory depression from opioids is usually not sufficient in a monitored animal to elevate carbon dioxide high enough to produce profound vasodilation or increased cerebral edema or bleeding. If morphine or any of the opioids is given to relieve pain in a patient with suspected head trauma, one should be aware of the potential for some opioid respiratory depression and prevent carbon dioxide levels from increasing by using a conservative opioid dose and maintaining ventilation and adequate oxygenation.

Opioids produce analgesia through their action on opioid receptors, but most opioids do not induce anesthesia or depress stimuli from other sensory organs. Therefore, animals given opioids may still respond to sound, cold, heat, taste, and visual stimuli. Although it has been previously reported that animals may display hypersensitivity to auditory stimuli, it is more likely that such response is part of the **dysphoria** (i.e., bad hallucination) that occurs sometimes with high opioid doses or in animals that are very sensitive to dysphoric effects of opioids. Because lower opioid doses are used today than previously, especially in species sensitive to dysphoria (e.g., cats and horses), the incidence of opioid-related dysphoria occurs far less than the incidence of discomfort and anxious behavior observed when an animal suddenly feels pain during anesthetic recovery. When true opioid dysphoria does occur, it is readily controlled with sedatives or tranquilizers.[5]

Hydromorphone and **oxymorphone** are two full μ agonists with a greater potency than morphine (i.e., they can achieve a set level of analgesia at a lower dose) but very similar to morphine is most other ways. These drugs have similar efficacy to morphine, meaning that the ultimate degree of analgesia that can be achieved is similar. These two drugs have the advantage of not stimulating vomiting to the same degree as morphine and causing less histamine release, hence less histamine-mediated vasodilation and risk for hypotension.

MYTHS AND MISCONCEPTIONS

The myth of morphine mania

For many years the generally accepted idea was that morphine and other opioids routinely produced excessive excitement and dysphoria ("morphine mania") in cats and horses, and therefore this drug was to be avoided. However, although the cat and horse do appear to be more prone to excitement from opioids, the older doses used in cats and horses were extrapolated from the dog, resulting in higher opioid concentrations in the horse and cat. For example, because a cat has a lower volume of distribution (see Chapter 3) than the dog, this means the drug injected is diluted to a lesser degree by tissue fluids than the equivalent dose injected into the dog, and hence the opioid concentration achieved in the cat is much higher, producing a greater effect.

The same dog dose given to a cat can result in 2.5 times higher concentration in the cat than the dog.[2] Such a high concentration is likely to produce excitement and dysphoria in the cat, especially if given as an IV bolus. Indeed, high IV doses of opioids predictably produce dysphoria in cats. At the same time, however, lower doses produce signs of euphoria (pleasant hallucinations or feelings) as indicated by increased purring, signs of affection, and kneading.[2]

Likewise, an equivalent dog dose in the horse would produce concentrations between 2.5 and 5 times that in the dog with the same expected dysphoric side effect. However, adjusting the dose downward allows the horse to tolerate the drug fairly, well and excitement is typically not observed.[2]

Note that as mentioned in the text, pain-free animals are more prone to dysphoria than are animals in pain. Because research on opioid effects on cats and horses was done in pain-free subjects, dysphoria was frequently reported. Clinical experience has shown, however, that cats and horses given opioids post trauma or postsurgery usually do not experience dysphoria or morphine mania.[5]

One quirky characteristic of hydromorphone is that it is cited as being the opioid that is more likely to cause drug-induced hyperthermia (i.e., increased body temperature) in cats after surgery than other opioids, although other studies have found that most opioids will increase the cat's body temperature mildly (up to 102.5° F).[6,7] The hyperthermia is usually transient (i.e., of short duration) and mild, typically not requiring medical intervention, although the authors of one study did take measures to cool some cats that they felt were too warm; none of those cats showed any abnormal clinical signs upon recovery.[7]

Fentanyl is a potent μ-agonist opioid with a greater potency than morphine but a shorter duration. Because of its short duration (30 min to 2 h, depending on the dose and route of administration), fentanyl needs to be given by a constant rate IV infusion (CRI), as a patch, and as a transdermal solution.[2] It shares the same effects as morphine but has less nausea and vomiting, and its strong mu effect actually decreases the vomiting response.[2]

Veterinarians have been using fentanyl as a human dermal patch ("skin patch") applied to a clipped and cleaned area on the body. Because the amount of fentanyl given to the animal is based on the surface area of the patch applied to the skin, small patches are used in cats and small dogs and increasingly larger patches are used in larger dogs. The patch should not be cut, as this will alter the rate at which the drug is released and cause evaporation of the alcohol-based gel in which the fentanyl is dissolved. Instead, if the patch is to be used on a small dog or cat or a geriatric animal that does not need much fentanyl, half of the patch's membrane that is exposed to the skin can be covered with tape to block half of the contact area and reduce the dose.[8]

Studies have shown that the amount of fentanyl absorbed via the patch varies widely from patient to patient based upon the thickness of the skin and the degree of blood perfusion to the area where the patch is located. It takes between 12 and 24 h after the fentanyl patch has been applied for fentanyl to reach therapeutic concentrations in the dog and 6 to 12 h in cats.[2,3] Because of the lag time, the patch should be applied the day before surgery, or if the trauma or injury has already occurred, another injectable opioid should be used during the first 12 to 24 h until the full analgesic effect of the fentanyl patch is achieved. The duration of analgesia provided by one patch is between 24 and 72 h in dogs (average around 48 h) and approximately 4 days in the cat.[2] This wide variability in achieved concentrations and duration explains why some animals may not have adequate analgesia, though others show signs of excessive sedation or other adverse effects of opioid drugs.

The patch is relatively easy to remove, and occasionally the adhesive on the patch irritates the skin; the animal should be carefully monitored for any signs of the patient licking the patch site or trying to remove the patch. Additionally, if the patch falls off by itself, it is important that it be located and disposed of properly to prevent the pet from eating it or curious children playing with it and absorbing the drug through their own skin. Finally, narcotic abusers may seek out discarded fentanyl patches because they know the patches are a source of opioid drug they can use. Thus, the veterinarian and veterinary technician need to be on guard for signs that any fentanyl patch is being diverted into the wrong hands.

! YOU NEED TO KNOW

Dangers From a Fentanyl Patch

Two Canadian adolescents died after using transdermal fentanyl patches. A 15-year-old girl was found in respiratory depression and unresponsive 21 h after the first application of a Duragesic 25 patch. In the other case, a 14-year-old boy was found in respiratory arrest 14 h after the patch had been first applied. Duragesic has been marketed in Canada for use in controlling chronic pain; however, the patch is not recommended for use in children younger than 18 years of age because of the risk of life-threatening respiratory depression.

What should be learned from this situation: Veterinary technicians must caution owners regarding the proper use and disposal of this patch medication.

Source:
From *Canadian Adverse Reaction Newsletter.* 2004;14(4);
Off label perils. *Compend Contin Educ Vet.* 2004;26(11):834.

Methadone and meperidine are both μ agonists used to a lesser degree than the other full agonist opioids previously listed but still are used enough in veterinary medicine that veterinary technicians need to be familiar with them. In addition to the μ-agonist effects, **methadone** blocks another receptor called the NMDA (*N-methyl-D-aspartate*) receptor. Blocking the NMDA receptor depresses the activity of parts of the brain, thus reducing some of the adverse opioid effects such as hypersensitivity or reaction to other sensory stimuli. Methadone is the full μ-agonist opioid least likely to produce vomiting, and it has little to no histamine release compared with other opioids.[8,9]

Meperidine (Demerol) is a weaker μ agonist than morphine and is said to produce analgesia that is about one fifth that of morphine.[3] It also has a short duration of action compared with the other opioids described and has more cardiac depressant effects than the other opioids. Because of the availability of newer opioids without meperidine's limitations, it is not used very widely today in veterinary medicine.

Buprenorphine is a partial μ agonist with moderately strong analgesic properties and is also a κ antagonist. Its degree of analgesia is more limited than morphine because of a ceiling effect, which means that, regardless of the dose given, the degree of buprenorphine analgesia will never reach that of morphine. Increasing the dose of buprenorphine does not increase the degree of analgesia but only extends the duration of the drug's effect. Thus, buprenorphine has less efficacy than morphine because the maximal analgesic effect of buprenorphine is less than morphine's maximal effect.

Buprenorphine is favored over butorphanol because it has a longer duration of activity (6–8 h) and is considered to be one of the least likely of these opioids to produce adverse effects.[5] The duration of buprenorphine is partially explained by its high affinity and tight binding to the μ receptor, thus prolonging its μ-agonist effect and delaying its breakdown. One of the other advantages listed for buprenorphine is its ability to be rapidly absorbed across the mucous membranes of the mouth, allowing the drug to be administered by spraying it into the mouth of a very aggressive or fractious cat. This is sometimes done with feral cats that have not been handled by humans instead of attempting to restrain the cat to give an IV or IM injection.[9]

In 2014, a form of buprenorphine was approved by the FDA for SQ injection specifically in cats (Simbadol). The label dose is one injection per day for up to 3 days, indicating that the analgesia persists for at least 24 h and, according to the manufacturer, can last up to 48 h. Because there is wide variability from cat to cat for the achieved plasma concentration of buprenorphine, some variability can be expected in observed clinical response. The manufacturer indicates that, because of risk of accidental injection of this opioid, the drug can only be administered by veterinarians and veterinary technicians.[10]

In 2022, the FDA approved a transdermal solution (Zorbium™) that forms a depot for slow release buprenorphine under the skin for feline postoperative pain. This dosage form is approved to be placed at the veterinary clinic/hospital only and provides analgesia within 30 min of application, and lasts for 4 days. Zorbium™ is weight based and available in a unit dose applicator. There is one prefilled tube for cats weighing 1.2 to 3 kg and a prefilled applicator for cats weighing greater than 3 kg up to 7.5 kg. The medication should be applied to the skin (do not clip the area) on the dorsal cervical region of the neck, being sure the skin is not damaged and the cat cannot reach the area. Use gloves to apply the buprenorphine and allow the area to dry for at least 30 min. The manufacturer recommends applying the medication to the cat 1–2 h before surgery. Once the area is dry the cat can be pet safely, so no risk to the owner, and can also be put in dorsal recumbency on a heating pad for surgery without compromising the medication.

Butorphanol (Torbutrol, Torbugesic) is a mixed agonist/antagonist opioid whose effects vary from weak partial μ-receptor agonist activity to μ-antagonist activity plus a strong κ-agonist effect.[1] Like buprenorphine, butorphanol has a ceiling effect; thus its maximum analgesia is less than the maximum analgesia provided by the full μ-agonist opioids.

Because butorphanol is a weaker analgesic than morphine and has a duration that is too short to last for many types of surgeries (30–60 min in the dog, 90 min in the cat[5,9]), it is not to be used alone as the sole source of analgesia but is one of the analgesics most commonly combined with other anesthetic, sedative, or analgesic agents to create a balanced anesthetic regimen. Because butorphanol is a partial agonist, it can be used to reverse some degree of the respiratory depressant effects of stronger, full μ-agonist drugs such as hydromorphone while providing some level of analgesia and sedation of its own. As described previously, this characteristic makes butorphanol a partial agonist/partial antagonist.

Although butorphanol has less respiratory depression than the stronger, full μ-agonist opioids, it has a strong cough suppression activity and is FDA approved for use as an antitussive in small animals.

Tramadol is a centrally acting analgesic that is often included with the opioid analgesics even though it likely has several mechanisms by which it reduces the perception of pain other than stimulation of opioid receptors. Tramadol itself has little analgesic effect, and its analgesic activity is dependent on successful metabolism to *O*-desmethyltramadol, usually abbreviated as M1 (metabolite #1). The M1 metabolite has a μ-agonist effect but also produces other effects by preventing the reuptake (thus prolonging the effect) of serotonin and norepinephrine (NE). It also blocks muscarinic cholinergic receptors that would normally respond to acetylcholine. Finally, the drug also stimulates α_2 receptors, which produces sedation and additional analgesia.[1,8] Thus, this drug's mechanism of action to produce analgesia and sedation is complex.

The efficacy and role of tramadol in veterinary medicine are still emerging. We know that dogs do not metabolize tramadol a great deal to the M1 metabolite, thus the degree of analgesia achieved in dogs should be classified as mild to moderate. Cats, on the other hand, do produce a good deal of M1 metabolite and thus should have a greater degree of μ-agonist analgesia.[2] The influence of the other mechanisms likely contributes to the total observed effect of analgesia and sedation.

Tramadol should not be used with behavioral drugs like tricyclic antidepressants or serotonin-reuptake inhibitors (see Chapter 9) because these drugs, like tramadol, also inhibit the reuptake of serotonin and can result in a toxic accumulation of serotonin producing serotonin syndrome.[2,8] There has been some suggestion that tramadol can elicit seizure activity in dogs, although the seizures produced were readily controlled.[1] It is also suspected that long-term use of tramadol in the dog causes a diminished analgesic effect over time.[1,2] This is a drug that

seems to have a role in veterinary medicine, but that role is still in the process of being clearly defined by clinical trials and evidence.

Opioid Antagonist Drugs

An advantage of using opioids for analgesia alone or in anesthetic regimens is that their effects are reversible with narcotic antagonists. These drugs reverse some of the effects of opioid narcosis by competing for sites on the μ and κ receptors. **Naloxone** (Narcan) is considered a pure narcotic antagonist because when it combines with μ and κ receptors, it has no intrinsic activity—meaning when the drug combines with the cell receptor, it produces no effect on the cell. If an animal has been sedated with an opioid agonist, then naloxone, if given in sufficient quantity to compete against the agonist for available receptor sites, should almost completely reverse the sedation, analgesia, and respiratory depression of potent opioids, such as hydromorphone, without producing sedation of its own. Naloxone has a more difficult time reversing the effects of buprenorphine because the buprenorphine molecule adheres tightly to the μ receptor, making displacement of the buprenorphine molecules by naloxone molecules difficult.

The complete reversal of an opioid analgesic can result in the animals suddenly becoming very aware of painful conditions or stimuli. Therefore, pure opioid antagonists such as naloxone are best used to reverse opioid overdoses. This is the reason why law enforcement and emergency first responders carry naloxone to reverse heroin overdose cases. In cases in which the veterinarian wants to partially reverse respiratory depression from strong opioid analgesics without losing all the analgesia, a partial agonist/partial antagonist such as buprenorphine or butorphanol is a better choice.

Although naloxone can reverse sedative and analgesic effects, it cannot reverse the emetic effects of apomorphine because the emetic effect results from dopamine receptor stimulation, not stimulation of opioid receptors.

TRANQUILIZERS AND SEDATIVES

Tranquilizers and sedatives produce a relaxed state, usually without producing significant analgesia (unless the drug specifically has analgesic properties). Although the terms "tranquilizer" and "sedative" are used interchangeably in the clinics, they have slightly different meanings and actions. A tranquilizer is a drug that is an anxiolytic agent (literally "breaks apart anxiety") or a drug used to calm a patient, whereas a sedative drug is one that makes an animal sleepy but really does not reduce the patient's anxiety or agitation. Because a strong tranquilizer can allow an animal to relax and appear to become sleepy (because it is less anxious), and because the effect of any tranquilizer or sedative can vary among species or even from patient to patient, the observed effects of tranquilizers and sedatives often overlap to some degree, thus generating the loose, interchangeable use of the terminology.

The veterinary technician should realize that although some sedatives may have a small degree of analgesia, tranquilizers are not analgesics. Thus, a tranquilized animal in a relaxed state is still quite capable of feeling pain and responding quickly and viciously to manipulations that elicit pain. Only if the animal is sedated so deeply that it begins to approach narcosis (i.e., a state of sleep from which an animal is not readily aroused) or is anesthetized will the animal's response to pain be decreased. Because owners and lay veterinary staff may be unfamiliar with this disconnect between relaxed appearance and ability to respond quickly and violently to a painful stimulus such as moving a broken bone, it is very easy for these individuals to be seriously injured when the animal suddenly appears to "wake up" and violently respond to the pain. Thus, the well-educated veterinary technician has the responsibility to use this knowledge to protect not only him- or herself but others as well.

Acepromazine

Acepromazine maleate is a phenothiazine tranquilizer that is often used to calm animals for physical examination, for transport, and as part of a preanesthetic regimen. They are classified in human medicine as major tranquilizers and hence are used as antipsychotic drugs. Unlike some of the sedatives discussed later, phenothiazine tranquilizers have no analgesic effect of their own, and tranquilized animals can feel and respond to pain very well.

Phenothiazine tranquilizers in general produce their tranquilizing effect by blocking dopamine receptors in the brain. Additional tranquilization comes from blocking alpha-1 (α_1), muscarinic cholinergic, and histamine (H1) receptors in the brain. Blocking these same receptors on the CRTZ and emetic center explains why acepromazine has antiemetic and antimotion sickness effects, especially in the dog (see Chapter 4).

Although phenothiazine tranquilizers are generally safe, in some situations they should be used with caution or not at all. **Phenothiazines** block the α_1 receptors found on smooth muscle cells that cause vasoconstriction of the precapillary arterioles (the small arteries that pass blood into the capillaries). Blocking α_1 receptors results in relaxation of smooth muscle and blocks the sympathetic nervous system's ability to increase arterial blood pressure through vasoconstriction. For this reason, phenothiazines should be used with caution or not used at all in animals with hypotension (decreased blood pressure) associated with shock, blood loss, or dehydration.[11]

A common but harmless effect of phenothiazine tranquilizers is protrusion of the nictitating membrane (i.e., the third eyelid) over the surface of the eye. The appearance of this fleshy membrane can be alarming to clients using the drug for the first time to control their dog's motion sickness. Obviously the appearance of the membrane also makes ophthalmologic examination more difficult.

Because acepromazine, and phenothiazine tranquilizers in general, block histamine (H1) receptors and thus have an antihistamine effect, these tranquilizers should probably not be given before skin testing for allergies, as they can interfere with the histamine response (i.e., the wheal and flare reaction) needed to identify those substances to which an animal is allergic.

It is known that the antidopamine effect of acepromazine produces behavioral changes in animals, including some inhibition of learned behaviors (e.g., having learned not to bite another animal in the home to defend its territory). Another effect noted, but not completely understood, is that occasionally some cats and dogs exhibit frenzied behavior when given acepromazine or other antidopamine-type drugs. There are anecdotal reports of cats becoming aggressive and hyperactive after acepromazine administration, and the drug insert lists this as a precaution. These reactions are unpredictable because this is considered an idiosyncratic reaction that is not dose related and cannot be predicted by an identifiable risk factor.

In stallions, phenothiazine tranquilizers may produce transient (a few hours) or rarely permanent penile prolapse, of which the latter would be devastating for the value of a breeding animal.

It was previously cautioned in the veterinary literature that acepromazine would reduce the threshold of seizures, increasing their frequency in dogs with a seizure history. In 2006, a survey conducted by Dr. Linda Shell for the Veterinary Information Network identified that 82% of the veterinarians surveyed believed that acepromazine should be avoided in epileptic dogs.[11] However, this belief has since been discounted because of a lack of clinical evidence to support this claim in veterinary patients. This precaution originated from experience with chlorpromazine in human medicine, but a similar phenomenon has not documented in veterinary medicine. Thus, we no longer consider acepromazine to be a significant risk for epileptic animals.

Benzodiazepine Tranquilizers

Benzodiazepines are a group of tranquilizers widely used for their calming and muscle-relaxing effects in veterinary medicine. Benzodiazepines can often be recognized by the "-epam" suffix in their nonproprietary names. They include **diazepam** (Valium), **zolazepam** (component of Telazol), **midazolam** (Versed), and **clonazepam** (Klonopin). Benzodiazepines produce their calming effect by enhancing the activity of gamma (γ)-aminobutyric acid (GABA), one of the more important inhibitory neurotransmitters found in the CNS of mammals. The benzodiazepine molecule attaches to the GABAA receptor (pronounced "gah-bah-A" receptor) located on an excitatory neuron and causes the GABA inhibitory neurotransmitter to bind more tightly with its receptor, opening chloride channels that flood the neuron cell with chloride and decrease the neuron's ability to depolarize when stimulated. By increasing GABA's inhibitory activity, benzodiazepine tranquilizers make the neurons less likely to depolarize when stimulated, the brain less active, and the animal appears to become less agitated and more relaxed. This same CNS inhibitory effect makes benzodiazepines effective anticonvulsants.

Like phenothiazines, the benzodiazepines do not produce analgesia. By themselves, benzodiazepines are not particularly strong tranquilizers. However, they do have the advantage of having minimal negative effects on the cardiovascular system, are excellent anticonvulsants, and produce CNS-mediated skeletal muscle relaxation. Thus, they are most often included in a balanced anesthetic regimen with opioid analgesics, other sedatives, and anesthetics to ease induction of anesthesia, cause skeletal muscle relaxation, and to promote a smooth, seizure-free recovery.

Unlike the phenothiazine tranquilizers, benzodiazepines have little effect on the brain's CRTZ and therefore are not useful in preventing motion sickness. In the unlikely event of a benzodiazepine overdose or if there is a need to shorten a prolonged recovery (especially in cats), these drugs can be reversed with the benzodiazepine antagonist drug **flumazenil.**

Diazepam was the first benzodiazepine developed and widely disseminated in human medicine as the trade name Valium. Although the generic form of the drug dominates the market today often packaged in bottles labeled only as "diazepam," the name "Valium" is still often used to describe this drug because this particular trade name is so ingrained in the veterinary vocabulary. Diazepam is one of the most common benzodiazepines given to veterinary patients as a component of a preanesthetic protocol, but it is also the drug of choice to control active seizures (see Chapter 9). As a component of an anesthetic protocol, diazepam counters muscle rigidity seen with some anesthetics and reduces some of the dysphoria and agitation associated with recovery from dissociative anesthetics like ketamine. One of the drawbacks to diazepam is that it is poorly soluble in water, which means that it does not mix well with many drugs or IV solutions.[11,12]

Midazolam is the other main benzodiazepine used as a preanesthetic tranquilizer. Almost everything said about diazepam applies to midazolam, with the exception that midazolam has greater affinity for the receptor, a greater potency (more effect for less dose), and compatibility with IV fluids and other water-based drug media. Midazolam is used with ketamine to reduce central excitatory effects and can be also used as an anticonvulsant.

Because of their stimulatory effects on the appetite center in the brain, diazepam and midazolam have been used in the past to increase the appetite of anorectic cats. However, because hepatic failure has been reported in cats given repeated oral dosages of diazepam, the potential benefit of appetite stimulation must be balanced against the risk of liver damage, and the risk has made this use for benzodiazepines less acceptable.

Zolazepam is incorporated with the anesthetic agent tiletamine into a commercially available sedative-analgesic combination product called Telazol. The tiletamine is a dissociative anesthetic like ketamine, and zolazepam reduces the central excitatory effect, just like diazepam and midazolam do for ketamine. Thus, veterinary practices may create a similar drug cocktail by combining diazepam or midazolam with ketamine. The combined product Telazol is used as a short-acting anesthetic in which only a moderate amount of analgesia is required.

Clonazepam is not commonly used as a preanesthetic drug because it is an orally administered benzodiazepine. However, it has been used in veterinary medicine as an adjunct (additional) drug added to phenobarbital to maintain long-term control of seizures in epileptic dogs.

Alpha-2 Agonists

α_2 Agonists are sedative analgesics widely used in small animal, equine, and large animal medicine and surgery. Unlike opioid analgesics, α_2 agonists are not controlled substances and do not require additional certification to purchase or use them. The drugs in this group include **xylazine** (Rompun), **detomidine** (Dormosedan), **medetomidine** (Domitor), **dexmedetomidine** (Dexdomitor), and **romifidine** (Sedivet).

The name of the group refers to the adrenergic α_2 **receptor** to which the drug attaches to produce its effect. These particular receptors are found on neurons that release norepinephrine (NE) and act as a safety mechanism to prevent excessive sympathetic nervous system effects. When NE is normally released from the neuron and produces its sympathetic nervous system effect on the target organ, some of the NE also combines with the α_2 receptor on the NE-releasing neuron, shutting down additional release of NE. When α_2-agonist drugs attach to and stimulate the α_2 receptors (Fig. 8.2), they decrease norepinephrine release within the CNS and in the peripheral nervous

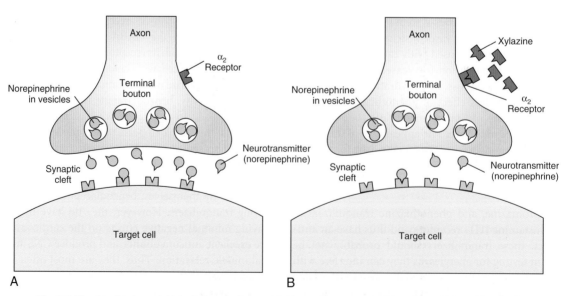

Fig. 8.2 The Mechanism of Alpha-2 Agonist Drugs. (A) Normally, norepinephrine (NE) is released and travels across the synaptic cleft to receptors on the target cell. After NE is released, some of the NE provides negative feedback to prevent further NE release by attaching to the α_2 receptor on the terminal bouton of the axon that released the NE. (B) When xylazine is present, it attaches to the α_2 receptors on the terminal bouton. This stimulates the α_2 receptor's negative feedback effect on the release of NE, decreasing its release and decreasing central nervous system excitation.

system, decreasing general CNS alertness and producing sedation. The degree of sedation with α_2 agonists is said to be more predictable than the tranquilization produced by benzodiazepines or phenothiazine tranquilizers.

α_2 Agonists are classified as sedative-analgesics; therefore in addition to the sedation described and unlike the tranquilizers described previously, α_2 agonists also decrease perception of painful stimuli. In horses, xylazine and detomidine are used to relieve pain associated with GI conditions such as colic. Although these drugs can be used to control visceral pain associated with intestinal disease, their analgesic effect on skin and superficial tissue (somatic, or nonvisceral, pain) appears to be less effective. It has been cautioned that the use of α_2 analgesia for equine colic (abdominal pain) may mask some of the outward clinical signs of pain that are used to determine the progression of colic or the need for surgical intervention to treat advanced colic.

In addition to the sedation and analgesia, this class of drugs also produces CNS-mediated skeletal muscle relaxation, which is helpful when used in conjunction with dissociative anesthetics (e.g., ketamine), which have poor muscle-relaxation capabilities.

Once a degree of sedation has been achieved with α_2 agonists, further administration will not produce a deeper depth of sedation or analgesia but will only prolong the duration of the drug and increase the incidence of side effects. Thus, like the partial μ agonists discussed previously, α_2 agonists have a *ceiling effect* that limits the maximum effect of the drug.[13]

Analgesia from α_2 agonists wears off before the sedation effect does. Thus, an animal sedated with an α_2 agonist may begin to respond to painful stimuli even though the animal appears to be still resting comfortably. This illustrates an important safety point made with the tranquilizers: a sedated animal may be quite capable of responding rapidly and violently to painful stimuli if there is no analgesic effect present. In addition, some veterinary sources state that although the animals appear sedated with α_2 agonists, they may actually startle more readily to loud noise or sudden touch. Horses sedated with these drugs may suddenly kick hard without warning, especially when xylazine is used.[13]

α_2 Agonists do have significant physiologic side effects on many body systems and therefore require the veterinary technician to evaluate the patient carefully before, during, and immediately after using these drugs. The veterinary technician needs to understand these physiologic changes so he or she can correlate the outward-appearing clinical signs with what is happening inside the animal because of the drug.

Xylazine produces vomiting in a significant percentage of cats by directly stimulating α receptors in the CRTZ. This is such a predictable occurrence in cats that xylazine is one of the drugs of choice to induce emesis after a cat has ingested a toxic substance. Dogs are less sensitive to this emetic effect because the canine CRTZ has fewer α receptors than the felines, but a significant percentage will also vomit with α-agonist drugs. The incidence of vomiting is less in the newer α_2-agonist drugs than the older drug, xylazine. Vomiting from an α_2 agonist can be reduced to some extent by the use of phenothiazine tranquilizers like acepromazine.

α_2 Agonists have a profound effect on the cardiovascular system. Initially the α_2-agonist activity in the brain depresses the neurons that normally send sympathetic nervous system impulses out to the rest of the body. Thus, there is a decrease in sympathetic tone, which allows a dominance of parasympathetic effects on the sinoatrial (SA) node. In the cardiovascular system this is manifested as bradycardia, which is felt as a slower pulse. The parasympathetic dominance on the atrioventricular (AV) node can slow conduction of the depolarization wave from the atria to the ventricles, resulting in first- or second-degree AV block appearing on the ECG (see Chapter 5 for further explanation of AV block).

At the same time that the CNS effects are occurring, the α_2 agonists are also stimulating the α_1 receptors on the peripheral arterioles, causing arteriolar vasoconstriction and elevating arterial blood pressure despite the bradycardia. So in phase I of α_2-agonist drug administration, the animals are usually **bradycardic** (slow heart rate) and hypertensive (elevated arterial blood pressure).

The degree to which the hypertension occurs during phase I depends on how selective the α_2-agonist drug is for just the α_2-receptor site over the α_1 receptor. The oldest drug, xylazine, has an α_2 to α_1 selectivity ratio of 160 to 1 or 160:1, meaning that 160 α_2 receptors will be occupied by the drug for every 1 α_1 receptor. Detomidine has an α_2 to α_1 ratio of 260:1, and medetomidine and dexmedetomidine both have a ratio of 1620:1. Thus, the newer drugs (detomidine, medetomidine, and dexmedetomidine) have far more selectivity to attach to α_2 receptors over the α_1 than xylazine so there should be fewer α_1 side effects. As phase I progresses, the responsiveness of the peripheral arteriole α_1 receptors will begin to lessen, allowing the smooth muscles to relax and the vasculature to begin to dilate. With the vasodilation, the arterial blood pressure begins to drop. Normally the drop in blood pressure would be detected by the **baroreceptors** ("baro," meaning pressure) in the large arteries and the hypotension compensated for by a reflex release of sympathetic nervous system signals from the CNS. But because the α_2 depression of the CNS sympathetic signals is still present from the drug, there is no compensatory sympathetic stimulation and no increased heart rate or increased force of contraction. Thus in phase II, the bradycardia remains but the arterial blood pressure drops and the animal becomes hypotensive (low blood pressure). The technician will feel the initial slow but firm pulse remain slow but become weaker.

Although atropine is often recommended for bradycardia or AV block from other causes (atropine blocks the parasympathetic receptor on the heart, reducing the effect of the parasympathetic dominance), its use with α_2 agonists is controversial. Reducing the parasympathetic effect would allow the sympathetic to dominate, but because the α_2-agonist drugs have suppressed CNS output of sympathetic signals, the response from atropine would be somewhat muted. Plus, the use of atropine with α_2-agonist drugs may generate cardiac arrhythmias, which may not justify atropine's use if the bradycardia and AV block do not pose a significant clinical risk to the patient.[13]

In cattle and other ruminants, xylazine increases the contractility of uterine smooth muscle. If given to pregnant ruminants in high doses, xylazine could have the potential to induce premature onset of parturition. Increased uterine pressure also occurs in pregnant mares and small animals but has not resulted in premature parturition or abortion and is considered to be safe to use in pregnant horses, dogs, and cats.

The α_2-agonist drugs inhibit the release of insulin from beta cells in the pancreas, reducing the ability of the body to move glucose from the blood into the tissues. The resulting hyperglycemia (elevated blood glucose) is transient and in healthy animals does not get high enough to produce glucosuria. Although there is no clear recommendation about the use of α_2-agonist drugs in diabetic patients, the use of these drugs in confirmed diabetics should be reason to more closely monitor blood glucose levels. This α_2-hyperglycemic effect may be dampened in animals that already have diabetes because of insufficient beta cell function.

Stress or fear in the animal before administration of the α_2 agonist may decrease the ability of these drugs to produce significant sedation quickly. Although α_2 agonists can prevent additional release of norepinephrine, they do nothing about the NE already in circulation from the stress or fear response. Therefore, the onset of sedation from the α_2-agonist drug is delayed until these levels of norepinephrine drop.

Xylazine was the first α_2-agonist drug used in veterinary medicine, and it found wide use in both large and small animals. There is significant dosing variation among species, with horses requiring half the equivalent dog dose to produce the intended effect, cattle requiring only 10% of the equivalent horse dose, and goats and sheep requiring even lower doses than cattle. Using a horse dose in a cow could potentially kill the cow. Swine require even higher doses than dogs and so are considered to be the most "resistant" species to xylazine. This wide species variation is not observed to the same degree in the newer α_2-agonist drugs.

In deep-chested dog breeds (e.g., great Danes, Doberman pinschers) or dog breeds predisposed to gastric distention, the use of xylazine has resulted in an increased risk for gastric distention. The mechanism is not understood but may be related to multiple factors, including the atonic effect (lack of tone) α_2 agonists have on the stomach. Dogs predisposed to bloat or with a previous history of gastric dilatation should generally not receive this drug.

Cattle are predisposed to rumen stasis (i.e., decreased rumen motility or rumen atony) from xylazine, which may result in subsequent development of gas bloat or tympany. In contrast to cattle's sensitivity to xylazine, swine appear to be quite resistant to its effects and require much higher dosages to produce any sedative effect. For this reason, α_2 agonists are usually not used in swine.

Detomidine (Dormosedan) is registered by the FDA for use in horses only but has some limited extra-label use in cattle and small ruminants. It is important to note that although xylazine dosing is listed as mg/kg, the doses for detomidine, medetomidine, and dexmedetomidine are often listed as mcg/kg (µg/kg). If listed as mg/kg, it is very important to notice the additional zero in the one-tenth place, such as 0.08 mg/kg, which would be equivalent to 80 µg/kg.

Generally it is reported that horses seem to kick less with detomidine than they do with xylazine. Because detomidine is more selective for alpha 2 receptors over alpha 1 receptors than xylazine, detomidine has less changes in arterial blood pressure.

Medetomidine (Domitor) is FDA-approved for use in dogs as a sedative analgesic for minor surgical procedures not requiring muscle relaxation. In postsurgical anesthetic recovery it is used to treat "emergent delirium" or the thrashing some dogs do when recovering from anesthesia. It may be used as a constant rate infusion in the intensive care unit (ICU) to reduce anxiety and provide some sedation and moderate analgesia. Even though medetomidine is approved only for use in dogs, the veterinary literature has extra-label medetomidine doses for cats and horses.

Dexmedetomidine (Dexdomitor) is FDA-approved for use in dogs and cats, and is considered to be a more "refined" drug than its predecessor, medetomidine. The "dextro" refers to one of two molecular configurations of medetomidine that exists as a "dextro" (right) or "levo" (left) medetomidine form. The dexmedetomidine form has been found to be the major biologically active form. So to enhance the effectiveness of medetomidine, which is a 1:1 blend of both dextro and levo forms, dexmedetomidine contains only the dextro form giving it greater potency than the blended medetomidine. Though more potent than medetomidine, the maximum analgesia and sedation of dexmedetomidine is similar and both drugs have the same ceiling effect. The levo form of medetomidine is thought to enhance the bradycardia and cardiac depression of the dextro form; thus removing the levo molecule from dexmedetomidine allows a higher cardiac output and less cardiac depression.

Romifidine (Sedivet) is FDA-approved in the United States for use in horses to facilitate handling, minor surgical procedures, and clinical examinations. It is used in Europe in dogs and cats and has been used to a limited extent as an extra-label drug in foals and cattle. It has similar cardiovascular, uterine, and blood sugar effects as the other α_2-agonist drugs, but is thought to have a longer-lasting sedation in horses.

Alpha-2 Antagonists

Some of the effects of α_2-agonist sedation can be reversed with α_2-antagonist drugs such as **yohimbine** (Yobine), **atipamezole** (Antisedan), and **tolazoline**. Atipamezole has replaced the use of yohimbine and tolazoline in small animal medicine and exotic animal practice because it is more selective for the α_2 receptor and therefore is more effective for reversal of detomidine, medetomidine, and dexmedetomidine, which are the α_2 agonists preferred for small animals and exotics. Yohimbine and tolazoline are less specific reversal agents and therefore are more commonly used to reverse xylazine.

It is important to remember that the sudden removal of analgesia by a reversal agent during anesthesia recovery and the return of pain may cause the patient to go into an emergent delirium. In addition, IV administration of these reversal agents may initially reverse the α_1 vasoconstrictive effect, causing a vasodilation that drops the arterial blood pressure. Normally, this drop in blood pressure would cause the CNS to release sympathetic signals to increase the heart rate and cause vasoconstriction again.

However, because it takes some time for the α_2-antagonist reversal agents to enter the brain and remove the α_2-agonist suppression of the sympathetic nervous system, there is a lag between when the α_1 block is reversed in the peripheral arterioles and when the α_2 block on the sympathetic nervous system block is removed. Without the compensatory sympathetic response to keep blood pressure up, blocking the α_1-agonist effect with an α_2-antagonist results in a much lower drop in arterial blood pressure and potential cardiovascular collapse in unhealthy animals. Therefore, the potential side effects of IV administration of α_2 antagonists should be considered before administering the dose.

ANESTHETICS

Anesthesia means "without sensation." A fully anesthetized animal or person cannot feel stimulations of pain, cold, heat, pressure, or touch. General anesthesia is the reversible loss of these sensations associated with unconsciousness, and local anesthesia is the reversible loss of sensation in a regional area of the body without loss of consciousness.

Anesthetics should not be confused with analgesics, which are compounds that decrease pain perception but do not necessarily cause total loss of all sensations. For example, opioid narcotics are analgesics because they decrease the perception of pain; however, they are not anesthetics because animals can usually still feel other sensations. However, a higher dose of an analgesic drug may induce narcosis, a state of sleep from which the patient is not easily aroused, and by producing a profound narcosis that higher dose may produce an anesthetic effect.

Sedatives or tranquilizers are not anesthetic agents; however, they enhance the effect of anesthetic drugs and decrease the amount of anesthetic drug needed by calming the animal or putting it into a state of relaxation or light sleep.

Injectable Anesthetics

Barbiturates are drugs that were historically used to induce anesthesia or provide primary anesthesia in limited situations. The use of propofol has largely replaced the use of the ultrashort-acting barbiturates for anesthesia induction, but longer acting barbiturates are still commonly used in euthanasia solutions.

The ultrashort-acting barbiturates are thiopental and **methohexital**. Thiopental is no longer available in the United States and methohexital, though available, has largely fallen out of use. **Pentobarbital** is the prototype for the short-acting barbiturates and was used in veterinary medicine as an anesthetic agent for short procedures when gas anesthetic agents are either unavailable or impractical. The long-acting barbiturates are represented by **phenobarbital**. Although phenobarbital has been used successfully for anesthesia in veterinary patients under conditions described for pentobarbital, a more common use of phenobarbital is as one of the anticonvulsant drugs of choice for long-term control of epilepsy in small animals.

Barbiturates have a number of unique characteristics related to redistribution, induction of metabolism, and production of local inflammatory reactions if not injected properly. Information about barbiturates is readily available from online sources or from veterinary anesthesiology texts. The nature of phenobarbital as an anticonvulsant will be discussed in the next chapter.

Propofol is an injectable anesthetic agent chemically unrelated to barbiturates and other injectable anesthetics but has some of the similar properties of barbiturates. Propofol is often used to induce anesthesia and has a very rapid recovery time compared with other induction agents. Its rapid recovery with minimal residual effects has made it a popular anesthetic agent for use in people and animals for short-duration diagnostic procedures. If you have had a short diagnostic procedure done on an outpatient basis in a human hospital (e.g., colonoscopy), you have likely had IV propofol.

The original propofol was produced as a drug dissolved in an emulsion of drug, egg lecithin, and soybean oil. Because of the organic nature of this emulsion, bacteria could grow and theoretically produce endotoxins if the propofol emulsion became contaminated. For this reason, it was required that unused propofol from a vial be discarded within 24 h after being opened. Lipid-free formulations of propofol have a longer shelf life and reduced risk for bacterial growth after contamination than the original propofol formulation with egg lecithin and soybean oil, and a veterinary form of propofol (PropoFlo-28) containing benzyl alcohol has a shelf life of 28 days once the vial has been opened.

Propofol (and barbiturates) work at the $GABA_A$ receptor site mentioned with the benzodiazepine tranquilizers. Instead of enhancing the GABA neurotransmitter's effect on the $GABA_A$ receptor like benzodiazepines do, propofol directly stimulates the $GABA_A$ receptor and produces the same effect that the inhibitory neurotransmitter would. When stimulated, the $GABA_A$ receptor opens chloride channels in the neuron to which it is attached, causing an inward flooding of negatively charged chloride ions and a negative interior charge change that makes it harder for the neuron to be stimulated to fire (see Chapter 5 on depolarization and repolarization). The net effect is suppression of neuronal activity in the brain, resulting in sedation or anesthesia.

In addition, propofol also inhibits the NMDA receptor mentioned with the opioid methadone. Inhibition of these receptors produces an anesthetic effect and is the major mechanism for anesthesia caused by the dissociative anesthetics discussed later.

Propofol is usually injected as an IV bolus to induce anesthesia, or as a CRI to provide anesthesia for less invasive or less painful procedures. Care should be taken not to inject the IV bolus too rapidly, as this will result in apnea (cessation of breathing). The incidence of apnea is closely correlated with the dose and the rate of administration, with rapid rates having a high risk for apnea. Some authors recommend giving the IV bolus dose in 25% increments every 30 s until the desired effect is achieved. Even with using a CRI intravenously and theoretically being able to titrate the dose to effect, apnea sometimes still occurs. The presence of opioid analgesics or other respiratory depressant drugs increases the apnea risk from propofol.

Fortunately, the apnea is transient due to the rapid metabolism of propofol to an inactive metabolite and the redistribution of the drug from the brain to other tissues. Redistribution is not the same as elimination and only represents relocating the drug to an area of the body that is less likely to produce adverse reactions. In the case of propofol, the IV-administered drug is initially quickly distributed to the brain where it produces anesthesia. However, during the first few minutes after injection the drug still in the blood is also being distributed to lesser perfused tissues like fat, causing drug concentrations in the blood to continue to fall. As the drug concentrations in the blood fall, propofol follows the concentration gradient and moves from the high concentrations in the brain to the lower concentrations in the blood. As propofol leaves the brain the degree of anesthesia decreases and the animal begins to wake up. Thus, redistribution of the drug from brain to blood to other less perfused tissues accounts for much of the short duration of anesthesia after an IV bolus is given or after the CRI is stopped.[14]

Propofol provides effective sedation but only minimal analgesic activity at dosages that do not induce full anesthesia. Even in an unconscious state, animals often respond to painful stimuli unless other analgesics such as opioids or α_2 agonists also are administered.

People receiving propofol sometimes report pain on injection; this may also occur in veterinary patients. The newer propofol products are formulated to have less pain on injection.[15]

Propofol decreases arterial blood pressure, producing systemic hypotension that is mostly caused by vasodilation. Propofol does decrease the heart rate, but most of the hypotension is due to the vasodilation. Patients who are already hypovolemic (e.g., from blood loss, significant dehydration) or geriatric will have more profound cardiovascular effects.[15]

Because propofol is a phenol type of chemical, cats cannot effectively conjugate and metabolize it, as well as other species, and therefore have the potential to develop Heinz body anemia if the propofol is given repeatedly on consecutive days. Another study in cats showed no significant changes in the red blood cells with repeated dosing of propofol, so we must conclude that this Heinz body anemia effect can vary from patient to patient.[14]

Ketamine and **tiletamine** are called dissociative anesthetics. They are short-acting injectable anesthetics that produce a rather unique form of anesthesia in which the animal feels dissociated (i.e., apart) from its body. This dissociative effect is thought to be associated with antagonism of the NMDA receptor mentioned previously with methadone and propofol. In this case there is a dissociation between two systems of the brain that results in a cataleptic state. *Catalepsis*, or catalepsy, is characterized by an appearance of being awake but being unable to respond to external stimuli.

In addition, ketamine and tiletamine cause central sympathetic nervous system activation, resulting in vasoconstriction, increased heart rate, increased arterial blood pressure, and increased work load on the heart. Healthy animals are tolerant of these effects, but animals with cardiovascular disease or those that are already tachycardic (i.e., have a fast heart rate) should probably not receive these dissociative anesthetic agents.

The analgesia provided by ketamine and tiletamine comes not only from the NMDA receptor antagonism but also from opioid agonist effects. Stimulating the μ- and κ-receptors produces significant analgesia. Ketamine and tiletamine produce good somatic (i.e., peripheral tissue) analgesia and are suitable for superficial surgery; however, they are much less effective in blocking visceral pain (i.e., organ pain) and should not be used alone as anesthesia for internal procedures.

Antagonism of the NMDA receptors by ketamine and tiletamine is thought to prevent the wind-up phenomenon in the spinal cord mentioned previously with the opioid drugs. NMDA receptor stimulation is part of the increased hypersensitization or wind-up process that occurs over the hours after an injury or trauma begins to send pain signals up the spinal cord. By using ketamine and tiletamine as part of the surgical anesthetic protocol, ketamine and tiletamine block NMDA receptors and prevent wind-up.

One of the advantages of dissociative anesthetics is that many reflexes (e.g., laryngeal, pharyngeal, corneal) are maintained. Thus, the animal may be able to better reflexly swallow, and normal respiratory responses to hypoxia (i.e., low oxygen) or elevated carbon dioxide are maintained. Even though ketamine does not cause significant respiratory depression, the respiratory rhythm is often altered so that the animal takes a long, deep inspiration, holds the breath momentarily, and then quickly exhales, producing a respiratory pattern referred to as an apneustic breathing pattern. Despite this apneustic breathing pattern the carbon dioxide concentrations and amount of air ventilated over time will be within normal limits.[15]

At the same time there are normal reflexes, there is a general lack of muscular relaxation (often increased muscle tone or rigidity) that would make manipulation of limb positioning or stretching of skeletal muscles (e.g., in orthopedic surgery to fix a broken bone) more difficult. α_2 Agonists or benzodiazepines can be given with the dissociative anesthetic to act as central skeletal muscle relaxants to counteract the "waxy rigidity" produced by ketamine or tiletamine.

In animals that are in the dissociative state from ketamine or tiletamine the eyes remain open and unblinking, which can dry the cornea. When using these drugs in a patient, the veterinary professional should apply an ophthalmic lubricant or ointment to prevent corneal damage.[16]

Ketamine and tiletamine are chemically related to another potential abuse drug with hallucinogenic activity called *phencyclidine* (also known as PCP, angel dust, and several other street names). Because of its similarity to phencyclidine, ketamine has gained popularity and is known on the streets as "Special K." Stolen or diverted ketamine is evaporated to a white powder and then inhaled by the abuser. Ketamine is classified as a C-III controlled substance; because of its abuse potential it should be stored and inventoried according to federal and state controlled substance storage laws and guidelines.

Ketamine is well absorbed through the mucous membranes of the mouth and nasal cavity. The drug is sometimes squirted into the mouth of a hissing, fractious cat (e.g., feral cats, cats not acclimated to human contact) to safely subdue the animal enough to handle it and properly anesthetize it. The bitter taste usually does produce copious salivation.[15]

Although dogs primarily remove ketamine through hepatic metabolism, cats depend on the kidney for ketamine elimination. Thus, cats with renal disease or male cats with urinary tract obstruction should not receive large doses of this drug. If used in these animals, renal function must be maintained to assure elimination of ketamine metabolites, and the animal should be closely monitored for signs of prolonged anesthetic effect.

Tiletamine is commercially packaged with the benzodiazepine tranquilizer zolazepam in the product Telazol. Like ketamine, tiletamine is a C-III controlled substance. The zolazepam tranquilizer reduces some of tiletamine's CNS excitation and side effects. The product is used for restraint or anesthesia for minor procedures lasting less than an hour in cats and less than 30 min in dogs.

As with ketamine, animals given tiletamine have open eyes (with the potential for corneal drying), poor muscle relaxation, and analgesia insufficient to prevent perception of visceral pain. The zolazepam in Telazol reduces CNS excitation and provides some degree of muscle relaxation. Tiletamine anesthesia lasts longer and produces better analgesia than ketamine; however, even when tiletamine is combined with zolazepam in Telazol, the drug should only be used for restraint or minor surgical procedures.

Etomidate is a short-acting anesthetic agent that works in a similar mechanism as the benzodiazepine tranquilizers (i.e., enhancing GABA effect on GABA$_A$ receptor). It is used primarily for induction of anesthesia, especially in patients with cardiovascular problems, because of etomidate's minimal negative effect on the heart (i.e., no change in heart rate, cardiac output, or arterial blood pressure). It does not have any significant analgesic effects and therefore should not be used alone as an anesthetic agent. Like the dissociatives, etomidate produces significant skeletal muscle tone that can be countered by using benzodiazepines because of their centrally acting muscle relaxant effect.

Alfaxalone (Alfaxan) is a unique drug that has been used for several years in the United Kingdom but only recently has been marketed in the United States. Alfaxalone is classified as a neurosteroid or neuroactive steroid, meaning it is similar to endogenous hormone-like steroids synthesized in the brain that alter the neuronal activity within the brain. There are many natural neurosteroids produced in the brain, but alfaxalone causes sedation and anesthesia by enhancing the effect of the GABA neurotransmitter on GABA$_A$ receptors, which opens chloride channels, allows negatively charged chloride ions to flood into the neuron, and makes it far harder for the excitatory neuron to depolarize. The net effect is inhibition of the brain and CNS depression.[15]

Although alfaxalone can produce cardiovascular depression at higher doses, at clinically relevant doses the cardiovascular parameters are very stable. However, at clinically appropriate doses, the drug label information indicates that 44% of the dogs and 19% of the cats experience apnea after induction. This apnea lasts on average 100 s for dogs and 60 s for cats.[4] Thus, intubation and maintenance of respiration may be necessary for the first minute or so after induction.

Like propofol, the IV administration of alfaxalone as an anesthetic induction agent should be slowly done over 60 s, with one quarter of the total dose administered every 15 s. Once anesthetic induction is achieved, the animal is either intubated and maintained on gas anesthesia, or it can be maintained with alfaxalone by CRI.

The manufacturer recommends insuring the animal recovering from alfaxalone anesthesia be kept quiet and not handled so as to avoid paddling, muscle twitching, or spontaneous muscle movements, some of which can be violent. These effects are transient and have no long-term effects.[8]

Inhalant Anesthetics

Inhalant, or gas, anesthesia is the administration of an anesthetic drug via the lungs that is absorbed from the alveoli into the blood and distributes to the brain to produce unconsciousness. Proper gas anesthesia requires administering enough of a potentially very dangerous drug to maintain a safe plane of surgical anesthesia while giving as little drug possible to avoid or minimize adverse effects. The technique to properly balance all aspects of anesthetic gas delivery is discussed in greater detail in veterinary and veterinary technology resources dedicated to anesthesia. The skill and technique for properly delivering gas anesthesia are too important and too extensive to be thoroughly covered in this text or any other text where gas anesthesia constitutes only a few pages of a much larger volume. The focus of this section will be on the key characteristics of the anesthetic drug itself.

Generally, injectable anesthetics are used initially to induce sedation or anesthesia, and then the anesthetized patient is maintained with gas anesthesia. The most common gas anesthetics used in veterinary medicine today include **isoflurane**, **sevoflurane**, and **desflurane**. These anesthetics are listed in order of their popularity and use in North America. A fourth gas agent, **nitrous oxide (N$_2$O)** will be briefly mentioned. Desflurane and nitrous oxide are used less than isoflurane and sevoflurane. Halothane, at one time the most commonly used gas anesthetic in veterinary medicine worldwide, was discontinued in North America in 1995, although it remains in use in some countries across the world.

Each anesthetic gas has a minimum alveolar concentration (MAC), which is the lowest concentration of drug that must be achieved in the alveoli to produce a safe level of anesthesia. The MAC serves as a means for measuring the potency (i.e., how much drug it takes to produce a given effect) of the gas anesthesia. The lower the MAC the less gas it takes to produce anesthesia and the more potent the anesthetic gas.

Because gas anesthetics are delivered by breathing, the suppression of breathing by injectable or gas anesthetics can affect the amount of anesthetic drug delivered into the body via the lungs. Therefore, the veterinary technician must be familiar with the effect each anesthetic gas has on respiratory rate, blood pressure, and other observable signs that indicate the depth of anesthesia.

Despite more than 150 years of inhaled anesthetic use, little is understood about how these drugs actually produce anesthesia. There is no common molecular structure found in all anesthetic agents, nor is there an identified receptor that can be identified that would accept all anesthetic gas agents. Anesthetic gases not only anesthetize common domestic animals, but they also anesthetize all vertebrates and even invertebrate animals. They also decrease movement of protozoa and inhibit the movement of plants that respond to touch. Thus, the only thing that can be said for sure about the mechanism of anesthetic gases is that they must affect some element found in all life processes.

One of the advantages of the current gas anesthetic agents is that they are not metabolized to any significant amount, and therefore they do not produce metabolites potentially toxic to the kidney or the liver. This reduces some of the clinical side effects and major concerns observed with older gases.

All gases depress the respiratory and cardiovascular systems based upon dose of the gas. There is variation among species and the type of anesthetic gas itself. Although older gases used to predispose the heart to generation of ectopic foci (see Chapter 5) and sudden appearance of arrhythmias, isoflurane, sevoflurane, and desflurane have little of this characteristic. This is not to say that arrhythmias never occur, but the effect of these gases on their appearance is far less than what can be ascribed to hypoxia during anesthesia or the influence of catecholamine release because of stress or fear.

It is important to remember that unconsciousness does not mean analgesia. Gas anesthetics do not provide analgesia, and the rapid recovery from gas anesthesia with isoflurane, sevoflurane, or desflurane can produce delirium and a somewhat stormy recovery because of the transition from unconscious state to sudden awareness, especially if the animal is in pain. Use of a tranquilizer or sedative to relieve anxiety plus appropriate use of analgesics to prevent sudden awareness of pain can smooth the recovery period from these gas anesthetics.

Isoflurane

The rapid, smooth induction of anesthesia and short recovery period of the inhalant anesthetic isoflurane (IsoFlo, Forane) signaled the demise of halothane use in veterinary practices. Unlike the newer inhalant anesthetics such as sevoflurane and desflurane, isoflurane has an odor described on the package insert as "mildly pungent, musty, and ethereal," which can make anesthesia induction with a mask on a conscious animal difficult because the animal may fight the mask and odor. Human anesthesiologists will "flavor" the smell with bubblegum, grape, and other more acceptable scents when used on children.

Isoflurane may have a greater cardiac stabilizing effect than the other gases, but all three of the modern gases are much more cardiac stable than the older gases. Isoflurane does produce vasodilation, which would decrease resistance to cardiac output and potentially drop the arterial blood pressure. However, in healthy patients any drop in blood pressure is usually easily corrected.

Sevoflurane

Sevoflurane (SevoFlo) is newer than isoflurane and runs second to being the most widely used gas anesthetic in veterinary medicine. It has a very rapid induction and recovery (even faster than isoflurane), good cardiac stability (does not predispose the myocardium to arrhythmias), and respiratory depression similar to that of isoflurane.

The rapid induction and recovery make sevoflurane a good anesthetic for outpatient procedures. Sevoflurane would also be good for cesarean sections because any anesthetic gas absorbed by the fetuses would be eliminated quickly and not depend on their immature livers to metabolize the drug. Because anesthetic recovery is so rapid with sevoflurane, the judicious use of tranquilizers and analgesics is important to smooth the transition from anesthesia to full awareness of all body sensations, including pain.

Like isoflurane, sevoflurane is minimally metabolized by the liver. However, sevoflurane does react with the carbon dioxide scavenger compounds commonly used in anesthetic machines (e.g., soda lime) and cause production of a chemical called compound A. The discovery of this compound and some data that showed it can be nephrotoxic in rats generated a great deal of concern around the mid to late 1990s. However, controlled studies in dogs administered sevoflurane for 3 h a day, 5 days a week for 2 weeks (30 h total) showed no evidence of nephrotoxicity. Other studies and investigations failed to uncover increased reports of nephrotoxicity linked to sevoflurane use in animals. At this point, there seems to be little support for concern over the generation of compound A.

Desflurane

Desflurane is the least used of the three anesthetic gases based upon its low potency (i.e., requires a higher MAC to produce equivalent anesthetic level to isoflurane and sevoflurane), its pungency (similar to isoflurane), and high cost. Desflurane also requires a special heated and pressurized vaporizer to turn the liquid desflurane into a vapor that can be inhaled. Once vaporized, the anesthetic gas has low solubility in the blood, which means that the gas can be quickly delivered from the alveolus to the brain without having to "fill up" the blood with gas first. This low solubility allows a more precise control over the depth of anesthesia by providing a closer correlation between adjustments made in the vaporizer delivery of the gas and the degree of anesthesia occurring in the brain.[17]

Other Anesthetic Gas
Nitrous Oxide

Nitrous oxide, also referred to as "laughing gas," is sometimes added to the inhaled anesthetic protocol or anesthetic cocktail to reduce the amount of the more potent gas or injectable anesthetic required to induce or maintain anesthesia. It is safe when used properly but has much weaker anesthetic qualities than other inhalant anesthetics and should never be used alone to provide surgical plane anesthesia in veterinary patients.

Nitrous oxide diffuses through the body very rapidly and enters gas-filled body compartments such as the stomach, rumen, and loops of bowel. When a gas diffuses into a compartment, it increases the overall pressure within that compartment. Under normal conditions, this causes no ill effects. However, if the animal has a distended rumen, twisted necrotic bowel, dilated stomach (gastric dilation), or gas-filled thoracic cavity (pneumothorax), the increased pressure from nitrous oxide diffusion can rupture devitalized tissue or compress adjoining structures. Therefore, nitrous oxide is contraindicated under these conditions.

At the end of surgery when the flow of inhalant anesthetic gas is stopped, 100% oxygen should be administered at a high flow rate as the animal recovers with the endotracheal tube in place. When the flow of nitrous oxide ceases at the end of a surgical procedure, nitrous oxide rapidly diffuses out of tissues into the blood and then into the alveoli, where it dilutes the oxygen concentration. If the flow of 100% oxygen has been turned off and the animal is receiving oxygen only from room air, which contains 15%–17% oxygen, the oxygen concentration in the lungs can be diluted enough by the nitrous oxide to produce hypoxia. This phenomenon, called diffusion hypoxia, or the second-gas effect, is the reason for maintaining a high rate of oxygen flow for at least 5 to 10 min after the end of nitrous oxide administration.

CENTRAL NERVOUS SYSTEM STIMULANTS

CNS stimulants are occasionally used to stimulate respiration in anesthetized animals or to reverse CNS depression caused by anesthetic or sedative agents. In addition to stimulant drugs used for therapeutic purposes, CNS stimulation may also be part of the mechanism by which toxicants produce their toxic effects. For example, the poison strychnine blocks a neurotransmitter's inhibitory activity, causing CNS excitatory mechanisms to dominate; theobromine, the component in chocolate, increases NE release and inhibits adenosine's inhibitory activity; caffeine, found in diet pills and some headache medications, has a mechanism of action similar to that of theobromine; and amphetamines or cocaine ingestion produces similar CNS stimulatory effects.

Methylxanthines

Caffeine and theobromine belong to a broad group of drugs known as methylxanthines, which include the respiratory bronchodilating drugs **theophylline** and **aminophylline** (see Chapter 6). Because chocolate toxicity in dogs is well known, veterinary technicians should be aware of facts surrounding this syndrome. The active ingredient in chocolate is **theobromine**. A 10-lb dog would have to ingest two or three candy bars of milk chocolate to ingest enough theobromine to produce toxicity. Fortunately, ingestion of that much chocolate by such a small dog would likely produce vomiting, thus decreasing the amount of theobromine absorbed.

A greater danger comes from ingestion of unsweetened baking chocolate, which usually contains up to 10 times the amount of theobromine per ounce compared with milk chocolate. Thus, a single ounce of baking chocolate could be enough to produce toxicity in a susceptible 10-lb dog. An additional source of theobromine intoxication in horses is cocoa bean hulls, which are sometimes used as stall bedding.

Treatment of chocolate toxicity is by induction of emesis and supportive care. Animals that ingest amounts of milk chocolate sufficient to cause toxicity usually vomit spontaneously and develop diarrhea. Removal of a large mass of chocolate by gastric lavage using a stomach tube can be difficult because the soft chocolate tends to form a ball within the stomach.

Doxapram

Doxapram (Dopram, Dopram-V) is a CNS stimulant that works primarily at the medulla of the brainstem to increase respiration in animals with apnea (cessation of breathing), bradypnea (slow breathing), or other conditions in which the respiratory rate and depth of ventilation (how deeply the patient breathes) need to be increased. The species most often receiving this are newborn calves and newborn foals.

Doxapram also stimulates other parts of the brain in addition to the medullary area, but this stimulation is significantly weaker. Doxapram should be used with caution in animals that are predisposed to seizures although there has not been any evidence to show conclusively that doxapram increases frequency of seizure activity in epileptic animals. The CNS stimulation is dose dependent; thus for animals with a history of seizures it would be prudent to avoid using higher doses of doxapram.

α_2 Antagonists (yohimbine, tolazoline, atipamezole) and opioid antagonists (naloxone) are considered to be CNS stimulants by way of reversing the sedative effects of their respective drug groups. These were discussed previously.

⬦ NERVOUS SYSTEM DRUGS

Analgesics, Anesthetics, Antagonists

Analgesics	Romifidine (Sedivet)
Opioid analgesics	α_2-Antagonists
Morphine	Yohimbine (Yobine)
Hydromorphone	Atipamezole (Antisedan)
Oxymorphone	Tolazoline
Fentanyl	
Methadone	**Anesthetics**
Meperidine	Injectable anesthetics
Buprenorphine	Barbiturates
Butorphanol (Torbutrol,	Methohexital
Torbugesic)	Pentobarbital
Tramadol	Phenobarbital
Opioid antagonist	Propofol
Naloxone (Narcan)	Dissociative anesthetics
	Ketamine
Tranquilizers and Sedatives	Tiletamine (Telazol)
Phenothiazine tranquilizers	Etomidate
Acepromazine	Alfaxalone
Benzodiazepine tranquilizers	Inhalant anesthetics
Diazepam (Valium)	Isoflurane
Zolazepam (Telazol)	Sevoflurane
Midazolam (Versed)	Desflurane
Clonazepam (Klonopin)	Other anesthetic gas agents:
Benzodiazepine antagonist	nitrous oxide
Flumazenil	
α_2-Agonists	**CNS Stimulants**
Xylazine (Rompun)	Methylxanthines
Detomidine (Dormosedan)	Theophylline
Medetomidine (Domitor)	Aminophylline
Dexmedetomidine (Dexdomitor)	Theobromine
	Doxapram (Dopram)

REFERENCES

1. Kukanich B, Papich MG. Opioid analgesic drugs. In: Riviere J, Papich M, eds. *Veterinary Pharmacology and Therapeutics.* Wiley-Blackwell; 2009:301–336.
2. Kukanich B, Wiese AJ. Opioids. In: Grimm KA, Lamont LA, Tranquilli WJ, et al., eds. *Veterinary Anesthesia and Analgesia: The Fifth Edition of Lumb and Jones.* Ames, IA: John Wiley & Sons; 2015:207–226.
3. Booth DM. Control of pain in small animals: Opioid agonists and antagonists and other locally and centrally acting analgesics. In: Booth DM, ed. *Small Animal Clinical Pharmacology and Therapeutics.* Philadelphia: Saunders; 2012.
4. Duke-Novakovski T. Opioids. In: Egger CM, et al., eds. *Pain Management in Practice.* Ames, IA: Wiley-Blackwell; 2013:41–68.
5. Grubb TL. Opioids, myths, magic and misconception. In: *Proceedings of the 2013 Western Veterinary Conference, Las Vegas, Nevada*; 2013.
6. Niedfeldt RL, Robertson SA. Postanesthetic hyperthermia in cats: a retrospective comparison between hydromorphone and buprenorphine. *Vet Anaesth Analg.* 2006;33(6):381–389.
7. Posner LP, et al. Effects of opioids and anesthetic drugs on body temperature in cats. *Vet Anaesth Analg.* 2010;37(1):35–43.
8. Accessed online: https://academic-plumbs-com.ezproxy.lib.purdue.edu/search?contentType=all&query Accessed on 06.12.2022.
9. Epstein ME. Opioids: Which, why, how and what's new? In: *Proceedings of the 2013 Western Veterinary Conference, Las Vegas, Nevada*; 2013.
10. Package insert for Simbadol, Abbott Laboratories/Zoetis United States, July 2014.
11. Shell L. Acepromazine and Seizures Survey; 2006. (website). www.vin.com/doc/?id=2992617&pid=8538. Accessed 06.04.2015.
12. Rankin DC. Sedatives and tranquilizers. In: Grimm KA, Lamont LA, Tranquilli WJ, et al., eds. *Veterinary Anesthesia and Analgesia: The Fifth Edition of Lumb and Jones.* Ames, Iowa: John Wiley & Sons; 2015:196–206.
13. Posener LP, Burns P. Sedative agents: Tranquilizers, alpha-2 agonists, and related agents. In: Riviere J, Papich M, eds. *Veterinary Pharmacology and Therapeutics.* Ames, Iowa: Wiley-Blackwell; 2009:337–380.
14. Posener LP, Burns P. Injectable anesthetic agents. In: Riviere J, Papich M, eds. *Veterinary Pharmacology and Therapeutics.* Ames, Iowa: Wiley-Blackwell; 2009:265–300.
15. Berry SH. Injectable anesthetics. In: Grimm KA, Lamont LA, Tranquilli WJ, et al., eds. *Veterinary Anesthesia and Analgesia: The Fifth Edition of Lumb and Jones.* Ames, Iowa: John Wiley & Sons; 2015:277–296.
16. Pawson P, Forsyth S. Anesthetic agents. In: Maddison JE, Page SW, Church D, eds. *Small Animal Clinical Pharmacology.* Philadelphia: Elsevier Health Sciences; 2008.
17. Steffey EP, Mama KR, Brosnan RJ. Inhalation anesthetics. In: Grimm KA, Lamont LA, Tranquilli WJ, et al., eds. *Veterinary Anesthesia and Analgesia: The Fifth Edition of Lumb and Jones.* Ames, Iowa: John Wiley & Sons; 2015:297–331.

SELF-ASSESSMENT

1. Fill in the following blanks with the correct item from the Key Terms list.

   A. _____ This term means a pain receptor.

   B. _____ This is the translation of physical stimulus into a depolarization within the pain receptor.

   C. _____ This is the modification of the pain signal from the pain receptor and the sensory nerve as the signal travels up in the spinal cord.

   D. _____ This is the type of anesthesia that produces overall unconsciousness.

   E. _____ This is the condition in which an area of the body becomes especially sensitive to any *painful* stimulation.

   F. _____ This is the condition in which an area of the body becomes especially sensitive to *any* sensation, not just pain.

   G. _____ This describes the process in which the spinal cord over time becomes more effective at transmitting pain signals up the spinal cord to the brain.

   H. _____ This term describes drugs derived as extracts from poppy seeds.

   I. _____ This term describes chemically synthesized opiate-like drugs.

   J. _____ The term that means a stuporous state from which an animal is not easily aroused.

   K. _____ This term describes the types of drugs that produce a stuporous state from which the animal is not easily aroused.

   L. _____ This term describes a drug made by combining an opioid drug with a tranquilizer or sedative.

   M. _____ These are the three opioid receptors of significance in veterinary medicine.

   N. _____ This term means a bad hallucination.

   O. _____ This term describes a type of drug (not a specific drug name) that can reverse some of the effect of a stronger drug but has some effect of its own.

   P. _____ This term describes a type of drug that combines with more than one type of receptor and produces an effect on each of the receptors.

   Q. _____ This term describes a type of drug that combines with more than one type of receptor but does not produce an effect on either receptor.

   R. _____ This term describes a type of drug that combines with one receptor and produces an effect and also combines another receptor but produces no effect.

   S. _____ This is the opioid receptor that produces most of the analgesia when stimulated by an agonist.

T. _____ This is the other opioid receptor most commonly involved with veterinary analgesic drugs that produces a more moderate level of analgesia than the other receptor that produces a stronger analgesia.

U. _____ This term is used to describe how much dose (mass of drug) it takes to produce a particular effect.

V. _____ This term describes the maximum effect a drug can have.

W. _____ This is the type of pain that originates from inflammation or trauma to organs.

X. _____ This is the type of pain that originates from the skin and superficial tissues.

Y. _____ This means an elevated body temperature.

Z. _____ This describes the phenomena wherein a drug effect increases in magnitude as the dose increases until, at some dose, the effect no longer increases, regardless of how much more the dose increases.

AA. _____ This is the type of drug (not a specific drug) that calms a patient's anxiety but does not necessarily make the patient sleepy.

AB. _____ This means to literally "break apart anxiety."

AC. _____ This is the type of drug (not a specific drug) that makes an animal sleepy but does not really do anything to relieve the anxiety.

AD. _____ This is the family of tranquilizers to which acepromazine belongs.

AE. _____ This is the receptor that is blocked in the brain by acepromazine to produce the tranquilization effect.

AF. _____ This term describes a type of adverse effect that is not dose related and cannot be predicted by any identifiable risk factor.

AG. _____ This is an important inhibitory neurotransmitter whose action is enhanced by the presence of benzodiazepine tranquilizers on the neurotransmitter's receptor.

AH. _____ This is the receptor to which diazepam and midazolam attach to produce their effects.

AI. _____ This is the receptor to which drugs like xylazine and medetomidine bind to produce their sedative/analgesic effects.

AJ. _____ These are receptors in the major arteries of the body that detect changes in arterial blood pressure.

AK. _____ This term means without sensation.

AL. _____ This is the type of anesthesia that produces a reversible loss of sensation in a regional area of the body without a loss of consciousness.

AM. _____ This is the receptor in the spinal cord to which drugs like ketamine and tiletamine attach to produce analgesia; also a site of action for propofol and methadone.

AN. _____ This describes the process by which an anesthetic is initially distributed to the brain, produces anesthesia, then diffuses back out of the brain to the blood and finally to other tissues.

AO. _____ This is the type of injectable anesthetic (not a specific drug) in which the animal feels apart from its body.

AP. _____ This is a term that describes the state of an animal or person where he or she appears to be awake but is unresponsive to external stimuli.

AQ. _____ This term means a fast heart rate.

AR. _____ This is a descriptive term for when an animal slowly breathes in and holds its breath for a moment before quickly expiring.

AS. _____ This is a type of drug (not a specific drug) that is similar to natural hormone-like compounds produced by the brain that alter neuronal activity in the brain.

AT. _____ This is the measurement by which the potency of gas anesthesia is measured.

AU. _____ This is a potentially nephrotoxic substance generated by sevoflurane reacting with the carbon dioxide scrubber materials in an anesthetic gas machine.

AV. _____ This is the phenomenon wherein nitrous oxide floods into the alveoli at the end of the anesthetic delivery and crowds out the oxygen, causing the animal to experience oxygen deprivation.

AW. _____ This is the term that means slow breathing.

AX. _____ This is the term that means cessation of breathing.

AY. _____ This is the term that describes a "pleasant hallucination" or feeling.

2. Fill in the following blanks with the correct drug from the Nervous System Drug list. When practicing these questions, write out the answers on a separate sheet, focusing also on the appropriate spelling of these drug names.

   A. _____ Prototype opioid by which all other opioid drugs are measured for potency.

   B. _____ Complex drug that is converted to a metabolite (M1) to produce its mu (μ) agonist analgesic effect but that also prevents reuptake of serotonin and norepinephrine (NE), blocks muscarinic receptors, and stimulates alpha-2 (α_2) receptors.

   C. _____ Opioid used a bit less in the United States than some of the others opioids; it is not only a μ agonist but also an N-methyl-D-aspartate (NMDA) antagonist.

   D. _____ Four tranquilizers classified as benzodiazepines.

   E. _____ Mixed strong kappa (κ)-agonist opioid that also has weak mu (μ)-agonist or μ-antagonist activity; ceiling effect; approved for use as a canine antitussive.

   F. _____ Gas anesthetic characterized by its pungent, musty odor.

G. _____ Opioid drug that should not be used with tricyclic antidepressants or serotonin reuptake inhibitors because of the potential to produce serotonin syndrome.

H. _____ First α_2-agonist drug with least specificity for α_2 over α_1 receptors.

I. _____ Opioid antagonist.

J. _____ Phenothiazine tranquilizer.

K. _____ Injectable anesthetic whose analgesia comes from μ- and κ-agonist activity but, more importantly, from NMDA antagonist activity.

L. _____ Benzodiazepine that is the drug of choice to control active seizures.

M. _____ Tranquilizer that causes the third eyelid to cover part of the eye as a harmless side effect.

N. _____ Potent μ agonist; very short duration requires administration by constant rate infusion (CRI), patch, or transdermal solution.

O. _____ Benzodiazepine not used as a preanesthetic but as an adjunct drug to maintain control of epileptic seizures in dogs.

P. _____ Three inhalant anesthetics.

Q. _____ Two opioid drugs that can be given to partially reverse the effects of a stronger μ-agonist opioid without totally reversing all of the analgesia or sedation.

R. _____ Two dissociative anesthetics.

S. _____ Family of central nervous system (CNS) stimulants that include caffeine, theophylline, and aminophylline.

T. _____ Benzodiazepine antagonist.

U. _____ Tranquilizer that can cause equine penile prolapse.

V. _____ The benzodiazepine combined with tiletamine in Telazol.

W. _____ The α_2-agonist drug limited to horses in the United States but used in dogs and cats in Europe.

X. _____ Sedative analgesic drug used as the drug of choice to make cats vomit.

Y. _____ Partial μ agonist and a κ antagonist; exhibits a ceiling effect; lasts longer than butorphanol because of its stronger affinity for the μ receptor.

Z. _____ Benzodiazepine that does not mix well with intravenous (IV) fluids or water-based liquid media of other drugs.

AA. _____ α_2 Agonist Food and Drug Administration (FDA) approved for use in horses; is more selective than xylazine for the α_2 receptor than the α_1 receptor but is less specific for the receptor than the newer α_2-agonist drugs.

AB. _____ IV anesthetic agent that often produces transient apnea and has a quick initial recovery due to redistribution of the drug.

AC. _____ Newer α_2 agonist composed of two different molecular configurations of the drug; used to treat emergent delirium.

AD. _____ Anesthetic that produces a state of catalepsy.

AE. _____ Three α_2 antagonists.

AF. _____ Which α_2 agonist may be associated with an increased risk for gastric distention in deep-chested dog breeds?

AG. _____ Which barbiturate is not used as much for its anesthetic properties as it is for long-term control of epilepsy seizures?

AH. _____ IV short-acting induction agent with rapid recovery time that makes it ideal for outpatient diagnostic or surgical procedures.

AI. _____ Gas anesthetic used less in veterinary medicine than the other two gas anesthetics because it requires a special heated and pressurized vaporizer.

AJ. _____ IV anesthetic agent that was originally made of drug dissolved in a media that could grow bacteria if contaminated; newer versions have much longer shelf life.

AK. _____ The α_2 antagonist that is preferred to be used over the other two α_2 antagonists for small animal and exotic animal use.

AL. _____ Newer α_2 agonist that is a more refined drug because it only contains one of the two molecular forms of this drug.

AM. _____ Injectable anesthetic that maintains reflexes and muscle tone, resulting in "waxy rigidity" of the patient.

AN. _____ Injectable anesthetic that causes patient to keep eyes open, requiring application of ophthalmic ointments to protect the cornea.

AO. _____ The dissociative anesthetic agent combined with zolazepam in Telazol.

AP. _____ This is the anesthetic in demand for abuse purposes; is evaporated into a white powder and inhaled or ingested; called "Special K."

AQ. _____ Neurosteroid injectable anesthetic.

AR. _____ Gas anesthetic that generates compound A.

AS. _____ CNS stimulant found in chocolate.

AT. _____ Laughing gas.

AU. _____ Opioid that has a greater potency than morphine but similar to morphine in most other ways; more likely to cause drug-induced hyperthermia in cats after surgery.

AV. _____ CNS stimulant drug that is not a methylxanthine; avoid using high doses in animals with seizure activity.

3. Indicate whether each of the following statements is true or false.

   A. The μ-receptor increases the release of neurotransmitters like acetylcholine, dopamine, and serotonin.

B. A local anesthetic would be used to block transduction of nerve pain.

C. Wind-up can occur only if the patient is conscious and aware of the pain.

D. An animal would be harder to arouse if it was in a state of narcosis versus a state of tranquilization.

E. Neuroleptanalgesics are gas anesthetics that produce light anesthesia and no analgesia.

F. A partial opioid agonist would have greater analgesic effect than a full opioid agonist.

G. A mu (μ)-opioid agonist drug would generally be expected to have greater analgesia than a kappa (κ)-agonist.

H. The ceiling effect refers to the maximum effect of a drug being lower compared to the maximum effect achievable by another strong agonist drug.

I. If Drug A produces surgical-level analgesia at 50 mg/kg and Drug B produces the same level of analgesia at 150 mg/kg, we would say that Drug B has greater potency than Drug A.

J. If Drug A produces a surgical plane of anesthesia at its maximum dose but Drug B produces a level of analgesia that is lower than that required for surgery at its maximum dose, Drug A has lower potency than Drug B.

K. Acepromazine makes seizure activity more likely in epileptic animals.

L. Acepromazine would be effective in reducing vomiting from motion sickness.

M. Diazepam would be equally effective as acepromazine in reducing vomiting from motion sickness.

N. Flumazenil reverses opioid respiratory depression.

O. α_2 Agonists are better at controlling somatic pain than visceral pain.

P. A heavily tranquilized animal will usually not feel pain.

Q. Initially an α_2-agonist drug will cause a bradycardia and hypotension, which will be followed later by a tachycardia and hypertension.

R. Cows are more sensitive to the effects of xylazine than horses.

S. The initial partial recovery from anesthesia shortly after an IV bolus of propofol is given is because of the rapid metabolism of the drug.

T. We would expect to see bradycardia in an animal given ketamine or tiletamine.

U. Doxapram is an opioid whose side effect includes respiratory depression.

4. Explain why buprenorphine would be preferred to naloxone for reversing the respiratory depression caused by hydromorphone in a dog that just had major orthopedic surgery to repair a complicated fracture.

5. How is the characteristic respiratory depression of opioids used for therapeutic purposes?

6. What side effects do opioids have on the gastrointestinal (GI) tract?

7. What does the pupil do in response to opioid administration? How does this vary with species? Is this a predictable response?

8. What effect do opioids in general have on the heart? Do these changes reduce the amount of blood actually pumped by the heart per minute? Why does morphine produce a drop in arterial blood pressure?

9. Why is it that opioids seem to be somewhat better at blocking dull, aching pain versus the more discrete, sharp pain associated with a surgical incision?

10. Why do animals vomit when given opioids? How does this vary depending on whether the animal is in pain or not when given the opioid?

11. Is morphine mania a real thing in cats?

12. If a small dog needs a smaller dose of fentanyl than can be provided by the smallest fentanyl patch, how can the patch be modified to accommodate the need for a lower dose?

13. Why does fentanyl need to be given by CRI instead of just a bolus IV dose?

14. What precautions must the owner of a pet with a fentanyl patch be educated about before the pet is sent home with the patch?

15. What is a transdermal solution of fentanyl? What precautions must be taken when the veterinary technician or pet owner applies this drug? What additional precautions must the owner take after the medication has been applied?

16. What does blocking an NMDA receptor do? What drugs utilize this mechanism to produce their intended effects?

17. Why should tramadol not be used with many behavioral modification drugs?

18. Why would acepromazine not be a good tranquilizer to use to calm a dog before an allergy skin testing procedure?

19. Phenothiazine's alpha 1 blocking effect has what effect on the body?

20. Stimulating a γ-aminobutyric acid A ($GABA_A$) receptor has what general effect on the nervous system? Increasing release of GABA neurotransmitter would be expected to have what effect?

21. Diazepam and midazolam are both capable of stimulating a cat's appetite. Why are they not used for that purpose anymore?

22. Why can the use of α_2-agonist drugs to treat equine colic actually interfere with the veterinarian's ability assess the progression of the colic condition?

23. A veterinary technician gave a dose of medetomidine to a dog to relieve pain from a pelvic fracture. The degree of analgesia provided did not seem to achieve the desired level. Should a second dose of medetomidine be given to increase the depth of analgesia?

24. What is the physiologic mechanism by which xylazine causes an initial bradycardia and hypertension?

25. As the initial effect of xylazine on the α_1 receptors decreases, what happens to the heart rate and arterial blood pressure?

26. What species are the most sensitive to the effects of α_2-agonist drugs?

27. Why will a frightened dog not become sedated very quickly when given α_2-agonist drugs?

28. How does the dose of a xylazine for a cow compare with that of a horse? What species is most resistant to the effects of α_2-agonist drugs?

29. Why is dexmedetomidine considered to be a more "refined" drug than medetomidine?

30. Does the apnea produced by normal doses of propofol usually require emergency intervention?

31. A German shepherd has a dislocated hip caused by being hit by a car. The veterinarian wants to manipulate the dislocated hip back into place. Why would dissociative anesthetics not be good anesthetic choices by themselves for this procedure?

32. A cat is in recovery from a 40-min procedure in which ketamine and an opioid were used as the only anesthetic agents. You notice the cat is squinting and its eyes seem painful. What might be a reason for this given the types of anesthetic agents that were used?

33. Is the generation of compound A considered to be a serious threat to normal kidney function in veterinary patients that have a single surgical procedure with sevoflurane?

34. Why must the oxygen flow rate on the anesthetic machine be turned way up at the end of any procedure in which nitrous oxide was used as an adjunct anesthetic gas?

35. A client telephones and asks if his 65-lb Siberian husky will become ill from the half of a milk chocolate bar it just stole off the kitchen table. Is this a potential health threat?

Drugs Affecting the Nervous System: Anticonvulsants and Behavior-Modifying Drugs

CHAPTER OUTLINE

OBJECTIVES

After studying this chapter, the veterinary technician should be able to:

- Utilize the correct terminology to describe seizure and convulsive activity.
- Explain the role of phenobarbital, diazepam (or other benzodiazepines), and bromides in controlling either status epilepticus or providing long-term control of epileptic seizures.
- Explain the idiosyncratic reactions seen with phenobarbital and what these reactions mean to the patient and the use of phenobarbital in the patient.

- Explain the mechanisms by which benzodiazepines and phenobarbital produce their anticonvulsant activity.
- Recognize the names of other anticonvulsant drugs that are sometimes used in veterinary medicine.
- Explain the general principles of how behavior-modifying drugs work.
- Give examples of drugs that are used to modify behavior that belong to the antipsychotic, the antidepressant, and the anxiolytic drug groups.
- Identify the behavior-modifying drugs that are specifically Food and Drug Administration (FDA) approved for use in veterinary medicine.

KEY TERMS

adjunct drug
alanine aminotransferase (ALT)
alkaline phosphatase (ALP)
anticonvulsants
antidepressant
antipsychotic
anxiolytic
clonic seizures
convulsions
cytochrome P-450 (CYP)
drug-induced hepatopathy
epilepsy
epilepsy of unknown origin
focal seizures
gamma (γ)-aminobutyric acid (GABA)

gamma (γ)-aminobutyric acid A (GABA$_A$) receptors
generalized seizures
genetic epilepsy
grain (measurement)
hyperthermia
hypoxia
ictus
idiopathic epilepsy
idiosyncratic adverse reaction
induced
limbic system
major tranquilizers
mixed-function oxidases (MFOs)
monoamine oxidase inhibitors (MAOIs)

neuropathic pain
polydipsic
polyphagic
polyuric
postictal phase
prodrome or prodromal phase
selective serotonin reuptake inhibitors (SSRIs)
serotonin syndrome
structural epilepsy
status epilepticus
therapeutic monitoring
tonic seizures
tonic–clonic seizures
tricyclic antidepressants (TCAs)

In addition to the central nervous system (CNS) effects associated with drugs used to calm animals, manage pain, or stimulate the CNS, two other groups of CNS-related drugs are also used in veterinary medicine. This chapter focuses on the mechanisms of action and problems encountered when using anticonvulsant drugs and drugs for modifying behavior.

ANTICONVULSANTS

Seizures are periods of excessive brain electrical activity that can appear outwardly as a variety of signs depending on what area of the brain is affected. Seizures can be generalized or focal depending whether one area of the brain or the entire brain is affected. Focal seizures may appear as muscle movement of one limb or area of the body and the animal typically does not lose consciousness. Generalized seizures, as would be expected, involve all of the body and often are associated with a loss of consciousness.

Convulsions are seizures that manifest themselves as spastic muscle movement caused by stimulation of motor nerves in the brain or spinal cord. Seizure convulsions are characterized as tonic seizures in which there is increased skeletal muscle tone resulting in stiffening of limbs, clonic seizures in which there is rapid contraction and relaxation of muscles, and the more common tonic–clonic seizures that used to be called "grand mal" seizures and consist of a rapidly alternating tonic seizures and clonic seizures.

Although seizures generally originate from the brain, seizure activity can also be caused by various pathologic states that only secondarily affect the brain and include conditions such as hypoxia (i.e., low tissue oxygen tension), hypoglycemia (i.e., low blood sugar level), and hypocalcemia (i.e., low blood calcium level). Toxicity from lead or strychnine; infectious diseases such as canine distemper; or conditions involving the CNS, such as hydrocephalus, brain neoplasia, and parasitic migration through the CNS may also precipitate seizures. Although the actual seizure activity itself may, in some cases, be treated with an anticonvulsant, the underlying problem must be corrected before seizure activity ceases.

Recurrent seizures originating from the brain are referred to as epilepsy and are characterized by sudden loss of motor control, unconsciousness, and tonic–clonic seizures of a relatively short duration (2–3 min). Beyond this definition of epilepsy, there is considerable debate about the terminology used to describe the origin of the epileptic seizure and how it manifests, with different authors choosing to use different descriptions Many definitions are adopted from standards for describing epilepsy in humans. Some of the more common terms are listed below:

- Idiopathic epilepsy is a term that literally translates into "cause of the epilepsy is unknown" and hence the term idiopathic is loosely applied to epilepsy in which there is no definitive cause identified after a diagnostic workup (i.e., a tumor, seizure-causing chemical, toxin, or disease was not identified).
- Status epilepticus refers to the state of being in the seizure activity and often is used to describe the condition of animals with prolonged seizure activity.

- Prodrome or prodromal phase refers to the signs that appear before the actual seizures. In human medicine this may be referred to as the *aura* because patients feel or *foresee* that they are about to experience a seizure. Animals may experience an aura or prodrome in which they seek out their owners, appear anxious, pace, or whine.
- Ictus is the seizure activity itself.
- Postictal phase occurs after the seizure activity has subsided. During this phase, which can last from seconds to hours, the animal may appear tired, confused, anxious, or even blind, depending on the nature and location of the seizure activity within the CNS and the type of seizure experienced.
- Genetic epilepsy is a term now preferred by some veterinarians to describe animals whose epilepsy is most likely traced to a breed or genetic predisposition.
- Structural epilepsy is a term used to describe epilepsy that can be attributed to identified lesions within the brain.
- Epilepsy of unknown origin is when the cause of the epilepsy (i.e., genetic origin or structural lesion in the brain) has not been identified.

Regardless of the descriptive terminology, drugs used to control seizures are called anticonvulsants. Most seizures associated with epilepsy, although frightening to the animal's owner, are usually not life threatening. However, prolonged seizure activity, such as occurs with toxicity or brain pathology, can result in hyperthermia (i.e., elevated body temperature) from prolonged muscle activity, hypoxia (i.e., low oxygen levels) from the inability to expand the chest because of prolonged thoracic muscle contractions, or severe acidosis (i.e., pH of the blood becomes more acidic) from the release of lactic acid from overworked muscles. Once status epilepticus is controlled with anticonvulsants the veterinarian must identify or rule out the cause of the seizure activity. Idiopathic epilepsy is often the default diagnosis after other causes have been ruled out.

The goal of seizure control with anticonvulsants is to find a balance between the needs of the animal and the emotional and practical limits of the owner. For example, a dog that has minor seizures twice a year with 6 months of normal behavior between episodes may not be a candidate for daily anticonvulsant therapy because the seizures themselves pose no significant risk to the animal and the amount of diligence to give medication on a daily basis is unrealistic for the owner's situation. On the other hand, if the client or family members are upset by even the occasional seizure (e.g., large dog in a household with small children) and they are willing to medicate the animal daily, the goal may be to use daily medication to eliminate seizures completely or reduce them to very mild ones of short duration and infrequent occurrence. Seizure activity in a horse or livestock animal usually warrants euthanasia because of the potential for injury to animal handlers and others near the animal during a seizure.

Phenobarbital

Phenobarbital is still the drug of choice given orally for long-term control of seizures in dogs and cats. This barbiturate is inexpensive and, because of its long half-life, may be given orally once or twice a day. It is fairly well established that phenobarbital acts by decreasing the likelihood of spontaneous depolarization in brain cells and reduces the spread of electrical activity throughout the brain from this seizure focus (i.e., the point of seizure origin) by enhancing the action of the gamma (γ)-aminobutyric acid (GABA) neurotransmitter. The result of these two effects is a decrease in seizure frequency and a lessening of the seizure severity.

For phenobarbital to be effective in controlling seizures caused by active underlying pathology, concentrations of the drug must continuously remain in the normal therapeutic range. Fortunately, phenobarbital is relatively slowly removed from the body, which requires only daily or twice-daily administration of the medication to maintain therapeutic concentrations. This dosing schedule is reasonable for most clients to maintain on a long-term basis.

Although the therapeutic range for phenobarbital is fairly well established for dogs and cats, the dosages required to achieve and maintain those therapeutic concentrations vary widely from patient to patient based upon the amount of drug needed to control the seizure focus and the wide variability in how the individual animal metabolizes the drug.

Phenobarbital is biotransformed by mixed-function oxidases (MFOs), a family of enzymes found primarily in the liver. The particular MFO enzyme involved with phenobarbital metabolism is called cytochrome P-450 (CYP) and was mentioned in Chapter 3 regarding metabolism of drugs in general, as many drugs are metabolized by this enzyme.

Mixed function oxidases can be induced by the repeated administration of phenobarbital, meaning that the number of MFO enzymes increases with repeated exposure to the drug and results in more rapid metabolism of the phenobarbital. As a result of induced metabolism, the concentrations of active drug in the blood will decrease as the body becomes more efficient at metabolizing the drug, decreasing the effectiveness of the phenobarbital dose, and allowing seizure activity to resume or worsen. This induced metabolism is the basis behind the drug tolerance and increased dose required to control seizures when barbiturates are initially used.

The half-life of elimination for these drugs varies widely in dogs and cats, reflecting the differences in the ability of the liver to convert the active drug to the more readily excreted metabolite. Canine half-lives from various studies range from 30 to 90 h, with feline studies showing a similarly wide range. Because of this wide range in metabolic rate and elimination half-life, two dogs of the same weight, age, and breed can require very different phenobarbital dosages to achieve the same drug concentrations in the blood. In addition, the phenobarbital half-life for the individual patient can change over time because of hepatic induction of the phenobarbital metabolism requiring the dose be increased to compensate. Cats have a lower therapeutic range for phenobarbital than dogs, consequently, phenobarbital dosages in cats are approximately half of those used in dogs.

Because plasma phenobarbital concentrations achieved with any given dose vary considerably from patient to patient, when an animal shows either signs of toxicity or the therapy is not adequately controlling seizures, the only way to be sure a dosage regimen is adequate is to check blood concentrations of phenobarbital (i.e., therapeutic monitoring). Without therapeutic monitoring, the veterinarian is unable to accurately know whether the patient's unacceptable seizure control is caused by inadequate dosing of phenobarbital or the disease itself becoming refractory (unable to be controlled) to the phenobarbital drug effects. Because higher doses of phenobarbital are associated with greater risk of adverse reactions including potentially fatal liver reactions, the time spent to determine the phenobarbital blood concentration allows the veterinarian to more intelligently adjust the phenobarbital dosage or select a different anticonvulsant drug.

Adverse Effects of Phenobarbital

When many animals are started on oral phenobarbital tablets to control epileptic seizure activity, they show signs of sedation and ataxia (i.e., they may wobble or stagger when walking). This is usually a temporary effect reflecting an initial high concentration of phenobarbital being achieved in the blood and body tissues. Owners need to be advised that these side effects should diminish over the first 2–3 weeks of therapy. Severe sedation or continuous ataxia that persists may be a sign of phenobarbital overdose; however, this can only be verified if therapeutic monitoring of phenobarbital plasma concentrations are determined by submission of a blood sample for testing.

Dogs or cats on phenobarbital may become polyphagic (i.e., increase in appetite), polydipsic (i.e., increase in drinking), or polyuric (i.e., increase in urination), although these signs appear far less frequently in cats. Phenobarbital appears to have an inhibitory effect on the release of antidiuretic hormone (ADH), a hormone that normally helps the body conserve water by reducing water loss through the kidneys as urine. With a decreased effect of antidiuretic hormone, the animal excretes more water (polyuria) and subsequently needs to drink more water to compensate. The polyuria and polydipsia tend to diminish with time, although some animals may show these signs to some degree the entire time they are on phenobarbital. These signs quickly disappear after the drug is discontinued.

Serum levels of liver-associated enzymes such as alkaline phosphatase (ALP) and alanine aminotransferase (ALT) usually increase after an animal has received phenobarbital for a few days. As long as the animal is otherwise acting normal and other liver parameters such as the serum bile acid levels (called *serum bile acids* or just *bile acids*) remain normal, the elevated ALT and ALP are most likely not indicative of liver disease but reflect a normal increase that is expected with phenobarbital administration. ALP does not appear to increase in cats as much as it does in dogs. The increased serum concentrations of ALT and ALP in animals as a result of phenobarbital administration return to normal a few weeks after phenobarbital therapy is discontinued.

Phenobarbital-induced hepatotoxicity or drug-induced hepatopathy (i.e., liver disease caused by drugs) is an idiosyncratic adverse reaction (i.e., the reaction cannot be predicted) and occurs relatively rarely in dogs but has not been reported in cats.[1] The cause is unknown and may be fatal if the condition is not recognized and treated early enough. The cause may be associated with metabolism of phenobarbital to hepatotoxic metabolites within the liver, the exposure to hepatotoxic drugs or other hepatotoxic compounds in the environment when the animal is on phenobarbital, or high doses and prolonged treatment with the drug.[2] However, because the reaction is considered idiosyncratic, no specific, repeatable cause has been identified. As stated earlier, the alteration of liver parameters other than ALT and ALP can help differentiate phenobarbital hepatotoxicity from the expected increased enzyme activity from phenobarbital use.

Occasionally a dog receiving phenobarbital becomes excitable or hyperactive instead of lethargic or sedated. This may occur at a subtherapeutic dose, and an increase in the dose of phenobarbital does not necessarily seem to decrease this effect until very high concentrations of phenobarbital are achieved. This idiosyncratic reaction to phenobarbital is not predictable and is not dose dependent. That is, as the dose increases, signs do not necessarily increase in severity. Often these animals need to be switched to a different anticonvulsant.

The dose of phenobarbital is often measured in grains, with 1 grain equaling approximately 60 mg. The apothecary scale conversion of grains to milligrams is technically 1 grain = 64.8 mg; however, today that conversion is typically rounded to 1 grain = 60 mg. Tablets are usually available in ¼-, ½-, and 1-grain sizes, which roughly correspond to 15, 30, and 60 mg, respectively. Tablets are also available in as 100-mg tablets that is roughly equivalent to 1.5 grains.

Because the mixed function oxidases (MFOs) are also responsible for metabolism of a number of other commonly used veterinary drugs, phenobarbital induction of this enzyme system can result in other drugs also being broken down more rapidly with a subsequent decrease in concentrations. Therefore, epileptic animals treated with phenobarbital may need to have the dose of any other drugs using the same metabolic pathway increased to compensate for their accelerated metabolism. A general rule is to always check drug resources for potential drug interactions when any additional drug is given to an animal already on phenobarbital.

Benzodiazepines

Benzodiazepine tranquilizers control seizures by rapidly penetrating the blood–brain barrier and enhancing the inhibitory effect of the CNS neurotransmitter GABA mentioned with phenobarbital. Because GABA helps counter the effect of stimulatory neurotransmitters in the brain, such as acetylcholine and norepinephrine, enhancing the GABA effect quiets the activity and excitability of the CNS.

Diazepam (Valium) is an older benzodiazepine tranquilizer but is still a commonly used drug of first choice for treatment of animals in status epilepticus. Other benzodiazepine tranquilizers considered for use as anticonvulsants include midazolam, clonazepam, lorazepam, and clorazepate.

Diazepam comes in oral (PO) and intravenous (IV) dose forms. Although diazepam is quite effective for a short time when given IV, it is far less effective when given PO especially in dogs. Approximately 2%–5% of the diazepam given orally to dogs actually makes it to the systemic circulation because of the significant liver metabolism from the first-pass effect (see Chapter 3 to review first-pass effect). Because the metabolites of diazepam have less anticonvulsant activity than diazepam itself (25%–33% less), the first-pass effect makes diazepam a relatively ineffective drug when given PO.[3] This rapid, efficient hepatic metabolism also explains diazepam's fairly short duration of activity when it is given intravenously.

Another reason why diazepam is not used to control seizure activity long term is that the body develops tolerance to the diazepam activity very quickly. In most dogs, tolerance is noticed within a week of starting diazepam treatment.[3] This tolerance plus the first-pass effect and short half-life limit diazepam's use in the dog to IV treatment for active status epilepticus but not as oral medication for long-term maintenance of seizure control.

Cats are less efficient at metabolizing diazepam than dogs; therefore, diazepam theoretically should remain available for longer in the cat than the dog and be more effective as an anticonvulsant for maintaining control on a long-term basis. However, a fatal idiosyncratic drug-induced hepatopathy has been reported in cats receiving low-dose diazepam for treatment of behavior disorders. For this reason, most clinicians are cautious about long-term use of diazepam in cats, and phenobarbital is still the drug of choice for long-term control of seizures in cats just as it is in dogs.

If diazepam is added to a bottle or bag of IV fluids as part of a constant rate infusion (CRI), the mixture should be inverted several times to more evenly distribute the diazepam in the solution because it does not mix well with most IV fluids. If an animal in status epilepticus cannot be administered diazepam IV, the drug can be administered per rectum. This has been suggested as a method by which an owner can safely administer diazepam to prevent a seizure in an animal that is showing prodromal signs of an epileptic episode or as a treatment to stop a prolonged epileptic seizure. A gel formulation of diazepam (Diastat) is available in the United States for per rectum administration.

Side effects of injectable diazepam are usually minimal compared with barbiturates or opioids. Because benzodiazepine tranquilizers are muscle relaxants, the drug can produce ataxia and weakness. Diazepam also may reduce the effects of training or learned behavior, potentially allowing more aggressive or territorial behaviors exhibited previously before training to manifest again. Because of this behavioral change and because diazepam does not have any analgesic properties, veterinary technicians must always remember that a relaxed animal on benzodiazepine tranquilizer is still quite capable of responding in an aggressive and dangerous manner if the technician causes pain or if a stimulus for aggressive behavior occurs.

The other benzodiazepines (**midazolam, clonazepam, lorazepam**, and **clorazepate**) have similar penetrability into the brain and can decrease seizure activity with a mechanism similar to diazepam. Midazolam has been used as a diazepam substitute for control of active seizures and was generally thought to be fairly equivalent in its action, although there was no consistent agreement among veterinarians on this point.

Some benzodiazepines like clonazepam and clorazepate come in a tablet form that can be used as an adjunct drug (i.e., second drug added to the main drug dosage regimen) to help control seizures on a long-term basis. However, all these benzodiazepines have problems with a significant first-pass effect when given PO and must be given multiple times a day to maintain therapeutic concentrations. As with diazepam, most animals develop a significant tolerance to the other benzodiazepine drugs within a relatively short period, limiting their long-term use for seizure control.

It has been reported that animals on benzodiazepines for an extended period of time exhibit signs of withdrawal if the medication is abruptly stopped. Signs include listlessness, decreased appetite, weight loss, fever, and even recumbency. Thus, if the drug is to be stopped after long-term use of these drugs, the patient's dose must be tapered off over several days or weeks, depending on the length of time the patient was on the drug.[4,5]

Bromides

Potassium bromide is a very old drug. Bromides were used in the 1800s to treat a wide variety of "nervous disorders." Today, **potassium bromide** and **sodium bromide** are used as adjunct therapies for dogs whose seizures are not well controlled by phenobarbital alone.[6]

Bromide is more of a chemical reagent than a drug. It has been formulated into an FDA-approved chewable tablet form that is available through regular pharmacies; bromide can also be mixed with different flavored liquids or made into other dose forms by compounding pharmacies.

The mechanism of action of the drug is not clearly defined; however, it may act like chloride ions to change the resting membrane potential of neurons, making them more difficult to depolarize (i.e., fire), or it may enhance the activity of GABA neurotransmitter as described with phenobarbital and the benzodiazepines.[3] Regardless of the mechanism, the net effect is a nervous system that is less likely to spontaneously discharge and produce a seizure.

Like phenobarbital, potassium bromide has a long half-life. Whereas phenobarbital's half-life is measured in hours, potassium bromide's half-life in the dog is 21–24 days. Clinically this is important because it takes potassium bromide 3–5 months to reach steady-state concentrations (the formula is "Steady state = 5 × half-life"; see Chapter 3 on steady state). To avoid this lag time between when the drug is first given and when it reaches therapeutic concentrations, a single large loading dose or multiple medium-sized loading doses can be given to establish concentrations within the therapeutic range. Once therapeutic concentrations are achieved, a smaller maintenance dose is then given to keep the concentrations within range.

Vomiting may occur even if the bromide dose produces blood concentrations within the therapeutic range. This appears to be a direct gastric irritation effect of the sodium or potassium salt on the stomach. Vomiting can be reduced by using a liquid formulation instead of a capsule, by dividing the prescribed dose into twice-daily or three-times-daily doses, and by trying different foods with the potassium bromide to see which are most effective at decreasing the vomiting.[7]

Bromides are not used in cats because they can produce a respiratory syndrome that resembles bronchial asthma. These respiratory effects are common enough to warrant avoiding the use of bromides for seizure control in cats.

Although some neurologists are trying to use bromides as solo anticonvulsants, most often they are used in conjunction with phenobarbital when phenobarbital by itself fails to adequately control seizure activity.[3,4] As an alternative, bromides may be used to lower the amount of phenobarbital required to control the seizure activity, thereby decreasing the risk for a phenobarbital drug-induced hepatopathy. Even if phenobarbital and bromide levels are within acceptable therapeutic concentrations, the combination of these drugs often produces excessive sedation or ataxia requiring the phenobarbital dose to be decreased when the bromide is added.

When bromide is added to the phenobarbital regimen, the veterinary technician plays an important role in educating the client on the importance of checking anticonvulsant blood concentrations; the expected side effects that may be observed at home; and the possibility for breakthrough seizure activity as dosages are adjusted.

Other Anticonvulsants

Because development of antiseizure medications in humans continues, these drugs will continue to be "borrowed" for clinical trials or reported anecdotally in veterinary medicine. Veterinary technicians will hear these drugs mentioned at conferences or may have a veterinarian who wants to try out one of these drugs on an animal that is not responding particularly well to phenobarbital or the phenobarbital/bromide combination for long-term seizure control. Therefore, the veterinary technician should be able to recognize the names of these other anticonvulsants and have a basic understanding of significant adverse effects.

Zonisamide

Although unavailable in Canada, the human antiseizure medication **zonisamide** has been increasingly mentioned in the veterinary literature in the United States as an orally administered capsule drug used in dogs that are refractory to other anticonvulsants. Zonisamide is actually a sulfonamide (like the sulfa antibiotics), which makes it unique among the anticonvulsants; however, its mechanism is unknown. Some veterinarians advocate this drug as a seizure control drug in dogs when seizures are fairly infrequent.[8] However, this is not a universally accepted opinion because so little is known about how the drug is handled by the body and the extent of its adverse reactions.

Levetiracetam (Keppra)

Levetiracetam is also advocated by some as a first-line drug for mild seizures of fairly low frequency because of its safety and availability in an oral tablet and injectable form throughout North America and Europe.[8] Others advocate it as an adjunct anticonvulsant to be used with phenobarbital or phenobarbital/bromide combinations.[4] It does not work by mechanisms previously cited (e.g., it does not enhance GABA), nor does it seem to interact with any known neurotransmitter, ion channel (e.g., the chloride channels associated with GABA receptor stimulation), or receptor. It might interfere with the release of neurotransmitters from neurons, thus decreasing the ability of neurons to communicate with each other across synapses. The immediate release formulation (IR) does need to be given every 8 h, which decreases likelihood of client compliance for consistently administering the medication on a reliable schedule. The sustained release (SR) formulation is commonly used to reduce administration to twice daily; however, neurologists commonly stabilize a patient with the immediate release formulation before transitioning to the sustained release formulation. This drug is commonly used for both dogs and cats and is reportedly well tolerated. This medication may be used alone or in addition to other antiseizure medications.

Gabapentin

Gabapentin was a drug favored as an adjunct drug in the late 1990s and early 2000s. However, it has fallen out of favor because it does not seem to be as effective as levetiracetam or zonisamide in helping to control refractory seizures in dogs.[1,8] It is available as a capsule and oral solution; however, the oral solution may contain xylitol, which should not be used in dogs because of xylitol's effect on blood sugar (hypoglycemia) and the liver (hepatic necrosis).[3] The drug itself seems to be well tolerated by both dogs and cats when used as an adjunct drug with phenobarbital, but its degree of seizure control is variable, and there are mixed reviews by veterinary authors about its overall effectiveness.

One of the functions gabapentin is still used for in veterinary medicine is to control neuropathic pain, which is pain that originates not from a nociceptor but from the pain neurons themselves depolarizing and sending pain signals that confuse the brain into thinking there is trauma or injury to the part of the body supplied by that particular pain sensory nerve.

Gabapentin is gaining popularity for its sedation effect on cats and dogs before stressful events, such as going to the veterinary clinic. Veterinarians will commonly prescribe gabapentin to be given the day before, and again 2 h before travel to relax the dog or cat before attending the veterinary visit.[9–11]

This medication is a controlled substance in many states, and or a reportable drug on prescription drug monitoring programs. This increased reporting is due to the fact that gabapentin, when combined with other drugs of abuse, increases the effects of those drugs. For this reason, gabapentin should be treated as a controlled substance in relation to how it is stored and inventoried.

Primidone

Primidone is an approved drug for use as an anticonvulsant in dogs. Although primidone has some anticonvulsant activity of its own, most of the drug's efficacy is attributable to primidone's metabolism to phenobarbital. The other primidone metabolite, phenylethylmalonamide, has weak anticonvulsant activity in dogs. Because the efficacy of primidone largely depends on its metabolism to phenobarbital, many clinicians simply give phenobarbital rather than primidone. The side effects and drug interactions of primidone are similar to those seen with phenobarbital. Long-term use of large doses of primidone has been implicated in drug-induced hepatopathy.

There are other human anticonvulsant drugs sometimes used in veterinary medicine not listed here, and it is likely that additional human drugs will continue to be considered for use in veterinary medicine. Most will have mechanisms similar to those described for the drugs presented in this chapter. The veterinary technician should remain current on anticonvulsant therapies and be able to answer questions related to the drugs and their side effects.

BEHAVIOR-MODIFYING DRUGS

Personality, emotions, and fears are the result of a complex, integrated balance (or imbalance) of a wide variety of chemical neurotransmitters. This complexity shows how readily normal brain function can be altered by even minor changes in concentrations of various neurotransmitters. Chapter 8 discussed how several of these neurotransmitters (e.g., acetylcholine, epinephrine, GABA) were altered to produce changes in brain function that resulted in the beneficial effects of anesthesia, sedation, tranquilization, or analgesia. Activity in the brain can be decreased by suppressing the release of norepinephrine (e.g., xylazine acting on α_2 receptors to decrease norepinephrine release) or enhancing the activity of inhibitory neurotransmitters like GABA (e.g., diazepam and other benzodiazepine tranquilizers). Brain activity can also be increased by the use of methylxanthine compounds such as caffeine from coffee or theobromine in chocolate. Thus, is it easy to see how an imbalance of neurotransmitters can result in clinical depression, behavior changes, old-age memory changes, self-destructive activities, or anxiety/fear. As society has come to recognize that signs of some of these human behavioral syndromes seem to occur in pets, an interest has developed in using the human mood-altering medications to control what are perceived to be similar syndromes in pets.

Without a doubt, the use of behavior-modifying drug therapeutics is a complex study of pharmacology and has a wide range of differing opinions about the best course of action for approaching pet behavioral problems. This section provides some basic terminology and mechanisms so that the veterinary technician may gain an entry-level understanding of what these drugs do and how they are proposed to modify behaviors of the animal. Dosages and drugs change continuously; for the most current information on any drug or its dose, the veterinary professional needs to consult a valid, current website with reputable experts cited as the information sources.

What Are Behavior-Modifying Drugs?

Essentially, behavior-modifying drugs change the concentrations of selected neurotransmitters in the brain with the intent of decreasing or enhancing a specific mental (neuronal) activity. These drugs all work by one of the following general mechanisms:

- Enhancing the release of either inhibitory or excitatory neurotransmitters
- Enhancing the binding (i.e., affinity) of neurotransmitters to their receptors
- Imitating the natural neurotransmitter and combining with the neurotransmitter's receptor to stimulate the receptor (i.e., agonist effect)
- Imitating the natural neurotransmitter and combining with the neurotransmitter's receptor to reduce or prevent stimulation of the receptor (i.e., antagonist effect)
- Prolonging the action of the neurotransmitter by decreasing the breakdown or slowing the rate of termination of the neurotransmitter itself

- Shortening the action of the neurotransmitter by enhancing its breakdown or termination

The net effect of these mechanisms is to either increase or decrease the action of a neurotransmitter and thus its activity in specific regions of the brain.

A variety of terms are used to describe behavior-modifying drugs; however, the three following terms capture the basic descriptions applied to behavior-modifying drugs used in veterinary medicine.

Antipsychotic drugs are also called major tranquilizers and include phenothiazine tranquilizers such as acepromazine. Even though veterinary patients do not express specific, identified psychoses, these drugs still play a role in treating behavior disorders in pets.

Antidepressant drugs, as the name implies, are mood-elevating drugs used in human therapy. In veterinary medicine, antidepressants are used for a number of behaviors in pets that are not necessarily associated with what we would call "depressed" behaviors.

Anxiolytic drugs are drugs that "lyse" anxiety or decrease fear responses and were discussed with the tranquilizers in Chapter 8.

Antipsychotic Drugs

Antipsychotic drugs include the **phenothiazine tranquilizers** like **acepromazine**. Other drugs in human medicine classified as antipsychotics are not commonly used in veterinary medicine because of their limited anxiolytic properties, abundant side effects, and spontaneous muscle movement caused by blocking dopamine receptors in the brain. The additional motor movements can sometimes be interpreted as seizure-related convulsions, but they are actually reflecting the neurotransmitter imbalance caused by these drugs blocking dopamine receptors.

Increased dopamine and the stimulation of dopamine receptors in parts of the brain involved with emotion (i.e., the limbic system) have been shown to result in abnormal behaviors. Thus, blocking dopamine receptors in this area of the brain allows other neurotransmitters to dominate and decreases the incidence of the abnormal behaviors related to emotions. Phenothiazine tranquilizers are also known to have a variety of effects on other receptors that may or may not contribute to a particular behavior. However, the dopamine-blocking (i.e., antagonist) effect does help explain the change in emotional behavior observed with animals on phenothiazine tranquilizers.

Generally, this class of drugs in veterinary medicine is used to decrease inappropriate behavioral responses to stimuli but has the disadvantage of reducing both normal and abnormal responses to the environment. In other words, these drugs are not very specific in their mechanism of action and produce their beneficial effects at the cost of calming all behaviors, including those behaviors that are not necessarily desirable to decrease.

Animals and people on these drugs tend to have less interest in their environment, have fewer emotional responses to stimuli, and have a depression of complex behaviors. Learned responses (but not instinctual responses) of avoidance to certain stimuli (e.g., audio reprimand, visual fear stimulus) are reduced with the use of phenothiazine tranquilizers. This is one reason why phenothiazines are used to control learned fear responses associated with thunderstorms, firecrackers, or other stimuli.

However, because phenothiazines do not suppress instinctual responses, treatment can sometimes result in uncovering of underlying inappropriate behaviors. For example, phenothiazines are generally not recommended for use in suppressing aggressive behavior problems. Some aggressive animals may have learned adaptive behaviors that have reduced their displayed natural aggression to fit into the social order in a human household or to avoid receiving negative reinforcement (i.e., punishment). If a phenothiazine tranquilizer is used to attempt to "tranquilize" the displayed level of aggression, the animal's learned response to control aggressive tendencies may be lessened, allowing the instinctual aggressive behavior to reemerge. The animal actually may become more aggressive and startle more readily in response to stimuli or situations. Thus, as with all drugs, an understanding of the limitations of the phenothiazines for behavior-modification therapy is important.

Antidepressant Drugs

Three classes of antidepressant drugs used in human beings have also found use in veterinary medicine: the tricyclic antidepressants (TCAs), the selective serotonin reuptake inhibitors (SSRIs), and the monoamine oxidase inhibitors (MAOIs). The TCAs are named for their chemical structure, and the latter two drug groups are named for the mechanisms by which they work.

Tricyclic antidepressants (TCAs) used in veterinary medicine are mostly human products; however, there is a veterinary version of **clomipramine** that is marketed as the FDA-approved veterinary product **Clomicalm**. Other TCA human products used in veterinary medicine include amitriptyline, doxepin, imipramine, desipramine, and nortriptyline.[12] All of these drugs work by decreasing the reuptake of serotonin and norepinephrine from the synaptic cleft (i.e., the space in the synapse between two communicating neurons), which allows the neurotransmitter to accumulate and prolongs its stimulatory activity.[13]

TCA drugs have been used effectively in humans to decrease excessive arousal and reduce anxiety; thus, they are used to treat generalized anxiety and separation anxiety behaviors in dogs and cats, decrease inappropriate spraying and excessive grooming in cats, and reduce excessive feather plucking in birds.[5] Clomipramine's FDA-approved indication is for treatment of obsessive-compulsive disorders in dogs. Obsessive-compulsive disorders are defined as behaviors that are repeated over and over again in the same way and appear to serve no real purpose. Because identification of a true obsessive-compulsive disorder is sometimes difficult to identify in animals (other than repeated licking, chewing, or grooming), a more common use for clomipramine is for treatment of separation anxiety and aggressive behaviors.

TCA drugs do not blunt the overall normal behavioral responses to environmental stimuli to the same degree that phenothiazine tranquilizers do, but they should not be used simultaneously with other antidepressant drugs like SSRIs or MAOIs because of the similar mechanisms of the drugs.

Before using any TCA, the most current warnings and precautions should be researched online from reputable websites. TCAs have many potentially adverse effects, and new information on veterinary patients is becoming available all the time. TCAs can cause severe reactions if used with certain other drugs or specific medical or disease conditions, the list of which is too long to be included here.

As with most of these behavior-modifying drugs, TCA drugs must be taken every day for the problem behavior to change. In addition, the response to the treatment will not be seen for several days because of the time it takes for the brain biochemistry to readjust to the drug's effect. In addition, it may take a few weeks for the drug to have its full effect, which means the evaluation of the treatment cannot be accurately performed until the animal has been taking the drug consistently for 2–4 weeks.[5]

Just like in human medicine, the individual patient's variable response to these drugs means that one TCA could work very well in Patient A but have poor results or even adverse effects at the very same dose for the same behavioral disorder in Patient B. Often dosages have to be adjusted or drugs changed until the right combination of drug and dose is found for a particular patient. The veterinary technician plays a key role in communicating this important point to the clients or pet owners so they do not get discouraged when the behavioral problem fails to disappear in a few days.

Selective serotonin reuptake inhibitors (SSRIs) are another class of antidepressants derived from TCA drugs; thus, they share part of the same mechanism described for TCA drugs but are more selective for blocking only serotonin reuptake instead of reuptake of both norepinephrine and serotonin like the TCAs do. Many of the names of human SSRI drugs are familiar from television advertisements: fluoxetine (Prozac), paroxetine (Paxil), sertraline (Zoloft), and fluvoxamine (Luvox).[13] **Reconcile** is the trade name for the FDA-approved version of **fluoxetine** for use in dogs to treat separation anxiety.[5]

Serotonin is a neurotransmitter identified as playing a significant role in determining mood and behavior. The SSRI drugs enhance the effect of the serotonin neurotransmitter by blocking its removal from the synaptic cleft. The serotonin remains for a longer period of time at its site of action, accumulates, and extends its effect.[5,14]

Like the TCA drugs, the SSRI drugs take a few weeks to produce their intended effect; in some patients there may be an initial increase in anxiety before there is a decrease in anxiety.[13] Benzodiazepine tranquilizers may be used initially to smooth the transition until the SSRI has a chance to change the brain chemistry and produce its beneficial effect. The types of behaviors for which these drugs have been used are similar to those of the TCAs and include obsessive-compulsive behaviors, anxiety, and aggression. Fluoxetine and sertraline have been used successfully in pets to specifically treat separation anxiety and the fear of people.

There is evidence that a lack of serotonin in the CNS is associated with excessively aggressive behavior.[5,14] Thus, SSRI drugs, which will increase the effect of serotonin, have been used in dogs to treat dominance-related (dog-to-people) aggression and dog-to-dog aggression.

The side effects of these drugs can be quite diverse. Some authors claim that SSRIs are safer than TCAs because SSRIs have a more specific action than TCA drugs. However, one major precaution is that MAOIs should never be used in combination with the SSRI drugs because the MAOI inhibits the breakdown of precursors for several catecholamine compounds, including serotonin. Thus, the combination of excessive production and release of serotonin by MAOI drugs and inhibition of serotonin removal from the synapse by SSRIs can produce a serotonin toxicity called serotonin syndrome. Serotonin syndrome is potentially fatal and characterized by hypertension (i.e., high arterial blood pressure), hyperthermia, tremors, seizures, and altered mental status.[4]

Monoamine oxidase inhibitors (MAOIs) work by inhibiting the enzyme monoamine oxidase, whose purpose is to catabolize (i.e., break apart) serotonin, dopamine, and norepinephrine. By inhibiting the enzyme, MAOI drugs allow additional accumulation of these neurotransmitters, stimulating the CNS in general. The only MAOI used to any extent in veterinary medicine is **selegiline**, also known as **deprenyl**. Selegiline comes in an FDA-approved form that is marketed as the veterinary product **Anipryl** for use in treating Cushing's disease (i.e., high corticosteroid hormone production) and for "canine cognitive dysfunction" (i.e., old-dog senility).

Selegiline use in dogs tends to inhibit the type of monoamine oxidase enzyme that usually catabolizes dopamine. Thus, unlike the phenothiazines, which block dopamine action and reduce its activity, MAOI drugs increase the amount of dopamine found in selected cells within the CNS and enhance the dopamine effect. Thus, those behavioral problems related to a decrease of available dopamine in selected areas of the brain may be successfully treated with MAOIs. Because old-dog dementia, a senility-like syndrome, is thought to involve a decreased amount of dopamine in parts of the brain, selegiline has been advocated for improving cognitive function.

Selegiline treats hyperadrenocorticism (Cushing's disease) that is caused by excessive production of adrenocorticotropic hormone (ACTH) from the pituitary gland. ACTH normally stimulates release of natural corticosteroids (i.e., cortisol) from the adrenal gland; in pituitary-dependent Cushing's disease, the adrenal gland is normal but is being overstimulated by excessive ACTH from the pituitary, giving the clinical signs of hyperadrenocorticism. See Chapter 13 for a more thorough description of normal corticosteroid production and control. Selegiline blocks the release of excessive ACTH by elevating dopamine levels in the area of the pituitary that creates a negative feedback inhibition that decreases ACTH production, subsequently decreasing cortisol production by the adrenal gland.

Anxiolytic Drugs

Anxiolytic drugs are tranquilizers belonging to the **benzodiazepine** group (e.g., **diazepam, clonazepam, chlorazepate, lorazepam**) discussed with anticonvulsants in this chapter and with tranquilizers in Chapter 8. Benzodiazepines work by facilitating stimulation of the GABA A (GABAA) receptors by the inhibitory neurotransmitter GABA, depressing the neurons of the CNS.

At low doses of diazepam the animals become more relaxed and less excitable. The actual reduction in anxiety (e.g., nervousness in social interactions) does not occur until moderate-level doses of diazepam are used. At high doses, the animals become quite sedated and ataxic and readily fall asleep.[5]

Diazepam and the other members of this group are not used as frequently for behavior modification as some of the other drugs because of their nonspecific activity and their interference with the animal's ability to learn behavior modification. Because behavior modification through training is considered essential to successfully changing unwanted behavior patterns, the use of diazepam may compromise this process.[5]

Though diazepam and the benzodiazepines can be used to reduce general anxiety without requiring behavior modification, they are not the best drugs to use in trying to reduce aggression in veterinary patients. If the pet's aggression is a direct response to anxiety, benzodiazepines may be useful in reducing the aggression. However, if the animal is currently less aggressive because anxiety or fear of punishment is holding that aggressive behavior in check, the use of benzodiazepines may remove that anxiety, allowing full expression of the underlying aggressive behavior.

As mentioned previously, tolerance develops to benzodiazepines with prolonged use, and withdrawal signs can appear in animals that have been on these drugs for more than a few days. The use in cats is limited by the concern over potentially fatal drug-induced hepatopathy that is an idiosyncratic (and therefore not predictable) reaction by the cat liver to the drug or its metabolites.

Trazodone

Trazodone is a serotonin antagonist/reuptake inhibitor that is a human drug commonly used to address anxiety and induce mild sedation in dogs, and less commonly in cats and horses. In dogs this medication is commonly used in the hospital to reduce anxiety, as well as postoperatively to help the dog stay calm if long term cage rest is required.[11,15] This medication has been shown to address anxiety in dogs more effectively than the phenothiazine tranquilizers; therefore, it is more commonly used than acepromazine for this indication.[11,15] This medication has a wide therapeutic index allowing veterinarians to start on the low end of the dosage range and titrate up to the desired effect. This medication does interact with many other drugs, the veterinary technician must be aware of these interactions to be able to effectively monitor the patient for these interactions. A good resource for these interactions is in the Plumb's formulary or the package insert. Trazadone can also be administered to cats prior to travel and horses requiring long term stall rest.

Other Behavior-Modifying Drugs

A wide variety of other medications have been used in an attempt to curb repetitive behavior, aggression, excessive vocalization or other anxiety behaviors, and self-destructive behavior. The list includes β-blockers (see Chapter 5), antihistamines, anticonvulsants (phenobarbital), buspirone (a nonspecific anxiolytic human drug that stimulates serotonin receptors directly), and even progestin drugs. The range of these drugs reflects the complexity of the pharmaceutical side of behavior modification. Unfortunately, many of these drugs have significant side effects that either limit their use or require close monitoring of the animal to avoid significant clinical complications.

The point to remember is that no "magic bullet" exists for behavior therapy. Behavior modification requires training techniques, persistence on the part of the pet owner, and *possibly* medication to assist with the behavior-modifying process. By understanding this point and being aware of the potential problems with using individual behavior-modifying drugs, the veterinary technician can help educate the client to have a realistic view of the capabilities and limitations of the behavior-modifying process.

NERVOUS SYSTEM DRUGS

Anticonvulsants and Behavior Modifiers

Anticonvulsants
Phenobarbital
Benzodiazepines
  Diazepam
  Midazolam
  Clonazepam
  Lorazepam
  Clorazepate
Bromides (sodium and potassium)
Other anticonvulsants
  Zonisamide
  Levetiracetam
  Gabapentin
  Primidone

Behavior-Modifying Drugs
Antipsychotics (phenothiazine tranquilizers)
  Acepromazine
Antidepressants
  Tricyclic antidepressants (TCAs): clomipramine (Clomicalm)
  Selective serotonin reuptake inhibitors (SSRIs): fluoxetine (Reconcile)
  Monoamine oxidase inhibitors (MAOIs): selegiline/deprenyl (Anipryl)
Anxiolytics
Trazodone
  Benzodiazepines
Diazepam
Clonazepam
Chlorazepate
Lorazepam

REFERENCES

1. Parent J. Feline epilepsy: recognition, evaluation, and treatment. In: *Proceedings of the American College of Veterinary Internal Medicine Forum, Nashville, Tennessee*; 2014.
2. Webster CR. Drug induced liver injury in the dog. In: *Proceedings of the American College of Veterinary Internal Medicine Forum, New Orleans, Louisiana*; 2012.
3. Boothe DM. Anticonvulsants and other neurologic therapies in small animals. In: Boothe DM, ed. *Small Animal Clinical Pharmacology and Therapeutics*. Philadelphia: Saunders; 2012:932–993.

4. Papich MG. Anticonvulsant drugs. In: Riviere J, Papich M, eds. *Veterinary Pharmacology and Therapeutics*. Ames, Iowa: Wiley-Blackwell; 2009:493–508.

5. Sherman BL, Papich MG. Drugs affecting animal behavior. In: Riviere J, Papich M, eds. *Veterinary Pharmacology and Therapeutics*. Ames, Iowa: Wiley-Blackwell; 2009:509–538.

6. Plumb DC. Plumb's Veterinary Drug Handbook. 8th ed. Ames, Iowa: Wiley Publishers; 2015. Accessed online: https://academic-plumbs-com.ezproxy.lib.purdue.edu/drug-monograph/ba9xQv20CJPROD?source=search&search. Accessed on 06.12.2022.

7. Baird-Heinz HE, Van Schoick AL, Pelsor FR, et al. A systematic review of the safety of potassium bromide in dogs. *J Am Vet Med Assoc*. 2012;240(6):705–715.

8. Parent J. Antiepileptic drugs in dogs: use and misuse. In: *Proceedings of the American College of Veterinary Internal Medicine Forum, Nashville, Tennessee*; 2014.

9. van Haaften KA, Forsythe LRE, Stelow EA, Bain MJ. Effects of a single preappointment dose of gabapentin on signs of stress in cats during transportation and veterinary examination. *J Am Vet Med Assoc*. 2017;251(10):1175–1181. https://doi.org/10.2460/javma.251.10.1175 [PMID: 29099247].

10. Erickson A, Harbin K, MacPherson J, Rundle K, Overall KL. A review of pre-appointment medications to reduce fear and anxiety in dogs and cats at veterinary visits. *Can Vet J*. 2021;62 (9):952–960 [PMID: 34475580; PMCID: PMC8360309].

11. Sinn L. Advances in behavioral psychopharmacology. *Vet Clin North Am Small Anim Pract*. 2018;48(3):457–471. https://doi.org/10.1016/j.cvsm.2017.12.011. Epub 2018 Feb 5. PMID: 29415813.

12. Wismer T.A.. Antidepressant drug overdoses in dogs (website). https://www.aspcapro.org/sites/default/files/e-toxbrief_0700.pdf. Accessed 06.03.2022.

13. Radosta L. Happy drugs: basic behavioral pharmacology. In: *Proceedings of the 2013 Central Veterinary Conference, Washington, DC*; 2013.

14. Boothe DM. Drugs that modify animal behavior in small animals. In: Boothe DM, ed. *Small Animal Clinical Pharmacology and Therapeutics*. Philadelphia: Saunders; 2012:903–931.

15. Kim SA, Borchardt MR, Lee K, Stelow EA, Bain MJ. Effects of trazodone on behavioral and physiological signs of stress in dogs during veterinary visits: a randomized double-blind placebo-controlled crossover clinical trial. *J Am Vet Med Assoc*. 2022;260 (8):876–883. https://doi.org/10.2460/javma.20.10.0547 [PMID: 35333743].

FURTHER READING

Overall KL. Rational use of behavioral medication for cats. In: *Proceedings of the 2012 Atlantic Coast Veterinary Conference*. Atlantic City, New Jersey; 2012.

SELF-ASSESSMENT

1. Fill in the following blanks with the correct item from the Key Terms list.

   A. _____ This term means a type of drug that is used to control seizure activity.

   B. _____ This describes the periods of excessive brain electrical activity.

   C. _____ This is a type of seizure that is limited to one limb or one area of the body.

   D. _____ This is a type of seizure in which the entire body is involved and often is associated with a loss of consciousness.

   E. _____ This is the outward manifestation of seizures involving spastic muscle movement.

   F. _____ This is the type of seizure in which there is increased muscle tone and stiffening of the limbs.

   G. _____ This is the type of seizure in which there is rapid contraction and relaxation of the muscles.

   H. _____ This term describes the condition in which there are recurring seizures originating from the brain and characterized by sudden loss of motor control, unconsciousness, and tonic–clonic seizures of short duration.

   I. _____ This is a type of epilepsy in which the cause of the disease is unknown.

   J. _____ This is the state of being in a seizure activity and usually describes a state of prolonged seizure activity.

   K. _____ This is the period of time just before the onset of seizure; often referred to as the "aura."

   L. _____ This is a term that describes the seizure itself.

   M. _____ This is the period of time immediately after the seizure has subsided in which the animal may appear tired, confused, or anxious.

   N. _____ This is a type of epilepsy in which the cause is assumed to be related to a breed or inherited predisposition.

   O. _____ This is a type of epilepsy in which there is an identified lesion in the brain that is causing the seizures.

   P. _____ This is a type of epilepsy that is idiopathic in nature in that the cause of the epilepsy has not been identified (no genetic origin and no structural lesion identified).

   Q. _____ This term means an elevated body temperature.

   R. _____ This means low oxygen levels.

   S. _____ This is the neurotransmitter that normally is inhibitory on the central nervous system (CNS) and is part of the mechanism by which phenobarbital acts.

   T. _____ This is a family of enzymes found in the liver and is involved with the metabolism of phenobarbital and a number of other drugs.

U. _____ This is a particular type of mixed-function oxidase (MFO) that is involved in phenobarbital metabolism.

V. _____ This means that the metabolism of a drug has been accelerated.

W. _____ This means increased appetite.

X. _____ This means increased drinking.

Y. _____ This means increased urination.

Z. _____ These two liver-associated enzymes are normally elevated when an animal is taking phenobarbital.

AA. _____ This term describes liver disease caused by drugs.

AB. _____ This is a type of adverse drug effect that is not dose dependent and cannot be predicted.

AC. _____ This is a nonmetric unit used to describe the concentration of phenobarbital found in a tablet.

AD. _____ This term refers to a second drug that is added to a dosage regimen to bolster the effect of the main drug.

AE. _____ This term describes a type of pain that originates from the nerves themselves as opposed to originating from trauma or injury detected by nociceptors.

AF. _____ This group of tranquilizers constitute some of the main drugs that are classified as antipsychotic drugs.

AG. _____ This group of behavior-modifying drugs are mood-elevating drugs.

AH. _____ This term is another term that describes tranquilizers or drugs that decrease fear responses or anxiety.

AI. _____ This is the part of the brain involved in the generation of emotions.

AJ. _____ These are the three drug groups classified as antidepressant drugs.

AK. _____ This is what MAOI stands for.

AL. _____ This is what SSRI stands for.

AM. _____ This is what TCA stands for.

AN. _____ This describes the group of clinical signs that result when there is a toxic accumulation of serotonin neurotransmitter.

AO. _____ This is the receptor to which the gamma (γ)-aminobutyric acid (GABA) neurotransmitter attaches.

AP. _____ This describes checking concentrations of phenobarbital in the blood and adjusting the dose based upon whether or not the concentrations are within the normal therapeutic range.

2. Fill in the following blanks with the correct drug from the Nervous System Drugs list. When practicing these questions, write out the answers on a separate sheet, focusing also on the appropriate spelling of these drug names.

A. _____ The orally administered drug of choice for long-term control of epileptic seizures.

B. _____ The anticonvulsant that is still the drug of first choice for control of active seizures or status epilepticus.

C. _____ The antidepressant drug that also is used to treat canine Cushing's disease.

D. _____ Name the four anxiolytic drugs.

E. _____ The anticonvulsant that is metabolized by cytochrome P-450 (CYP) and increases the metabolism of any other drug that uses the same liver enzyme.

F. _____ The two types of antidepressants that, if given together, produce serotonin syndrome.

G. _____ The anticonvulsant to which tolerance develops within a week or so after therapy is started; has a history of causing a potentially fatal drug-induced hepatopathy in cats.

H. _____ Antidepressant drug that blocks the enzyme that normally breaks down dopamine, serotonin, and norepinephrine.

I. _____ The anticonvulsant with a very long half-life that is used as an adjunct therapy in animals not well controlled with phenobarbital alone.

J. _____ Phenothiazine tranquilizer that is an antipsychotic drug.

K. _____ The anticonvulsant that enhances the action of GABA and induces its own metabolism.

L. _____ Behavior-modifying drug that works by blocking reuptake of both norepinephrine and serotonin.

M. _____ Behavior-modifying drug that works by blocking reuptake of serotonin only.

N. _____ The anticonvulsant that often produces vomiting as a side effect because of the salt to which it is attached; often requires the use of a loading dose because of the long lag time between when therapy is started and steady state is achieved.

O. _____ The anticonvulsant that normally increases levels of alkaline phosphatase (ALP) and alanine aminotransferase (ALT).

P. _____ The Food and Drug Administration (FDA)-approved tricyclic antidepressant (TCA) drug for use in dogs (list both the nonproprietary name and trade name).

Q. _____ The FDA-approved selective serotonin reuptake inhibitor (SSRI) drug for use in dogs (list both the nonproprietary name and trade name).

R. _____ The FDA-approved monoamine oxidase inhibitor (MAOI) drug for use in dogs (list both the nonproprietary name and trade name).

S. _____ The anticonvulsant sometimes measured in grains, as well as milligrams.

T. _____ Behavior-modifying drug that works by blocking dopamine receptors in the brain.

U. _____ The short-acting anticonvulsant with strong first-pass effect that renders it fairly useless when given orally (PO).

V. _____ The drug that is FDA approved for use to treat "canine cognitive dysfunction" or old dog senility.

W. _____ The anticonvulsant that has an idiosyncratic reaction in which the animal becomes excited, anxious, or hyperactive instead of sedated.

3. Indicate whether each of the following statements is true or false.

   A. Convulsions are changes in electrical activity in the brain, and seizures are the motor movements that result from that electrical activity.

   B. The violent shaking types of seizures seen in a dog with epilepsy would be classified as tonic–clonic seizures.

   C. Idiopathic epilepsy and epilepsy of unknown origin essentially are the same thing.

   D. Excessive release of GABA would result in CNS stimulation and seizures.

   E. If a drug is metabolized by the same CYP that metabolizes phenobarbital, the use of that drug in an animal already on phenobarbital would likely require an increase in the drug's dose to compensate for the effect of phenobarbital on the drug's metabolism.

   F. Cats require a higher dose of phenobarbital to produce a similar degree of seizure control compared with dogs.

   G. The increase of ALP and ALT liver enzymes in a patient on phenobarbital indicates the animal's liver is damaged by the phenobarbital.

   H. One quarter of a grain equals 30 mg.

   I. Generally, diazepam is more effective when given orally than when injected intravenously (IV).

   J. Diazepam does not mix readily with most IV fluids.

   K. One of the advantages of potassium bromide is that a change of dose results in a rapid corresponding change in bromide concentrations in the blood.

   L. A drug that enhances the effect of gamma-aminobutyric acid (GABA) would cause CNS depression.

   M. Phenobarbital is normally metabolized to primidone for most of its anticonvulsant activity.

   N. Phenothiazine tranquilizers work by stimulating dopamine receptors in the brain.

   O. SSRI antidepressant drugs are considered more specific in their mechanism of action than the TCA antidepressant drugs.

   P. As a general rule, TCA dosages (mg/kg) tend to be the same across all patients of the same species.

   Q. Fluoxetine comes in a form approved for use in the dog.

   R. Decreased serotonin levels in the brain correlate with overly aggressive behavior.

   S. Selegiline (Anipryl) is an MAOI drug.

   T. Benzodiazepines would be among the drugs classified as anxiolytics.

   U. Benzodiazepines are generally very effective for long-term control of seizure activity even if used just by themselves.

   V. After a few weeks of having a patient on phenobarbital, the dose typically needs to be decreased to compensate for changing levels of phenobarbital in the blood.

   W. Phenothiazine tranquilizer drugs may cause inappropriate aggressive behaviors of animals to emerge.

   X. TCAs have an advantage over phenothiazine tranquilizers such as acepromazine because they do not suppress overall behavior as much as phenothiazines do.

   Y. An increased presence of the dopamine neurotransmitter has been associated with a senility-like syndrome in dogs.

   Z. Diazepam reduces anxiety by decreasing the amount of the neurotransmitter GABA.

   AA. There is no simple "magic bullet" for behavior therapy.

4. If a dog needs 1.5 grains of phenobarbital per day, how many milligrams of drug is this?

5. Mr. Smith comes in to get a refill on his dog's heartworm medication and mentions to you that his teacup poodle, who was diagnosed with idiopathic epilepsy last week and started on a low dose of phenobarbital, is pacing, acting anxious, panting, and not sleeping through the night as he used to. Normally phenobarbital tends to produce ataxia, sedation, wobbly gait, and lethargy for the first few days. Is this change in behavior likely from the drug even though it is the opposite of what is typically seen?

6. In looking over the blood results for Mr. and Mrs. Johnson's dog who has been on phenobarbital for 3 weeks, you see that the complete blood count and most of the blood chemistry profile results are within the reference range (i.e., within normal limits). However, ALP and ALT levels are higher than normal. You remember from your medical nursing and clinical pathology courses that an increase of these enzymes in the blood means that they are getting into the blood from the liver and can indicate injury to, or disease in, that organ. You also remember that anticonvulsant drugs can cause liver problems; yet the veterinarian does not seem concerned about this. Should he or she be?

7. Potassium bromide often causes vomiting. How can the incidence of vomiting be reduced?

8. Which would cause animals to become more tranquilized: a drug that blocks destruction of GABA or a drug that occupies a GABA receptor but has no intrinsic activity?

9. Why would continued seizures be more of a concern in an animal that is outside on a hot July day compared with a cool October day?

10. Mr. Wang wants to know why his dog needs to have the phenobarbital dose adjusted 3 weeks after starting the medication. "Did you not correctly give the dose the first time?" he asks. How do you respond?

11. The veterinary assistant who helped you and the veterinarian control status epilepticus in a dog using diazepam wonders why you do not send the dog home on the same drug. "The drug stopped the seizures, so why wouldn't you just use the same drug to keep seizures from happening again at home?" she asks. How do you respond?

12. Why do bromides need a loading dose to get started even though phenobarbital does not?

13. The veterinarian has a large, 135-lb male German shepherd that was previously trained as a sentry dog for guarding a government facility. The dog is showing increasingly aggressive behavior toward the owner when the owner comes around its food dish. When asked by the owner if tranquilizers will help, the veterinarian states that "it might actually make him more aggressive." What does the veterinarian mean by that? How can that happen with a tranquilizer?

14. What happens if you give two antidepressant drugs like fluoxetine (Reconcile) and selegiline (Anipryl) to the same canine patient at the same time?

Antimicrobials

OBJECTIVES

After studying this chapter, the veterinary technician should be able to:

- Describe the meaning of characterizing terms that describe antimicrobials: -cidal, -static, concentration-dependent, time dependent, etc.
- Explain in detail how resistance develops and emerges from bacterial populations, why this is of concern to human health, and what can be done to reduce the emergence of resistant bacteria.
- Describe the basic mechanism of action, key characteristics of the drug group, and the clinically significant disadvantages or adverse reactions for each of the key veterinary drugs described.

- Explain the role bacterial antibiotics play in treating heartworm disease and controlling protozoa like coccidia and giardia.
- Explain how kidney damage can be avoided when using aminoglycosides.
- Identify what drugs are best to use to treat intracellular bacteria like *Rickettsia, Chlamydia,* and *Mycoplasma* and why.
- Explain the difference between azole antifungals and amphotericin B as far as mechanism of action, degree of toxicity, and time to onset of antifungal activity.
- Explain the clinical differences between the azole antifungals described.

KEY TERMS

absolute contraindication
aerobic
anaerobic
antibiotic
antimicrobials
aplastic anemia
bactericidal
bacteriostatic
beta (β)-lactam
β-lactamase
β-lactamase–resistant

β-lactam ring
breakpoints
cephalosporinase
chelate
concentration-dependent drugs
cross-reactivity
cross-resistance
culture and sensitivity/ culture and
   susceptibility
crystalluria
deep/systemic mycoses

dermatophyte
DNA gyrase
empiric therapy
enteric sulfa
enterohepatic circulation
fungicidal
horizontal transmission of
   resistance
hypersensitivity
intermediate resistance or
   susceptibility

keratoconjunctivitis sicca
leukopenia
liposomal form (amphotericin B)
maximum tolerated dose (MTD)
messenger RNA (m-RNA)
minimum bactericidal concentration (MBC)
minimum inhibitory concentration (MIC)
methicillin-resistant *Staphylococcus aureus* (MRSA)
nephrotoxic
nystagmus
ototoxic
pathogens
penicillinase

plasmid
porins
postantibiotic effect
potentiated
pyoderma
pyogenic
relative contraindication
residue
resistant
ribosome
selection pressure
spectrum of activity

superinfection
superficial mycoses
suprainfection
susceptibility
teratogenic effects
time-dependent drugs
thrombocytopenia
transfer RNA (t-RNA)
urticaria
vertical transmission of resistance
virucidal
wolbachia

Antimicrobials are drugs that kill or inhibit the growth of microorganisms, or microbes, such as bacteria, protozoa, viruses, and fungi. The term antibiotic is often used interchangeably with the term antimicrobial, but antibiotics specifically describe a natural substance produced by one microorganism that suppresses growth of another microorganism. The classic example is the penicillium mold growing on a culture plate that was observed to kill or suppress bacterial growth around the mold and led to the discovery of the antibiotic penicillin. Today most antimicrobials, even antibiotics that were once manufactured from cultures of growing molds or microorganisms, are now chemically synthesized, so the distinction between antimicrobial and antibiotic has blurred even further. In veterinary medicine, "antibiotics" is the term generally applied to any antimicrobial that inhibits or kills bacteria, although, as will be shown in this chapter, even that definition is blurred sometimes to include activity against protozoa or fungal agents.

TABLE 10.1 Time-Dependent vs Concentration-Dependent Drugs

Bacteriostatic Drugs (Time-Dependent)	Bactericidal Drugs (Time-Dependent)	Bactericidal Drugs (Concentration-Dependent)
Must maintain concentrations constantly above the minimum inhibitory concentration (MIC)	Must maintain concentrations constantly above the MIC	Must achieve a concentration high above the MIC
Chloramphenicol*	Cephalosporins	Aminoglycosides
Lincosamide/clindamycin*	Penicillin family	Fluoroquinolones
Macrolides		
Sulfonamides		
Tetracycline family		

*Can be bactericidal for susceptible bacteria.

TYPES OF ANTIMICROBIALS

An antimicrobial can be classified according to the type of microorganism it fights (i.e., the drug's spectrum of activity) and whether it kills the microorganism or only prevents it from replicating and proliferating. The suffix *-cidal* denotes drugs that kill the named microorganism (e.g., bactericidal, fungicidal, virucidal). The suffix *-static* denotes drugs that inhibit replication but do not directly kill the microorganism (e.g., bacteriostatic and *fungistatic*). Drugs generally have the potential to both kill and inhibit pathogens (i.e., disease-causing organisms) with lower concentrations or shorter treatment durations producing a sublethal inhibiting effect, and higher concentrations or longer treatment durations producing the death of the pathogenic organisms.

Bacteriostatic drugs temporarily inhibit the growth of bacteria, but once the drug is removed the organism can begin to multiply again. Therefore, drugs that only inhibit replication (-*static* drugs) depend more on a functional immune system to ultimately defeat the organism than -*cidal* drugs, which kill the pathogen outright. This is why people or animals with compromised immune systems (e.g., cats with feline immunodeficiency virus infection, animals who receive cancer chemotherapy) or patients with severe bacterial disease usually require drugs that are -*cidal* to treat the infections (Table 10.1).

Disinfectants and antiseptics are antimicrobial chemicals that kill a variety of pathogens. Because they are applied to the surface of the body or on inanimate objects, they are discussed separately in Chapter 11.

GOAL OF ANTIMICROBIAL THERAPY

The goal of antimicrobial therapy is to kill or disable pathogens without killing the host. Unfortunately, many animals die each year because of side effects or inappropriate administration of antimicrobials. Successful administration of antimicrobials requires the following conditions:

- The microorganism must be susceptible to the antimicrobial drug.
- The antimicrobial must be able to reach the site of infection in high enough concentrations to kill or inhibit the microorganism.
- The animal must be able to tolerate the required high concentrations of the drug.

Factors such as client compliance (client faithfully following the dosing instructions), ease of administration, convenient dosage interval, dose form, and cost also influence drug selection.[1] However, the three bulleted conditions listed must be met before any other factors are considered.

Susceptibility, Resistance, Intermediate, and Breakpoints

Because bacterial strains vary in their susceptibility to different antimicrobials, it is recommended to obtain a sample from the infection site and isolate and culture (grow) the bacteria obtained to determine to which antimicrobials the particular bacterial strain is sensitive. This process of identification and drug susceptibility testing is commonly referred to as culture and sensitivity or culture and susceptibility.

The culture and sensitivity testing can determine the susceptibility of a bacterial strain to certain drugs by determining how much drug it takes to inhibit or kill the bacteria. When a culture and sensitivity is done, the bacteria are exposed to increasing concentrations of drug to determine the lowest concentration that inhibits the growth of the cultured bacteria. The lowest drug concentration needed to inhibit bacterial growth is called the drug's minimum inhibitory concentration (MIC) for that bacterial strain (Fig. 10.1).

Although knowing the drug's MIC for a particular bacteria strain is very useful, it may be that the required concentration for bacterial inhibition is too high to be tolerated by the body, which means that drug cannot be administered systemically to treat the infection. The highest concentration of a drug that can be tolerated by the animal before significant toxicity signs or adverse effects occur is called the maximum tolerated dose

(MTD) concentrations. Thus, for a drug to be used systemically to treat an infection, the drug's MIC for the cultured bacteria needs to be lower than the concentrations of the MTD for a drug. If the MICs determined for the bacteria isolated and cultured from the infection site are higher than the drug's MTD concentration, the bacteria are considered to be resistant to that particular drug. If the cultured bacteria have an MIC for a drug that is a much lower concentration than the drug's MTD concentration, the cultured bacteria are considered to be *susceptible* to that particular drug.

Because bacteria can develop resistance to individual antimicrobials, it is not unusual for the same bacteria to be susceptible to some antibiotics but completely resistant to others. For example, a strain of *Staphylococcus* bacteria may be highly sensitive to the antibiotic gentamicin but quite resistant to penicillin. In this example, the *Staphylococcus* strain would have a relatively low MIC for gentamicin compared with gentamicin's limiting MTD concentration inside the patient. However, penicillin's tolerated MTD concentrations for the patient would be below the penicillin MIC needed to be obtained to successfully inhibit this particular *Staphylococcus* strain.

Sometimes a bacterial strain is not classified as being either clearly resistant or clearly susceptible to a particular drug but is classified as having an intermediate resistance or susceptibility. In this case, the MIC of the bacteria for this particular drug is still below the MTD concentration and hence susceptible to inhibition by the drug. However, the bacteria's MIC for the drug is very close to the MTD concentration, and the drug concentrations achieved at the actual infection site may or may not be sufficient to inhibit the bacterial growth. Thus, for infections classified as having intermediate susceptibility the factors influencing the

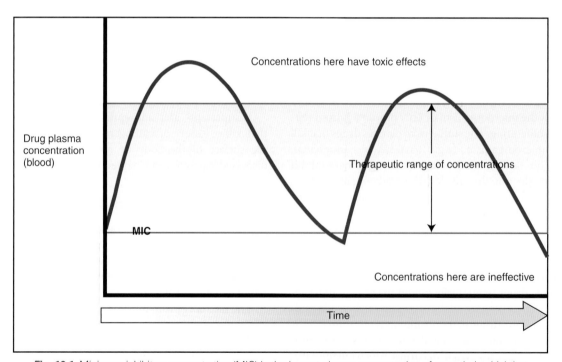

Fig. 10.1 Minimum inhibitory concentration (MIC) is the lowest plasma concentration of an antimicrobial that effectively exerts antimicrobial action. Levels below this are ineffective, and levels exceeding the therapeutic range are toxic.

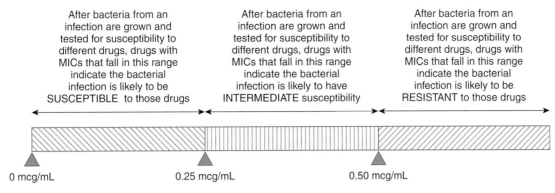

After bacteria from an infection are grown and tested for susceptibility to different drugs, drugs with MICs that fall in this range indicate the bacterial infection is likely to be **SUSCEPTIBLE** to those drugs

After bacteria from an infection are grown and tested for susceptibility to different drugs, drugs with MICs that fall in this range indicate the bacterial infection is likely to have **INTERMEDIATE** susceptibility

After bacteria from an infection are grown and tested for susceptibility to different drugs, drugs with MICs that fall in this range indicate the bacterial infection is likely to be **RESISTANT** to those drugs

0 mcg/mL   0.25 mcg/mL   0.50 mcg/mL

Breakpoints listed in a national standard for one specific bacterial species

Fig. 10.2 Breakpoints mark a drug's MIC that differentiates between when a bacterial strain is considered susceptible, intermediate susceptible, or resistant to that particular drug.

delivery of the drug to the infection site may ultimately determine whether or not the drug is effective against the cultured bacteria residing at that infection site.[2]

Who determines the magic MIC at which a bacterium is classified as resistant, intermediate, or susceptible for a particular drug? There are internationally recognized laboratories or governing bodies that set the standards for predicting the susceptibility for bacterial species to different antibiotic drugs based upon thousands of bacterial cultures and susceptibility testing. These recognized entities identify the theoretical breakpoints that should differentiate MICs that indicate a bacterial strain is susceptible to a drug from a bacterial strain with intermediate susceptibility or bacteria that would be resistant to the drug (Fig. 10.2).[2] For example, after testing thousands of bacterial samples the international standard setting organization determined that a particular bacterial species would have its growth inhibited and be considered susceptible to a particular drug if the isolated bacteria from an infection had an observed MIC less than 0.25 mcg/mL. Based upon the same testing of thousands of bacterial samples, this organization also determined that any bacteria of this bacterial species having an observed MIC greater than 0.50 mcg/mL would not be inhibited by tolerable concentration of drug and therefore any bacteria with an MIC greater than 0.50 mcg/mL would be designated as being resistant to the drug. In this example, if the actual bacteria from the animal's infection were cultured and the MIC determined for that bacteria to a particular drug, a determined MIC drug concentration of 0.35 mcg/mL for this isolated bacteria would fall squarely in the intermediate susceptibility category. If the MIC required of this drug to inhibit the bacteria found in the patient's infection had been determined to be 0.15 mcg/mL, the bacteria would be considered very susceptible to the drug. If, however, the MIC had been found to be 0.75 mcg/mL for the bacteria isolated from the patient, then the drug concentration needed to inhibit the bacteria would be above the concentration able to be tolerated by the patient and this bacteria would be considered to be resistant to the inhibitory effects of the drug.

Even if a culture and sensitivity indicates that the bacteria at the infection site are susceptible (sensitive) to a particular antimicrobial, unless the antimicrobials can reach the infection site at the needed concentrations to inhibit the bacteria (i.e., the MIC is actually achieved at the infection site itself), the antimicrobial will be ineffective. In other words, the antimicrobial must be able to be absorbed from the administration site and distributed to the site of infection in sufficient quantity to produce concentrations in excess of the MIC to do any good.

One other term sometimes used to describe the ability of a drug to actually kill, vs inhibit the growth of, a bacterial species is the minimum bactericidal concentration (MBC). Typically the MBC is a higher concentration than the MIC because the bacteria are not just being held in a static condition but are actually being killed by the drug directly. Though it is important to conceptually understand what is meant if the MBC is mentioned, from a position of determining bacterial susceptibility to a drug using breakpoints, the MIC is the concentration typically used.[2]

RESISTANCE OF MICROORGANISMS TO ANTIMICROBIAL THERAPY

Bacteria and other microorganisms have developed the ability to survive in the presence of antimicrobial drugs designed to kill them. This acquired resistance is a significant concern in human and veterinary medicine because it means that antibiotics that previously were effective in treating certain bacterial infections are no longer effective. Because misuse of antibiotic drugs can potentially facilitate the emergence of resistant bacteria, there is increased scrutiny by the federal and state health authorities over how antibiotics are used in veterinary medicine. It has been shown fairly conclusively over the past 15 years that there is a strong correlation with the widespread use of veterinary antibiotics in food animal medicine and the emergence of bacteria that are resistant to those drugs. Although this is bad news for veterinary patients, it also means that human patients who acquire these same resistant bacteria may not be successfully treated with standard antibiotic treatments.[2]

The Centers for Disease Control and Prevention (CDC) has a National Antimicrobial Resistance Monitoring System (NARMS) that works with state and local health departments, the Food and Drug Administration (FDA), and the US Department of Agriculture (USDA) to track changes in bacterial susceptibility and resistance in the United States. The results of the NARMS reports has continued to increase the concern that misuse of veterinary antibiotics may play a role in overall development or emergence of resistant bacteria.[3]

Today's veterinary technician needs to be very aware of this public health concern and has an obligation to work with the veterinarian and others who administer antibiotics to help assure that veterinary antimicrobials are used appropriately and safely so as to reduce the emergence of more resistant bacterial species.

How Does Bacterial Resistance Occur?

Typically resistance occurs as a result of a genetic mutation in the deoxyribonucleic acid (DNA) of bacteria. Millions of mutations occur daily in bacteria all over the world; however, the vast majority of these mutations have no significant effect on the bacterial function or the mutation may be detrimental instead of helpful to the bacteria causing the bacteria to die out and taking the genetic mutation with them. However, if only one of the billion or trillion spontaneous mutations results in a beneficial mutation and resistance developing in a single bacterium, when that bacterium proliferates it will give rise to an entire strain of resistant bacteria. The passing of this resistant genetic trait to the daughter cells and all subsequent generations of the original bacterium is called vertical transmission of resistance.

Bacteria do not just transfer resistance-encoded DNA to their offspring, but they also transfer resistance to other unrelated bacteria by sharing a piece of DNA called a plasmid through a process referred to as the horizontal transmission of resistance. Horizontal resistance occurs when some bacteria make physical contact with another bacterium and transfer the plasmid-containing resistant DNA across the cell membrane. Others can pick up DNA with resistant genes left in the environment after the death and lysis of another bacterial cell. Still others can receive resistant DNA by a bacterial virus called a *bacteriophage* that transfers DNA from one bacterium to another. The bottom line is that once a bacterium acquires resistance-conferring genes in its DNA, the DNA is spread rapidly among other bacteria of the same species and to other bacteria in unrelated species.

In some cases, the resistant genes code for a pump that grabs the antibiotic when it enters the bacteria and pumps it out before it has a chance to damage the bacterium. Other bacteria will develop enzymes capable of digesting and destroying the antibiotic molecule. Some bacterial genetic changes can modify the receptor molecule where the antibiotic would normally attach, making it impossible for the antibiotic to attach to the site that would damage the bacterium. Another mechanism can change the outer layers of the bacterium, preventing the antibiotic from physically entering the bacterium and blocking it from reaching the target site within the bacterial cell. Often resistant bacteria will develop more than one resistant mechanism, creating a multi-drug resistant bacterial strain.[4,5]

Selective Pressure, Resistance, and Clinical Disease

Although the presence of resistant bacterium increases the odds that the bacterial strain will survive in the presence of some antibiotics, it does not necessarily mean the animal is actually going to break with an clinical infection that is resistant to antibiotic treatment. The patient's immune system, the bacterial competition for limited available resources, and other environmental or host factors may limit bacterial proliferation and keep the bacterial population below the number needed to produce clinical disease.

As shown in Fig. 10.3, if a low antibiotic dose is administered, only the weakest bacteria are going to be inhibited or die while all those bacteria that are more resistant to the drug will survive. The bacteria that survive have been "selected" because of their inherent genetic makeup or some other advantage over the weaker bacteria. After the weaker bacteria have been eliminated, there are fewer bacteria to compete for resources, and these selected more resistant bacteria can proliferate and dominate the bacterial population. This elimination of weaker bacteria by low dose or inappropriate administration of antimicrobial drugs is how selection pressure causes a resistant population of bacteria to emerge.[2,4]

The same thing can occur if the antibiotic is not used long enough. On day 1 of treatment with an antibiotic, only the weakest bacteria are going to be killed. On day 2, the next most susceptible bacteria will die. On day 3, most of the weaker bacteria have been selected for destruction, and the overall population count of bacteria is considerably smaller. At that point, the animal is feeling much better and the owner stops the antibiotic. Unfortunately the population of remaining bacteria have been

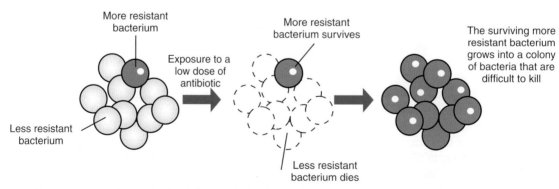

Fig. 10.3 Mechanism by which small doses of an antimicrobial can select for emergence of more resistant strains of bacteria.

selected for their resistant characteristics, and, unless they are eliminated by the immune system, these bacteria can proliferate and create an infection that is now resistant to the drug previously used.

Thus, selection pressure does not create mutations or speed up the rate at which mutations occur; it only helps resistant

CLINICAL APPLICATION

Time-Dependent vs Concentration-Dependent Effects

Even if an antimicrobial drug achieves drug concentrations in excess of the minimum inhibitory concentration (MIC) at an infection site, other variables may prevent the drug from eliminating the bacterial infection. For example, bacteriostatic drugs such as sulfonamides, tetracycline, and lincosamides will not kill the susceptible bacteria at the infection site but will only inhibit their reproduction. If the bacteria are only inhibited from further division by the bacteriostatic drug, once the antimicrobial drug concentration drops below the MIC the bacteria will begin to divide and proliferate again, unless they are killed by the animal's immune system. Therefore, to be most effective, bacteriostatic drugs must be present continuously at the infection site at concentrations above the MIC so the bacteria stop proliferating and so the immune system can destroy the bacterial infection. Drugs that are required to remain at high concentrations at the infection site continuously are said to be *time of contact* dependent, or just *time dependent*, to be effective in eliminating bacterial infections.

This time-dependent characteristic of antimicrobial drugs can also apply to bactericidal drugs. For example, the beta (β)-lactam drugs kill bacteria by preventing proper formation of the bacterial cell wall during replication. Because β-lactam interference with wall formation only occurs when the bacteria are dividing, penicillins or cephalosporins must be present at the site in concentrations that exceed the MIC continuously to catch the bacteria at the time of their cellular division. The point to remember is that significantly increasing the peak drug concentration well above the MIC for β-lactam drugs like penicillins or cephalosporins does not, by itself, necessarily increase the effectiveness of these antimicrobials unless the drug concentrations remain above the MIC continuously.

In contrast to the time-dependent bactericidal agents, *concentration-dependent* bactericidal agents must either achieve a peak drug concentration far exceeding the MIC or maintain a high level of concentration for a longer period of time to be maximally effective. For example, for gentamicin or amikacin to be truly effective, the peak drug concentration at the site of infection must be 8–10 times higher than the MIC for the bacteria. However, this high peak concentration does not have to be maintained, and the drug concentrations can drop rapidly once the high peak concentration is attained. When aminoglycosides achieve this single high peak concentration and then concentrations drop, bacteria will continue to die even after the drug concentrations have dropped below the MIC. This continued killing effect in the absence of drug concentrations above the MIC is called the *postantibiotic effect*, and it is a concentration-dependent effect.

What should be learned from this situation: It is critical to follow the recommended dose regimen exactly in order to attain drug concentrations either at sufficiently high levels or for sufficiently long periods of time required to destroy the bacterial infection. Failure to follow the dose exactly may mean that the time-dependent or concentration-dependent characteristic of the drug is not achieved and the bacteria are allowed to survive, creating selection pressure that can allow a resistant population of bacteria to emerge. Table 10.1 lists the antibiotics that are time-dependent or concentration-dependent.

bacteria proliferate and emerge into a clinical disease that is resistant to treatment.[1] If clients do not follow the instructions to treat their animal with antibiotics, they can facilitate the emergence of resistant bacterial populations. See Clinical Application: Time-Dependent vs Concentration-Dependent Effects for another example of how lack of client compliance can result in selection pressure and emergence of resistant populations.

To reduce the emergence of resistant populations of bacteria, the appropriate antimicrobial dose must be used, and the full duration of treatment must be completed. By understanding how bacterial resistance can be cultivated, the veterinary technician can better educate the owner on the rationale for completing all of the antibiotic in the manner prescribed by the veterinarian.

Resistance and Drug Residues

A residue is the presence of a drug, chemical, or its metabolites in animal tissues or food products, resulting from either administration of that drug or chemical to an animal or contamination of food products during food processing. As discussed in Chapter 3, food animal drugs must be withdrawn and the treatment stopped a specific number of days before the animal can be slaughtered for human food or the food products (e.g., eggs, milk) can be sold. The withdrawal time allows enough time for the drug to be excreted from the body and tissue concentrations to drop below the required government-mandated limit. It is important to ensure that only very low drug residues remain in human food because most antimicrobial residues are not degraded by cooking or pasteurization and therefore can persist in the food products and eventually be ingested by human consumers.[2]

Exposure to low levels of antimicrobials in ingested food can potentially cause two effects in human beings: an allergic reaction (hypersensitivity) to the antimicrobial or selection for resistant bacteria in the intestinal tract. For example, if a farm family harvested their own cows for food and the meat contained antibiotic residues, the family would consume a low level of antibiotic over several days or weeks, killing off the most susceptible (sensitive) bacteria in their gastrointestinal (GI) tracts and leaving only the more resistant bacteria to grow and proliferate. This change in gut flora (i.e., the composition of bacteria and protozoa in the intestinal tract) could result in diarrhea or more severe signs of systemic disease, depending on which species of bacteria survived and proliferated.

Because of the public's concern over drug residues and the responsibility that veterinarians and veterinary technicians have in maintaining food safety, veterinary professionals must take the time to educate food animal producers on the appropriate use of antimicrobials and withdrawal times, label all dispensed medications with clear instructions for proper administration and withdrawal times, and be strong advocates for adhering to mandated withdrawal and residue avoidance regulations.

CLASSIFICATION OF ANTIMICROBIALS BY THEIR MECHANISM OF ACTION

Antimicrobials work by different mechanisms to kill or inhibit bacteria and other microorganisms. Antimicrobials generally exert their effects at five sites in microorganisms: the cell wall, cell membrane, ribosomes, critical enzymes or metabolites, and nucleic acids.

Antimicrobials can inhibit or kill bacteria by interfering with formation of the bacterial cell wall during bacterial cell division. Normally, the bacterial protoplasm draws water into the bacterium by osmosis, producing a tendency for the bacterial cell to swell. The intact bacterial cell wall keeps the bacterium from bursting in much the same way that placing a balloon in a rigid container during inflation confines the balloon and prevents it from overinflating and bursting. Antimicrobials that interfere with bacterial cell wall formation only work while the wall is forming during bacterial cell division. Once the bacterial cell wall is constructed, it is not readily affected by antimicrobial drugs. Thus, drugs that target the bacterial cell wall are most effective against actively dividing bacterial colonies, and anything that slows bacterial division (e.g., bacteriostatic drugs) can reduce the effectiveness of these drugs. Penicillin and cephalosporins are antimicrobials that act by disruption of new wall formation.[5]

Antimicrobials can also damage the bacterial cell membrane, making this barrier leaky, which would allow either antimicrobial drug molecules to more readily enter the bacterium or vital cytoplasmic components to escape. Unlike drugs that act on the developing bacterial cell wall, antimicrobials that target the cell membrane can exert their effect on both dividing or static (i.e., nondividing)

bacteria. Polymyxin B is a common ingredient in topically applied first aid creams and is an example of an antibiotic that works by this mechanism.

Antimicrobials can inhibit essential protein synthesis in pathogenic microorganisms such as bacteria and fungi. Just like mammalian cells, these pathogens manufacture essential proteins from the amino acids floating in their cytoplasm. See Fig. 10.4 for a depiction of protein synthesis. A strand of messenger ribonucleic acid (m-RNA) enters the nucleus, copies a segment of the genetic code that contains the code for a particular protein, and then carries the copy out into the cellular cytoplasm. The m-RNA combines with a specialized organelle called the ribosome that acts like a protein-producing factory. As the m-RNA strand is fed into the ribosome, the code on the m-RNA is "read" and a signal is sent for a transfer RNA (t-RNA) molecule holding a particular amino acid to enter the ribosome, attach to the m-RNA, and connect the amino acid to an adjacent amino acid in a specific sequence. By stitching together these amino acids in a specific order, a functional protein molecule is produced.

Some antimicrobial drugs work by disrupting production of essential proteins by combining with the ribosome and interfering with the m-RNA or the ability of the t-RNA to get the amino acids to the ribosome. By blocking production of these essential proteins, the cell either stops dividing or dies. In some cases, it is a lack of essential proteins that damages the cell membrane and causes it to leak. Some antimicrobials that act by combining with ribosomes and disrupting protein synthesis include lincosamides, macrolides, tetracyclines, and aminoglycosides.[6,7]

Other antimicrobial drugs may interfere with critical enzymes needed by pathogenic bacteria to produce essential nutrients or

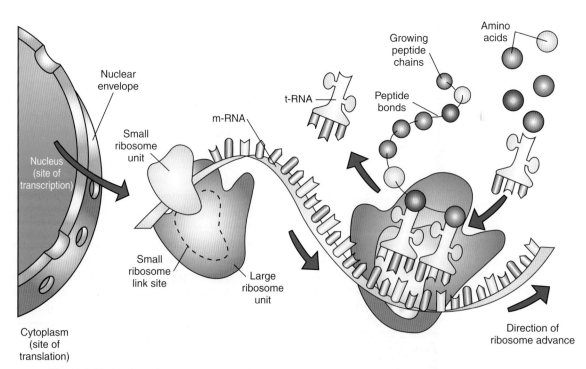

Fig. 10.4 Mechanism of protein synthesis by a cell. The messenger RNA (m-RNA) comes out of the nucleus and is run through a ribosome where it codes for specific transfer RNA (t-RNA) to temporarily attach to the m-RNA and transfer the amino acid they were carrying to the growing protein chain before formed by the ribosome.

substances they need to survive. Alternatively, antimicrobials may leave the critical enzymes alone but bind with key intermediate compounds produced by the enzymes, rendering these compounds worthless to the bacterium. Either mechanism results in a bacterium that is unable to function properly. Sulfonamide antibiotics work primarily by this mechanism.[8]

Finally, antimicrobials can interfere with the production of bacterial nucleic acids (RNA and DNA), altering the ability of the cell to divide or produce critical proteins needed by the cell. Though this mechanism can be very effective in killing a pathogen, there is always a concern about the potential for the antimicrobial to also attack the mammalian DNA of the host animal or person. For that reason, antimicrobials that work by attacking DNA are scrutinized closely for any potential effect on mammalian DNA before they are allowed to be used. Some antifungal drugs work in this manner and have the capability to produce fetal abnormalities in pregnant animals receiving the drug. However, newer antibiotics disrupt DNA function by interfering with the enzymes needed for DNA to function or replicate but do not disrupt the DNA sequence itself. In addition, these newer antimicrobials attack specific types of molecular structures found only in bacteria and not found in mammalian cells.[9] Both of these safeguards make these newer drugs much safer to use and reduce the risk for mutations or birth defects in the veterinary patient. The newer antibiotics that work through this mechanism include the fluoroquinolones (e.g., enrofloxacin, orbifloxacin).

CLASSES OF ANTIMICROBIALS

Every year new veterinary antimicrobial products are marketed for use against bacteria or other pathogens. Occasionally these drugs are brand-new classes of antibiotics, but more often they are simply repackaged versions of older drugs placed in a new dosage form or with an expanded target of microbes. Because of the constant stream of new antibiotics entering the veterinary medical market, keeping up with the new drugs can seem overwhelming. However, by understanding the basics of how each general class of antimicrobials works, the overall spectrum of activity for each class or group, and the mechanisms behind the key side effects, the veterinarian or veterinary technician should possess the necessary background to quickly understand what a new drug should be able to do and how it will work.

Penicillins

Penicillins are among the most commonly used antibiotics in veterinary medicine and can usually be recognized by their -cillin suffix in the drug name. Because of a particular ring-like structure in their chemical composition, penicillins are also called *beta-lactam*, or β-lactam, antibiotics in reference to their β-lactam ring. The other major group of antibiotics with a β-lactam ring are the cephalosporin antibiotics.

The most frequently used penicillins in veterinary medicine include the natural **penicillin G**; the broad-spectrum aminopenicillins, which include **ampicillin** and **amoxicillin**; the *penicillinase-resistant* or β-lactamase–resistant penicillins **cloxacillin, dicloxacillin, oxacillin,** and **methicillin**; and the extended-spectrum penicillins, including **ticarcillin, carbenicillin,** and **piperacillin**. Several other penicillins are used in human medicine but rarely in veterinary medicine because of cost and lack of FDA approval for use in animals.

Penicillins are generally effective against many Gram-positive bacteria and a lesser number of Gram-negative bacteria. Penicillins identified as broad-spectrum or extended-spectrum are effective against a wider range of bacteria than the natural penicillins or penicillinase-resistant penicillins.[5] Though general guidelines for whether a particular penicillin is effective against a particular Gram-positive or Gram-negative bacteria are useful in a broad sense, the emergence of resistant bacteria still requires a culture and sensitivity test be performed on bacteria in an infection site to more accurately identify if a particular antimicrobial will be effective or not.

Penicillins are bactericidal and work primarily by attaching to and blocking the bacterial enzymes needed to assemble the cell wall during bacterial cell division, making the resulting wall more structurally unstable and making the bacterium more prone to lysis from osmotic imbalances. Different penicillins affect different wall-building enzymes, which partially explains why one type of penicillin might be more effective against a bacterial population than another type. Methicillin-resistant *Staphylococcus aureus* (MRSA) is a bacterial strain found on the skin that has acquired resistance to all penicillins, including the extended-spectrum penicillin called *methicillin*. MRSA bacteria are resistant because the targeted wall-building enzyme to which penicillin attaches changes its molecular shape and in so doing makes the penicillin drugs unable to dock with and disrupt the enzyme. Therefore, the wall-building enzyme continues to function, and the bacterial cell wall forms normally. Without interference from any penicillin, MRSA bacterial infections can more readily proliferate and spread from patient to patient at home or in a hospital environment (e.g., nursing home).[5,1]

Because the cell wall assembly only occurs during cell division, penicillins are only effective against an actively dividing colony of bacteria. Thus, if a bacteriostatic antimicrobial (e.g., sulfonamide antibiotic) is used in conjunction with penicillin, the bacteriostatic effect would inhibit division of the bacteria, decreasing the opportunity for penicillins to prevent cell wall formation. A broad generalization of this concept is likely the reason for the erroneous statement that "no bactericidal antimicrobial should be used simultaneously with a bacteriostatic antimicrobial." Instead, a more accurate statement would be that "bacteriostatic antimicrobials should not be used simultaneously with β-lactam antibiotics" because the β-lactam antibiotics need the bacterial colony to be actively replicating. Bacteriostatic drugs can still be used effectively with other bactericidal drugs as long as those bactericidal drugs kill bacteria by disrupting protein synthesis or blocking essential enzymes.

Penicillin Pharmacokinetics

Penicillins are generally well absorbed from injection sites and the GI tract, with the exception of penicillin G, which is readily inactivated by gastric acid and so should never be given orally (PO). Penicillins are generally well distributed to most tissues in the body. However, because penicillin molecules are hydrophilic at body pH, they typically will not reach therapeutic concentrations in the globe of the eye, the brain, or the prostate gland because of the cellular barriers between the tissue and the blood supply. Although meningitis (i.e., inflammation of the meninges, membranes covering the brain) makes the blood-brain barrier more permeable and allows more drug molecules, including penicillins, to enter the central nervous system (CNS), even then the penicillins usually do not achieve concentrations within the CNS sufficient to significantly inhibit or kill bacteria.[5]

Most penicillins are excreted by the kidney intact without being metabolized. Not only are penicillins filtered by passive diffusion at the renal glomerulus but also they are actively transported (secreted) by the renal tubules into the forming urine. Because of the active secretion, the penicillin accumulates to much higher concentrations in the urine than is found in the blood, and thus urine concentrations of penicillins will exceed the MIC for many bacteria found in the kidneys, bladder, or genitourinary tract. This is why penicillins are commonly used to treat bacterial cystitis (i.e., urinary bladder inflammation caused by bacterial infection).

Penicillin Group Spectra of Activity and Resistance

There are general rules that can be applied to make an educated clinical guess as to which antimicrobial should be effective based upon the veterinarian's experience and knowing how the drug has performed historically in other patients with a similar infection. Based upon this historical data and experience, the veterinarian can predict whether the bacteria present are likely to be Gram positive or Gram negative or if they are aerobic (i.e., require oxygen) or anaerobic (i.e., do not require oxygen). Based upon the predicted Gram-positive/Gram-negative and aerobic/anaerobic characteristics of the bacteria in the infection, the veterinarian can make an educated guess about what antimicrobial drug should be effective. The selection of a particular antimicrobial drug before the results of a culture and sensitivity test are returned is referred to as *empiric treatment*, or implementing empiric therapy.[5] Often broad-spectrum antibiotics are used initially until the culture and sensitivity test results are returned, at which point a narrower spectrum antibiotic can be selected.

Each penicillin group has a slightly different bacterial spectrum. As a general rule, most penicillins are more effective against Gram-positive bacteria than Gram-negative bacteria. Unlike Gram-positive bacteria where the cell wall is readily accessible to penicillin drug molecules, Gram-negative bacteria have an outer capsule that penicillins can only penetrate by slipping through special capsule openings or porins (like pores). Some Gram-negative bacteria become resistant to penicillin drugs by genetically decreasing the size of the porins, making them too small to allow penicillin molecules to pass, preventing the drug from reaching the bacterial cell wall.[4,5] *Pseudomonas* is a particularly resistant Gram-negative bacteria commonly found in otitis externa (i.e., outer ear infections in dogs) or necrotic tissue, and only the most aggressive extended-spectrum penicillins (e.g., **ticarcillin**, **carbenicillin**) are likely to have much chance to be effective against this bacterial strain.

Although general guidelines based upon historical medical data exist for which bacteria are likely to be sensitive or resistant to penicillins (or any antimicrobial), the only way to determine for certain if a penicillin will work is to perform a culture and sensitivity test on the specific bacteria found in the infection.

Generally, if a strain of bacteria develops resistance to one type of penicillin, the bacteria will often also be resistant to many of the other penicillins. This phenomenon is known as cross-resistance.[2] Some bacteria, especially staphylococci, acquire resistance to many penicillins by producing an enzyme that attacks the penicillin's β-lactam ring, damaging the drug molecule and rendering the penicillin ineffective. These bacterial enzymes are called *β-lactamases* or penicillinases if they specifically attack penicillins, and almost all penicillin drug molecules are susceptible to this bacterial enzyme. Thus, development of bacterial β-lactamase would confer bacterial cross-resistance to many penicillin drugs.

There is one group of penicillins that is not affected by bacterial β-lactamase enzymes, and this group includes **oxacillin**, **dicloxacillin**, **cloxacillin**, and **methicillin**. These penicillins are often used in treatment of bovine mastitis or other infection sites in which β-lactamase–producing staphylococci have historically been found. Although these drugs are able to kill β-lactamase–producing staphylococci, their overall spectrum of activity against bacterial strains is far less (narrower) than the spectra of the more common penicillins like amoxicillin or ampicillin. Thus, the use of β-lactamase–resistant penicillins is usually limited to infections in which β-lactamase is likely to be produced by the bacteria.

Penicillin drugs that are normally inactivated by β-lactamase can be chemically protected from the enzyme if they are combined with another compound producing a stronger modified, or potentiated, penicillin that is resistant to the β-lactamase enzyme. **Clavulanic acid** (potassium clavulanate) and **sulbactam** are added to penicillin drugs such as amoxicillin or ampicillin to produce a potentiated penicillin compound capable of withstanding bacterial β-lactamase enzymes. Clavulanic acid has a β-lactam ring like penicillin so it can combine with the β-lactamase enzymes instead of the penicillin blocking the active enzyme site, and preventing the bacterial enzyme from combining with and destroying the penicillin molecule. By "sacrificing" itself and tying up the β-lactamase, clavulanic acid allows the penicillin to survive to attach to the cell wall enzymes and prevent normal cell wall formation.[5]

Precautions for Use of Penicillins

Compared with many other antibiotics, penicillins are quite safe drugs primarily because they target bacterial cell walls and mammalian cells only have cell membranes, not cell walls. The most common type of adverse reaction to penicillin drugs are hypersensitivity reactions (allergic reactions), which can manifest in a variety of clinical signs from a mild skin rash and hives to life-threatening anaphylactic shock. The severe anaphylactic reactions are more common with injectable penicillin products than with oral products and usually require aggressive emergency treatment, including administration of epinephrine and corticosteroids. Less severe drug reactions include skin rashes (urticaria or hives), swelling of the face, swelling of lymph nodes, hematologic changes (eosinophilia, neutropenia), and fever. If an animal exhibits hypersensitivity to one type of penicillin, the animal is likely to react adversely to other penicillin drugs, a phenomenon called cross-reactivity.

The mild signs of hypersensitivity can potentially progress to more severe clinical signs with repeated exposure to the same drug. Thus, it is important that the veterinary technician note in the patient's medical record and notify the veterinarian any clinical signs observed or reported by the client after the animal has been released that could possibly be evidence of a mild reaction to the drug. If this is not done and the animal receives a second injectable dose of the drug, the hypersensitivity reaction could be much more severe or life-threatening.

When given orally, penicillins may destroy beneficial Gram-positive bacteria residing in the lumen of the intestinal tract, allowing more pathogenic (i.e., disease-causing) bacteria, which are generally more penicillin resistant, to proliferate. This condition, called superinfection or suprainfection, can produce severe diarrhea that can result in death in some species such as guinea pigs, ferrets, hamsters, and rabbits. Other species in which penicillins must be used with caution include snakes, birds, turtles, and chinchillas.

Because penicillins are readily available to food animal producers, the importance of observing withdrawal times for penicillins and all other antimicrobials should be emphasized. Because selected penicillins are used to treat or control mastitis in cattle, dairy milk is frequently tested for the presence of penicillins. If a dairy producer administers penicillin and fails to observe the mandated withdrawal time between the last dose administered and when milk from the cow can be shipped to market again, the single cow with the contaminated milk could end up ruining an entire truckload of milk when the milk manufacturer tests for antibiotic contamination. In such cases, the source of contamination is traced back to the particular animal and the dairy producer generally ends up purchasing the entire bulk storage tank of unusable contaminated milk.

Considerations for Specific Penicillin Groups

As mentioned previously, there are four basic groups of penicillin drugs: the natural penicillins, the aminopenicillins, the penicillinase-resistant or β-lactamase–resistant penicillins, and the extended-spectrum penicillins. By understanding the penicillin group characteristics, when new penicillin drugs are made available to veterinary medicine the veterinary technician can better understand what the new drug does by knowing to which penicillin group it belongs.

Natural penicillin is the penicillin that is the same as the penicillin produced by mold (like the green mold found on bread) and includes **penicillin G**. Penicillin G is considered to have a narrow spectrum of activity compared with most of the other penicillins, and many bacteria are now resistant to this penicillin. As mentioned previously, it is always administered by injection because it is largely inactivated by the acidic stomach environment if given orally. Penicillin G is available in three injectable forms: an aqueous solution, which is penicillin complexed with potassium or sodium (e.g., penicillin G sodium); a

suspension form in which the penicillin G is combined with **procaine**; and a longer-acting suspension form in which the penicillin G is combined with **benzathine**. Only the aqueous forms of penicillin G sodium or potassium can be given intravenously (IV). This form can also be given subcutaneously (SQ) and intramuscularly (IM). Procaine penicillin G has been used with another antibiotic, novobiocin, as an intramammary infusion (i.e., administered via a plastic syringe with blunt applicator tip) in cows with mastitis.

The addition of procaine and benzathine to penicillin G delays absorption of the antibiotic from IM or SQ injection sites, extending the duration of drug activity. **Procaine penicillin G** usually provides adequate concentrations for 24 h, and **benzathine penicillin G** produces effective blood concentrations for 3–5 days. A disadvantage of the extended duration of the procaine and benzathine forms is that the initial peak plasma concentrations right after injection of the drug will not be as high as those attained after injection of the rapidly absorbed aqueous form, and the concentration over the duration of the extended absorption will fluctuate up and down because of variability of absorption from hour to hour. Fig. 10.5 illustrates the extended-duration penicillin G drugs.

It is important to note that procaine is also a local anesthetic. Therefore, it may be prohibited for use in horses at some race tracks because of the potential to make the horse less responsive to pain. Because a single injection of procaine penicillin G may make the horse test positive for procaine for as long as 2 weeks, the veterinarian working with competition horses must know the local regulations (race track or local ordinances) governing the use of procaine in race horses.

Ampicillin and **amoxicillin** are the **aminopenicillins** and have a wider effective spectrum against Gram-negative bacteria than penicillin G because of their ability to more readily move through the porins in the outer membrane of Gram-negative bacteria and reach the target sites on the Gram-negative bacterial cell wall. Like penicillin G, they are still susceptible to destruction and inactivation by β-lactamase.

Because aminopenicillins are not inactivated by gastric acid like penicillin G is, aminopenicillins are available in oral forms (capsules, coated tablets, and liquid suspension), as well as injectable forms. Oral amoxicillin is less affected than ampicillin by the presence of food in the GI tract; however, if possible the pet should be given the aminopenicillins on an empty stomach (if the animal can tolerate it). Although amoxicillin by itself is susceptible to destruction by β-lactamase, it is also available in combination with clavulanic acid (e.g., Clavamox, Augmentin), which protects the aminopenicillin against bacterial β-lactamase destruction.

The injectable ampicillin and amoxicillin forms can be formulated into a **trihydrate** form (e.g., amoxicillin trihydrate) to form a slow-release suspension that will prolong the absorption of aminopenicillins in a similar manner to the way procaine did with penicillin G.

The **β-lactamase–resistant penicillins** include **cloxacillin, dicloxacillin, oxacillin,** and **methicillin** and are naturally resistant to the effects of this bacterial enzyme (they do not require clavulanic acid or sulbactam). As previously mentioned, their

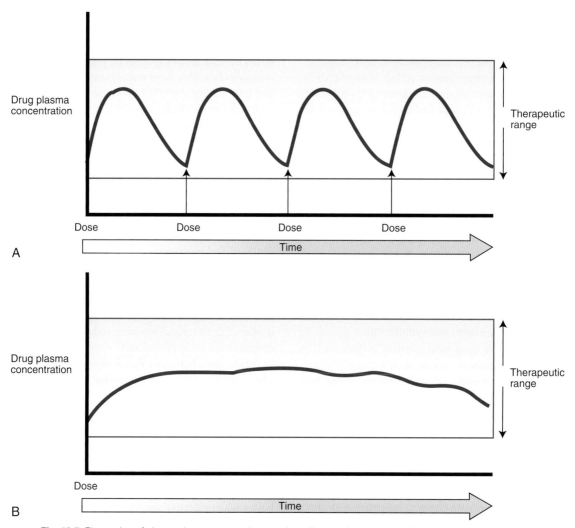

Fig. 10.5 Fluctuation of plasma drug concentrations produced by standard parenteral formulations and extended-absorption formulations of penicillin. (A) Penicillin concentrations after parenteral administration. (B) Penicillin concentrations when combined with procaine or benzathine.

overall spectrum of antibacterial activity is slightly less than that of the natural penicillins and the aminopenicillins because they do not penetrate the outer membrane of Gram-negative bacteria and thus cannot readily access the target sites on the Gram-negative cell wall. If Gram-positive *Staphylococcus* bacteria are resistant to methicillin, the infection would be called methicillin-resistant *S. aureus* or MRSA and all members of this antibiotic group would be ineffective against this bacterial strain.

β-Lactamase–resistant penicillins are most commonly used to treat staphylococcal osteomyelitis (i.e., bone infections), staphylococcal pyoderma (i.e., skin infections), and staphylococcal mastitis (available as intramammary teat infusion syringes).

The **extended-spectrum penicillins** include the human medications **ticarcillin, piperacillin,** and **carbenicillin** and have a wider spectrum than the other penicillins. These drugs are expensive and hence are not used very often in day-to-day veterinary practice. Unlike the other penicillins, these extended-spectrum penicillins are able to readily penetrate the outer membrane of Gram-negative bacteria, including *Pseudomonas,* and therefore

are sometimes referred to as "antipseudomonal penicillins." To enhance their effectiveness, the extended-spectrum penicillins are sometimes combined with other bactericidal antimicrobials like the aminoglycoside antibiotics (e.g., amikacin, gentamicin) to produce a synergistic effect that is greater than the antibacterial activity of either drug alone. However, these extended-spectrum penicillin drugs are still susceptible to β-lactamase enzymes, which is why some of these drugs are combined with clavulanic acid (e.g., ticarcillin plus clavulanic acid is Timentin). Because these drugs are considered "specialized" drugs to be held in reserve, they are most commonly used to treat severe, resistant Gram-negative infections in small animals.

Cephalosporins

Cephalosporins are bactericidal β-lactam antimicrobials that, like the penicillins, function by disrupting bacterial cell wall formation during cellular division. The *ceph-* or *cef-* prefix in the nonproprietary drug name identifies most members of this group, with *cef-* generally being used on the more recently discovered cephalosporins.

Cephalosporins are classified by generations according to when they were first developed. First-generation cephalosporins are primarily effective against Gram-positive bacteria such as *Streptococcus* and *Staphylococcus*. First-generation drugs are less effective against Gram-negative bacteria than the second- or third-generation cephalosporins. Cephalosporins are more resistant to the degradation by bacterial β-lactamase than most penicillins, and therefore they are more effective against *Staphylococcus* species of bacteria than the penicillin drugs.

Although second-generation cephalosporins are more effective against more Gram-negative bacteria than the first-generation drugs, they are generally less effective against Gram-positive cocci species (*Staphylococcus* and *Streptococcus*) than the older drugs. The same is true for third-generation cephalosporins, some of which are even effective against Gram-negative *Pseudomonas*. Thus, each generation of drug has gained some advantage over the previous generation but has lost some advantages as well. This general shift of spectrum from Gram-positive bacteria to more Gram-negative bacteria as the generations advanced is a general guideline because within each generation there are some drugs with spectra of activity that do not necessarily fit this rule. Again, culture and sensitivity testing for a specific infection will better help identify the appropriate definitive antimicrobial treatment.

In addition to FDA veterinary-approved cephalosporin drugs, some human cephalosporin drugs are also used in veterinary medicine.

First-generation cephalosporins used in veterinary medicine:
- cefadroxil (veterinary product), trade name Cefa-drops
- cephapirin (veterinary product), trade name Cefa-Lak/Cefa-Dri
- cephalexin (human product), trade name Keflex
- cefazolin (human product), trade name Kefzol

Second-generation cephalosporins:
- No veterinary products approved for use in veterinary medicine.
- Human products generally not used

Third-generation cephalosporins used in veterinary medicine:
- cefovecin (veterinary product), trade name Convenia
- cefpodoxime (veterinary product), trade name Simplicef
- ceftiofur (veterinary product), trade name Naxcel or Excenel

There are cephalosporins classified as fourth-generation and fifth-generation drugs, but none of those are used in veterinary medicine. The third-generation cephalosporins are often selected for initial empiric therapy (i.e., before the culture and sensitivity results come back) because of their broad spectrum of activity.

Mechanism of Action for Cephalosporins

Cephalosporins are β-lactam antibiotics with bactericidal mechanisms similar to those of penicillins. The cephalosporins bind to and inhibit enzyme(s) responsible for the formation of bacterial cell walls, causing a loss of the cell wall integrity. The loss of rigidity prevents the cell wall from maintaining the bacterium's osmotic balance and causes the bacterium to swell with water and lyse more easily with osmotic changes. Because more than one enzyme is involved in bacterial cell wall formation, the difference in spectra of activity for cephalosporins can be partially explained by the different affinities (i.e., attraction or ability to bind to) each cephalosporin has for the different cell wall–forming enzymes.

Like penicillins, cephalosporins are only effective against rapidly dividing bacterial colonies. Because cephalosporins are most effective against a population of bacteria that is rapidly dividing, simultaneous use of bacteriostatic antibiotics may reduce the efficacy of cephalosporins.

Because cephalosporin molecules have a β-lactam ring, they are susceptible to β-lactamase enzymes produced by bacteria but less so than the penicillins. Some β-lactamase enzymes may render cephalosporins ineffective without adversely affecting penicillin drugs. These bacterial β-lactamases specific for cephalosporins over penicillins are referred to as cephalosporinases.

Like penicillins, cephalosporins do not readily pass through the blood-brain barrier and therefore are not the drug of choice to treat bacterial infections of the CNS. β-Lactam antibiotics generally pass through the placental membranes of pregnant females to enter fetal tissues and can also pass into the animal's milk after systemic administration. Like penicillins, cephalosporins can achieve high concentrations in urine because most of the drug is excreted by both glomerular filtration and active secretion that pumps drug into the renal tubules, and therefore these drugs can be effective in treating renal or urinary tract bacterial infections.

Precautions for Use of Cephalosporins

Cephalosporins, like penicillins, are considered safe antimicrobials because mammalian cells do not have cell walls. Also similar to penicillins is the potential for cephalosporins to produce hypersensitivity reactions. However, the incidence of hypersensitivity reactions to cephalosporins is much lower than that of penicillins. Hypersensitivity reactions can cause fever, rashes, eosinophilia, and anaphylaxis. If an animal has evidence of hypersensitivity reaction to penicillins, the animal should also be considered a potential risk for hypersensitivity reactions to cephalosporins, and vice versa, because of cross-reactivity that has been reported between these two β-lactam drugs.

Superinfection caused by overgrowth of pathogenic bacteria may be associated with oral administration of first-generation cephalosporins. In addition, orally administered cephalosporins may cause anorexia, vomiting, and diarrhea by a mechanism not entirely understood (perhaps direct irritation of gastric mucosa).

Aminoglycosides

Aminoglycosides are a powerful group of antimicrobials used in veterinary medicine to combat a variety of serious, usually Gram-negative, aerobic bacterial infections. Aminoglycosides used in veterinary medicine include **gentamicin**, **amikacin**, **neomycin**, **kanamycin**, **tobramycin**, and **apramycin**. With the exception of amikacin, aminoglycosides can be identified by the *-micin* or *-mycin* suffix in the chemical or nonproprietary name. Note that many trade or proprietary names (not chemical or nonproprietary names) of tetracyclines also use the -*mycin* suffix; drugs with these trade names should not be confused with aminoglycosides. Of the aminoglycosides, amikacin and gentamicin are the two most commonly used in veterinary medicine.[7]

Mechanism of Action

Aminoglycosides are bactericidal through their action on the bacterium's ribosomal production of essential proteins. Because the ribosome is located within the bacterial cytoplasm, aminoglycosides must be transported through the bacterial cell membrane (which is inside of the cell wall) to exert their effects. Unfortunately aminoglycosides are highly ionized at body pH, making them hydrophilic and thus unable to diffuse across the bacterial cell membrane by passive diffusion. Thus, aminoglycosides must be actively transported by a carrier into the bacterium. This active transport mechanism requires oxygen, so for this reason aminoglycosides are only effective against bacteria that live in oxygen-rich environments (i.e., *aerobic bacteria*) and are totally ineffective against bacteria that live in an environment that lacks oxygen (i.e., *anaerobic bacteria*). The use of cell wall–inhibiting antibiotics such as penicillins enhances the ability of aminoglycosides to enter, and subsequently kill, the bacterial cell. Once taken up by the aerobic bacterium, the aminoglycoside combines with the ribosome and prevents normal synthesis of protein from amino acids. The effect on the ribosomes is bactericidal.[7]

Contemporary thinking is that once-daily dosing of aminoglycosides is equally effective and much safer than the older approved twice-daily and three times–daily dosing regimens.

Although the half-life of aminoglycosides is typically short (2–5 h) and concentrations with once-a-day dosing drop well below therapeutic concentrations a few hours after the dose is given, the drug continues to produce a postantibiotic effect that extends the drug's killing activity for the full 24 h between doses regardless of the low antibiotic concentrations. To produce a strong postantibiotic effect, the drug must achieve a very high peak concentration, even though it drops rapidly after the peak. This means that unlike β-lactam antibiotics that need to be "on site" continuously to be bactericidal and therefore are time-dependent drugs, the aminoglycosides just need to hit a critically high peak concentration for a short period of time and therefore are considered concentration-dependent drugs.[4,7]

Although some cross-resistance occurs between members of the aminoglycoside family, it is not as common as with the penicillins. For example, some strains of *Pseudomonas* bacteria are resistant to gentamicin but sensitive to amikacin. Bacterial resistance is attributable to destructive enzymes produced by the bacteria or inability of the aminoglycoside to cross the cell wall or cell membrane.

Pharmacokinetics of Aminoglycosides

As mentioned previously, aminoglycosides are hydrophilic at most physiologic pH levels and therefore are usually administered parenterally (SQ, IM, or IV). Injection into the peritoneal (i.e., abdominal) cavity or the pleural (i.e., thoracic) cavity results in equally rapid absorption. If aminoglycosides are administered by mouth (PO) absorption across the GI tract wall would be severely limited. The few aminoglycosides used orally are intended to remain in the intestinal tract and not be absorbed to any significant extent. Neonates, animals with intestinal hypomotility (i.e., slow gut movement), and animals with hemorrhagic or necrotic intestinal disease absorb greater amounts of aminoglycosides administered orally and thus are potentially at greater risk of systemic side effects from the absorbed aminoglycoside drug.

Although aminoglycosides are not well absorbed across intact skin, they are well absorbed through denuded or abraded skin, or when used to irrigate surgical sites. Thus, applying a bandage soaked in aminoglycoside to a degloving injury (i.e., where the skin is traumatically removed from the paw) may result in a significant amount of drug being absorbed through the subcutaneous tissue. The hydrophilic aminoglycoside molecules do not penetrate the blood-brain barrier of the brain or the globe of the eye to any significant degree. Aminoglycosides are not secreted to any great degree into the respiratory tract, but if administered by inhalation (e.g., aerosol administration with a nebulizer), high concentrations can be achieved on the surface of the lining of the respiratory tract without significant increases of concentrations in the underlying tissues.

CLINICAL APPLICATION

Topical Application Induces Renal Failure

A 4-year-old cat had a large draining abscess over the lumbar region from an attack by a dog 4 weeks previously. *Pseudomonas* susceptible to gentamicin was cultured from the wound. The wound was lavaged with a gentamicin solution twice within 24 h. The cat was anesthetized and the wound cleaned. The cat recovered uneventfully from anesthesia. Gentamicin was administered subcutaneously (SQ) at 2.2 mg/kg q12h, starting 12 h after the wound was lavaged.

Three days later the cat showed signs of elevated blood urea nitrogen (BUN) and creatinine, both signs of decreased renal function. The urine specific gravity, which is a measure of the degree to which the kidney is capable of concentrating urine, was 1.008. In an animal that is somewhat dehydrated, the urine specific gravity should reflect a more concentrated urine (e.g., a specific gravity of greater than 1.035), which indicates the body is conserving or retaining water by not allowing the water to enter the urine. Because the kidneys are responsible for diluting or concentrating the urine under the control of antidiuretic hormone and aldosterone, the failure of the kidneys to concentrate urine appropriately suggested renal failure. The urine sediment contained red blood cells, white blood cells, and granular casts.

Because gentamicin *nephrotoxicosis* was suspected, the gentamicin was stopped and intravenous (IV) fluids begun at a rate of 6 mL/kg per hour. Ampicillin was used in place of the more nephrotoxic gentamicin. Unfortunately, the signs of renal toxicosis continued to worsen. The BUN and creatinine levels continued to climb even though IV fluid administration should have decreased these parameters. Despite the fluids, diuretics (furosemide), and other drugs designed to increase blood flow to the kidney, the urine output decreased. At the owner's request, the cat was euthanized.

Necropsy showed severe necrosis (i.e., cell death) of the proximal convoluted tubule of the kidney, one of the major sites where gentamicin and other aminoglycosides are taken up from the plasma by active transport. Serum samples

Continued

previously obtained from the cat 7–8 h after the second flushing of the wound with gentamicin showed a gentamicin concentration of 58.07 µg/mL. This concentration would have reflected the amount of drug in the body before the SQ administration of the drug had been started. Serum samples that had been taken at 80 and 96 h after the wound flushing showed concentrations of 10.43 and 13.13 µg/mL, respectively. The serum sample at 96 h post wound flushing was 24 h after the last SQ dose of gentamicin had been administered.

Gentamicin plasma (blood) concentrations should typically drop below 2.0 µg/mL at the low point after drug administration to reduce the risk for nephrotoxicosis. With the combination of gentamicin flushed directly into the wound (10 mL of gentamicin had been infused into the wound sites) and subsequent SQ administration of the gentamicin at a dose that would normally be well tolerated by a cat, gentamicin never had the chance to drop below the critical 2.0 µg/mL, making the conditions ideal for developing aminoglycoside nephrotoxicosis. In this case the nephrotoxicosis was not reversible and the animal was euthanized.

What should be learned from this situation: Although aminoglycosides cannot cross intact skin or intact intestinal tract very readily, a break in the barrier (in this case flushing the wound directly with the drug) can allow the hydrophilic molecules to be absorbed quite well, achieving significant concentrations in the plasma. The only way that nephrotoxicosis can be prevented with aminoglycosides is to allow the plasma concentrations to drop low enough to allow the intracellular drug to passively diffuse out of the cell. The persistent plasma concentrations greater than 2 µg/mL because of the drug in the wound site and injected SQ did not allow the plasma concentrations to drop low enough for back-diffusion of gentamicin from the kidney cells to the plasma to occur. The end result was overaccumulation of drug inside the kidney cells and permanent damage to the kidneys. Thus, veterinary technicians and veterinarians must remember that topically applied aminoglycosides should be considered the same as SQ-administered drugs if the skin barrier is broken.

In contrast to their inability to passively diffuse into the brain or eye, aminoglycosides are actively pumped into the cells of kidneys and the inner ear where they can accumulate to very high concentrations. This accumulation is thought to contribute to the nephrotoxicity and ototoxicity produced by frequent doses of aminoglycosides.

Aminoglycosides are eliminated almost exclusively by glomerular filtration in the kidneys. Because the molecules are in the hydrophilic state in the forming urine of the renal tubules, minimal drug resorption occurs in the loop of Henle and most of the drug is excreted in the urine. This efficient elimination helps explain the short half-life of aminoglycosides (usually 1–2 h depending on the species) in animals with normal renal function. Because these drugs are almost exclusively eliminated by the kidneys, any decrease in renal function from old age, dehydration, shock, or kidney disease can slow elimination and increase half-life, prolong high plasma drug concentrations, and increase the risk of nephrotoxicity or ototoxicity. Conversely, anything that increases renal perfusion could potentially speed up the elimination of the aminoglycosides and shorten the half-life. When interpreting the measured plasma concentrations of an aminoglycoside drug and its elimination half-life, the presence of IV fluid therapy or factors that cause temporary decreased renal perfusion will artificially skew the half-life and observed concentrations,

making a simple recommendation for dosage change based on the concentrations more difficult.

Precautions for Use of Aminoglycosides

Aminoglycosides are potentially nephrotoxic (i.e., toxic to the kidney) and ototoxic (i.e., toxic to the inner ear) even at normal doses if the drug is given for an extended period of time. Therefore, anyone who administers these drugs or monitors their effects in an animal should be aware of the way these drugs act in the body.

As previously mentioned, cells of the inner ear and kidney actively take up aminoglycosides from the blood/plasma, which causes the drug to accumulate within the cells so much that they produce toxicity. Only by lowering the concentration of drug outside the cell can the amount of drug being pumped into the cells be reduced. Also, the accumulated drug within the cell may have some weak opportunity to leave those cells by passive diffusion that moves drug molecules across a membrane from high concentrations (inside the cell) to low concentrations (in the plasma or blood). Because aminoglycosides are hydrophilic and do not readily pass through cell membranes by passive diffusion, any diffusion requires a steep concentration gradient from inside to the plasma. Thus, a very low plasma/blood concentration during the dosing interval is essential to preventing accumulation and toxicity.

A dosage regimen can facilitate achieving the very low plasma concentration by extending the dose interval (i.e., the time between doses) so that more time is allocated for the drug plasma concentrations to drop very low. Failure to allow the plasma concentrations to drop low enough, such as the delivery of aminoglycosides by a constant rate infusion (CRI) or multiple doses during a 24-h period, would mean a greater accumulation of drug within the renal or otic cells and a more significant risk for nephrotoxicosis and ototoxicosis.

It was stated previously that aminoglycosides should not be used in animals with compromised kidneys because aminoglycosides are eliminated via the kidneys. However, sometimes they need to be given to a neonate foal whose renal function is less than normal. In these situations the normal dose (mass of drug) is given to attain the high peak concentration necessary for bactericidal activity and the postantibiotic effect, but the interval between injections is lengthened to allow more time for the decreased renal elimination ability to get rid of the drug and achieve very low plasma concentrations (Fig. 10.6).

An early sign of aminoglycoside nephrotoxicity is the appearance of casts or increased protein in the urine. In the absence of aminoglycoside plasma concentration measurements, daily urinalyses of high-risk patients for the presence of casts and protein may provide some early indications of impending nephrotoxicity. By the time elevated blood urea nitrogen (BUN) and creatinine levels are detected on a blood chemistry panel, 70%–75% of the kidney function has already been compromised to some degree. However, aminoglycoside nephrotoxicity may be reversible if the drug is withdrawn soon enough or the dosage interval is lengthened to reduce drug accumulation before extensive renal tubular necrosis (actual cell death) has occurred.

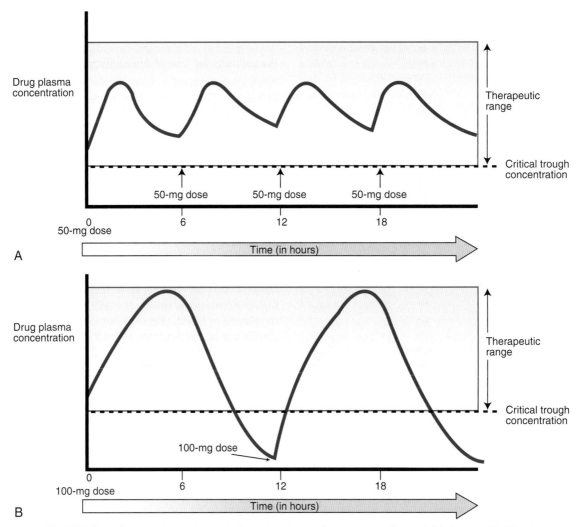

Fig. 10.6 Extending the dosage interval allows the plasma drug concentration to fall below a critical level. (A) Fifty milligrams of aminoglycoside given q6h: trough concentration does not decrease enough to prevent nephrotoxicity. (B) Same daily dose with 100 mg of aminoglycoside given q12h: trough concentration is low enough to decrease risk of nephrotoxicity.

Aminoglycoside use resulting in ototoxicity can cause deafness in affected animals. Although deafness is not necessarily a devastating disability in many household pets (most animals can adapt), deafness can end the usefulness and investment in service dogs who are trained to assist impaired people, work with law enforcement, or perform other critical tasks in which hearing commands or being able to respond to environmental auditory stimuli is essential to being able to do their jobs.

Ototoxicity also often affects balance (the vestibular system of the inner ear), so again service and working dogs can be rendered completely ineffective if unable to maintain their balance. Cats are apparently highly sensitive to the vestibular toxic effects of aminoglycosides and may circle, fall over, or display repetitive, rapid eye movements (i.e., **nystagmus**) as a result of toxic aminoglycoside administration. Therefore, the benefits of aminoglycoside administration must be weighed carefully against the potential risks in these types of animals.

Neomycin appears to be the aminoglycoside with the greatest potential for inducing nephrotoxicity in animals and people if it is systemically absorbed. However, neomycin is not used as an injectable, and it is poorly absorbed from the intestinal tract when given PO per approved label use for diarrhea treatment, thus limiting its nephrotoxic risk under normal circumstances. Nephrotoxicity from gentamicin use has been reported in other nondomestic species, including exotic animals, wildlife, and birds.

Although aminoglycosides are quite effective against many aerobic bacteria, the presence of cellular debris at the infection site (pus) can block aminoglycosides from reaching the bacteria in the infection site. Cellular debris is composed of ruptured cells and cell contents, including the nucleic acids of ribosomes. As previously stated, aminoglycosides attach to the nucleic acids of ribosomes in bacteria to produce their bactericidal effect. If an aminoglycoside enters an infection site that contains a significant amount of cellular debris, the drug tends to bind to the nucleic acids in the cellular debris; therefore, less drug reaches and is absorbed into the bacteria. Thus, **pyogenic** (pus-producing) infections, such as abscesses or topical infections with necrotic tissue must be cleaned or flushed thoroughly to remove cellular debris before applying aminoglycosides.

As previously mentioned, aminoglycosides require oxygen to be taken up by the bacteria. Therefore, anaerobic conditions such as abscesses, deep puncture wounds, deep cavities in the mouth or gums, and the colon would be areas in which an otherwise excellent aminoglycoside antibiotic would be rendered essentially ineffective.

Because aminoglycosides are such important drugs when used appropriately, and because aminoglycosides also have the potential to produce very serious side effects or be inactivated when used inappropriately, the veterinary professional must carefully consider the dosage regimen and the physiologic or pathologic conditions that exist in the patient at the time the drug is administered.

Fluoroquinolones or Quinolones

Quinolones, or fluoroquinolones, are a group of bactericidal antimicrobials that are continually expanding in human and veterinary medicine and in some cases have replaced aminoglycosides for treating serious aerobic Gram-negative bacterial infections.[9]

The majority of fluoroquinolones can be identified by their -floxacin suffix in the nonproprietary name. The first quinolone introduced to veterinary medicine in North America in the late 1980s was **enrofloxacin** (Baytril). Since that time **marbofloxacin** (Zeniquin), **orbifloxacin** (Orbax), **difloxacin** (Dicural), **pradofloxacin** (Veraflox), and **danofloxacin** (Advocin) have been approved as veterinary drugs. **Ciprofloxacin**, a human drug that gained public attention with the emergence of the bioterrorism threat of anthrax, and **ofloxacin**, a human ophthalmologic antibiotic, are two other quinolones cited in veterinary literature for use in animals. There are other fluoroquinolones used in human medicine that from time to time appear in veterinary literature. However, the ones listed here are the most frequently mentioned.

Enrofloxacin, **marbofloxacin**, and **orbifloxacin** are all approved for use in the dog and cat, and **difloxacin** is approved for use in dogs. **Pradofloxacin** is unusual in that it was developed for use only in cats in the United States but has been used in both dogs and cats in Europe. **Danofloxacin** (Advocin is its trade name) is one of the few quinolones still allowed to be used in food animals because of concern that fluoroquinolone antimicrobial use in food animals could be facilitating the emergence of resistant bacteria that could infect humans. However, danofloxacin's use is limited to beef cattle only (not dairy cattle or veal) for treatment of bovine respiratory disease. It has been used extra-label in goats and horses not used for human food. Note that there are currently no quinolones approved and labeled for use in horses, so all use of quinolones in horses is extra-label. No quinolones can be used in any horse intended for human food and any extra-label use of fluoroquinolones in any food animal is prohibited by law in the United States.

Mechanism of Action

In bacteria, the DNA molecule must be tightly coiled to be properly stored within the bacterial cell. The enzyme DNA gyrase (also called *topoisomerase II*) facilitates the unwinding of DNA strands so they can be recoiled into tight supercoils. Quinolone antimicrobials interfere with DNA gyrase, preventing bacterial DNA supercoiling and subsequently disrupting DNA function; this rapidly kills the bacterium. Quinolones do not disrupt mammalian cell function because bacterial and mammalian DNA gyrases are different; hence, quinolones are considered safe drugs to use.[9]

The fluoroquinolones have the advantage over β-lactam antibiotics in that they are effective in treating skin, respiratory, and urinary infections caused by both Gram-negative bacteria like *Pseudomonas, Klebsiella, Escherichia coli,* and *Salmonella* species, as well as Gram-positive bacteria including β-lactamase–producing *Staphylococcus*. Enrofloxacin's activity against *Pseudomonas* is considered to be superior to gentamicin's activity and on par with some of the more powerful aminoglycosides. Although quinolone-resistant *Pseudomonas* has emerged, quinolones and some third-generation cephalosporins are the only orally administered antibiotics considered to have effectiveness against *Pseudomonas*. In spite of this impressive spectrum of activity, veterinary-approved quinolones are not consistently effective against some common Gram-positive *Streptococcus* species. Therefore, quinolones are not recommended for use in streptococcal infections. Many MRSA *Staphylococcus* bacteria have developed a pump that removes quinolones once they enter the bacterium, thus preventing the drug from killing the bacterium and making the MRSA resistant to quinolone antimicrobials. As stated previously, concerns over development of resistant bacteria have prompted regulations that prevent any extra-label use of quinolones in food animals.

Because of quinolone's effectiveness against *Salmonella* species and *Pseudomonas,* these drugs are commonly used to treat bacterial infections in reptiles and other species where these two bacteria are commonly found in captive habitats.

Like aminoglycosides, quinolones are concentration dependent, meaning they must achieve a single, high peak concentration but do not have to remain at the infection site to continue to have bactericidal activity. Additionally, like aminoglycosides, quinolones are not effective in anaerobic environments and therefore are only effective against aerobic bacteria.

Pharmacokinetics of Quinolones

Some variability in the absorption of oral quinolone products occurs across species. Orally administered quinolones are absorbed almost 100% from the intestinal tract of dogs and cats. Absorption of oral quinolones is far more variable in horses and ruminants. Although young calves can adequately absorb orally administered enrofloxacin, bioavailability is less than 20% after oral administration in mature ruminants. Adult horses seem to absorb quinolones well after oral administration, but foals do not. Unlike some penicillins, enrofloxacin absorption after oral administration is not significantly affected by food; food only slightly delays the onset of absorption.

Most modern quinolones are highly lipophilic and accumulate in high concentrations in the kidneys, liver, lungs, bone, joint fluid, aqueous humor of the eyeball, and respiratory tissues. Concentrations of quinolones in the urine typically exceed plasma concentrations (some sources say they exceed concentrations by several hundred times); thus, they are present at concentrations that far exceed the MIC for susceptible organisms in the urinary tract. This explains why quinolones are one of the drugs of choice for treating urinary tract infections.

Quinolones also produce 4–10 times higher concentrations inside macrophages and neutrophil cells than the surrounding plasma.[9] Thus, when these inflammatory cells move into a site of infection or inflammation, they carry the drug with them, delivering high concentrations to the bacteria causing the infection. This is the mechanism by which quinolones achieve such high concentrations in the skin of animals with pyoderma (i.e., infection of the skin involving pus), making them drugs of choice for this condition. This mechanism also explains the effectiveness of quinolones in treating bacterial respiratory disease. As a general rule, most antibiotics cannot penetrate the prostate gland, but quinolones can accumulate in the prostate at concentrations two to three times that of plasma, and therefore it is one of the few antimicrobials that effectively treats prostate infections.

Each quinolone has a slightly different route of elimination. Enrofloxacin is mostly eliminated by the kidney; however, up to one fourth of the enrofloxacin is also metabolized to ciprofloxacin, which in turn is metabolized to inactive metabolites. Difloxacin is almost exclusively metabolized by the liver to inactive metabolites and thus would not be as effective in treating urinary tract infections as enrofloxacin because of how little drug is excreted into the urine. Marbofloxacin, orbifloxacin, and the rest of the quinolones are eliminated by a combination of liver and renal routes.

Ten percent to 40% of enrofloxacin is actually metabolized to **ciprofloxacin** for part of enrofloxacin's antibacterial activity. Hence, it makes sense that the human ciprofloxacin drug can also be used in an extra-label manner in small animal medicine for similar types of infections for which enrofloxacin might be indicated.[10]

Precautions for Use of Quinolones

Although quinolones are considered very safe drugs, they can adversely affect developing joint cartilage. During periods of rapid growth in dogs, high doses of fluoroquinolones may cause bubble-like lesions to form in the joint cartilage. Because this cartilage is the weight-bearing surface in joints, concern exists about the potential for joint degeneration and arthritic changes as the animal grows older. Although these reported bubble-like changes occurred only after administration of five times the normal dose, the manufacturer label still states that enrofloxacin is contraindicated for use in small- and medium-sized dogs between the ages of 2 and 8 months. The veterinary professional must remember that large-breed dogs have periods of rapid cartilage and bone development that extend well beyond 8 months; therefore, use of quinolones is contraindicated for up to 12 months in large breeds and 18 months in giant breeds. Some authors state that in clinical practice such use of fluoroquinolones is **relatively contraindicated** under these conditions, meaning that if the young animal is going to die if not given the fluoroquinolone, then the drug should be given despite the concern over the potential future impact on the joints.

Relative contraindications are a way of suggesting that the drug *may* be given if the benefit outweighs the risk as opposed to absolute contraindication where the drug should not be given under certain conditions, period (e.g., patients identified as having allergic hypersensitivity to penicillins and therefore should not be given penicillins).

Although enrofloxacin has been used in horses (extra-label use), studies have not been done to look for similar articular cartilage changes in this species. Thus, avoiding this drug in young horses might be prudent because of the unanswered question about the potential of cartilage damage in this species.

Apparently quinolone absorption can be significantly reduced if administered orally with antacids or sucralfate (ulcer treatment medication; see Chapter 4). In human beings, the absorption of orally administered quinolone can be reduced by up to 90% with concurrent administration of sucralfate. As a rule, concurrent use of quinolones with any drug or compound with two or three positive charges (e.g., iron, magnesium, calcium) or with sucralfate should be avoided completely or their administration separated from each other by at least 4 h.

Some evidence supports the warning against using quinolones in animals that are prone to seizures. At high doses, quinolones can inhibit the inhibitory neurotransmitter gamma-aminobutyric acid (GABA), allowing overexcitement of the CNS. In instances described in the literature as rare or infrequent, quinolones have precipitated seizure activity in animals predisposed to seizures. Therefore, the benefits of quinolone use should be weighed against the possibility of producing seizures before using these antibiotics in epileptic animals.

Although the initial 1997 dose of enrofloxacin for cats was labeled at 5–20 mg/kg once daily or divided twice daily, dosages of greater than 20 mg/kg in cats were discovered to potentially cause mild to severe changes in the retina, in some cases resulting in blindness. In 2000, the manufacturer issued a notice to veterinarians that the dose of enrofloxacin for cats would be reduced from a range of 5–20 mg/kg to a single dose of 5 mg/kg. Although this blindness phenomenon has not been reported extensively for other fluoroquinolones, there have been some anecdotal reports of blindness suspected to be associated with other quinolones and reports of blindness in cats on enrofloxacin at doses less than the currently recommended 5 mg/kg. The blindness reported may be temporary or permanent and is more often associated with higher doses than lower doses. However, because of the idiosyncratic nature of this retinal degeneration veterinarians still cannot predict which cat will be affected because many cats do tolerate higher doses without apparent changes to retinal function.

Indiscriminate use of quinolones for routine infections in which other older drugs could be equally effective has been implicated as a factor in the development of bacterial resistance against this group of drugs. Quinolones play a very important role in combating human bacterial infections; therefore, there is increasing concern that bacterial resistance observed in animals could readily transfer to resistant bacteria in people and pose a significant threat to human medical treatments. This increased bacterial resistance is thought to be particularly likely if the resistant bacteria are consumed or contacted from contaminated animal produces being used as human food. It was from this concern that the ban on the extra-label use of quinolones in any food-producing animal, including the quinolones that were originally approved for use in poultry, was enacted. With the continuing concern over the effect of drug residues in human food, quinolones will not likely be approved on a large scale for livestock use in the near future. It is conceivable that a ban on quinolone antibiotics could also be extended to other antimicrobials used in food-animal production in the future severely limiting the treatment options available to the veterinarian. Therefore, today's veterinary technician needs to understand what is driving this concern and government regulation, the mechanism by which resistance occurs, and what steps the veterinary profession and livestock producers need to take to limit further emergence of resistant bacteria.

Tetracyclines

Tetracyclines are a group of bacteriostatic antimicrobials that have been used in veterinary medicine for many decades, especially in food animal production. Tetracycline drugs can usually be recognized by the -cycline suffix of the nonproprietary name. Although many drugs belong to the tetracycline family of antimicrobials, the tetracycline family of drugs can be divided into two general classes of drugs[1]: the older, hydrophilic drugs and[2] the newer, lipophilic drugs. The older drugs include **tetracycline** (the individual drug, not the drug family) and **oxytetracycline**, and the newer and more lipophilic drugs include **doxycycline** and **minocycline**. Doxycycline and minocycline are used more frequently in animals today because of their longer half-life, broader spectra of antibacterial action, and better penetration of tissues than the older tetracyclines.[6]

Many microorganisms previously susceptible to tetracyclines are now resistant to most of the older tetracyclines so these drugs have fallen out of favor as a first-line drug for general infections. However, tetracyclines as a family have unique properties including the ability to accumulate within mammalian cells and reach organisms that hide within mammalian cells. The newer tetracycline drugs are among the first drugs of choice for treating diseases caused by *Chlamydia* species, *Mycoplasma* species, *Rickettsia* species, and spirochete bacteria. The common diseases caused by these organisms for which tetracyclines are among the first choice include:

- Rocky Mountain spotted fever caused by *Rickettsia rickettsii*, an intracellular parasitic type of Gram-negative bacteria
- Potomac horse fever caused by the rickettsia organism *Neorickettsia risticii*
- Lyme disease caused by the spirochete type of bacteria *Borrelia burgdorferi*
- Leptospirosis caused by the spirochete species *Leptospira*
- Mycoplasma pneumonia caused by intracellular organisms of the *Mycoplasma* species that are special bacteria that do not have a cell wall
- Chlamydial infections caused by *Chlamydia* species bacteria in cats and birds
- *Wolbachia* bacteria that live within canine heartworms and contribute to canine heartworm disease

Wolbachia is a Gram-negative, intracellular organism that lives symbiotically within, and is dependent on, the worms of canine heartworm disease (*Dirofilaria immitis*). Within the past few years it has been discovered that the *Wolbachia* bacteria likely contributes to the lung disease and possibly renal disease that occurs secondarily to heartworm infection. It has been shown that the *Wolbachia* bacteria also contribute to the health of the heartworm and that the viability of heartworms diminishes significantly if the *Wolbachia* bacteria are eliminated by doxycycline or minocycline. Doxycycline is now recommended as part of an initial treatment of heartworms in dogs by the American Heartworm Society (2014 report).[11] This will be discussed in greater detail in Chapter 12.

Mechanism of Action

Tetracyclines as a class bind to bacterial ribosomes and prevent t-RNA from linking to the ribosome, thereby disrupting protein synthesis. In contrast to the aminoglycosides, which also bind to ribosomes and disrupt protein synthesis in a slightly different way, tetracyclines inhibit bacterial cellular function and division but do not cause immediate bacterial destruction. Because tetracyclines are usually bacteriostatic, they depend on a functional immune system to help them overcome a microbial infection.

Tetracyclines do not bind to the mammalian ribosomes of domestic animals and pets as readily as they do with bacterial ribosomes. Therefore, at normal dosages mammalian cells are not significantly affected by tetracyclines. However, at higher dosages protein synthesis in mammalian cells may also be affected.

Pharmacokinetics of Tetracyclines

The two groups of drugs in the tetracycline family differ in their lipophilic/hydrophilic nature, and hence they have different abilities for absorption from the GI tract and differ in their abilities to penetrate cellular barriers to distribute to the brain, prostate, and other protected compartments. Generally, doxycycline and minocycline are more lipophilic and therefore more readily absorbed from the GI tract than oxytetracycline or tetracycline. The hydrophilic nature of tetracycline and oxytetracycline makes them less able to passively diffuse across the GI tract wall and be absorbed, and their hydrophilic nature makes them more readily able to chelate with (i.e., bind to and precipitate out of solution) the mineral ions with divalent cations (i.e., ions with two positive charges): calcium (Ca^{2+}), magnesium (Mg^{2+}), iron (Fe^{2+}), and copper (Cu^{2+}).

If oxytetracycline or tetracycline is administered by mouth with a meal that includes dairy products, such as milk or cheese, or other foods high in divalent cations or trivalent cations (i.e., three positive charges), much of the drug may be chelated in the gut and not absorbed. In addition to milk and cheese, other common items that can chelate tetracyclines include iron supplements, oral antacids (Mg^{2+}), and antidiarrheal products that contain kaolin, pectin (Kaopectate), or bismuth subsalicylate (Pepto-Bismol). In contrast to oxytetracycline or tetracycline, doxycycline's absorption is only reduced by approximately 20% in the presence of most of these products, which is not clinically significant in most cases.

Oxytetracycline is the more commonly used injectable tetracycline because of its good absorption from IM injection sites. In contrast to oxytetracycline, tetracycline is erratically absorbed from IM injection sites and therefore produces more reliable concentrations when administered by mouth. Oxytetracycline injectable is also commonly marketed in a longer acting form as LA-200, which is administered with a longer dose interval of 2 or 3 days.

Once absorbed into the systemic circulation, tetracyclines are distributed to most tissues and can reach significant concentrations in saliva and bronchial secretions. Because tetracycline and oxytetracycline are hydrophilic, they do not achieve significant concentrations in the CNS or penetrate mammalian cells to reach intracellular pathologic organisms nearly as well as doxycycline or minocycline. Because of its penetrability, doxycycline is preferred over tetracycline and oxytetracycline for treatment of CNS signs associated with borreliosis (i.e., Lyme disease).

Oxytetracycline and tetracycline are excreted by a combination of renal filtration and, to a lesser extent, the liver. Because renal elimination is a fairly important excretion pathway for these two drugs, any change in kidney function such as renal disease or decreased renal perfusion (i.e., reduced blood flow) may reduce elimination and allow accumulation of drug in the body unless the dose is decreased. Oxytetracycline and tetracycline are partially excreted by the liver into the intestine where they are chelated with intestinal contents and excreted with the feces.

Doxycycline and minocycline are largely excreted by the liver into the intestine. Once excreted into the intestine, doxycycline may be reabsorbed because it chelates less with the intestinal contents and its lipophilic form more readily passes across the GI tract wall than oxytetracycline or tetracycline. Once reabsorbed, doxycycline can enter systemic circulation and effect infections until it is again removed by the liver. As discussed in Chapter 2, this is called enterohepatic circulation. Because doxycycline does not depend on glomerular filtration for elimination, its dose does not necessarily have to be reduced in animals with impaired kidney function.

Precautions for Use of Tetracyclines

The major problems with tetracyclines relate to their binding with calcium and other divalent cations. Tetracycline and oxytetracycline chelate with the minerals of developing tooth enamel and dentin, imparting a yellow, mottled discoloration if given when teeth are developing. Because the discoloration is permanent if incorporated into the adult tooth dentin and enamel, the veterinary professional should be careful not to administer tetracycline from 4 to 16 weeks of an animal's life while the adult teeth are developing. Although doxycycline can potentially cause the same discoloration effect on the teeth, it does not bind as well to the calcium in the tooth and has less of a color to cause discoloration than the more water-soluble oxytetracycline or tetracycline. In addition to combining with tooth dentin and enamel, tetracyclines also combine with the calcium in bones and at very high doses may slow bone development in young animals.[6]

Because tetracycline drugs are bacteriostatic antimicrobials, they may interfere with the efficacy of the β-lactam drugs penicillin and cephalosporin. The β-lactams can only inhibit the bacterial cell wall when the cell is dividing; therefore β-lactam antibiotics require an actively growing bacterial colony to exert their antibacterial action. These two group of drugs are not generally used together for that reason.

Tetracyclines are not considered effective against anaerobic bacteria and will not eliminate *Pseudomonas* infections even though some of these drugs do have activity against other Gram-negative bacteria.

As with other broad-spectrum antimicrobials, orally administered tetracyclines can produce superinfections from reducing populations of some beneficial GI tract flora (i.e., bacteria) and allowing overgrowth of pathogenic bacteria in the gut. In ruminants, high oral doses can kill off significant numbers of normal ruminal flora, resulting in ruminoreticular stasis (i.e., decreased rumen inactivity) and possibly bloat. In dogs, even if superinfections do not occur, diarrhea, vomiting, and anorexia are commonly reported and most likely caused by the direct irritation of the GI mucosa by orally administered tetracyclines. Cats tolerate tetracyclines even less and may show fever, depression, or abdominal pain. Because doxycycline absorption is not adversely affected to any significant degree by the presence of food in the intestines, food may be given with doxycycline to decrease some of these GI side effects.

Doxycycline powder from a broken capsule or a partially chewed tablet may adhere to the esophagus, injuring the tissues and causing inflammation and eventually forming scar tissue with the potential to create a stricture (i.e., narrowing) of the esophagus. The doxycycline hyclate formulation of doxycycline is thought to be more of a risk for esophagitis and erosion because of its highly acidic nature.[6] Esophageal damage and stricture formation have been reported in cats given oral doxycycline "dry" without any liquid, which allows the medication to stick to the esophageal lining. Studies have shown that giving a few teaspoons of water after the oral doxycycline dosing markedly reduces adhesion of doxycycline dose form to the esophagus and improves the successful movement into the stomach. Therefore, it is important that pet owners understand the importance of giving several milliliters of water to the cat immediately after the oral doxycycline is given.

IV injections of relatively small doses of doxycycline in horses have resulted in cardiac arrhythmias, collapse, and death. These signs have been observed in other species receiving rapid IV injections of normal doses of oxytetracycline and have resulted in low heart rate, electrocardiogram (ECG) abnormalities, and hypotension. Horses, however, appear to be especially susceptible to the arrhythmia effect from doxycycline to the point where the arrhythmia can cause sudden death. Oral administration of doxycycline in horses does not produce this same effect.[4,6]

It has been previously reported in the literature that expired tetracycline and oxytetracycline can decompose to form a nephrotoxic compound that results in reduced ability by the kidney to reclaim glucose from the urine, resulting in glucosuria. However, though Fanconi's syndrome was reported in the past in veterinary and human patients, it does not occur with the currently available formulation of tetracycline drugs.[6]

Sulfonamides and Potentiated Sulfonamides

Sulfonamides (sulfa drugs) are bacteriostatic antimicrobials that were the first antimicrobials used on a widespread basis in human and veterinary medicine. Because they have been in use for so long, many strains of bacteria have become resistant to them. To increase the efficacy of sulfonamides and convert them from bacteriostatic to bactericidal drugs, they are sometimes combined with other compounds such as **trimethoprim** and **ormetoprim** to *potentiate* (i.e., increase) their antibacterial effects.

Some of the more common sulfonamides and their potentiated combinations used in veterinary medicine include **sulfadimethoxine** (also combined with the potentiating compound ormetoprim in the veterinary drug Primor), **sulfadiazine** (also combined with the potentiating compound trimethoprim in the veterinary drug Tribrissen), **sulfamethoxazole** (also combined with trimethoprim in the human drug Septra or Bactrim), and **sulfasalazine** (Azulfidine, used for its antiinflammatory effect in inflammatory bowel disease). Other sulfonamides are used in veterinary medicine for poultry, food animals, and even aquaculture (fish).[8]

Sulfonamides are sometimes described as enteric or systemic sulfas in reference to the location of their site of action. The site of action for an enteric sulfa such as sulfasalazine is within the intestinal tract, and therefore the drug is designed to not be absorbed into the body to any great extent. In contrast, systemic sulfas are intended to be absorbed from the intestinal tract into the body to access many internal tissue sites and treat systemic infections.

Mechanism of Action

Bacteria need to synthesize folic acid from raw materials to survive. The folic acid they create is then used in protein and nucleic acid metabolism. Sulfonamides disrupt this essential process by inactivating a key enzyme involved in synthesis of folic acid. The potentiating compounds trimethoprim and ormetoprim also produce a bacteriostatic effect by interfering with a different enzyme in this same metabolic pathway. Separately, sulfas and trimethoprim and ormetoprim are bacteriostatic, but when combined into a potentiated sulfonamide drug they attack this essential metabolic pathway at two different locations to produce a bactericidal effect.[8]

The spectrum of action for potentiated sulfonamides is broad and includes Gram-positive bacteria, Gram-negative bacteria, protozoa organisms (e.g., intestinal coccidia, *Toxoplasma* organisms that cause toxoplasmosis, and *Sarcocystis neurona*, the organism of equine protozoal myeloencephalitis, or EPM). Although many bacteria are resistant to sulfonamides today, many of the commonly encountered protozoa in veterinary patients are still susceptible.

Unlike other sulfonamides, **sulfasalazine** is not commonly used for its antimicrobial effect; rather, it is used for its antiinflammatory effect in the colon to treat colitis. When sulfasalazine is given orally, less than one third of the drug is absorbed. The remainder stays in the bowel lumen, where it passes into the colon and is transformed by colonic bacteria into another sulfonamide (sulfapyridine) and an aspirin-like antiinflammatory drug (aminosalicylic acid). As discussed in Chapter 4 and as will be discussed in Chapter 13, the aspirin-like antiinflammatory compound inhibits prostaglandin formation, which in turn decreases colonic inflammation and hypersecretion associated with large bowel inflammatory disease.

Pharmacokinetics of Sulfonamides

With the exception of the enteric sulfonamide sulfasalazine, sulfonamides and their potentiated forms are well absorbed from the GI tract of monogastric (i.e., single-stomach) animals like the dog and cat. In ruminants the trimethoprim component of potentiated sulfas may be trapped in the rumen after oral administration and degraded to some degree, thereby reducing the amount of trimethoprim absorbed. Oral absorption for horses and ruminants varies a great deal based upon diet and the age of the animal. The drug insert included with the sulfonamide antibiotic should provide details on the effectiveness of the drug given the age of the animal and its current diet.

Generally, sulfonamides exist in a nonionized lipophilic form at body pH and therefore are well distributed throughout the body, including the pleural fluid (fluid within the thorax), peritoneal fluid (abdominal fluid), synovial fluid (joint fluid), and ocular fluid (fluid within the eye). Like the quinolones, most sulfonamides readily traverse the blood-prostate barrier and enter the prostate gland. Sulfonamides cross the placenta and have the potential to attain concentrations that are therapeutic or toxic to the fetus. Sulfonamides can also pass into the milk of nursing females. Because of their lipophilic nature, sulfa drugs also penetrate the blood-brain barrier and achieve significant concentrations in the CNS and the cerebral spinal fluid (CSF).[8]

Sulfa drugs vary in the degree to which they are excreted intact in the urine or metabolized by the liver before being excreted by the kidneys. Several sulfonamides are both filtered by the glomerulus and actively secreted into the renal tubules, achieving significant concentrations in the urine. This is one of the reasons sulfonamides are used to treat urinary tract bacterial infections.

In the potentiated compounds, the sulfonamide component and the potentiating compound (e.g., trimethoprim, ormetoprim) usually have different half-lives of elimination and different patterns of distribution. Trimethoprim is fairly quickly eliminated from the plasma; however, it may remain within some tissues for a longer time than its short half-life indicates. The pharmacokinetics of ormetoprim in domestic animals has not been well described. Clinically these pharmacokinetic differences between the sulfonamide and its potentiating compound are important because the bacteriocidal effect will only be achieved if both compounds penetrate the infection site together and achieve concentrations above the MIC for the bacterial species involved. This may be the reason some clinicians administer trimethoprim-sulfonamide products twice daily, even though once-daily use is recommended.

Precautions for Use of Sulfonamides

One of the more common reactions to sulfonamides in dogs is decreased tear production, resulting in keratoconjunctivitis sicca (KCS, or "dry eye"). Dogs with sulfonamide-induced KCS will suddenly begin to accumulate mucoid or crusty matter around the eye, show signs of ocular discomfort by rubbing the face or pawing at the eyes, and develop a dull appearance to the surface of the cornea. A veterinarian should immediately examine any dog treated with sulfonamides who begins to show these signs to determine whether tear production has been reduced. In the past, many cases of sulfonamide-induced KCS could not be reversed. Fortunately there is a cyclosporine ophthalmic ointment (Optimmune) that is available that will restore production of near-normal levels of tears. However, affected dogs must be treated with cyclosporine for the rest of their lives.

Other reactions associated with sulfonamides include skin reactions, which are manifested as pruritus (i.e., itching), swelling of the face, and hives. Additional hypersensitivity reactions can manifest as liver necrosis and liver failure. Doberman pinschers are cited by some authors as being more susceptible to sulfonamide hypersensitivity (allergic) reactions than other breeds.[12]

Thrombocytopenia (decreased platelets), leukopenia (decreased white blood cells), and anemia have been reported in dogs and cats on sulfonamides. The mechanism of action for these toxic side effects is not well understood. Animals who are on high doses or prolonged duration of therapy with sulfonamide appear to be more susceptible to these effects, but they can apparently also occur at most dosages and relatively short duration of therapy.

Some sulfonamides or their metabolites may precipitate in the kidney if an insufficient volume of urine is being formed (i.e., when the animal is dehydrated) or if the urine becomes acidic. The resulting crystalluria (crystals in the urine) can damage the renal tubules. The older sulfonamides and sulfadiazine are more prone to precipitation and crystal formation than the newer compounds. Although this adverse effect is now considered rare with the modern sulfonamides, pets on sulfonamides should have adequate water at all times (e.g., outdoor pen watering system is working or watering pan does not get overturned by the pet).

Salivation with oral administration of sulfonamide drugs in cats is common and profuse if the tablet is broken while administering the drug. The veterinary technician should work with the client to show how best to administer the drug without the tablet becoming lodged in the back of the throat or mouth or broken by the cat chewing on the tablet.

Unlike the systemically absorbed sulfonamides, the enteric sulfa **sulfasalazine** potentially poses a risk to cats because they cannot metabolize absorbed salicylates, as well as dogs. As mentioned previously, sulfasalazine is metabolized by GI bacteria to sulfapyridine and an aspirin-like aminosalicylic acid (salicylic acid or salicylate). If the salicylate compound is absorbed in sufficient amounts to overwhelm the cat's ability to metabolize the

CLINICAL APPLICATION

Skin Eruptions in Dogs on Sulfonamides

Case 1: A 5-year-old male miniature schnauzer was treated with oral trimethoprim-sulfamethoxazole at a dose of 24 mg/kg b.i.d. Eight days into treatment he developed pustules over most of the trunk. The trimethoprim-sulfamethoxazole was discontinued and cephalexin (cephalosporin antibiotic) 25 mg/kg t.i.d. and prednisone 0.5 mg/kg b.i.d. were begun. No significant improvement occurred after 1 week. At this point, the dog had a fever of 104.4°F and many ulcerative lesions on the neck, chest, axillary (armpit), and inguinal (groin) areas, covering an estimated 35% of the dog's body. Crusts and alopecia (hair loss) were evident on most other areas of the body. Skin scrapings were negative for parasites and skin fungus (dermatophytes). Bloodwork (complete blood count, blood chemistry profile) showed mild changes consistent with inflammation and the use of corticosteroids (increased serum alkaline phosphatase level). Biopsy suggested lesions consistent with a drug-induced condition (erythema multiforme).

The dog was treated with IV fluids to compensate for fluids lost from the open lesions and chlorhexidine (Nolvasan) whirlpool baths b.i.d. to reduce bacterial infection in the skin. The fever came down, no further lesions appeared, and existing lesions began to improve within 3 days of starting whirlpool baths. The dog was discharged 7 days after initiation of therapy with instructions to continue the chlorhexidine baths for an additional week. Most skin lesions were healed 2 weeks after the dog went home.

Case 2: A 10-year-old castrated male golden retriever with a long-term skin problem was put on trimethoprim-sulfamethoxazole at an oral dose of 22 mg/kg b.i.d. to combat the *Staphylococcus* bacteria cultured from the skin. The skin responded well initially; however, 12 days after starting the sulfa drug the dog stopped eating, developed a fever (105.8°F), and developed itchy skin lesions all over the body. Skin biopsies were taken and submitted for histopathology. Based on the history a tentative diagnosis of drug eruption (skin lesions from drug administration) was made. The trimethoprim-sulfamethoxazole was stopped and 0.2 mg/kg of oral prednisolone given b.i.d. for 4 days. Oral cephalexin (Keflex) was given at 23 mg/kg t.i.d. for 3 weeks. Eight days after stopping the sulfonamide, no new lesions had formed and existing lesions were covered with crusts (healing).

Case 3: A 7-year-old castrated male mix-breed dog with a 3-year history of recurrent episodes of skin inflammation with infection was presented to the referral hospital after treatment with trimethoprim-sulfamethoxazole failed to improve the skin condition as it had in the past. The skin in the axillary areas was without hair (alopecia) and roughened. Reddened papules of 1½ to 3 in. were present on the trunk and abdomen. Skin scrapings and fungal cultures were negative. Biopsies were taken. Based on biopsy and clinical appearance, a tentative diagnosis of drug eruption was made. The potentiated sulfonamide was stopped and the dog bathed with a 3% benzoyl peroxide shampoo every 5 days for 3 weeks. After 1 week most of the lesions had resolved.

What should be learned from these cases: Veterinary technicians must be aware of the dermal manifestation of drug eruption (skin reactions to drugs) so that if a client calls and mentions a change in the skin condition after starting the antibiotic, the veterinary technician will report this information accurately to the veterinarian for follow-up to determine whether a drug reaction has occurred. Failure to properly report this information or to dismiss it as "normal" for a dog or cat with "bad skin" could result in the dermatitis becoming progressively worse and potentially endangering the animal's life from opportunistic pathogens that thrive on severely damaged skin.

Abstracted from case report: Medleau L, et al. Trimethoprim-sulfonamide-associated drug eruptions in dogs. *J American Animal Hospital Association*. 1990;26:305–311.

drug, it can accumulate and produce salicylate (i.e., aspirin) toxicity. Therefore, sulfasalazine must be used cautiously in cats or animals with aspirin hypersensitivity.

Regardless of which sulfonamide is used, veterinary professionals should know how to recognize the signs of an adverse reaction to sulfonamides and advise animal owners in advance of possible side effects to prevent the serious complications caused by an adverse reaction.

OTHER ANTIMICROBIALS USED IN VETERINARY MEDICINE

Lincosamides

Lincosamide antibiotics include **lincomycin**, **clindamycin** (Antirobe), and **pirlimycin** (Pirsue). These drugs are bacterial protein inhibitors and can be bacteriostatic or bactericidal, depending on the concentrations attained at the infection site. Lincomycin is approved for use in a variety of species, including dogs, cats, swine, and poultry, but clindamycin is only approved for use in dogs. Pirlimycin is approved for use only in dairy cattle as a mammary infusion for mastitis. The lincosamides in general are effective against many aerobic, Gram-positive cocci. However, **clindamycin** is different from the other lincosamides in that it also has good efficacy against many anaerobic bacteria, which makes it an effective drug for use in deep pyodermas (i.e., skin infections), abscesses, dental infections, bite wounds, and osteomyelitis caused by *S. aureus*.[4,13]

Because lincosamides are generally metabolized in the liver and then excreted in the urine or bile, severe liver or renal disease can prolong the half-life of elimination and necessitate reducing the dose to prevent toxicity.

Because pirlimycin is used in dairy cattle, withdrawal times for milk and tissue residues are important. According to the manufacturer's package insert, current recommendations for milk withdrawal are 36 h after the last treatment, and withdrawal time for tissue residues (for slaughter purposes) is 9–21 days after the last treatment, depending on the number of treatments received.

Lincosamides in general are contraindicated for use in animals who rely on fermentation for part of their digestion of food because these drugs can alter the GI tract flora, allowing *Clostridium* bacteria to proliferate and produce toxins that can result in diarrhea and, in severe cases, death. This would include rabbits, hamsters, chinchillas, guinea pigs, horses, and ruminants. Even in approved species like dogs and cats, vomiting, diarrhea, and bloody diarrhea may occur from overgrowth of pathogenic bacteria caused by killing of competing anaerobic bacteria in the intestinal tract.

Macrolides

The macrolide antibiotics are a broad class of chemically related bacteriostatic drugs that primarily are used to treat Gram-positive bacterial respiratory disease. The specific macrolide drugs used in veterinary medicine include the human drugs **erythromycin** and **azithromycin** (Zithromax), and the veterinary drugs **tilmicosin** (Micotil), **tylosin** (Tylan), and **tulathromycin** (Draxxin). Tilmicosin, tylosin, and tulathromycin are all approved for livestock use, and the human products erythromycin and azithromycin are used in small animals. Tylosin is also occasionally used in dogs and cats extra-label particularly for a chronic diarrheal syndrome in dogs as mentioned in Chapter 4.[13]

Macrolides work by inhibiting bacterial protein synthesis and share similar spectra of antibacterial activity and bacterial cross-resistance. Because the spectrum of activity is similar to penicillin, the macrolides are often used as penicillin substitutes in animals or people allergic to penicillin.

Erythromycin, and the other macrolides, are effective in treating respiratory infections because they accumulate in respiratory secretions and thus are delivered to the surface of the respiratory tract where the bacterial infection typically starts (bacteria are breathed in and land on the surface of the respiratory epithelium). Erythromycin is similar in molecular structure to motilin, a compound found in the intestinal tract that stimulates intestinal motility. Thus, in human beings and to a lesser degree in veterinary patients, erythromycin can cause intestinal cramping, abdominal pain, and diarrhea. In healthy dogs, erythromycin doses too low to have an antimicrobial effect have been used to increase stomach motility in the normal direction, increase the speed of gastric emptying, and to therapeutically reduce stomach acid reflux into the esophagus. Erythromycin use in horses may cause diarrhea but stops after the drug is discontinued and usually does not result in a fatal diarrhea.[13]

Azithromycin is a human macrolide derived from erythromycin but has a slightly broader spectrum of activity than erythromycin. Like erythromycin, it accumulates in significant concentrations in the respiratory tract by being incorporated into respiratory secretions. In addition to Gram-positive bacteria, azithromycin is also effective against *Mycoplasma* organisms, a bacterial strain found in pneumonia and feline respiratory disease; thus this drug has been used for persistent respiratory diseases that do not respond to other first-line antibiotics.[11,13]

Tilmicosin (Micotil) is a macrolide approved for SQ administration for treatment of bovine respiratory diseases. The drug concentrates well in lung tissues and is especially effective against the organisms that cause bovine respiratory disease complex. The drug is highly irritating if given IM and can cause death in some species if given IV. Horses, swine, primates, and human beings are much more sensitive to the cardiotoxic effects of tilmicosin and can exhibit tachycardia (rapid heart rate) and potentially fatal arrhythmias.

Deaths in livestock handlers from accidental injection of Micotil have been reported in the toxicology, agricultural, and livestock literature. In a case described in a publication from the National Agricultural Safety Database, a cattleman accidentally injected himself with Micotil after being knocked down by a charging cow. In this case, the cattleman died 1 h after injection from cardiac arrest. In another case reported in the *Journal of Toxicology,* the subject was attempting to inject a steer when he accidentally injected himself in the forearm.[14] Clinical signs did not appear for 5 h, at which point severe chest pains occurred. In this case the injected individual survived.

In addition to these reports, there are hundreds of other accidental injections reported that did not result in any injury to the person injected. Thus, the arrhythmia reaction is fairly rare, but there is no antidote for the drug once injected. Because tilmicosin can potentially be dangerous to human beings, veterinary professionals must be especially careful to prevent accidental injection into human beings by not carrying uncapped syringes loaded with the drug, carrying no more of the drug than needed for one animal (do not use multidose syringes or put multiple doses in one syringe), and taking precautions to prevent contact of the drug with the eyes. A physician should be contacted immediately in cases of accidental human injection or contact with the eyes.

Note: There have been reports of tilmicosin being used as a suicide drug. Therefore, it is important that this drug be tightly controlled even though it is not a Drug Enforcement Administration (DEA)-designated Controlled Substance.

Tylosin (Tylan) has historically been used was to promote growth (feed to weight conversion) in cattle, swine, and chicken. It has a wide variety of other approved uses such as treating infectious bovine keratoconjunctivitis (IBK) or "pink eye" (*Moraxella bovis*), swine dysentery (diarrhea), respiratory disease in cattle and pigs, and other diseases in poultry. In pigs it plays an additional role in reducing a bacteria-mediated arthritis and reducing a chronic intestinal disease called porcine proliferative enteritis (PPE). Note that according to the manufacturer's package insert, Tylan has been approved for treating a bacterial infection in honey bees.[13]

Tylosin requires a somewhat prolonged withdrawal time of 2 (for pigs) to 3 weeks (for cattle) and should not be used in lactating animals because residue can appear in the milk for even longer periods of time. Tylosin is not approved for use in dairy cattle.

As mentioned in Chapter 4, tylosin is used in middle-aged, larger breed dogs to treat a chronic diarrhea syndrome of unknown origin that has been labeled a "tylosin responsive enteritis." The underlying cause of this syndrome is unknown, but tylosin has been shown to control the diarrhea but not necessarily provide a permanent cure.

Tulathromycin (Draxxin) is the newest of the macrolides used frequently in veterinary medicine to treat livestock diseases. The manufacturer claims that a single injection can provide therapy for bovine respiratory disease for up to 14 days. Like tylosin, it is also effective against bovine IBK or pink eye and is recommended for treatment of a bacterial infection of cattle hooves called *interdigital necrobacillosis*, or more simply, *bovine foot rot*.

Metronidazole

Metronidazole (Flagyl) is a bactericidal antimicrobial that is also effective against protozoa that cause intestinal disease, such as *Giardia* (giardiasis), *Entamoeba histolytica* (amebiasis), *Trichomonas* (trichomoniasis), and *Balantidium coli* (balantidiasis). Although no approved veterinary form of metronidazole exists, human formulations are used for treatment of protozoal infections of the large bowel in dogs and cats and enteric bacterial infections caused by anaerobic bacteria in horses, dogs, and cats.

Because metronidazole has been used successfully in common domestic species, it is also being used to treat anaerobic infections in avian and reptilian species. Resistance to metronidazole by *Giardia* and some bacteria is beginning to be noticed and reported in the veterinary scientific literature.

The exact mechanism of action of metronidazole is not known, but it may be metabolized to a form that can disrupt synthesis of DNA and nucleic acids. The metabolic process by which metronidazole is converted to its active form can only occur under conditions of low oxygen; therefore, metronidazole is only effective against anaerobic bacteria and has minimal effectiveness against aerobic bacteria. For that reason, metronidazole is often selected for use in the lumen of the intestinal tract or for soft tissue infections that form anaerobic conditions (e.g., deep puncture wounds).

As mentioned in Chapter 4, metronidazole has been reported to produce some reversible transient neurologic side effects, including loss of balance, head tilt, nystagmus (rapid, repeated horizontal, vertical, or circular eye movement), disorientation, and even tremors and seizures. These effects are observed more frequently in animals receiving an overdose; however, they have also been observed in animals treated with recommended doses for long periods of time. The observed neurologic effects usually disappear within a few hours to days after the drug is stopped.

Chloramphenicol and Florfenicol

Chloramphenicol is an antimicrobial that is bacteriostatic at low concentrations but may become bactericidal at higher dosages. It works by binding to ribosomes in sensitive bacteria and disrupting bacterial protein synthesis. However, chloramphenicol can also disrupt mitochondrial function in bone marrow cells of mammals temporarily damaging production of bone marrow cells, or it can produce a more serious and fatal aplastic anemia in human beings. The fatal aplastic anemia (decreased production of red blood cells, white blood cells, and platelets) reported in humans has not been reported to occur in animals exposed to chloramphenicol. Even though the aplastic anemia in humans is rare and idiosyncratic (i.e., it cannot be predicted), the risk for it has resulted in chloramphenicol use in any food animals to be completely banned.

In the past, chloramphenicol was used widely because of its excellent ability to penetrate tissues, including the prostate gland, globe of the eye, and CNS, and its effectiveness against intracellular organisms like *Rickettsia*, mentioned with the tetracycline drugs. But because of the concern over exposure of chloramphenicol to those administering it (e.g., handling capsules of chloramphenicol powder or breaking tablets), the use of the drug declined a great deal. More recently, chloramphenicol has made a slow comeback and is cited more frequently in the veterinary literature for treatment of diseases in which the infection resides in areas of the body difficult to access (e.g., globe of the eye, brain, prostate).

In dogs, most of a chloramphenicol dose is metabolized by glucuronide conjugation in the liver, and very little drug is excreted unchanged into the urine. Because cats and very young animals of other species are deficient in the glucuronide pathway, they poorly metabolize chloramphenicol in the liver and thus are more likely to accumulate the drug than the dog if the dose is not decreased significantly. Neonates (especially neonatal kittens) can easily develop chloramphenicol toxicosis because of their poor hepatic function.

When handling chloramphenicol powder in capsules or tablets or while mixing the powder into a suspension, veterinary technicians must avoid repeated contact with or inhalation of the powder. Precautions include washing hands after handling capsules or tablets, avoiding inhalation of chloramphenicol powder, and using care when breaking chloramphenicol tablets or opening capsules.

Florfenicol (Nuflour) is a newer antibiotic related to chloramphenicol but with some significant differences that enable this drug to be safely used in cattle for bovine respiratory diseases such as shipping fever or pneumonia. Like chloramphenicol, florfenicol is bacteriostatic, disrupts protein synthesis at the bacterial ribosomes, and penetrates tissues fairly well. Unlike chloramphenicol, florfenicol is approved for use in cattle and, according to the manufacturer's literature, lacks the chemical component that makes chloramphenicol toxic to human bone marrow. Florfenicol is approved for IM injection administered as two injections 48 h apart or SQ at a higher dosage as a one-time dose. The drug has a 38-day withdrawal time if administered as a single SQ injection dose, but only a 28-day withdrawal time if administered as two IM doses at half the dose of the SQ injection. Because insufficient data are available regarding florfenicol's effect on bovine reproduction, pregnancy, and lactation, the drug should not be used in cattle of breeding age. The veterinary technician should thoroughly read the drug information on this and any new drug before use.

Rifampin

Rifampin is a bactericidal or bacteriostatic antimicrobial belonging to the class of antimicrobials known as rifamycins. It is used almost exclusively in horses (especially young foals) and almost always is used simultaneously with an aminoglycoside, a β-lactam, or doxycycline antibiotic because of fairly widespread bacterial resistance to rifampin alone. Interestingly, rifampin may act synergistically (i.e., enhance the effect) with an antifungal drug called **amphotericin B** (see later, Antifungals), making it an effective agent against some fungal agents like *Histoplasma*, *Aspergillus*, and *Blastomyces*.

Rifampin suppresses formation of the RNA chain by inhibiting an RNA polymerase enzyme needed by bacteria to synthesize RNA. Like quinolones, rifampin only affects bacterial RNA polymerase and does not disrupt the function of mammalian RNA polymerases.

Rifampin imparts a reddish-orange color to urine, tears, sweat, and saliva. Owners of animals being treated with rifampin should be informed of this change so they are not unduly alarmed. The plasma may also look red and resemble hemolysis (lysis of the red blood cells releasing hemoglobin); however, the red blood cells are intact. Because real hemolysis can be a threat to the kidneys and requires additional treatment with IV fluids, it is important to differentiate the red plasma from rifampin from the red/pink plasma of hemolysis.

Bacitracin

Bacitracin is an antibiotic that works similarly to penicillins and cephalosporins in that it inhibits the formation of bacterial cell walls. Bacitracin has the potential to produce nephrotoxicity; therefore, its use is confined to topical antibiotic preparations or ocular (i.e., ophthalmic) preparations, sometimes in conjunction with neomycin (an aminoglycoside) or polymyxin B (an antibiotic effective against *Pseudomonas* bacteria).

ANTIFUNGALS

This group of antimicrobial drugs was developed to be effective against many of the fungal organisms that cause superficial mycoses (i.e., fungal skin infections) such as ringworm, and the deep or systemic mycoses (i.e., fungal infections within the body) such as histoplasmosis, blastomycosis, cryptococcosis, coccidioidomycosis, candidiasis, sporotrichosis, and aspergillosis. Because most antifungal drugs have potentially severe side effects, veterinary technicians must be aware of the correct procedures for safe handling, administration, storage, and disposal of antifungals.

Amphotericin B

Amphotericin B is a potent antifungal drug for treatment of the deep mycoses. Amphotericin is administered parenterally, primarily intravenously, but doses also exist for SQ administration. Amphotericin is not given by mouth because it is poorly absorbed from the GI tract. Once absorbed, amphotericin B reaches the fungal elements and binds to and damages a specific molecule called *ergosterol* that is a major component of the fungal cell membrane. The resulting damage creates holes in the fungal cell membrane and allows critical cellular components to leak from the fungal cell, producing a fungicidal or fungistatic effect depending on the concentration of drug achieved at the fungal infection site. One of the significant advantages of amphotericin B over the imidazole antifungal agents (discussed later) is the rapid onset of fungicidal activity (hours) compared with the imidazoles (days).

Amphotericin can cause several serious side effects by combining with cholesterol in mammalian cell membranes and producing a similar toxic effect as that observed with fungal cell membranes. These side effects manifest as nephrotoxicosis (kidney toxicity), fever, anorexia, and nausea. Of these side effects, nephrotoxicosis is the most common and most significant. Most canine patients (some studies say more than 80%) show some degree of nephrotoxicosis after amphotericin B administration. Nephrotoxicosis occurs because of amphotericin's strong vasoconstrictive effects on the renal blood supply (this results in poor circulation, tissue hypoxia, and kidney cell death) and its direct toxic effect on the cell membranes of the renal tubules (primarily the distal convoluted tubule). Renal function tests (including BUN, creatinine, and urinalysis) should be closely monitored before and during treatment with amphotericin B so the degree of renal damage can be evaluated. Renal damage is dose related; therefore, more renal damage occurs with high doses or prolonged dosing of amphotericin.

Although some sources state that the nephrotoxic effect of amphotericin can be blunted by administration of IV fluids to maintain renal blood flow, the IV fluids do not prevent damage to the kidney. Depending on the extent to which amphotericin B harms the kidney cells, the nephrotoxicosis may be reversible or irreversible. Even if the kidney damage is irreversible, if the extent of the damage is limited the animal can still have adequate renal function after conclusion of the amphotericin treatment.

Within the past few years a new formulation of amphotericin B has been created in which the drug itself is encapsulated in a lipid "capsule" that reduces the nephrotoxicity of the amphotericin B. This new form, called a liposomal form, is thought to better deliver the drug directly to the fungal element membrane, where the amphotericin B is released and attaches to the fungal membrane, instead of attacking cholesterol molecules in the mammalian cell membrane. Though more expensive than the older, conventional form of amphotericin B, the liposomal form is becoming more widely accepted in veterinary medicine because of its less toxic side effects.

Azoles: The Imidazole Derivatives

Azole antifungal agents, also called *imidazole derivatives*, are composed of two groups (imidazoles, which contain two nitrogen atoms, and triazoles, which contain three) and include several compounds such as **ketoconazole**, **itraconazole**, **fluconazole**, **miconazole**, **voriconazole**, and **clotrimazole**. Of these drugs, ketoconazole is the prototype imidazole. Ketoconazole, itraconazole, voriconazole, and fluconazole are typically administered orally, whereas miconazole and clotrimazole are applied topically. Other azole drugs borrowed from human medicine occasionally appear in the veterinary literature, and they can typically be identified by their *-azole* suffix.

Nearly all deep or systemic mycoses in animals today are treated with these drugs or with amphotericin B. Because imidazole derivatives have fewer side effects than amphotericin B, they are often used as the first drug of choice for the long-term treatment of most deep fungal agents, except the ones that are rapidly growing where the quicker onset of amphotericin would be preferred. Several of the azoles are also used to treat superficial dermatophytosis (i.e., "skin plants") and yeast infections.

The imidazole derivatives interfere with the enzyme that synthesizes ergosterol, a key component of fungal cell membrane mentioned with amphotericin's mechanism of action. Without the ergosterol molecule, the fungal cell membrane damage results in membrane leakage. Unlike amphotericin's rapid onset of action on the fungal cell, imidazoles usually take 5–10 days of treatment before they become fungicidal.

The older systemic azoles, like ketoconazole and itraconazole, need an acidic pH in the GI tract to be absorbed when given PO. Hence, these drugs should not be given at the same time as antacid drugs like H_2 blockers or local antacids like Tums or Rolaids. They will also bind to GI protectant drugs like sucralfate (see Chapter 4).

Although the azoles do not produce nephrotoxicosis like amphotericin, they do have their own adverse reactions that must be monitored in patients receiving these drugs. GI side effects are the most common adverse reaction with the imidazole derivatives, with ketoconazole probably being the least tolerated of the azoles. Vomiting is more commonly associated with higher doses of the azoles, occurs more commonly in cats than dogs, and can be reduced by splitting the daily dose into small individual doses given more frequently.

Ketoconazole is the prototype azole antifungal and has been replaced to some degree by the newer imidazole drugs. Ketoconazole has been reported to have teratogenic effects (i.e., creates birth defects) in the pregnant dog, producing mummified fetuses and stillbirth puppies at birth. Additionally, ketoconazole can interfere with the cytochrome P450 (CYP) enzyme that converts progesterone to testosterone, resulting in decreased testosterone levels. Thus, ketoconazole should not be used in male dogs that are used in an active breeding program.

This same inhibition of CYP can also interfere with conversion of basic sterol molecule into cortisol by the adrenal gland, reducing the production of cortisol by the adrenal cortex. This inhibition has been occasionally used therapeutically to control the overproduction of cortisol by adrenal tumors in canine Cushing's disease (i.e., hyperadrenocorticism). Although ketoconazole is not a drug of first choice for controlling Cushing's disease, it is a less expensive way to control the disease compared with the other drugs that actually destroy the adrenal tumor.

Hepatotoxicity has been reported with ketoconazole use. This reaction is idiosyncratic, meaning that it is not dose related and its occurrence is unpredictable. Animals on ketoconazole should have liver parameters checked periodically to monitor liver function. However, it is important to remember that selected liver enzymes (e.g., alanine aminotransferase) on the serum chemistry profile will normally go up in many animals put on ketoconazole without there being any liver damage. Thus, as long as the other liver enzymes on the chemistry profile have not increased and the animal does not show any other signs of liver injury or failure, the treatment protocol for the ketoconazole does not need to be changed.

Itraconazole is a more potent antifungal than ketoconazole and generally more effective than ketoconazole or fluconazole against *Aspergillus* fungus. It has fewer GI side effects compared with ketoconazole, but it can produce vomiting in cats and dogs at higher doses. Itraconazole can still impair testosterone production, and hepatic side effects, including hepatotoxicity, have been reported. Neither ketoconazole nor itraconazole penetrate cell membranes very well; hence these drugs are not used for fungal infections involving the globe of the eye or the brain. Itraconazole does bind well to proteins in the tissues, however, resulting in prolonged accumulation of the drug in the areas of the skin and nail bed where superficial mycoses typically reside. Itraconazole is one of the drugs of choice for treating guttural pouch mycosis in horses, a fungal infection of the pharyngeal area of the throat often caused by *Aspergillus*.

Fluconazole is also more potent than ketoconazole but thought to be slightly less effective against deep mycoses than itraconazole. Unlike ketoconazole and itraconazole, fluconazole does not require an acidic GI tract pH to be absorbed when given orally and thus can be used with antacid drugs. Fluconazole also penetrates the CNS better than ketoconazole or itraconazole and thus is one of the drugs of choice for treating mycotic meningitis (i.e., fungal infection of the brain) and ocular mycoses. GI side effects still occur and are dose related, but hepatotoxicity is far less frequently reported. In fact, if an animal is suspected to have early signs of hepatotoxicity while on ketoconazole or itraconazole, the animal is often switched to fluconazole as an alternative. Unlike the other drugs, fluconazole is excreted mostly by the kidney and achieves therapeutic concentration in the urine. Therefore, fluconazole is a drug of choice for treating fungal cystitis (i.e., fungal infections of the bladder).

Clotrimazole and **miconazole** are recommended for use with topical yeast infections, superficial dermatophytes (i.e., "skin plants") and, in the case of clotrimazole, for use as an intranasal infusion to treat nasal aspergillosis. Clotrimazole is included in some veterinary otic medications along with aminoglycoside antibiotics and glucocorticoid antiinflammatory drugs. Miconazole is likewise confined to topical applications and is found in lotions, sprays, and as an ingredient in an over-the-counter (OTC) equine shampoo.

Griseofulvin

Although it has been replaced by itraconazole to some extent, griseofulvin is a fungistatic drug used primarily to treat infections from *Trichophyton* and *Microsporum* species of dermatophytes found superficially on dogs, cats, and horses. These fungi usually infect the skin, hair, nails, and claws, causing the condition known as ringworm.

Griseofulvin is the only FDA-approved drug for systemic administration (as opposed to topical administration) to treat superficial fungal diseases in veterinary patients. While griseofluvin is effective against dermatophytes when given systemically, it is ineffective if given topically because it does not penetrate the skin sufficiently to reach the dermatophytes. Griseofulvin is limited to use against those fungal agents that have an energy-dependent active transport uptake mechanism capable of pulling griseofulvin into the fungal cell, and because only dermatophytes have such a mechanism (as opposed to the deep mycoses or yeasts), the use of griseofulvin is limited to the superficial mycoses.

Griseofulvin is available as an oral microsized powder (for horses) or as tablets. To be absorbed from the GI tract, the particles of griseofulvin must be very small, and the medication must be given with fatty foods. Griseofulvin products are produced in "microsized" and "ultramicrosized" formulations, indicating the relative size of the drug particles. Because the ultramicrosized formulation is smaller, it is better absorbed than the microsize formulation when given with a fatty meal. Because these two formulations are absorbed to different extents and have different bioavailabilities, the dosage must be adjusted when switching from one formulation to the other.

Griseofulvin works by impairing microtubules that make up the structure of the fungal cell and provide a major part of the mechanism by which a replicating cell divides in half. By impairing the microtubule function, griseofulvin only inhibits the fungal agent and does not immediately kill, slowing the rate at which the fungus is eliminated from the body. The onset of antifungal activity is also slow because griseofulvin accumulates in the deepest part of the skin where the youngest cells are located and only reaches the more superficial layers where the

dermatophytes live when these young skin cells carry the drug toward the surface over the span of 2–3 weeks. Griseofulvin is still one of the antifungal drugs used for treating dermatophytes that infect the nails because, unlike most of the other antifungals, griseofulvin becomes incorporated into the keratin that comprises the nail and therefore is delivered to the dermatophyte infection site.

Griseofulvin is metabolized by the liver and conjugated with glucuronide. Cats are slow to conjugate any drugs with glucuronide, so they eliminate griseofulvin slowly. The slow rate of elimination predisposes cats to accumulate a toxic level of the drug unless the drug dose is appropriately titrated for the cat. For this reason, doses of griseofulvin for cats are lower than for dogs.

Griseofulvin is reportedly teratogenic in cats at high doses, producing cleft palates and other skeletal, skull, and nervous system defects in kittens of queens treated during gestation. Therefore, griseofulvin is contraindicated for use in pregnant animals. More common side effects of orally administered griseofulvin include anorexia, vomiting, and diarrhea. Although more severe effects such as anemia and leukopenia have been reported, these are rare at normal dosages.

Terbinafine

Terbinafine is a widely marketed antifungal for treating toenail fungus in humans (Lamisil). For nail-associated dermatophytes it must be given orally because topically applied forms of the drug will not penetrate the nail sufficiently to deliver the drug. There are topically applied ointment or powder forms that are used for superficial skin dermatophytes not associated with the toenails or hooves. Although there is less veterinary experience with this drug than with the azoles, terbinafine it is showing up in the veterinary literature as a treatment alternative for selected superficial dermatophytosis, including *Aspergillus*. Terbinafine works by a different mechanism than the azole antifungals but still produces its antifungal effect by damaging the fungal cellular membrane. Like griseofulvin, systemically administered terbinafine concentrates well in the upper-most layers of the skin where the dermatophytes reside. Side effects are similar to those observed with the azole antifungals (i.e., GI upset, low risk of hepatotoxicity).

Nystatin

Nystatin is a topical antifungal often included with topical antibiotic/corticosteroid ointment used in veterinary medicine. Nystatin has an antifungal mechanism that is similar to amphotericin B, but nystatin is considered to be very nephrotoxic. Thus, nystatin use is strictly limited to topical application.

Other antifungal agents sometimes seen in veterinary medicine include flucytosine (5-fluorocytosine [5-FC]), which is used synergistically with amphotericin B to enhance its antifungal activity; potassium or sodium iodine, which are inexpensive ingredients in antifungal shampoos; and lufenuron, which is an antiparasitic ingredient in flea medications like Sentinel. Lufenuron has been widely promoted on the Internet for control of ringworm in catteries or households with many cats. Lufenuron's mechanism for decreasing viable flea eggs is to interfere with a compound called chitin that is found in the exoskeleton of insects and the egg-tooth of flea larva. Chitin is also found in the cell wall of fungal elements, and hence lufenuron is thought to be potentially antifungal for that reason. Clinical studies on the effectiveness of lufenuron in controlling superficial dermatophytosis or ringworm in cats has not clearly shown there is any benefit for use in multicat households to decrease the incidence of ringworm. Veterinary technicians should be aware of this widely spread rumor and counter the inaccurate information about the efficacy of lufenuron in curing ringworm in cats.[15,16]

ANTIMICROBIAL DRUGS

Penicillins
Natural penicillins
  Penicillin G
Aminopenicillins
  Ampicillin
  Amoxicillin
β-Lactamase–resistant
  Cloxacillin
  Dicloxacillin
  Oxacillin
  Methicillin
Extended spectrum
  Carbenicillin
  Ticarcillin
  Piperacillin
Penicillin adjuncts
  Clavulanic acid
  Sulbactam
  Benzathine
  Procaine
  Trihydrate

Cephalosporins
First generation
  Cefadroxil (Cefa-Drops)
  Cephapirin (Cefa-Lak, Cefa-Dri)
  Cephalexin (Keflex)
  Cefazolin (Kefzol)
Third generation
  Cefovecin (Convenia)
  Cefpodoxime (Simplicef)
  Ceftiofur (Naxcel, Excenel)

Aminoglycosides
Gentamicin
Amikacin
Kanamycin
Neomycin
Tobramycin
Apramycin

Quinolones (Fluoroquinolones)
Enrofloxacin (Baytril)
Marbofloxacin (Zeniquin)
Orbifloxacin (Orbax)
Difloxacin (Dicural)
Pradofloxacin (Veraflox)
Danofloxacin (A180)

Ciprofloxacin
Ofloxacin

Tetracyclines
Tetracycline
Oxytetracycline (LA-200)
Doxycycline
Minocycline

Sulfonamides
Sulfadiazine (Tribrissen)
Sulfadimethoxine (Primor)
Sulfamethoxazole (Septra, Bactrim)
Sulfasalazine (Azulfidine)

Sulfonamide-Potentiating Compounds
Trimethoprim
Ormetoprim

Other Antimicrobials
Lincosamides
  Lincomycin
  Clindamycin (Antirobe)
  Pirlimycin (Pirsue)
Macrolides
  Erythromycin
  Azithromycin (Zithromax)
  Tilmicosin (Micotil)
  Tylosin (Tylan)
  Tulathromycin (Draxxin)
Metronidazole (Flagyl)
Chloramphenicol
Florfenicol
Rifampin
Bacitracin

Antifungals
Amphotericin B
Azoles: imidazole derivatives
  Ketoconazole
  Itraconazole
  Fluconazole
  voriconazole
  Miconazole
  Clotrimazole
Griseofulvin
Terbinafine
Nystatin

REFERENCES

1. Boothe DM. Treatment of bacterial infections. In: Boothe DM, ed. *Small Animal Clinical Pharmacology and Therapeutics.* Philadelphia: Saunders; 2012:270–356.
2. Boothe DM. Principles of antimicrobial therapy. In: Boothe DM, ed. *Small Animal Clinical Pharmacology and Therapeutics.* Philadelphia: Saunders; 2012:128–183.
3. CDC. National Antimicrobial Resistance Monitoring System for Enteric Bacteria (NARMS). In: *Human Isolates Final Report, 2013.* Atlanta, Georgia: USD Department of Health and Human Services, CDC; 2015.
4. Boothe DM. Antimicrobial drugs. In: Boothe DM, ed. *Small Animal Clinical Pharmacology and Therapeutics.* Philadelphia: Saunders; 2012:189–261.
5. Papich MG, Riviere JE. Beta lactam antibiotics: Penicillins and cephalosporins. In: Riviere JE, Papich MG, eds. *Veterinary Pharmacology and Therapeutics.* Ames, Iowa: Wiley-Blackwell; 2009:865–894.
6. Papich MG, Riviere JE. Tetracycline antibiotics. In: Riviere JE, Papich MG, eds. *Veterinary Pharmacology and Therapeutics.* Ames, Iowa: Wiley-Blackwell; 2009:895–914.
7. Papich MG, Riviere JE. Aminoglycoside antibiotics. In: Riviere JE, Papich MG, eds. *Veterinary Pharmacology and Therapeutics.* Ames, Iowa: Wiley-Blackwell; 2009:915–944.
8. Papich MG, Riviere JE. Sulfonamides and potentiated sulfonamides. In: Riviere JE, Papich MG, eds. *Veterinary Pharmacology and Therapeutics.* Ames, Iowa: Wiley-Blackwell; 2009:835–864.
9. Papich MG, Riviere JE. Fluoroquinolone antimicrobial drugs. In: Riviere JE, Papich MG, eds. *Veterinary Pharmacology and Therapeutics.* Ames, Iowa: Wiley-Blackwell; 2009:983–1012.
10. Plumb DC. *Plumb's Veterinary Drug Handbook.* 8th ed. Wiley Publishers; 2015.
11. Online access: https://academic-plumbs-com.ezproxy.lib.purdue.edu/drug-monograph/MkBhdO3gtmPROD?source=search& searchQuery Accessed 06.12.2022.
12. Current Canine Guidelines for the Prevention. Diagnosis, and Management of Heartworm Infection in Dogs. Wilmington, Delaware: American Heartworm Society; 2014.
13. Papich MG, Riviere JE. Chloramphenicol and derivatives, macrolides, lincosamides, and miscellaneous antimicrobials. In: Riviere JE, Papich MG, eds. *Veterinary Pharmacology and Therapeutics.* Ames, Iowa: Wiley-Blackwell; 2009:945–982.
14. Von Essen S, Spencer J, Hass B, et al. Unintentional human exposure to tilmicosin. *J Toxicol.* 2003;41(3):229–233.
15. Davis JL, Papich MG, Heit MC. Antifungal and antiviral drugs. In: Riviere JE, Papich MG, eds. *Veterinary Pharmacology and Therapeutics.* Ames, Iowa: Wiley-Blackwell; 2009:1013–1045.
16. Boothe DM. Treatment of fungal infections. In: Boothe DM, ed. *Small Animal Clinical Pharmacology and Therapeutics.* Philadelphia: Saunders; 2012:364–393.

SELF-ASSESSMENT

1. Fill in the following blanks with the correct item from the Key Terms list.

A. _____ This term means a type of compound that is produced by one microorganism that suppresses the growth of another.

B. _____ This is a broad term that means a type of compound that kills or inhibits the growth of any type of microorganism: bacteria, fungus, protozoa, or virus.

C. _____ This term means "kills bacteria."

D. _____ This term means "kills fungi."

E. _____ This term means "kills viruses."

F. _____ This term means "inhibits, but does not kill, bacteria."

G. _____ This term describes any organism that causes disease.

H. _____ This term describes the testing done to grow bacteria and then identify the specific antibiotics that will be effective in inhibiting or killing that bacteria.

I. _____ When a bacterial strain can be inhibited or killed by a particular drug, the bacteria is said to be this to that drug.

J. _____ This term means the lowest concentration of a drug needed to stop the bacterium from dividing.

K. _____ This term describes the dose of the drug that results in the highest drug concentrations allowed without significant toxic or adverse effect.

L. _____ If the minimum inhibitory concentration (MIC) for a drug used against a bacterial strain is higher than the maximum tolerated dose (MTD) for the drug, this term is applied to that bacterial strain to indicate the effectiveness of the drug.

M. _____ If the MIC for a drug used against a bacterial strain is only slightly lower than the MTD for the drug, this term is applied to that bacterial strain to indicate the effectiveness of the drug.

N. _____ If the MIC for a drug used against a bacterial strain is much lower than the MTD for the drug, this term is applied to that bacterial strain to indicate the effectiveness of the drug.

O. _____ This term describes the MICs for a drug at which the bacteria would go from being classified as susceptible to being classified as intermediate, or from being classified as intermediate to resistant.

P. _____ This term describes the minimum concentration of drug needed to kill a bacterium.

Q. _____ This term means the transferral of resistant genes from a parent bacterium to the daughter bacteria when the parent bacterium divides.

R. _____ This term means the transferral of resistant genes from one bacterium to another unrelated bacterium of the same species or even a different species.

S. _____ This describes the small piece of deoxyribonucleic acid (DNA) that is transferred from one bacterium to another and in so doing confers genetic resistance to drugs.

T. _____ This is the process by which drugs or other processes can eliminate only the weakest bacteria in an infection, allowing the strongest and most resistant bacteria to survive and proliferate into a resistant infection.

U. _____ This term refers to the small amount of drug left in tissue or food products after administration of a drug.

V. _____ This term is applied to an animal that has an allergic reaction to a drug.

W. _____ This is the ribonucleic acid (RNA) that transports a copy of the DNA code from the nucleus to the ribosome.

X. _____ This is the RNA that transports amino acids to the ribosome so they can be linked together to form a protein.

Y. _____ This is the central structural component of any penicillin or cephalosporin molecule.

Z. _____ This term describes any *Staphylococcus* bacterial strain that is resistant to a particular extended-spectrum antibiotic. It is a term that denotes strong bacterial resistance to many drugs.

AA. _____ This term describes the type of bacteria that require oxygen to survive.

AB. _____ This term describes the type of bacteria that do NOT require oxygen to survive.

AC. _____ This term describes the type of treatment a veterinarian selects before all diagnostic test results have been returned and is based upon an educated guess of what drug should be effective in an infection based upon how this drug has performed historically in other similar types of infections.

AD. _____ These are the small channels in the outer capsule of Gram-negative bacteria that allow some antibiotics to gain access to the interior of the bacteria.

AE. _____ This is an enzyme produced primarily by *Staphylococcus* bacteria that destroys both penicillin and cephalosporin drugs.

AF. _____ This is an enzyme produced primarily by *Staphylococcus* bacteria that destroys only penicillin drugs.

AG. _____ This is an enzyme produced primarily by *Staphylococcus* bacteria that destroys only cephalosporin drugs.

AH. _____ This term means to enhance the killing power of one antibiotic by adding an additional drug to it.

AI. _____ Another word for "hives."

AJ. _____ This term means that being hyper-sensitive or reactive to one drug makes it likely that you will be hypersensitive or reactive to a second drug or the same family.

AK. _____ This term describes what happens when an orally administered antibiotic kills some bacteria in the gastrointestinal (GI) tract, which allows surviving pathogenic bacteria to proliferate and produce severe diarrhea.

AL. _____ This refers to the phenomenon where an antibiotic can have bactericidal effects long after the drug concentration at the site of infection has dropped well below therapeutic concentrations.

AM. _____ This is the term used to describe those antibiotics that require the drug to continu-ously achieve concentrations above the MIC at the site of the infection for the drug to work.

AN. _____ This is the term used to describe those antibiotics that require the drug to achieve a very high peak drug concentration well above the MIC for a short period of time for the drug to work.

AO. _____ This term means "poisonous to the kidney."

AP. _____ This term means "poisonous to the inner ear."

AQ. _____ This term refers to the repetitive rapid eye movements that occur when an animal has vestibular disease or toxicity and feels experi-ences a spinning sensation.

AR. _____ This term means "pus producing."

AS. _____ This is the enzyme that quinolone antimicrobials target for their site of action.

AT. _____ This is the term that describes a pus infection of the skin.

AU. _____ This is the bacteria that lives within canine heartworms.

AV. _____ This term describes when a drug combines with an ion and precipitates out of solution.

AW. _____ This is the movement of a drug excreted into the GI tract that is reabsorbed back into the body, passes to the liver, and is once again excreted into the GI tract.

AX. _____ This is the type of sulfonamide anti-biotic (not a specific drug name) that is designed to remain in the lumen of the GI tract and not be absorbed systemically.

AY. _____ This is the side effect of sulfon-amides called "dry eye."

AZ. _____ This term means "decreased platelets."

BA. _____ This term means "decreased white blood cells."

BB. _____ This term means "the appearance of crystals in the urine."

BC. _____ This term means that "the produc-tion of bone marrow red blood cells, white blood cells, and platelets is decreased."

BD. _____ Dermatophytes are this type of mycosis.

BE. _____ Histoplasmosis, blastomycosis, cryptococcosis, and aspergillosis are all this type of mycosis.

BF. _____ This term describes the special type of lipid capsule surrounding a drug molecule that can reduce the toxicity of some drugs like amphotericin B.

BG. _____ If a drug is capable of creating birth defects, it is said to have this kind of an effect.

BH. _____ This term means "skin plants."

2. Fill in the following blanks with the correct drug from the Antimicrobial Drug list. When practicing these questions, write out the answers on a separate sheet, focusing also on the appropriate spelling of these drug names.

A. _____ Name the natural penicillin.

B. _____ Family of drugs that is the treat-ment of choice for Lyme disease.

C. _____ Name the three extended-spectrum penicillins mentioned in this text.

D. _____ The antibiotic that is relatively contraindicated to be given in dogs during their rapid growth phase for fear of damage to the articular cartilage.

E. _____ The enteric sulfa used to treat inflammatory bowel disease.

F. _____ Antibiotic very similar to another antibiotic that is banned from food animal use, but this antibiotic is actually FDA approved for use in food animals to treat respiratory disease; well known for its excellent ability to penetrate many tissues.

G. _____ Name the two amino penicillins.

H. _____ Antibiotic family that causes keratoconjunctivitis sicca.

I. _____ What drugs cause yellowing of the teeth dentin and enamel if given to a young animal?

J. _____ If this is added to penicillin G, it extends the duration of the drug for 3–5 days.

K. _____ Name the three third-generation cephalosporins most used in veterinary medicine.

L. _____ What drug can get stuck in a cat's esophagus and cause inflammation and possibly stricture of the esophagus?

M. _____ Sulfa antibiotic that can cause aspirin-like toxicosis in cats.

N. _____ Type of β-lactam antimicrobial that serves as a measurement for drug resistance in *Staphylococcus* bacteria.

O. _____ Group of antibiotics classified according to generations; no second-generation form is used in veterinary medicine.

P. _____ Group of antibiotics recognized by the -*mycin* or -*micin* suffix.

Q. _____ Antibiotic completely banned from use in any food animal because of its ability to cause aplastic anemia in humans.

R. _____ Two tetracycline family drugs that are hydrophilic and strong chelators of calcium.

S. _____ Name the four first-generation cephalosporins most used in veterinary medicine.

T. _____ Group of antibiotics known for nephrotoxicity and ototoxicity.

U. _____ The group of antibiotics that work by inhibiting DNA gyrase.

V. _____ The group of antibiotics that are β-lactams but are not penicillins.

W. _____ Name the four sulfonamide antibiotics that are most commonly used in veterinary medicine.

X. _____ Group of antibiotics recognized by the -*cillin* suffix.

Y. _____ The fluoroquinolone first associated with blindness in cats.

Z. _____ Family of drugs that is the treatment of choice for treating *Wolbachia* bacteria.

AA. _____ Group of antibiotics recognized by the -*cef* or -*ceph* prefix.

AB. _____ Ciprofloxacin is the metabolite of what other fluoroquinolone?

AC. _____ This is added to ampicillin or amoxicillin to prolong the duration of these drugs.

AD. _____ Group of antibiotics recognized by the -*cycline* suffix.

AE. _____ The group of antibiotics that work by inhibiting formation of the bacterial cell wall.

AF. _____ Name the four β-lactamase–resistant penicillins.

AG. _____ This antibiotic has been used as a suicide drug.

AH. _____ Horses are very sensitive to the intravenous (IV) administration of this drug and IV administration has produced fatal arrhythmias; other species are not as sensitive to the cardiac effects.

AI. _____ Two compounds added to amoxicillin or other penicillins to increase their effectiveness against bacterial β-lactamase.

AJ. _____ Name two compounds added to sulfas to potentiate their effects.

AK. _____ Two tetracycline type drugs that are lipophilic and do not chelate calcium very much.

AL. _____ Lincosamide antibiotic that is distinguished from the rest of the lincosamides because of its ability to kill anaerobic bacteria.

AM. _____ Family of drugs that is the treatment of choice for *Chlamydia* infections in cats and birds.

AN. _____ Type of penicillin that cannot be given by mouth because it is denatured by stomach acid.

AO. _____ Cattle antibiotic for pink eye and respiratory disease that is also effective in treating chronic intestinal disease of unknown origin in dogs.

AP. _____ Name the five macrolide antibiotics most commonly used in veterinary medicine.

AQ. _____ What antibiotic is now recommended for use as an initial treatment of canine heartworm disease?

AR. _____ If this is added to penicillin G, it extends the duration of the drug for 24 h.

AS. _____ This antibiotic is very effective against anaerobic bacteria, plus many protozoa including *Giardia*.

AT. _____ Macrolide antibiotic that can cause fatal arrhythmias in humans if they are accidentally injected with the drug.

AU. _____ Antibiotic used exclusively in horses but always used with another antibiotic because of resistance; turns plasma, urine, and tears reddish-orange in color.

AV. _____ Antifungal that is very nephrotoxic.

AW. _____ Prototype azole antifungal drug; teratogenic; used sometimes to control the effects of Cushing's disease caused by an adrenal tumor.

AX. _____ Azole antifungal that is the drug of choice for treating guttural pouch mycoses in horses; fewer side effects than ketoconazole.

AY. _____ Azole antifungal that does not require acidic pH in the GI tract to be absorbed; penetrates tissue, so is used to treat mycotic meningitis and ocular mycoses.

AZ. _____ Two azole drugs used specifically to treat dermatophytes; are added to otic preparations and equine shampoo.

BA. _____ Azole antifungal that, unlike other azoles, is excreted by the kidney and therefore is used to treat mycotic cystitis.

BB. _____ Antifungal taken systemically but only effective against fungi that have an active transport mechanism capable of taking the drug into the fungal cell.

BC. _____ Antifungal that has to be given orally with a fatty meal and comes in "microsized" and "ultramicrosized" preparations.

BD. _____ Topically applied antifungal that is very nephrotoxic if given systemically; added to many antibiotic and corticosteroid ointments in veterinary medicine.

3. Indicate whether each of the following statements is true or false.

A. For a bacteria to be susceptible to a particular drug, the MTD concentration would need to be higher than the MIC.

B. The minimum bactericidal concentration (MBC) is typically lower than the MIC.

C. The transfer of genetic code from one bacteria to another by physical contact would be an example of vertical transmission of resistance.

D. Selection pressure increases the number of bacterial mutations and hence increases resistance.

E. Aminoglycosides, fluoroquinolones, and penicillins are all concentration-dependent antimicrobials.

F. Bacteriostatic antibiotics are more dependent on an intact immune system than bactericidal antibiotics.

G. Penicillins should not be used at the same time as other bacteriostatic antibiotics.

H. Amoxicillin is primarily excreted by the liver.

I. Penicillin G and the aminopenicillins are especially effective against *Pseudomonas* bacteria.

J. If a bacterial strain is resistant to one member of the penicillin family, it is likely resistant to many other members.

K. Oxacillin by itself can kill β-lactamase–producing bacteria, but amoxicillin by itself cannot.

L. The overall spectrum of activity for dicloxacillin and cloxacillin is much broader than for ampicillin or amoxicillin.

M. Clavulanic acid prolongs the duration of penicillin to 3–5 days.

N. If an animal shows signs of hypersensitivity to one penicillin, it should be assumed the animal is also hypersensitive to all other penicillins.

O. Penicillins given orally are especially effective for treating GI problems in guinea pigs, ferrets, and rabbits.

P. Procaine extends the duration of penicillin G longer than benzathine.

Q. Penicillin G is more susceptible to gastric acid than amoxicillin.

R. First-generation cephalosporins are generally more effective against Gram-positive bacteria and less effective against Gram-negative bacteria than the third-generation cephalosporins.

S. Amikacin and gentamicin are both very effective in inhibiting anaerobic bacteria.

T. Aminoglycosides are most effective if given as a constant rate infusion (CRI) so that the drug is present at the infection site continuously.

U. Aminoglycosides are absorbed rapidly across the skin when applied topically.

V. To reduce the incidence of nephrotoxicity in aminoglycosides, it is important that the dose be decreased so that the peak drug concentration be decreased well below its normal high concentration.

W. Aminoglycosides are an important antibiotic in treating abscesses because they can reach their target site on bacteria without being interfered with by the presence of pus.

X. Because enrofloxacin interferes with DNA, it also creates a significant risk for birth defects if given to pregnant animals.

Y. Large-breed, young and growing dogs need to avoid the use of fluoroquinolones until later in their lives than medium- or small-breed, young and growing dogs.

Z. Enrofloxacin was associated with blindness secondary to the eyes drying out and damage occurring to the cornea.

AA. It is against the law to use quinolones extra-label in food animals.

AB. Fluoroquinolones penetrate the central nervous system (CNS) better than the aminoglycosides.

AC. If oral tetracyclines are used at the same time as oral antacid medications, the problem with chelation can be avoided by switching from calcium-based antacids to magnesium-based antacids.

AD. Tetracyclines in general are synergistic with and enhance the bactericidal activity of penicillins.

AE. Doxycycline penetrates the CNS better than oxytetracycline.

AF. Sulfadimethoxine is an enteric sulfonamide, and sulfadiazine is a systemic sulfonamide.

AG. Sulfonamides are one of the drugs of choice for protozoa like the causative organism for toxoplasmosis or equine protozoal myeloencephalitis (EPM).

AH. Sulfasalazine is the sulfonamide that can produce an aspirin toxicosis in cats.

AI. Clindamycin is very effective against anaerobic bacteria.

AJ. Macrolide antibiotics are very effective in treating respiratory disease.

AK. Accidental injection of tilmicosin into a human almost always produces a fatal arrhythmia.

AL. The neurologic side effects sometimes seen with metronidazole are irreversible in most veterinary patients.

AM. Fluconazole is more nephrotoxic than amphotericin B.

AN. The liposomal form of amphotericin B has fewer side effects than the conventional form.

AO. Azole antifungals begin working faster than amphotericin B.

AP. Azole antifungals increase the production of testosterone and have the potential to cause an animal to be overly aggressive.

AQ. Antacids enhance the absorption of drugs like ketoconazole and itraconazole.

AR. Clotrimazole and fluconazole are both drugs primarily applied topically as shampoos and otic preparations.

AS. When changing the griseofulvin dose form from microsized to ultramicrosized, the dose would probably need to increase.

4. A culture and sensitivity test comes back that indicates the MIC of Drug A needed to inhibit the bacteria is 10 mcg/mL. If the breakpoint for susceptible/intermediate is 4 mcg/mL and the breakpoint for intermediate/resistant is 16 mcg/mL, should this drug be used to treat this infection assuming the drug can be delivered sufficiently to the infection site?

5. Match the mechanism of action with the particular drug.
   A. Disrupts cell wall formation
   B. Damages cell membrane
   C. Interferes with essential protein production
   D. Interferes with production of essential nutrients or compounds
   E. Interferes with normal DNA replication or function
   ____ amoxicillin
   ____ minocycline
   ____ enrofloxacin
   ____ cefovecin
   ____ polymyxin B
   ____ sulfadiazine
   ____ gentamicin
   ____ penicillin G
   ____ doxycycline
   ____ tilmicosin
   ____ orbifloxacin
   ____ oxacillin
   ____ sulfadimethoxine
   ____ erythromycin
   ____ amikacin

6. To adjust the dose of an aminoglycoside so that it poses less risk for nephrotoxicity, the dose should be _____ (increased, decreased, remain the same) and the dose interval should be _____ (increased, decreased, remain the same).

7. What are the early signs of kidney injury from aminoglycosides that can appear before the blood urea nitrogen (BUN) and creatinine levels go up on the blood chemistry profile?

8. Why should oral tetracycline capsules not be given to a nursing calf?

9. A dog is being treated with sucralfate for gastric ulcers secondary to an overdose of the owner's arthritis medication. Because of the risk for infection from the gastric ulcer, the veterinarian is going to use enrofloxacin as a safe-guard against secondary bacterial infections. What is the problem with this?

10. Why must fluoroquinolones be used with caution in animals with a history of epileptic seizures?

11. Why is doxycycline used to help treat heartworm disease in dogs?

12. Why are tetracyclines the drugs of choice for treating *Rickettsia,* spirochetes, *Mycoplasma,* and *Chlamydia* infections?

13. What precaution must be given to the owner of a cat that is to be given oral doxycycline capsules?

14. What is the problem with doxycycline use in horses?

15. What makes penicillins and sulfonamides so great for use in treating bacterial cystitis?

16. The veterinarian is talking on the phone to an owner of a dog that was treated in the hospital 2 days ago and was sent home on sulfadiazine medication for a low-grade bacterial cystitis. The owner mentions that the dog seems to be squinting a bit this morning and there is "matter" in the corner of the eyes. The veterinarian tells the owner to bring the dog in right away. What is the problem the veterinarian suspects?

17. Lincosamides are generally great drugs but they cannot be used in rabbits, hamsters, chinchillas, or guinea pigs. Why?

18. Chloramphenicol and florfenicol are almost identical drugs. Why is one banned from use in food animals but the other is Food and Drug Administration (FDA) approved for use in food animals?

19. Why would an antifungal drug be prescribed to a patient with an adrenal tumor?

Disinfectants and Antiseptics

OBJECTIVES

After studying this chapter, the veterinary technician should be able to:

- Describe what would constitute the ideal disinfectant.
- Describe the challenges for effective disinfectant or antiseptic use, including the role of biofilms.
- Explain the terms used to describe the characteristics of disinfecting agents.

- Describe the common disinfectant/antiseptic compounds used in veterinary medicine as far as their mechanisms of action, spectrum of activity against pathogens, and significant limitations or precautions.

KEY TERMS

antiseptics
bactericidal
biguanides
biofilm
coagulum
cytotoxic
disinfectants
enveloped virus
fungicidal

germicides
halogens
high-level, intermediate-level, and low-level disinfectants
iodophor
microbicidal
microbiostatic
nonenveloped virus
nosocomial infections
protozoacidal

sanitizers
scrubs
spore form
sporicidal
sterilizers
surfactant
vegetative form
virucidal

Disinfection as a general term refers to the destruction of pathogenic microorganisms. Disinfection is important in maintaining the health of all animals whether on a farm, in a veterinary hospital, in a research facility, or in a breeding colony. However, disinfection is often taken for granted until there is an outbreak of an infectious disease within the hospital or facility. In 2008, the *Journal of the American Veterinary Medical Association* reported the results of a survey of 38 large veterinary teaching hospitals that indicated 82% of the hospitals had reported an outbreak of a hospital-associated infection (i.e., originating within the teaching hospital), and 32% of the surveyed hospitals had to close areas of the hospital to contain the outbreak.[1] While more recent published scientific studies are lacking, anecdotal evidence reported by veterinarians supports the fact that

hospital-associated infections are a constant battle in veterinary clinics and hospitals. This highlights the importance of appropriate infection control protocols, which veterinary technicians are often the leaders in the implementation of these practices.

Disinfection of hospital equipment and premises is especially important because of the natural selection for resistant strains that occurs when populations of microorganisms are exposed to low concentrations of antimicrobial chemicals. Nosocomial infections, which are infections acquired during a period of hospitalization, are especially difficult to control because any organism that can survive the routine cleaning, sterilization of instruments, use of antiseptic on patients, and widespread application of disinfectants must be a very tough, resistant organism.

In addition, some bacteria, such as the *Pseudomonas* species, are highly resistant to disinfection and antiseptics because of their ability to produce and immerse themselves in a **biofilm**. These bacteria attach to living tissue, implants, or catheters and begin to exude a microscopic glycocalyx material made of protein, deoxyribonucleic acid (DNA), and polysaccharides (referred to as "slime") in which the bacteria can proliferate protected from the disinfecting agents. Biofilm is of great concern if it forms on metal bone implants (e.g., plates and internally placed pins or screws) used to immobilize broken bones. If a surgically placed metal implant becomes infected with biofilm-producing bacteria, the infection prevents bone healing and the implant usually has to be surgically removed. Other common sites for creation of biofilm or nosocomial infections in a patient are the urinary tract (associated with the use of infected or contaminated urinary catheters), respiratory tract (associated with improperly disinfected endotracheal tubes), surgical sites (improper surgical prep or contaminated instruments), wounds (failure to clean bandages or areas around the wound site), and intravenous (IV) catheter insertion sites (failure to use adequate aseptic technique when inserting the catheter).

No one wants a perfectly healthy animal to come into their veterinary hospital or clinic for routine vaccinations or a wellness check-up only to have it break out with a very serious disease a few days later that was acquired in the veterinary hospital. Thus, disinfection is something we as a veterinary profession must be vigilant to maintain, and to do that properly, veterinary technicians need to understand the characteristics and limitations of the commonly used antiseptics and disinfectants.

TERMINOLOGY DESCRIBING DISINFECTING AGENTS

With literally hundreds of disinfecting products available to the veterinary professional and the general public, sorting through all the options and selecting a disinfecting agent that is most applicable to the needs of a particular clinical situation, housing facility (e.g., an animal shelter), or research unit can be overwhelming. Thus, disinfecting agents are often chosen because

"that's what we've always used" or an appealing price or sales pitch. A better approach is to identify the types of agents that pose the most threat to the patients or staff, the degree of organic material present in the areas to be disinfected, the speed of action of the agents to be targeted, the method of application, any safety concerns, and the cost. To start understanding these compounds, it is important first to understand the terminology commonly used to describe them.

The terminology used to describe disinfecting agents can be confusing. In addition to the scientific terminology, many vague terms are frequently used by the general public or the marketing agency that promotes the sale of the product. The terms *antiseptic* and *disinfectant* describe compounds with slightly different characteristics and uses. **Antiseptics** are chemical agents that kill or prevent the growth of microorganisms on living tissues. **Disinfectants** are chemical agents that kill or prevent the growth of microorganisms on inanimate objects such as surgical equipment, floors, and tabletops.[2] Disinfectants typically are more potentially toxic to veterinary patients, staff, or clients because they are intended for use on nonliving tissue and hence may be a more concentrated form of an antiseptic or may have chemical characteristics that produce irritation or tissue damage. Although the distinction between the two terms is often blurred by those who do not understand the difference, the veterinary technician needs to understand the delineation between the two: antiseptic is for living tissues; disinfectant is for inanimate objects.

Some disinfectants are listed as **high-level, intermediate-level, and low-level disinfectants**, a designation that generally refers to the ability of the disinfectant to kill pathogens with different levels of susceptibility. In general, **vegetative bacteria** (i.e., actively growing bacteria not in a spore state) and **enveloped viruses** (i.e., viruses surrounded by a thin, phospholipid/protein envelope used to enter a host cell) are usually very susceptible to disinfectants or antiseptics and therefore could be killed by low-level disinfectants.[2] The envelope around the enveloped virus does not protect the virus but is an essential component of the virus and is readily disrupted by detergents and disinfectants (Fig. 11.1). Enveloped viruses include the canine distemper virus (paramyxovirus), feline herpesvirus, rabies (rhabdovirus),

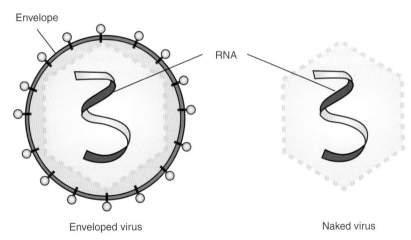

Envelope

RNA

Enveloped virus   Naked virus

Fig. 11.1 Enveloped and nonenveloped (naked) virus particles.

influenza virus (orthomyxovirus), and poxviruses (e.g., smallpox, cowpox). Nonenveloped viruses (i.e., "naked" virus core without a surrounding lipid envelope), bacteria or fungi in their spore form, and protozoal oocysts (i.e., cyst containing the zygote of the protozoan parasite) are all difficult to kill and would require high-level disinfectants.[2] Nonenveloped viruses in veterinary medicine include canine parvovirus, feline panleukopenia virus (it is a parvovirus), feline calicivirus, and papillomavirus (produces warts).

Antiseptics and disinfectants are sometimes described as sanitizers or sterilizers. The difference refers to the degree of microbial destruction achieved. Sanitizers are chemical agents that reduce the number of microorganisms to a "safe" level without eliminating all microorganisms. Sterilizers are chemicals or other agents that destroy all microorganisms. Most disinfectants and antiseptics tend to be sanitizers because sterilization is something only attained on inanimate objects, like surgical instruments after being treated with high-pressure steam or chemicals in an autoclave.

Many household cleaning products are advertised as germicides. A germicide is any chemical agent that kills microorganisms, but because microorganisms include viruses, bacteria, protozoa, and fungi, the term *germicide* is too nonspecific and should not be used by veterinary professionals.

The veterinary professional should know against which organisms the antiseptic or disinfectant is effective. Many sources describing the relative effectiveness of different compounds on various pathogens are available on the Internet that include charts that can be printed out and displayed as a reference in the hospital or research unit. A partial example adapted from the Center for Food Security and Public Health at Iowa State University is shown in Table 11.1.

The terminology used to describe the disinfectant chemical gives an idea of what pathogens it is most likely to be effective against. Bactericidal chemicals kill bacteria, virucidal chemicals kill viruses, fungicidal chemicals kill fungi, protozoacidal chemicals kill protozoa, and sporicidal chemicals kill microbial spores. Unlike some antimicrobials used in living organisms, disinfectants need to be microbicidal rather than microbiostatic because inanimate objects do not have an immune system to eliminate organisms not killed, and disinfectants must therefore completely eliminate all microorganisms on their own.

If a disinfectant is described as **sporicidal**, this means the chemical is capable of killing the pathogen when it is in its resistant or dormant state. Bacteria and fungi can exist in two forms: an actively growing vegetative form or a more static **spore form**. Bacterial spores are designed to be able to survive in a dormant state for years to decades so that under appropriate growing conditions they can switch to the vegetative form and begin multiplying again. For example, *Clostridium tetani*, the bacterial agent of tetanus, and *Bacillus anthracis*, the bacterial agent of anthrax, have been shown to exist as spores buried in the ground for decades, only to be reactivated on exposure to appropriate conditions of temperature, moisture, and aerobic or anaerobic environment. Because these spores are capable of surviving extreme environmental conditions for years, they are also resistant to the majority of disinfectants. Therefore, the possibility of the spores carried into the veterinary hospital environment or contaminating surgical procedures in the field means that sporicidal disinfection plays an important role in proper veterinary care.

TABLE 11.1   Antimicrobial Spectrum of Disinfectants*

Pathogen	Alcohol	Aldehydes	Biguanides	Halogens: chlorine	Halogens: iodine	Oxidizers	Phenols	Quaternary ammonium
Gram-positive bacteria	++	++	++	+	+	+	++	++
Gram-negative bacteria	++	++	++	+	+	+	++	+
Pseudomonas	++	++	+/−	+	+	+	++	−
Enveloped virus	+	++	+/−	+	+	+	+/−	+/−
Nonenveloped virus	−	+	−	+	+/−	+/−	−	−
Fungal spores	+/−	+	+/−	+	+	+/−	+	+/−
Parvoviruses	?	+	?	+	?	+/−	?	−
Bacterial spores	−	+	−	+	+	+	−	−
Coccidia	−	−	−	−	−	−	+	−
Prions	−	−	−	−	−	−	−	−

*Removal of organic material must always precede the use of the disinfectant.
Key: ++, highly effective; +, effective; +/−, limited effectiveness; −, not effective; ?, insufficient data.
Source: Adapted from *The Antimicrobial Spectrum of Disinfectants Table.* Ames, Iowa: The Center for Food Security and Public Health, Iowa State University; 2010.

APPROPRIATE USE OF DISINFECTING AGENTS

The commonly held concept of what constitutes adequate disinfection often ignores the importance of thorough cleaning with soap and rinsing to remove organic material and debris before application of the disinfectant. Many of the disinfectants and antiseptics used in veterinary medicine are inactivated if they contact organic material and hence they would do little to reduce pathogens in the environment or on the patient. Ignoring the basic principles of disinfection results in poor reduction of pathogenic microorganisms and the potential for the spread of disease regardless of how otherwise effective the disinfectant or antiseptic agent might be.

Cleansers, which are detergents or surfactants, must be used before application of the disinfectant to remove the organic material referred to earlier.[3] In environmental conditions such as animal wards or runs, this often means using power washers or other methods to remove dirt and feces from cracks and crevices in the holding area. Cleansers, soaps, and detergents are classified as anionic, cationic, and nonionic. By themselves, these products may have some antibacterial activity depending on the product and how they are used.

Common soaps are anionic cleansers and work well to liquify or solubilize (i.e., dissolve) dirt, fat, and microorganism membranes (which are made of phospholipids) so that they can be washed away. This latter point emphasizes the reason for rinsing a cleansed site thoroughly: otherwise the organic material will remain at the site and potentially interfere with the disinfectant that is applied after cleaning. Solubilizing (dissolving) cell membranes of bacteria can make soaps bactericidal against Gram-positive bacteria. However, the same anionic characteristic allows minerals like calcium (Ca^{2+}) found in hard water (i.e., tap water from wells that has not been run through a water softener to remove some minerals) to combine with the soap and inactivate its antibacterial characteristics. Quaternary ammonium compounds, which are cleansers also used as disinfectants, will likewise bind to anionic soaps, rendering both compounds ineffective.[3] This emphasizes again the need to rinse a cleansed site thoroughly before applying the antiseptic or disinfectant.

Cationic soaps and detergents are less recommended for use because they combine readily with proteins, fats, and phosphates and therefore will be easily inactivated by the presence of serum, blood, and tissue debris.[4] The combined disinfectant and cleanser quaternary ammonium mentioned earlier is an example of a cationic cleanser, and hence it is used more as a disinfectant than a cleanser; it must be applied to a surface that has been thoroughly cleaned. The older quaternary ammonium compounds were also inactivated by hard water, but the more recently used ones are less so and more effective in killing fungi, bacteria, and viruses.[3]

After thorough cleansing and rinsing, environmental surfaces should be allowed to dry thoroughly. Most pathogens prefer a moist environment and can persist for hours or days in a damp area of a kennel run or housing facility. It has been documented that hospital areas can be thoroughly cleaned, disinfected, and rinsed, but the pathogens can still survive if allowed to accumulate in small pools of water around drains, corners of housing units, uneven surfaces of concrete or flooring, or small cracks in partitions or floors.[5] Allowing sufficient time for all surfaces to thoroughly dry is essential.

SELECTING AN APPROPRIATE DISINFECTING AGENT

After cleaning and rinsing, the disinfectant can be applied. Selecting the appropriate disinfectant often means the difference between killing pathogens or allowing them to survive and proliferate.

Following are the characteristics of the ideal disinfecting agent:
- **Broad-spectrum antimicrobial activity.** A single disinfectant that could destroy all viruses, bacteria, and other pathogens would be ideal. Realistically, the chemicals used in most disinfectants often leave certain groups of pathogens untouched. Therefore, the veterinary professional should know the various disinfectants' spectra of antimicrobial activity to select the appropriate one for use against the microorganisms most likely to inhabit the site of application.
- **Nonirritating and nontoxic to animal and human tissue.** Many strong disinfecting agents for use on inanimate objects are irritating or toxic, especially those with a broad spectrum of antimicrobial activity. Several disinfecting agents can cause toxicity if accidentally ingested; the mist from the application is inhaled, if too much is applied to the skin or mucous membranes of the patient, or if prolonged contact occurs with the skin of the person applying the agent or the patient (e.g., animal lying in a cage that is not properly rinsed). Even approved antiseptics designed for use on living tissues can be cytotoxic (i.e., cell-killing) if applied in inappropriate concentrations or to open wounds. Veterinary technicians should be aware of the potential dangers that disinfectants pose to themselves and animals under their care.
- **Easily applied to inanimate objects and without causing corrosion or stains.** Concentrated hydrochloric acid could certainly destroy the microorganisms on the surface of a surgery table. However, the corrosive action of the acid would damage the table surface and create minute crevices in which contaminants and microorganisms could accumulate. Also, some antiseptic or disinfecting agents contain dyes that stain porous or easily marked surfaces.
- **Stable and not easily inactivated.** Most disinfecting agents take several seconds or minutes to reduce the population of microorganisms to safe levels. If during that time the agent is in contact with cellular debris, blood, or other organic materials, it may be inactivated by these contaminants and therefore cannot sufficiently reduce the number of microorganisms. The same is true for some surgical antiseptics when they make contact with soap residue left over from the scrubbing of the skin before application of the antiseptic. Ideally, a disinfecting agent should not lose its potency or effectiveness when in storage for an extended time.
- **Inexpensive.** Because disinfecting agents are used to such a great extent in veterinary medicine, these agents must be economical and affordable. Although this is an important consideration in selecting a disinfectant, it should not be the most important criterion.

The ideal disinfectant or antiseptic has yet to be discovered. Each disinfecting agent currently in use in veterinary medicine lacks one or more of the ideal characteristics listed earlier. However, by being aware of the deficiencies of any given disinfectant and matching its strengths with the given task, technicians can select the appropriate agent.

TYPES OF DISINFECTING AGENTS

Alcohols

Alcohol is most commonly used as part of an aseptic technique to disinfect surgical sites, injection sites, and sites with low-disinfectant requirements. Advantages of alcohol include its low cost, general lack of toxicity when applied topically, and bactericidal activity against Gram-positive and Gram-negative bacteria. However, technicians should be aware that alcohol is ineffective against bacterial spores. In addition, alcohol must be applied in sufficient quantities and remain in contact with the skin or site for 1–3 min to be effective against bacteria (several minutes are required for fungi). Therefore, a cursory swipe with an alcohol-soaked swab on an animal's skin, especially if the skin is encrusted with dirt or feces, does little to disinfect an injection site.

Although many alcohols can reduce some pathogens, **ethyl alcohol** and **isopropyl alcohol** are among the most common antiseptics applied to skin. The difference between the two alcohols is that ethyl alcohol has slight better virucidal activity, but isopropyl alcohol has slightly better bactericidal activity.

Alcohol's main mechanisms of action against pathogens are by solubilizing (i.e., dissolving) lipid membranes and by denaturing (i.e., altering structure) of proteins. For enveloped viruses, this means alcohol destroys the vital lipid envelop these viruses need to enter the host cells. For bacteria the alcohol will denature either the pathogen's surface proteins or essential metabolic proteins needed by the pathogen to survive. Nonenveloped viruses, like canine parvovirus, will be largely unaffected by the alcohol disinfection.

Ethyl alcohol and isopropyl alcohol are readily available as 70% alcohol concentrations, although higher concentrations are also available that must be diluted to 70% prior to use. Alcohol concentrations work best at a concentrations of 70%–90%, but concentrations in excess of 95% are less effective because very high alcohol concentrations lack the water needed to effectively denature the proteins of the pathogen and produce the disinfection.[6]

Alcohol has no cleaning ability (it does not act like a soap) and therefore should not be used to cleanse the site or equipment of fecal matter, blood, mucus, urine, or other organic debris.[4] Organic debris dramatically reduces the effectiveness of both ethyl and isopropyl alcohol. In addition, blood left on instruments will denature if soaked in alcohol and will become more tightly adhered to the equipment or instruments being disinfected. Thus, any piece of equipment soaked in an alcohol bath but contaminated with fecal material or cellular debris will not be properly disinfected.

Of all the antiseptic agents, alcohol produces the largest and fastest reduction in bacterial counts within 1–3 min of contact.[3,4] For this reason, hand sanitizers typically have alcohol as their preferred antiseptic. Because alcohol evaporates so quickly, and because alcohol also dehydrates the skin surface to which it is applied, hand sanitizers typically incorporate the alcohol into a gel form to reduce evaporation and provide glycerin to retain water in the skin. Repeated application of alcohol without moisturizers removes some of the skin's lipid component and dehydrates the skin cells and after repeated alcohol application can result in dry, flaky skin and pruritus (i.e., itchiness).

Unlike some other antiseptics, alcohol should not be applied to open wounds because it causes pain and may also facilitate survival of pathogens. Open wounds usually contain a serum exudate that is rich in protein. Alcohol denatures the structure of this protein, causing it to form a superficial barrier, or coagulum (Fig. 11.2). This coagulum may seal in or protect underlying bacteria, thereby preventing topical disinfectants from reaching the organisms. The infection could then spread to underlying tissues.

Although it seems obvious, some people forget that alcohol is very flammable. Therefore, alcohol liquid must not be present on tissue in which electrocautery or laser surgery is to be performed. In addition, it is good practice to remove any bottles or containers of alcohol from the location where the cautery or laser is being used. In addition, prolonged contact with alcohol can corrode metal surfaces and degrade rubber gaskets or

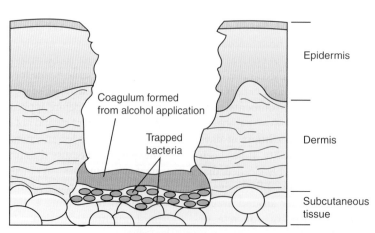

Fig. 11.2 Application of alcohol to an open wound can create a coagulum, trapping bacteria beneath it.

certain plastic tubing. Therefore, any instruments soaked in an alcohol bath should be examined to make sure plastic or rubber is not a component of the instrument.

Because alcohol is not virucidal against naked (nonenveloped viruses) or bacterial spores, and because it is inactivated in the presence of organic debris, alcohol is not recommended for high-level disinfection (where a strong disinfecting agent is needed).

Halogens: Chlorine Compounds

Chlorine compounds belong to a larger group of compounds known as halogens. They are classified as intermediate-level disinfectants because they can kill the vegetative forms of bacteria, algae, fungi, and both enveloped and nonenveloped viruses, including parvovirus. Chlorine ions liberated from the disinfecting compounds kill the pathogens by denaturing protein structure and chemically inactivating essential enzyme systems needed by the pathogen. Despite this wider spectrum of activity than many disinfectants, chlorine is not effective against bacterial spores.[4]

Chlorine disinfectants are most commonly available as **sodium hypochlorite** (formula = NaOCl) found in common, inexpensive household bleach and often referred to by the particular proprietary name Clorox. As might be expected, contact with high concentrations of sodium hypochlorite bleach can cause bleaching of colors and fabric deterioration. Chlorine is also corrosive to most metals, except high-quality stainless steel, and if left in contact for an extended period of time can pit or damage metal tabletops or surfaces, providing reservoirs for debris accumulation and proliferation of pathogens.

The pungent vapor of the liberated chlorine gas has been reduced over the years but is still sufficient to irritate the eyes and other exposed mucous membranes if the compounds are used in a poorly ventilated area. Mixing chlorine with other acidic cleansers (e.g., acetic acid or vinegar) can generate toxic amounts of chlorine gas, and mixing chlorine with ammonia-containing household cleansers can produce a very poisonous gas called chloramine. Therefore, sodium hypochlorite should not be mixed with anything except water.

Failure to adequately rinse a chlorine-disinfected surface on which an animal subsequently rests can result in skin irritation. Because of the skin irritation, chlorine products should not be used as antiseptics.

Although chlorine is the most commonly used disinfectant for fighting enteric viruses such as parvovirus, it is readily inactivated in the presence of any organic material such as feces, blood, and pus. The free chlorine ion needed to denature the pathogen proteins combines instead with the organic material, significantly reducing the availability of chlorine to react with the pathogen. Therefore, any site for chlorine disinfection should be thoroughly cleaned and rinsed before application of sodium hypochlorite bleach. In addition, the chlorine solution should remain in contact with the site for several minutes to ensure adequate destruction of pathogens. According to the Oregon State University Biological Safety bulletin, a 10% bleach solution left in contact with the site for 10 min at room temperature should produce adequate disinfection.[7] At lower temperatures, a longer period of contact would be needed to achieve the same degree of disinfection.[3]

Sodium hypochlorite solutions are not very stable after they have been diluted because the chlorine evaporates into the air, reducing the quantity of free chlorine available for disinfection. In addition, exposure to light breaks down the disinfecting compound. Thus, prepared dilutions of sodium hypochlorite for disinfecting dairy equipment, animal housing, and hospital flooring should be prepared fresh daily.[3,6]

So-called color-safe or color-fast bleaches do not contain sodium hypochlorite at all but instead contain concentrated hydrogen peroxide. Hydrogen peroxide is discussed later with the oxidizing agents, but it is not effective against many pathogens killed by sodium hypochlorite or "regular" bleach. Therefore, when disinfecting a parvovirus-contaminated surface or any other equipment, it is important that color-safe bleach products (which also go by the trade name Clorox) should not be confused with the sodium hypochlorite products.

Halogens: Iodine Compounds and Iodophors

Iodine compounds and iodophors are most commonly used as topical antiseptics before surgical procedures or for aseptic disinfection of tissue. Like chlorine, iodine compounds are also classified as halogens. They are bactericidal, virucidal, fungicidal, and sporicidal because of the free iodine, which diffuses into the pathogen cell and disrupts metabolism and protein structure and synthesis.[3]

These topical antifungal agents are quite effective against the dermatophytes that cause ringworm. Iodine is potentially effective against bacterial spores if the iodine solution remains moist and in contact with the site for more than 15 min. Although iodine can be inactivated by organic material, especially blood, to some degree, it is still considered to be better at maintaining its antiseptic activity in the presence of organic material than chlorines.

The older preparations of free iodine included such products as tincture of iodine or topical iodine solutions. These free-iodine compounds provided intermediate-level disinfection but were irritating to the tissues and painful on open wounds and delayed healing of tissues. Because of the tissue irritation, the use of these older products has largely been discontinued in veterinary medicine for antisepsis.

Instead of free-iodine compounds, iodophors are used instead, which are far less irritating and provide a longer duration of antiseptic or disinfecting action. An iodophor is a combination of molecular iodine and a carrier molecule that releases the iodine over time, prolonging the antimicrobial activity. The most common iodophor is iodine complexed with polyvinylpyrrolidone, or PVP, a combination more commonly known as **povidone-iodine**. Ovidone-iodine provides a low level to intermediate level of disinfection that is slightly less than that of the older free-iodine solutions because less free iodine is available from the iodophor at any given moment during the slower release process.

When combined with a detergent or nonionic surfactant (i.e., soaplike compounds that break the surface tension of water and allow easier interactions between organic material and chemicals), iodophors are often referred to as surgical scrubs. Surgical scrubs are designed to clean dirty surgical sites by solubilizing dirt and organic material and providing some low-level disinfection. Iodine solutions are iodine antiseptics without the added surfactant, so a povidone-iodine product without surfactant would be a solution.

It is important to distinguish between iodophor solutions and scrubs. The presence of the scrub soap is not appropriate for any use inside the body, and if such a need for iodine antiseptics is indicated (e.g., flushing an abscess), a solution without detergent must be used. Conversely, the detergent in surgical scrubs plays an important role in cleansing the skin before surgery. Neither form should be used in the peritoneal cavity because of the irritation and trauma caused by the free iodine; high concentrations of iodine should be avoided on denuded skin because of the potential for significant irritation and systemic absorption of iodine.

Because some iodine and iodophor preparations exist in concentrated forms, technicians should always check the container label to see whether dilution of the product is required before applying it to living tissue. Like with some other disinfectants, higher than recommended concentrations of iodine in iodophors are actually less effective than diluted iodophor concentrations because the free iodine is not released as readily at higher than recommended concentrations.[3]

Although less corrosive to inanimate surfaces than chlorine compounds, higher concentrations of iodine compounds can also be corrosive to metal if left in contact for an extended period.

Biguanides: Chlorhexidine (Nolvasan, Virosan, Hibistat)

Chlorhexidine, a member of a class of antiseptics known as biguanides, is one of the most commonly used disinfectant and antiseptic compounds in veterinary medicine. Chlorhexidine is used for a variety of purposes including cleaning cages, treating teat infections in cattle, surgical preparation as a scrub, and maintaining oral hygiene in companion animals. Its wide range of uses is likely related to its low tissue irritation and its bactericidal (both Gram positive and Gram negative) and fungicidal properties.[4] Chlorhexidine is not considered effective against nonenveloped viruses like parvovirus and has debatable effectiveness against the enveloped viruses.[3] Therefore, it is best to consider chlorhexidine as having little effect against most viruses encountered in veterinary medicine.[4]

Chlorhexidine works by damaging the cell membrane of the pathogen, lysing the cell. It remains more active than chlorine or iodine in the presence of organic material, including blood, but thorough cleansing of the application site is still recommended for it to achieve maximal effectiveness. Some chlorhexidine products are combined with a detergent to be used as a scrub. But combining chlorhexidine with other cleaning products is not advised because chlorhexidine can be inactivated by anionic and nonionic detergents, soaps, and the minerals in hard water. If used as a postscrub disinfectant it is important to thoroughly rinse the surface free of any soap residue before applying chlorhexidine.[4] Saline solutions added to chlorhexidine cause it to precipitate, but apparently this does not affect the antimicrobial properties.[3,4]

Chlorhexidine binds to the outer surface of the skin and appears to have some residual activity for up to 24 h if left in contact with the site. It is not irritating to the skin and can be incorporated into gauze wound dressings for antisepsis.[3] Additionally, chlorhexidine also binds preferentially to the surface of the oral mucous membranes and the teeth; hence, it has been marketed as an oral antiseptic to be used in conjunction with dental procedures.[3]

As an external ear preparation, chlorhexidine is considered to be quite safe, but if the compound gains access to the middle ear it is considered to be ototoxic.[3,4] Therefore, chlorhexidine should be used cautiously in severe otitis externa (ear canal infections) because of the possibility of chlorhexidine accessing the middle ear through a damaged or perforated tympanum (ear drum).

Aldehydes: Glutaraldehyde

Glutaraldehyde is a high-level disinfecting chemical sterilizer with a wide spectrum of activity against bacteria, viruses, fungi, and bacterial spores. It has a similar chemical structure to formaldehyde but with less of the irritation and none of the potential carcinogenic effects. Glutaraldehyde is used primarily as a disinfectant on equipment that cannot be heat sterilized, such as endoscopes, but has also been widely used to cold-sterilize clinical instruments (e.g., the product called Cidex).[4,8]

One of glutaraldehyde's advantages is its ability to kill bacteria normally protected from disinfectants by biofilm. As mentioned previously, biofilm is generated by bacteria when they attach to a surface (such as within the joint or box hinge of a surgical instrument, or in crevices of an endoscope) and develop a glycocalyx "shell" around themselves. Glutaraldehyde is able to penetrate the biofilm and reach the bacteria, plus cause the bacterial colony to detach from the surface of the instrument and be flushed away.

Glutaraldehyde 2% solutions are not inactivated by organic debris, and it is effective in the presence of hard water. Temperature has a significant effect on glutaraldehydes, as does pH, so it is important that cold-sterilization baths or solutions used to clean endoscopes are kept at room temperature and at neutral to alkaline pH. For example, glutaraldehyde is sporicidal at an alkaline pH (above 8) but generally not at an acidic pH.

As mentioned previously, glutaraldehyde is chemically related to formaldehyde, the noxious-smelling preservative most often associated with older preserved animal or tissue specimens. Glutaraldehyde still shares some of the tissue irritation, odor, and corrosion characteristics of formaldehyde; therefore, the technician should take precautions when working with this compound by wearing safety goggles and gloves, and working in a well-ventilated area. Any equipment, like endoscopes, disinfected with glutaraldehyde must be thoroughly rinsed with sterile water before use in or on living tissue.

Oxidizing Compounds: Hydrogen Peroxide, Peroxymonosulfate

Oxidizing compounds work primarily by denaturing proteins and lipids of microorganisms; however, they can potentially have similar effects on mammalian cells, and for that reason the use of different agents sparks continued debate.

Hydrogen peroxide as a commonly available 3% solution has historically been used to debride (i.e., remove) necrotic tissue and kill bacteria. But it is weakly bactericidal and probably provides most of its benefit by removing devitalized tissue to make the environment less suitable for bacterial growth. Although the foaming action of oxidizing agents in wounds is dramatic, these compounds are not virucidal and may actually damage tissue that is healthy or marginally viable. For that reason, 3% hydrogen peroxide has fallen out of favor as an antiseptic on tissues.

Although hydrogen peroxide as a liquid antiseptic is largely ineffective, a variant on hydrogen peroxide has been successfully marketed as a proprietary compound called "accelerated hydrogen peroxide" for use as a disinfectant. The accelerated hydrogen peroxide contains a lower concentration of hydrogen peroxide (0.5%), surfactants that break down the surface tension of water and allow penetration, wetting agents that allow liquids to spread out over a surface, and a chelator. It has been incorporated into commercial disinfectant products under the Clorox trade name and others. The manufacturer claims strong bactericidal, virucidal, along with some fungicidal activity for these products. Although targeted toward human hospital facilities, this product is finding its way into animal shelter facilities and veterinary hospitals.[5]

Peroxymonosulfate is another oxidizing agent that has been used to disinfect pools and hot tubs but has also been formulated with potassium to be used as a surface disinfectant.[4] Potassium peroxymonosulfate (PPMS) marketed as Trifectant comes mixed with a surfactant, organic acids, and buffers in a dry powder or tablet form that has to be dissolved in water. The manufacturer claims that it is virucidal, including against nonenveloped viruses, bactericidal, and fungicidal, even in the presence of organic material and hard water. The powder formulation is said to have no environmental residue problems and has low toxicity if applied topically or swallowed. Additional information on Trifectant specifically is available from the manufacturer, Vetoquinol USA.

Phenols (Lysol)

Phenols are a part of a larger group of related compounds found in mouthwashes, surface disinfectants, and many household disinfectants such as Lysol, pine oil, and similar cleansers. Phenol compounds are quite effective against Gram-positive bacteria but generally ineffective against Gram-negative bacteria, viruses, fungi, and spores. Phenols are not as easily inactivated by organic material as detergents, quaternary ammonium compounds, and chlorine solutions. However, because phenols are more toxic if taken into the body and because they have a slower onset of action than povidone-iodine or chlorhexidine, they are not commonly used as antiseptics for preparing surgical sites in veterinary medicine.

Although most household phenols are generally safe if used on inanimate surfaces, prolonged contact with concentrated solutions may damage the skin. For example, bird perches disinfected with phenols may cause lesions on the feet of birds. Dermal ulceration has been reported in reptiles kept in cages that are consistently disinfected with phenols. Dogs may develop skin lesions when runs are cleaned with phenols and not adequately rinsed. Phenols themselves are hard to adequately rinse from surfaces, especially slightly porous surfaces, and therefore tissue irritation from contact with residues are a common problem. Ingestion of phenols can result in severe liver damage.

Triclosan is a phenol that has been incorporated into a variety of soaps, disinfectants, deodorants, shampoos, medical

supplies, and even some plastics to decrease bacterial growth. Although widely found in household cleansers, phenols are sparingly used in veterinary medicine.[3,4]

Quaternary Ammonium Compounds

Quaternary ammonium compounds, or "quats," are cleansing agents (cationic surfactants) with germicidal activity, used in veterinary medicine to disinfect the surfaces of floors, walls, and vehicles utilized in livestock and egg-laying operations.[3,4] They are not used as antiseptics because the active ingredients bind to gauze and cotton commonly used to apply antiseptics to skin or tissue, and the Centers for Disease Control and Prevention (CDC) no longer recommends them for antisepsis.[3] The major quaternary ammonium compound used in veterinary medicine is **benzalkonium chloride,** which is the key ingredient in the disinfectant Roccal-D.

Quaternary ammonium compounds are effective against Gram-positive bacteria, but they are ineffective against bacterial spores and have poor efficacy against fungi and Gram-negative bacteria. Although quaternary ammonium compounds can destroy enveloped viruses, they are ineffective against nonenveloped viruses such as parvovirus. They act rapidly at the site of application and normally are not irritating to the skin or corrosive to metals.

Quaternary ammonium compounds readily bind to organic materials, rendering them less effective against many pathogenic microorganisms within or under such debris. Thus, thorough cleansing of a site before application of a quaternary ammonium compound is essential for adequate reduction of microbial populations. Because quaternary ammonium compounds are inactivated by contact with other detergents and soaps, the application site cleaned with soap or other surfactant must be rinsed thoroughly to remove residue before the quaternary ammonium antiseptic is applied. Finally, hard water reduces the antimicrobial activity of quaternary ammonium compounds. Therefore, proper cleansing, rinsing, and drying of the site before the application of the quaternary ammonium compound are essential to maintaining its effectiveness.

Other Disinfecting Agents

A veterinary technician may come across many other disinfecting agents in veterinary practice or research. The ones listed in this text constitute the majority of compounds routinely used. However, the veterinary technician must understand the benefits and drawbacks of any disinfecting or antiseptic agent used in the veterinary facility to avoid contamination of surgical sites, instruments, or hospital equipment. The following agents are occasionally used or are used less now than they were previously. Because they still are used, and sometimes used inappropriately, the veterinary technician should be aware of them.

Ethylenediamine tetraacetic acid (EDTA) and Tris buffer are two products that can be compounded and used together to irrigate ear infections, wounds, or fistulas infected with *Pseudomonas.* They are considered effective against a fairly narrow spectrum of Gram-negative bacteria and *Staphylococcus aureus.*

Acetic acid is sometimes used as a 0.25% solution to kill *Pseudomonas* organisms, as well as a variety of other Gram-positive and Gram-negative bacteria. Vinegar solution is primarily acetic acid and is sometimes recommended for yeast infections in otitis externa (i.e., ear inflammation caused by bacterial or yeast infections). Because better products are available that have greater efficacy and less tissue irritation, acetic acid is not often recommended today for use in veterinary medicine.

DISINFECTANTS AND ANTISEPTICS

Alcohols
Ethyl alcohol
Isopropyl alcohol

Halogens
Chlorine compounds
    Sodium hypochlorite
Iodine and iodophors
    Povidone-iodine

Biguanides
Chlorhexidine

Aldehydes
Glutaraldehyde

Oxidizing Compounds
Hydrogen peroxide
Peroxymonosulfate

Phenols
Triclosan

Quaternary Ammonium Compounds
Benzalkonium chloride

Ethylenediamine Tetraacetic Acid (EDTA) and Tris Buffer
Acetic Acid

REFERENCES

1. Benedict KM, Morley PS, Van Metre DC. Characteristics of biosecurity and infection control programs at veterinary teaching hospitals. *J Am Vet Med Assoc.* 2008;233(5):767–773.
2. Burgess BA. Is there a role for the veterinarian in cleaning and disinfection? In: *Proceedings of the 2014 American College of Veterinary Internal Medicine Conference, Nashville, Tennessee*; 2014.
3. Heit CH, Riviere J. Antiseptics and disinfectants. In: Riviere J, Papich M, eds. *Veterinary Pharmacology and Therapeutics*. Ames, Iowa: Wiley-Blackwell; 2009:819–834.
4. Boothe HW. Disinfectants, antiseptics, and related biocides. In: *Small Animal Clinical Pharmacology and Therapeutics*. Philadelphia: Saunders; 2012:425–433.
5. Hurley KF. Cleaning and sanitation in animal shelters. In: *Proceedings of the 2013 Wild West Veterinary Conference, Reno, Nevada*; 2013.
6. Dvorak G. Disinfection 101. The Center for Food Security and Public Health, Iowa State University. http://www.cfsph.iastate.edu/Disinfection/Assets/Disinfection1017.pdf. Accessed 06.01.2022.
7. Oregon State University Research Office. Fact Sheet/Disinfection Using Chlorine Bleach. Corvallis, OR: OSU Biological Safety; 2011.
8. University of Colorado Environmental Health and Safety. Environmental Health and Safety Guidance Document for Disinfectants and Sterilization Methods. Boulder, Colorado: University of Colorado, Anschutz Medical Campus; 2013.

SELF-ASSESSMENT

1. Fill in the following blanks with the correct item from the Key Terms list.

   A. _____ These are infections that are acquired during a period of hospitalization.

   B. _____ This is a microscopic glycocalyx material that surrounds and protects bacteria that attach to implants, catheters, and living tissue from the effects of most antiseptics or disinfectants.

   C. _____ This term describes chemicals that kill or prevent growth of microorganisms on living tissues.

   D. _____ This term describes chemicals that kill or prevent growth of microorganisms on the surface of inanimate object such as equipment, floors, and tabletops.

   E. _____ These are the three levels that describe the disinfecting capability of a compound.

   F. _____ This term applies to bacteria that are in the state of actively growing.

   G. _____ These types of viruses are surrounded by a thin membrane that is used by the virus to enter a host cell.

   H. _____ These types of viruses are considered to be naked viruses without any kind of outer membrane surrounding them.

   I. _____ This is the form of bacteria in which the bacterium is not actively growing and is very difficult to kill with disinfecting agents.

   J. _____ This term describes any type of disinfectant that completely removes or destroys all microorganisms.

   K. _____ This term describes any type of disinfectant that reduces the number of microorganisms to a safe level but does not completely eliminate them all.

   L. _____ This vague term refers to cleaning products that kill microorganisms but does not state which type of microorganism it kills.

   M. _____ This term means "kills bacteria."

   N. _____ This term means "kills viruses."

   O. _____ This term means "kills protozoa."

   P. _____ This term means "kills fungi."

   Q. _____ This term means "kills spores."

   R. _____ This term translates to "capable of killing microbes."

   S. _____ This term means that it will keep microbes from duplicating but will not kill the microbes directly.

   T. _____ Chlorine and iodine are examples of these.

   U. _____ This term describes a combination of iodine with another carrier molecule that releases the free iodine over a prolonged period of time.

   V. _____ These are chemical compounds that are soaplike in that they make it easier for interaction between organic material and disinfecting chemicals.

W. _____ This term describes antiseptics, like iodine, combined with a soap, detergent, or surfactant to effectively clean dirt and organic material off the site.

X. _____ The family of chemicals to which chlorhexidine belongs.

Y. _____ This combines with proteins on an open wound and forms a layer of altered proteins that can act as a barrier to disinfecting agents reaching the location of the bacteria on the skin or in a wound.

Z. _____ This term means that something is capable of destroying living mammalian (host) cells.

2. Fill in the following blanks with the correct drug from the Disinfectants and Antiseptics list. When practicing these questions, write out the answers on a separate sheet, focusing also on the appropriate spelling of these drug names.

A. _____ The low-cost, low-toxicity antiseptic used to disinfect surgical sites, injection sites, and low-level disinfecting sites; must remain in contact with the skin for 1–3 min to be effective against bacteria.

B. _____ Type of disinfectant that is very effective against nonenveloped viruses; is corrosive to metal (except stainless steel); and can have a pungent odor and be irritating to the skin.

C. _____ Disinfectant commonly used as a cold-sterilization liquid for instruments; temperature dependent to work the best; it is a tissue irritant that requires the use of safety goggles, gloves, and working in a well-ventilated area.

D. _____ Group of antiseptics that is used in common household cleaners like Lysol and also found in mouthwashes and surface disinfectants.

E. _____ Should not be applied to open wounds because it forms a coagulum that can prevent antiseptic agents from reaching bacteria under the coagulum.

F. _____ Sodium hypochlorite is an example of this type of disinfectant.

G. _____ A commonly used topically applied antiseptic that is safe to use as an external ear treatment but can be ototoxic if it gains access into the middle ear via a perforated ear drum.

H. _____ Very effective disinfectant that has the ability to penetrate biofilms to kill bacteria and to cause the bacteria to become unattached to the underlying equipment or tissue.

I. _____ Antiseptic and disinfectant that is used for cleaning cages, treating teat infections in cattle, and maintaining oral hygiene; only causes low levels of tissue irritation; and sticks to the surface of teeth and oral tissues.

J. _____ Often incorporated with glycerins or moisturizers because repeated use removes some of the skin's lipid components and dehydrates skin cells, making the skin dry and flaky.

K. _____ Agent of choice for disinfecting runs contaminated with parvovirus.

L. _____ Disinfectant group to which chlorhexidine belongs.

M. _____ Halogen that is not only bactericidal but also effective against dermatophytes like ringworm.

N. _____ Antiseptic/disinfectant compound that is inactivated by anionic and nonionic detergents and soap, along with minerals in hard water; binds to outer surface of skin and has residual activity for 24 h.

O. _____ Antiseptic that comes in two principal forms; effective against enveloped viruses but not nonenveloped viruses; does not kill spores; works best when slightly diluted with water to 50%–70%; has no cleaning ability.

P. _____ Type of halogen commonly incorporated into surgical scrubs.

Q. _____ High-level disinfecting agent used primarily to sterilize equipment that cannot be subjected to heat (e.g., endoscope); component of Cidex disinfectant product.

R. _____ Type of disinfectant agent found in regular bleach.

S. _____ This group of antiseptics and disinfectants contains hydrogen peroxide and peroxymonosulfate.

T. _____ Soaking instruments in this antiseptic will cause any blood on the instruments to become denatured and adhere more tightly to the instrument; used in hand sanitizers as preferred antiseptic.

U. _____ This topically applied disinfectant is hard to rinse off from surfaces or bird perches and contact with the residues can cause development of skin lesions or tissue irritation; not as easily inactivated by organic material as the halogens.

V. _____ Disinfectant that is also a cleansing agent and can act as a surfactant to disrupt dirt and organic material from surfaces; benzalkonium chloride is an example.

3. Indicate whether each of the following statements is true or false.

A. The presence of biofilm aids the disinfectant in reaching the bacteria by actively transporting the compounds into the bacteria.

B. To disinfect a surgery table, use a disinfectant. To disinfect a surgery site on an animal, use an antiseptic.

C. Enveloped viruses are more difficult to kill than nonenveloped viruses.

D. A sterilizer disinfectant would eliminate more of the pathogens than a sanitizer disinfectant.

E. A germicide kills bacteria but not viruses.

F. The spore form is the actively dividing form of bacteria.

G. Cleaning the disinfectant site with soap or surfactant is preferable but does not play that important of a role in overall disinfection.

H. As a general rule, the presence of blood, dirt, or feces reduces the effectiveness of a disinfectant or antiseptic.

I. Alcohols work by destroying lipid virus envelopes and denaturing proteins.

J. A thermometer used to take the temperature of a dog with parvovirus would be appropriately disinfected with alcohol.

K. A 95% ethyl alcohol solution would be more effective against pathogens than a 70% ethyl alcohol solution.

L. Alcohol is not a very good choice for cleaning dirt, blood, or fecal material from a site to be disinfected.

M. Because of alcohol's quick action, a 5-s alcohol swabbing of an injection site just before administering an injection should provide adequate bactericidal disinfection.

N. Alcohols are effective at reducing bacteria in open sores because of the way they denature protein.

O. Sodium hypochlorite is another name for common bleach.

P. Color-safe bleaches are simply a lower concentration of chlorine than regular bleaches.

Q. Adding vinegar or acetic acid to chlorine is recommended because it will increase its killing activity against pathogens.

R. Adding household ammonia cleanser to chlorine will produce a little more smell, but the extra killing activity justifies the inconvenience.

S. One of the major advantages of chlorine over other disinfectants is that it is effective against canine parvovirus, and it is not inactivated by fecal material, dirt, or blood to any great degree.

T. Diluted preparation of chlorine disinfectant should be made fresh every day.

U. Iodophors are slightly less effective against pathogens than the older free-iodine tinctures and solutions.

V. Povidone-iodine is a free-iodine form of antiseptic.

W. Iodine scrubs are used more in flushing abscesses than iodine solutions because scrubs contain surfactants that break down barriers to allow the iodine to penetrate better.

X. Iodine is a biguanide.

Y. Chlorhexidine an effective disinfectant against canine parvovirus.

Z. Chlorhexidine should not be diluted with hard water.

AA. Chlorhexidine adheres to skin, the surfaces of teeth, and the mucous membranes of the mouth.

AB. Endoscopes should be cleaned in glutaraldehyde.

AC. Glutaraldehyde is not very effective against bacteria that have generated a biofilm.

AD. Chlorhexidine is more of an odor, tissue irritation, and corrosion risk than glutaraldehyde.

AE. Peroxymonosulfate is the ingredient in accelerated hydrogen peroxide.

AF. Phenols are an ingredient in the disinfectant called Trifectant.

AG. Phenol residues are more of a problem in cages and perches than peroxymonosulfate.

AH. Triclosan is a phenol disinfectant.

AI. Benzalkonium chloride is a halogen.

AJ. Most Lysol-brand household disinfecting cleaners have phenol disinfectants in them.

AK. Quaternary ammonium compounds are better suited as antiseptics than disinfectants.

AL. Ethylenediamine tetraacetic acid (EDTA) and Tris buffer are used to treat ear infections and wounds infected with *Pseudomonas*.

AM. Acetic acid is vinegar.

4. Identify the following viruses as being enveloped or non-enveloped. Then identify them as easy to kill or difficult to kill with low- or intermediate-level disinfectants or antiseptics.
   - Rabies virus
   - Feline calicivirus
   - Canine distemper
   - Canine parvovirus
   - Feline herpes virus
   - Cow pox virus
   - Feline panleukopenia

5. Why does the veterinarian insist that you do a more thorough job of rinsing the surgical preparation site with alcohol or sterile water after cleaning the site with a surgical soap and before applying the final antiseptic application?

6. What are the five characteristics of the ideal disinfecting agent?

7. You are reading the insert of a new disinfectant, and you see a statement that identifies the disinfectant as a cytotoxic agent. This sounds good because that means it will kill more things and that is what you want in a disinfectant. Or is it?

Antiparasitics

CHAPTER OUTLINE

OBJECTIVES

After studying this chapter, the veterinary technician should be able to:

- Describe the characteristics of the ideal antiparasitic drug or compound.
- Use the appropriate terminology to describe the type of antiparasitic product, its spectrum of activity, and whether it kills or expels the parasite.
- Summarize the mechanism of action of macrolides, the role of P-glycoprotein (P-gp) in causing macrolide toxicity, and the characteristics and uses of the main avermectin and milbemycin compounds used in veterinary medicine.
- Describe the mechanism of action for the benzimidazoles, their role in parasite control, how their application differs from the macrolides, and the characteristics of the main benzimidazoles used in veterinary medicine.
- Describe the mechanism and the major characteristics of pyrantel antinematodals.

- Describe the two anticestodals used in veterinary medicine, their mechanism of action, and the differences in their spectra of activity.
- Describe how the different stages of heartworm disease are treated, what drugs are used, what risks are involved, what species of animals are treated and which are not, and the role of *Wolbachia* in the pathology of the disease and treatment.
- Describe the common veterinary antiprotozoal drugs, their characteristics (e.g., spectrum, method of activity, limitations), and any significant side effects or contraindications.
- Describe the challenges with ectoparasiticides and the four basic mechanisms of action into which all modern insecticides fit.
- Explain why organophosphates (OPs) and carbamates are still used in animal care, how they work, how clinical signs of toxicity would appear in host animals, and how toxicity is treated.

- Describe how pyrethrins and pyrethroids all work, what the role of synergists are, what pyrethroid toxicity would look like in host animals, what pyrethroids are most likely to cause toxicosis, and the characteristics of the main pyrethroids used as ectoparasiticides.
- Describe the mechanism for amitraz, what it is used for specifically, what species it causes toxicity in, and what precautions need to be taken to avoid toxicity or death in animals or humans.
- Describe the macrolides that are used for their ectoparasiticide activity.
- Explain the mechanism by which fipronil works, what it is used for, and precautions that must be taken when using the compound.
- Describe what neonicotinoids are, how they work, what two compounds are the most commonly used neonicotinoids in veterinary medicine, and for what purposes are they used.
- Explain what a spinosyn is, how it works, what two spinosyn compounds are used in veterinary medicine, how they are used, and precautions that must be taken when using them with ivermectin.
- Describe how isoxazoline compounds work, what two compounds are currently used that are isoxazolines, and any major precautions that need to be taken when using these products.
- Explain what indoxacarbs are, what makes them unique, why they are safe for use in most species, and how are they being used in veterinary medicine.
- Describe what insect growth regulators (IGRs) are, how insect development inhibitors (IDIs) are different from juvenile hormone analogs (JHAs), what compounds are used in veterinary medicine and whether they are an IDI or JHA, and the inherent limitations of these products when trying to control fleas.
- Describe the repellents used in veterinary medicine, their uses, and the precautions that must be exercised with their use.

KEY TERMS

ABCB1 (ATP-binding cassette type B1)
acetylcholine
acetylcholinesterase
adulticide
anthelmintic
anticestodal
antinematodal
antiprotozoal
antitrematodal
beta (β)-tubulin
caval syndrome
cestocides
chitin
coccidiocidal
coccidiostats
crystalluria
Dirofilaria immitis
ectoparasites
ectoparasiticides
emboli
endectocides
endoparasites

Environmental Protection Agency (EPA)
Food and Drug Administration (FDA)
gamma (γ) aminobutyric acid (GABA)
giardiasis
glutamate
heartworm-associated respiratory disease (HARD)
heartworm preventives
insect development inhibitors (IDI)
insect growth regulators (IGRs)
infective third-stage larvae (L3)
intima (arterial)
juvenile hormone analog (JHA)
macrolides
macrocyclic lactones
MDR1 (multiple drug resistance 1)
microfilaricide
miosis (pupils)
monoamine oxidase (MAO)
muscarinic cholinergic receptors
mydriasis
neuromuscular junction (NMJ)

nicotinic cholinergic receptors
ovicidal
P-glycoprotein (P-gp)
parasiticide
proglottids
pruritus
repellent
RiskMAP
scolex
selective toxicity/selectively toxic
sequestration
SLUDDE
synergists
taeniacides
teratogenic effects
vermicide
vermifuge
Wolbachia
Wolbachia surface protein (WSP)

Veterinarians have a wide array of products for use against internal parasites (e.g., gastrointestinal [GI] tract worms, protozoa, heartworms, and worms found elsewhere in the body) and external parasites (e.g., fleas, ticks, mites, and other arthropods). The importance of these products is partially to relieve suffering and disease in the animal but also to prevent transmission of disease to humans. In this latter, capacity veterinarians and veterinary technicians play an important role in helping to protect animals and citizens of their own communities through knowledge and proper application or dispensing of these antiparasitic products.

CHALLENGES WITH VETERINARY ANTIPARASITIC COMPOUNDS

There are a wide variety of antiparasitic chemicals and compounds, some of which are legend compounds (i.e., prescription or by order of the veterinarian), but others are over-the-counter (OTC) and available almost everywhere, from the smallest local grocery stores to the nearest mega retailer. To complicate matters, two governmental agencies regulate these products. The Food and Drug Administration (FDA) controls products that are either administered internally (i.e., orally, injectables) or absorbed significantly into the body if administered topically. FDA products are considered to be drugs and contain the legend on their label that requires dispensing by or on the order of a veterinarian. In contrast, any products that are applied topically and not absorbed to any great extent systemically are considered pesticides (e.g., flying insect sprays) and therefore are regulated by the Environmental Protection Agency (EPA). Because the EPA does not require their products to be regulated, other than very toxic insecticide applications that can only be used by regulated pest-control operators, topically applied veterinary products are sold OTC or available through the mail.

Several new parasiticide (they kill parasites) products are launched every year and, depending on the product and the manufacturer, the release may be accompanied by a media blitz to promote the product. Product manufacturing companies spend millions to entice consumers to purchase an OTC product on their own while shopping for groceries or other daily living supplies. However, legend products that can only be obtained through veterinarians are not protected from direct-to-consumer marketing by expensive advertisements that end with the using the phrase borrowed from their human drug counterparts: "Ask your veterinarian aboutum …." In addition to the traditional medium of television and all its permutations, the Internet is full of strong marketing messages that promise much to consumers seeking relief for their pets and themselves. Thus, veterinary professionals must spend a good deal of time and energy to stay up with the most recent products released, what they actually can and cannot do, and sometimes counter or bring into perspective the information the public is being told about the product.

Because veterinarians and veterinary technicians have a responsibility to protect pet and animal owners from diseases potentially transmitted to humans via animal internal or external parasites, they often must be equally as aggressive with information to avoid consumers opening themselves to the possible injury or illness because of inadequate parasite control. For example, some zoonotic diseases passed by parasites from animals to humans can be especially devastating to people who are immunocompromised because of disease, medications, or therapies for autoimmune diseases. Such individuals may believe that they are adequately protecting themselves by purchasing an antiparasitic product they saw strongly marketed in the media, when in actuality the product may not control key parasites that pose the greatest threat to their health. A veterinary professional would be able to identify this gap in parasite protection and advise the animal owner otherwise, but if they never get the opportunity to talk to the owner, the veterinary professional's advice will be unheard.

Even people who do not have special needs or conditions are at increased risk for disease because parasite exposure can cause parasite-transmitted diseases if they do not purchase the appropriate product. Parasites can be found in almost any environment regardless of how clean that environment may appear to the untrained eye. GI tract worms can infect humans through accidental ingestion of the parasite eggs from fecal-contaminated soil, other worms can migrate into the skin of humans sunbathing on a sandy beach where a parasite-infected dog defecated, or pet owners can be exposed to bacterial infections by being bitten by an external parasite brought into the house by the pet. External parasites like ticks and fleas can transmit Lyme disease, Rocky Mountain spotted fever, bubonic plague, and other diseases. Thus, control of parasite populations is a critical aspect of the veterinary professional's responsibilities that affects all people who own animals or are in contact with animals.

Because the veterinary technician is often the person communicating with clients and animal owners, it is especially important that the veterinary technician understand common parasites, their life cycles, the threat they pose to animals and humans, and what current products are effective (and which are not) against the parasites.

KEEPING CURRENT WITH NEW PRODUCTS

As stated previously, many products are released each year, and it can seem daunting to keep up with all of the products available and what the marketing media is saying about these products. However, in analyzing the new products it is common to find that many contain "old" compounds or chemicals that have been available and used in veterinary medicine for decades. Others will combine two "old" products together into a "new" formulation, and others will take a new product and combine it with an older one to expand the number of parasites controlled. Other products will use an "old" product but package the delivery system into a "new" product that claims to be "easier" or more "cost effective" to apply. Finally, there have been some breakthroughs that have brought genuinely new compounds to market. But even then, the new compounds often share a resemblance chemically or through their mechanism of parasite control with an older compound.

Therefore, the information presented in this chapter represents an overview of the key antiparasitic chemicals or agents that are incorporated into the plethora of OTC or veterinary products available for use in 2015. As with other drugs discussed in this text, the names used to describe the compounds are the nonproprietary names to reduce the numbers of compounds to be remembered. Although as a general rule students and veterinary professionals are strongly encouraged to use nonproprietary names for drugs in communicating to each other and clients, for antiparasitic compounds the veterinary professional really must know both the nonproprietary name (the active ingredient) and the proprietary or trade name. The trade name is so heavily entrenched in the public culture and media that it is the only product name that the client is going to recognize.

However, by knowing the nonproprietary name for the active ingredient, the veterinary professional can sort through all the products and identify which brand names actually contain the same basic active ingredient. By understanding the fundamental uses and limitations for each of these nonproprietary named antiparasitic compounds, the veterinary technician should be able to understand how "new" antiparasitic products or "new" combinations of multiple products work without having to learn an entirely new compound.

Although this chapter will provide a good foundation for understanding these compounds, it is still the responsibility of the veterinary technician and veterinarian to continue to educate themselves about the latest released antiparasitic products through journal articles, advertisements in veterinary trade publications, and information available at veterinary medical and veterinary technology conferences and conventions. Many drug companies choose to launch new products at the major veterinary conventions to gain a wider exposure for potential sales; hence these major conventions are good places to learn about the most recent products available.

PRINCIPLES AND TERMINOLOGY OF ANTIPARASITIC USE

If one believes the marketing advertisements on modern antiparasitic compounds, it would be easy to believe that these products readily remove all important parasites, easily, safely, and practically without thinking. However, intelligent decisions about which products to use need to go beyond the aggressive marketing pitch, attractive financial incentive offers, or comfort with a particular product that has always worked in the past. Therefore, when selecting an appropriate antiparasitic compound for use, the following characteristics of the ideal parasiticide should be considered:

- **Selective toxicity.** Selective toxicity means that the antiparasitic compound should be highly toxic to the parasite but should have little adverse effect on the host's tissue and the person applying or administering the product.
- **Economical.** An economical yet effective product is most desirable for treatment of parasitism. Economics is one of the most critical factors in selection of a parasitic control agent in livestock production, where the cost of a product used on the animals must be weighed against the potential economic return on the investment. Economics plays a much smaller role in equine or small animal parasite control.
- **Effective against all parasite stages with one application.** Ideally, internal antiparasitic drugs should kill all the adult parasites and any migrating larvae or immature forms with a single treatment. If a compound only kills adult worms living in the lumen of the GI tract but fails to kill the migrating larvae that are moving through the rest of the body, the larvae will form new adult worms in a few weeks to continue the infection. Likewise, external antiparasitics should be effective with one treatment or very convenient to reapply to assure client compliance and effective disruption of the parasite life cycle. Failure to break the life cycle means the animal is highly likely to be reinfected in a few weeks.
- **Safe for old, very young, pregnant, or debilitated animals.** This population of animals typically does not metabolize or eliminate toxic compounds (the parasiticides) and younger, healthy animals with fully functioning organs. For pregnant animals, any chemical or drug used must take into consideration exposure of the compound to the fetus and any potential teratogenic (i.e., birth defect–generating) effects or detrimental effects on the pregnancy itself.
- **Does not induce resistance in the target parasite.** Like antibiotics, there has been increasing concern about resistance of parasites to antiparasitic agents. This issue has been controversial in heartworm prevention medications and antiparasitic

compounds used in equine or livestock products. Although resistance is sometimes difficult to document (e.g., owner noncompliance with proper application of the product is always a confounding factor in trying to prove whether resistance exists or not), it has been documented in several internal and external parasite species. Selective pressure (see Chapter 10) resulting in emergence of resistant, mutated parasites has been documented. Therefore, any product available OTC or through veterinarians should be highly effective to avoid the development of parasite resistance.

Other desirable characteristics include a fragrant odor or lack of offensive odor (in external antiparasitics) and environmental safety (i.e., product breaks down quickly in the environment and does not enter the ground water aquifer).

Unfortunately, no single antiparasitic product incorporates all these ideal features, although over the years products have become much safer for the animal owner, the animal, and the environment and more selectively effective against disease-causing parasites. Veterinary professionals should still understand the specific needs of the animal and client, the environment in which the product will be used, and the characteristics and limitations of the antiparasitic product to make a rational, economical, and safe recommendation.

Today's veterinary clients are savvier about their animals' health. Therefore, by explaining the reason behind the specific interval for dosing the product, the proper application method, the site for the product application, and any changes in the environment the client needs to make to break the life cycle (e.g., cleaning up dog feces in the yard), client compliance with the instructions will be enhanced, increasing the odds of breaking the parasite life cycle and successfully controlling the parasitic infection.

INTERNAL ANTIPARASITICS

Although many discussions about parasites break them down into internal or external parasites, many compounds today are capable of killing both. These types of compounds are called endectocides, so named for their ability to kill some endoparasites (internally living parasites) and some ectoparasites (externally living parasites). This section discusses compounds used to kill or control parasites that reside primarily inside the body; however, some of the reagents will also be discussed in "External Antiparasitic" section

Terminology Used to Describe Internal Antiparasitics

Various terms are used to scientifically describe internal antiparasitics, along with terminology used by marketing firms to promote a particular product. To sort through the sometimes confusing terminology and better understand the effects, targeted parasitic species, and the limitations of a particular product, the veterinary technician should master the basic descriptive terminology.

Anthelmintic is a general term used to describe compounds that kill various types of helminths, or internal parasitic worms. Anthelmintics may also be described as a vermicide that kills the worm, or as a vermifuge, which only paralyzes the worm and often results in passage of live worms in the feces. Most products today are vermicidal and result in death and digestion of internal parasites. In many cases, no evidence of intact worms is seen in the stool of the infected animal after the worms have been killed.

Antinematodal compounds are anthelmintics used to treat infections of nematodes, or roundworms. The use of the term *roundworms* can be confusing because it is also often used to describe a subset of nematodes found in the GI tract of animals that are large enough to be observed passing in the stool like spaghetti (e.g., *Toxocara* species, *Toxascaris* species). This subset of nematodes is also sometime referred to vaguely as "ascarids." All nematodes are technically roundworms whether they fit into this subset or not because when cut in cross section, they are round in appearance. To avoid confusion when using the term *roundworm*, the specific species name of the nematode (e.g., *Toxocara, Toxascaris*) should be used in describing the parasites. The classification of worms that fit into nematodes is very large, and because one antinematodal does not kill all nematodes, knowing the specific parasite names is important for selecting the appropriate antinematodal to use.

Anticestodal compounds, or cestocides, treat infections of cestodes, which are tapeworms or segmented flatworms. Anticestodals are sometimes referred to as taeniacides, an older term that takes its name from the *Taenia* species of tapeworm. Again, a particular cesticidal drug may not be effective against all species of tapeworms commonly encountered in veterinary practice. Therefore, the veterinary technician should carefully read the package insert to determine the drug's spectrum of anticestodal activity.

Antitrematodal compounds treat infections of trematodes, which are flukes or unsegmented flatworms, including *Paragonimus*, *Fasciola*, and *Dicrocoelium* parasites. Antiprotozoal compounds treat infections of protozoa, which are single-celled organisms such as *Coccidia*, *Giardia*, and *Toxoplasma*. Coccidiostats are antiprotozoal drugs that specifically inhibit the growth of *Coccidia*. Many antibiotics like the sulfonamides and the fluoroquinolones also have antiprotozoal properties.

Many of the parasiticides today have a broad spectrum of activity. Drugs that are antinematodal may also be anticestodal and have additional effectiveness against external parasites. Thus, the classification of drugs as antinematodal vs anticestodal, or internal parasiticide vs external parasiticide, has blurred in the past few years (e.g., the endectocides). Thus, many of these products mentioned in one category (i.e., antinematodal, anticestodal, internal parasiticide, external parasiticide) will be mentioned in multiple sections.

ANTINEMATODALS

Avermectins and Milbemycins (the Macrolides)

Thanks to the 1976 discovery that a *Streptomyces* bacterium growing near a golf course in Japan possessed a broad range of parasiticide and insecticide properties, a group of revolutionary new, safer compounds with broad spectra of activity became available to the veterinarian in the 1980s. This group includes the **avermectins** (i.e., **ivermectin**, **selamectin**, **doramectin**, and **eprinomectin**) and the **milbemycins** (i.e., **milbemycin oxime** and **moxidectin**). Interestingly, the milbemycins had been discovered and were being used against agricultural pest insects for at least 3 years before the avermectins were discovered in Japan. It was only when it was discovered that the structurally similar avermectins had excellent activity against a wide variety of internal parasites that the milbemycins were then developed for use as anthelmintics. Thus, even though they were discovered first, milbemycin did not hit the veterinary market until well after the first avermectins, specifically the ivermectin products, were already well established as internal parasiticides.

To keep the multitude of compounds and their uses straight, the veterinary professional must remember that ivermectin (e.g., Heartgard, Ivomec, Iverhart, Zimecterin for horses), selamectin (e.g., Revolution), milbemycin (e.g., Interceptor, Sentinel, Trifexis, MilbeMite otic), moxidectin (e.g., ProHeart 6, Cydectin for cattle, Quest for horses), doramectin (e.g., Dectomax for use in livestock), and eprinomectin (e.g., Eprinex and LongRange for use in cattle) are all structurally similar and have similar mechanisms of action. The macrocyclic ring found in each of these compounds gives rise to the collective name for the group as the macrolides or macrocyclic lactones. Thus, when hearing these various terms (i.e., macrolides, avermectins, or milbemycins), remember they are all members of the same set of commonly used veterinary products.

The macrolides, like most of the modern antiparasitic drugs, are neurotoxins. Most of today's antiparasitics target specific receptors on neurons to selectively enhance or inhibit the activity of specific neurons or to enhance or inhibit the effect of the neuron's neurotransmitter. Thus, mechanisms of action for antiparasitic drugs usually involve a specific type of neuronal receptor or a specific neurotransmitter.

For the macrolides, the mechanism of action inside the insect or parasite is primarily through stimulation of a receptor site for the neurotransmitter glutamate. The glutamate neurotransmitter in invertebrates normally stimulates the glutamate receptor, which opens a channel in the cell membrane that allows negatively charged chloride ions to flow into the cell. The negative charge that is carried into the cells by the chloride ions makes the inside of the cell more negatively charged. As described in Chapter 5 (about cardiovascular drugs), for a neuron or muscle to depolarize (i.e., fire), the charge inside the cell must become more positive from its resting state until it reaches a threshold charge level, at which point sodium channels open up, allowing a flood of positively charged ions to enter, making the inside of the cell very positive. If negative chloride ions have flooded into the cell as a result of stimulation of the glutamate receptor, the inside of the cell is more negative than normal, meaning the resting charge (called the resting membrane potential) is farther away from the charge level needed to cause depolarization. The net result is that the neuron or muscle cannot depolarize and there is paralysis of the muscle or no firing by the neuron.

In parasites, this glutamate receptor–stimulated muscle paralysis affects the pharyngeal muscles (i.e., they cannot swallow) and the muscles associated with movement (i.e., they cannot move). Internal parasites starve to death or, if located in the

GI tract, are moved away from their infection site and die. The absence of these glutamate receptors in tapeworms and flukes explains why the macrolides are largely ineffective against most members of these parasite classes.

Although macrolides as a group are considered to be very safe compounds with a fairly selective toxicity and wide therapeutic index (see Chapter 3), they do produce a well-documented toxicity in susceptible animals or those that receive an overdose of the medications. When such toxicities occur in mammals, they are not mediated through glutamate receptors on the muscles or peripheral nerves because mammals do not have glutamate receptors in these locations. Instead, avermectins and milbemycins can combine with another receptor for a transmitter called gamma (γ)-aminobutyric acid (GABA), which, like glutamate, causes an opening of chloride channels and subsequent inhibition of neurons in the CNS (primarily brain). The GABA neurotransmitter and receptor were key components of the mechanism of action of the benzodiazepine tranquilizers and other drugs like propofol (see Chapter 8).

Fortunately, the GABA receptors targeted by avermectins and milbemycins are located within the CNS and therefore "safely" protected from exposure behind the blood-brain barrier. Still lipophilic drugs can readily diffuse through the blood-brain barrier and could potentially gain access to the GABA receptors in mammalian brains, producing toxicity. So why does toxicity not occur in animals every time a macrolide is administered?

In addition to the cellular membrane part of the blood-brain barrier, another component of the barrier is the presence of a special protein pump called P-glycoprotein (P-gp), whose function is to move drugs from the brain side of the blood-brain barrier back into the blood. Therefore, even though macrolides can diffuse from the blood across the tight cellular membrane of the blood-brain barrier and enter the brain, the P-gp pumps them back into the blood before they can combine with GABA receptors on neurons in the brain. It is important to note that P-gps are also found in the liver, where they transport drug from the blood into the bile for hepatic excretion, and also exist in the cells lining the GI tract, where they move selected drug molecules from the GI tract wall cells back into the lumen of the gut.

Because the effectiveness of the blood-brain barrier against macrolides is so dependent on the P-gp pump, anything that impairs the P-gp effectiveness allows macrolides to accumulate within the brain, increasing the risk for toxicity. There are two ways that this can happen: the P-gp can be inhibited by other drugs or the P-gp itself can be defective.

Although the list of drugs that inhibit P-gp includes a few drugs used in veterinary medicine (e.g., calcium channel blocker antiarrhythmics, cyclosporine immunosuppressant, antifungal agents ketoconazole or itraconazole), toxicity from macrolides because of less effective P-gp pumping originates mostly from defective production of the P-gp itself. Collies and other related breeds have a genetic defect in the gene that codes for their P-gp. This gene is called the MDR1 (multiple drug resistance 1) gene because it produces the P-gp found on the surface of cancer cells that pump out any antineoplastic drug that makes it into the cancer cell, making the cancer cell resistant to the drugs. This same gene has been more recently called the ABCB1 (ATP-binding

TABLE 12.1 Frequency of Breeds Affected by MDR1 Mutation as Listed on the Washington State University College of Veterinary Medicine Website	
Breed	Approximate Incidence of MDR1 Mutation
Collie	70%
Long-Haired Whippet	65%
Australian Shepherd	50%
Silken Windhound	30%
Shetland Sheepdog	15%
English Shepherd	15%
German Shepherd	10%
Old English Sheepdog	5%
Border Collie	<5%

MDR1, Multiple drug resistance 1.
Adapted from Veterinary Clinical Pharmacology Laboratory, College of Veterinary Medicine, Washington State University: *Breeds Affected Table (Website)*. http://vcpl.vetmed.wsu.edu/affected-breeds; accessed 01.07.15.

cassette type B1) gene for the type of protein it produces. Animals that have the MDR1 genetic defect produce P-gp that is either partially or totally impaired. Without functional P-gp pumps in the blood-brain barrier, drugs like the macrolides can gain access to the GABA receptors in the neurons of the brain and inhibit their ability to depolarize. Non-Collie breeds now show sensitivity to macrolide drugs, and genetic testing is available to determine whether a dog has this MDR1 genetic defect. See Table 12.1 for frequency of MDR1 mutation in dogs as measured and reported by the Washington State University College of Veterinary Medicine.

Macrolide toxicity because of genetic defect or from a very high dose of the macrolide that overwhelms the P-gp defensive mechanism produces signs associated with CNS depression. Thus, the animals hypersalivate, vomit, become ataxic, stagger, and progress to depression, unresponsiveness, bradycardia, mydriasis (i.e., pupil dilation), loss of menace response (i.e., do not respond to a hand moving toward the eye), and coma. Prolonged seizures have been reported in some dogs along with miosis (i.e., pupillary constriction), but it was thought that these may occur in animals secondary to brain injury caused by brain hypoxia (i.e., low oxygen). There is no antidote for avermectin or milbemycin toxicosis, and the persistent nature of these macrolides can require that the animal be kept alive in a comatose or severely depressed state for days to weeks before the effects of the drug wear off. See Clinical Application for a couple of cases of ivermectin toxicosis.

To kill most parasites, only small concentrations of macrolides need to be present in the tissues or fluid compartments where the parasite lives. The lipophilic nature of macrolides explains how avermectins and milbemycins can readily penetrate many tissues and persist at low, but still effective, concentrations for a long period of time. In addition to internal parasites, macrolides are effective against mites, sucking lice, and feeding ticks when administered systemically by oral or

CLINICAL APPLICATION

Ivermectin Toxicosis in Two Australian Shepherds

Case 1: A 10-month-old male Australian shepherd presented to a veterinary hospital 24 h after having received 4000 µg of a cattle ivermectin preparation. The dog was reluctant to move, was salivating profusely, had slowed respiration and heart rate, and had a subnormal temperature. On neurologic examination, the dog was poorly responsive to stimuli and had head bobbing, facial muscle twitches, and pinpoint, nonresponsive pupils. Reflexes in the limbs were normal to exaggerated. Complete blood count and serum biochemistry profiles were within reference ranges. Based on the history of exposure and clinical signs consistent with central nervous system (CNS) depression, including depression of brainstem control centers (respiratory, cardiovascular, temperature), a presumptive diagnosis of ivermectin toxicosis was made.

The dog was treated with supportive care. Intravenous (IV) fluids were given to maintain hydration, ophthalmic ointment was applied to both eyes to prevent drying of the cornea and corneal ulceration formation, supplemental heat was provided to maintain the body temperature, and the dog was turned over every 4 h to prevent decubital ulcers (pressure sores, or bed sores, on the skin). Glycopyrrolate (an anticholinergic drug) was given to help reverse the low heart rate by reducing the parasympathetic nervous system effect on the heart. Glycopyrrolate was chosen over atropine because atropine penetrates the brain and could produce unwanted side effects in the CNS, whereas glycopyrrolate does not appreciably penetrate the blood-brain barrier.

Unlike drugs that are excreted by the body through the kidney, ivermectin is metabolized and excreted by the liver. Therefore, the administration of IV fluids to increase the urine production (diuresis) was not instituted because it would not facilitate the removal of the hepatically eliminated ivermectin.

Over the next 10 days the dog slowly increased motor control. Because the dog was unable to feed itself, a gastrostomy (gastro, meaning stomach; stoma, meaning hole) tube was placed through the stomach and body wall so food gruel could be placed into the stomach by the tube. By day 8 the dog could stand if helped. Vision returned on day 10. On day 11, the dog was able to walk with a wobbly gait (i.e., ataxia) and was sent home with its owners.

The owners reported behavior changes after the dog went home. He became aggressive toward a companion cat, would try to nip the owners, and snapped at objects near his head. These behavior changes had disappeared by the time the dog was returned to the veterinary hospital on day 19 to have the gastrostomy tube removed. At day 19, the dog was clinically normal without any residual neurologic or physical signs.

Case 2: A 3-year-old female Australian shepherd also showed similar clinical signs after being fed 7600 µg of an equine ivermectin preparation. In this case, the respiratory depression was more profound, and, in addition to the other supportive measures, the dog had to be maintained on ventilator-assisted oxygen (positive-pressure ventilation) to keep blood oxygen concentrations within acceptable limits. This dog was on a ventilator until day 11 after ingestion and eventually recovered 21 days after administration of the ivermectin.

What should be learned from these cases: In both of these cases, the dogs showed signs shortly after being given 167 and 340 µg/kg of ivermectin. Small animal heartworm preventive medication typically has approximately 6 µg/kg (0.006 mg/kg) of ivermectin. Therefore, it would take ingestion or administration of a significant volume of small animal products to achieve the doses administered to these two animals. However, because the ivermectin preparations that were ingested were labeled for use on livestock and horses and thus had relatively high concentrations of the drug, ingestion of only a small volume of product produced severe toxicosis.

Because there is no antidote and toxicosis can result in a prolonged period of recovery, it is a wise investment of time to educate horse owners or others using the concentrated formulations of ivermectin to ensure that the product is kept away from dogs that might chew the container or ingest spilled or discarded product.

---

injection routes because they can penetrate into the tissues and the tissue fluid where these parasites are located or where they feed. Unfortunately, the lipophilic nature of macrolides and their penetration into milk means no injectable macrolides can be used in actively milking dairy cattle because of milk contamination for an extended period of time.

Despite their inherent lipophilic nature, topically applied macrolides are often formulated to reduce their ability to penetrate deep into the skin, where the drug might be absorbed systemically.

Macrolides are excreted intact by the liver into the feces. One benefit of this is that feces from treated livestock or horses can kill flies or fly larvae that contact the feces. Part of the efficient excretion of the drug from the blood into the bile of the liver is because of the presence of P-gp molecules in the liver that actively secrete macrolides into the bile, which then flows into the duodenum. However, because macrolides are lipophilic, they readily move across the GI tract wall; if not removed by the P-gps in the cells lining the GI tract, the macrolides will reenter systemic circulation (enterohepatic circulation, see Chapter 3). The enterohepatic circulation in conjunction with the persistence in the tissues explains the long-lasting effect of these drugs in the body.

Because macrolides are excreted intact into the feces, significant concentrations of the antiparasitic compound can accumulate in the feces. Dogs that have a habit of eating horse feces can ingest a significant dose of the avermectin or milbemycin that was administered to the horse a few days before, and, if the dog is a Collie-related breed or has the MDR1 gene mutation and ineffective P-gp, this could be sufficient drug to produce potentially severe toxicity. Thus, horse owners should be vigilant in collecting and properly disposing of horse manure in a way that dogs do not have access to it for at least 4 days after the macrolide was administered to the horse.[1]

Within the past few years the question of resistance of parasites to avermectins and milbemycins has been raised. A strain of heartworm isolated in Georgia (the MP3 isolate) was found to have increased resistance to several of the macrolide heartworm preventives when used prophylactically as a prescribed single dose but was susceptible to three consecutive monthly doses. Still, the studies concluded that there are pockets of resistant heartworms, but the degree to which the resistance exists is still not known.[2] This will be a topic in veterinary medicine that will continue to evolve over the next few years.

Ivermectin

Ivermectin was the first macrolide to be available for use in veterinary medicine. Its wide spectrum of activity includes everything from heartworms and intestinal parasites to external parasites. In addition, veterinarians have used the drug for many extra-label (not FDA approved) applications. It was, and still is, quite common to see ivermectin listed in the veterinary literature as an experimental or extra-label treatment for internal and external parasites in a wide variety of exotic animals, wildlife, avian species, and nonconventional household pets (e.g., hedgehogs, snakes, other reptiles). Many dosages also exist for use of ivermectin in dogs and cats to treat extra-label parasites such as demodectic mange, ear mites, microfilariae of the heartworm, and a wide variety of less frequently seen internal parasites. As long as the use of the drug is in compliance with extra-label drug use requirements in animals, including those animals intended for use as human food, these uses are mostly considered prudent and acceptable.

Because of its spectrum and success in treating parasites, ivermectin is incorporated with other anthelmintics to produce parasiticides with a wider spectrum of activity. For example, Heartgard Plus is a combination of ivermectin for prevention of heartworm disease and pyrantel pamoate, an effective drug for control of intestinal ascarids (i.e., roundworms). Iverhart Max has the same ingredients as Heartgard Plus but expands the spectrum to tapeworms by also incorporating another drug, praziquantel. Other combination drugs are currently available and others are likely to be released in the future. By understanding what each drug in the combination does separately, the veterinary technician can more easily understand the spectra and potential side effects of these combination drugs.

As with most other avermectins, ivermectin requires very small concentrations to be effective against parasites. For example, the normal dose of ivermectin needed to prevent heartworm infection in dogs is measured in micrograms of drug, or about 0.006 mg/kg of body weight. At that dose, even Collies with MDR1 mutation and poorly functioning P-gp should be able to tolerate the drug; toxicity reported in such Collies is about 0.1 mg/kg (16 times the 0.006-mg/kg dose needed to prevent heartworms), and death has been reported with a dose of 0.2 mg/kg (32 times the preventive dose). Even though the effective dose of these drugs are well above the doses that produce toxicity even in Collies with MDR1 mutations, the manufacturers warn that Collie-related breeds should be observed for signs of ivermectin toxicosis for 8 h after administration of the monthly heartworm preventive. Typically, ivermectin toxicity in dogs is not associated with use of small animal products, but more commonly reported with the accidental exposure to large animal products (e.g., ingesting discarded equine paste syringes) or the extra-label use of large animal products in small animals (e.g., using large animal ivermectin injectable to kill heartworm microfilariae).

Selamectin

Selamectin (Revolution) is an avermectin type of macrolide that entered the veterinary market after ivermectin and milbemycin oxime. It was targeted as a broad-spectrum endectocide approved for use as a heartworm preventive that is also effective against several GI tract worm parasites and external parasites, principally fleas, ear mites, sarcoptic mange, and one tick species. Unlike ivermectin, which is available primarily as oral or injectable dosage forms, selamectin was approved as a monthly topical application in both dogs and cats.

The topical application route first used in small animals for selamectin has since been adopted by newer antiparasitics for its convenience. Dogs absorb only about 4% of the applied drug systemically, but cats, because of the different thickness of their skin, absorb closer to 74%.[1] Because of the greater absorption of the drug in cats than dogs, selamectin is also approved in the cat to remove the hookworm *Ancylostoma tubaeforme* and the cat roundworm *Toxocara cati*. Although selamectin can kill roundworms in dogs and lungworms in cats, the drug is not approved for these indications.[1]

Toxicity in breeds with MDR1 mutation is rare because of the route of administration and, in the dog, the relatively low amount of drug absorbed systemically. Multiple studies show that the topical application retains its effectiveness as a heartworm preventive even after the pet is bathed. Thus, there should be little concern if the animal goes swimming or is exposed to rain after application of the compound to the skin at the back of the neck. Oral contact with the compound produces hypersalivation and vomiting, but topical application overdoses of 10 times the prescribed amount do not seem to produce significant signs in dogs or cats other than hypersalivation.[1]

Livestock Macrolides: Doramectin and Eprinomectin

Doramectin (Dectomax) is available as both an injectable and topical "pour-on" approved for use in cattle and swine, whereas **eprinomectin** is approved for use as a topical application in cattle (Eprinex) and as a subcutaneous (SQ) injectable for beef cattle (LongRange) that provides 100–150 days of antiparasitic activity. Both products are approved for use against a variety of internal parasite worms, as well as grubs, lice, and mange. Although doramectin is reported to be free of toxic signs in cattle at 25 times the recommended dose, the manufacturer states that use of doramectin in other species may result in severe adverse reactions, including death in dogs. Both drugs have specific indications and restrictions for their use even within cattle species (e.g., restricted use in lactating cattle of a certain age or veal calves). Therefore, the veterinary professional should know and comply with the restrictions applied to the drugs and should communicate to the livestock producer the importance of compliance with these restrictions to prevent drug residues.

Milbemycin Oxime

As previously stated, milbemycin is the name for the family of macrolide antiparasitic compounds that include milbemycin oxime and moxidectin. Milbemycin oxime was originally used against agricultural insects (mites) and was only looked at for its antinematodal activity after the antinematodal activity of avermectins became known.

Although dosages exist for milbemycin oxime use in everything from heartworm preventive in cats to treatment of demodectic and sarcoptic mange, the FDA-approved uses for the orally administered milbemycin tablets (e.g., Interceptor, Sentinel, Trifexis) are for heartworm prevention for dogs and cats, treatment/control for hookworms and roundworms in dogs and cats and whipworms in dogs, and as a topically applied treatment of ear mites in cats (e.g., MilbeMite Otic). The latter indication reflects its original use against agricultural mites. Milbemycin oxime has shown some promise in treatment of demodectic mange that is resistant to other mange medications. Milbemycin oxime works by the same mechanism as the avermectins and appears to have a similar pattern of safety when used at appropriate doses for macrolide-sensitive Collies. One source states that milbemycin oxime is nontoxic to Collies up to 20 times the regular dose.[1] Because milbemycin is used as a heartworm preventive, it will be discussed in greater detail in that section.

Moxidectin

Moxidectin (Cydectin, Quest, Advantage Multi, ProHeart 6), like other members of this group, has a wide range of potential uses. The list of parasites for which moxidectin is indicated in cattle (as a pour-on) and horses (as an oral gel) includes intestinal parasites, mites, cattle grubs, horse stomach bots, lice, flies, and nematodes living in other parts of the body. Moxidectin is available as an OTC equine product and therefore has been widely used by the lay public for a spectrum of parasites well beyond the approved label uses. Still, there are very few reports of moxidectin toxicity in horses. One clinical case report described three foals that had been administered moxidectin doses far exceeding the recommended dose. Clinical signs were consistent with overdose signs seen with ivermectin: CNS depression that progressed to coma. Moxidectin is not approved for use in horses younger than 4 months. Two of the three foals in this moxidectin toxicity case report were less than 2 weeks old, with the third foal being a 4-month-old miniature horse foal.[1]

For dogs, moxidectin is available as both an injectable for 6 or 12-month heartworm preventative and hookworms (ProHeart 6 and ProHeart 12) and as part of a topically applied combination product with imidacloprid (Advantage Multi) that is approved for heartworm prevention, treatment and control of common GI tract nematodes (e.g., roundworms, hookworms, whipworms), and treatment of sarcoptic mange and fleas. The combination product of moxidectin (Advantage Multi) is the only antiparasitic product that is FDA approved for eliminating the circulating microfilariae young of heartworm in dogs.

The injectable ProHeart 6 was originally released in 2001, but in 2004 the manufacturer voluntarily recalled the product because of FDA concerns over reported excessive adverse drug reactions. After additional testing, it was found that some residues left in the product from the manufacturing process had the capability of producing an allergic type of immune reaction that was thought to be tied to the severe reactions and death from the drug. After this compound was removed from the manufacturing process, the reports of adverse reactions in the overseas market where the drug was still being used declined significantly, and in 2008 ProHeart 6 was relaunched in the United States. When it was reintroduced into the US market, ProHeart 6 had more narrowed restrictions on the age of dogs to which the drug could be administered and mandated additional record keeping and client information/consent requirements. However, with the continued improved safety record since the rerelease, these additional restrictions were lifted in 2013. In 2019, ProHeart 12 was approved by the FDA as the first 12-month heartworm preventative.

Although the ProHeart 6 and 12 injectables provide protection against heartworm infection, they do not clear an infected dog of either the adult heartworms or the circulating microfilariae young. Also, although the moxidectin in ProHeart 6 and 12 kills adult and migrating larvae of the hookworm, they do not prevent reinfection of hookworm for the full 6 or 12 months depending on the product that is used.[1] Both of these injections are required to be administered in the office by a trained veterinarian or veterinary technician.

Benzimidazoles

Like the macrolides, benzimidazoles are a rather large collection of antiparasitic drugs developed in the 1960s from the prototype compound thiabendazole. These drugs were used in both human beings and animals, especially livestock, for treatment of a wide variety of nematodal infections. Because of the greater spectra of activity of newer anthelmintics and endectocides, this group has decreased in popularity for veterinary use. However, the relatively low cost of the drugs still makes them attractive for livestock operations, and paste products are often incorporated into rotating treatments for horses.

All the benzimidazoles act by attacking special proteins in the parasite's cells called β-tubulin. β-Tubulin is involved in a wide variety of cellular functions including cell division and maintaining cell shape, cell motility, cell secretion, and intracellular transport.[3]

By interfering with the function of β-tubulin, benzimidazoles disrupt the normal cellular function and eventually kill the parasite. Although mammalian cells also have β-tubulin, it is different from the parasite's β-tubulin, preventing benzimidazoles from binding as readily to the mammalian β-tubulin and hence providing a wide safety margin and selective toxicity for this class of antiparasitics.[3] The action of benzimidazole on the parasite's cells usually takes up to 24 h to kill the cells, and it may take multiple exposures to the drug over 3 or more days for some benzimidazoles to achieve their optimal killing effect on the parasite.[3] Therefore, some dosage regimens of benzimidazoles require the pet owner or livestock producer to administer the drug on consecutive days.

The β-tubulin mechanism of action is generally safe for mammalian cells for the reasons stated previously. However, rapidly dividing mammalian cells in the fetus may be affected by benzimidazoles because of the cells' dependence on properly functioning β-tubulin to make the microtubules that aid cellular division. Teratogenic effects (i.e., birth defects) have been noted at very high doses of selected benzimidazoles (e.g., 4 times the normal dose) when given early in pregnancy, especially to sheep. Teratogenic effects ranged from malformation of the limbs to abortion. Thus, some, but not all, benzimidazoles are contraindicated for use in some species during early pregnancy. The package label or drug insert for the individual drugs will provide more specific details.

Benzimidazole compounds can usually be recognized by the -azole suffix of the chemical name. In addition to the prototype

thiabendazole, other benzimidazoles used in North America include **fenbendazole** (Panacur, Safe-Guard), **oxibendazole** (Anthelcide EQ), **albendazole** (Valbazen), and **febantel** (Drontal Plus). Other benzimidazoles besides these are used in the United Kingdom, Australia, and other countries. Many of these products are formulated as pastes and solutions for use in control of equine intestinal parasites. Most also have applications in cattle and other food animals but little application today in companion animals, with the exception of febantel combined with the anticestodal drug praziquantel and the antinematodal pyrantel in the drug Drontal Plus.

Thiabendazole is the prototype drug for this group of antiparasitics, and like other members of this drug family, it has a wide range of activity against ascarids and strongyles in horses, cattle, sheep, and goats.[1,3] Because of the age of the product, parasitic resistance to this drug has been documented, limiting its use in equines and livestock.[1] The drug is safe when used at recommended dosages and rarely causes significant side effects, although the dying parasites may produce an inflammatory reaction. In addition to its antiparasitic activity, thiabendazole is unique in that it has some antiinflammatory and antifungal activity. For this reason, thiabendazole is sometimes added to otic (i.e., ear) medications (e.g., Tresaderm) and topical products.[4]

Fenbendazole (Panacur and Safe-Guard for dogs, horses, and livestock) has a wide spectrum of activity against nematodes and a variety of other parasites. Fenbendazole is effective against a limited number of species of tapeworms (*Taenia pisiformis* in the dog) but should not be used as a general cestocide (i.e., tapeworm-killing compound) unless the particular species of tapeworm has been identified. In horses and livestock, it is administered once as an oral paste, oral solution, or granules added to the feed, whereas in the dog it is given as granules that must be mixed with food for 3 consecutive days. The manufacturer states that repeated administration is required with continued exposure to parasites (e.g., grazing in infected fields). Extra-label dosages exist for livestock, exotics, and small "pocket pet" animals.

Oxibendazole (Anthelcide EQ) has long been used as an equine dewormer to control both large and small strongyles, large roundworms, pinworms, and threadworms.[3] It is administered as a paste in a syringe adjusted for the estimated weight of the animal. Because horses in fenced pastures are typically reexposed to parasites as they graze, the manufacturer recommends repeat treatment every 6–8 weeks.

Albendazole (Valbazen) is used to treat livestock with a spectrum of activity that includes intestinal nematodes, lungworms, trematodes (flukes), cestodes, and protozoa. It is one of the benzimidazoles that is thought to have the potential for teratogenic effects, and it has been linked to bone marrow suppression because of its effect on rapidly dividing cells. Therefore, although albendazole is still used in livestock, it should not be used during the first 30–45 days of pregnancy because of the potential for teratogenic effects. These dates vary with the species of animal to which the drug is given. The manufacturer's information will list the specific date with the given species. Like most of the benzimidazoles, ivermectin and modern anticestodals have largely supplanted the need for albendazole in companion animals; however, some products still exist and are still used in livestock because of their antiparasitic spectrum, especially against protozoa, and their relatively low cost.

Febantel (Drontal Plus) is a little different from the other benzimidazoles in that it is a "prodrug," meaning that it must be converted by metabolism to the active form of the drug, which in this case is fenbendazole and oxibendazole.[1] Febantel is not available as a stand-alone antiparasitic but instead is combined with pyrantel (an antinematodal) and praziquantel (an anticestodal).

Pyrantel

Pyrantel anthelmintics (Strongid, Nemex, Exodus) are highly effective antinematodals and considered very safe. They are marketed as **pyrantel pamoate** and a more water-soluble salt, **pyrantel tartrate**. Although pyrantel products are labeled for use against common nematodes in dogs and horses, dosages exist in the veterinary literature for many species treated by veterinarians. Pyrantel mimics the effect an excessive release of acetylcholine would have on nicotinic acetylcholine receptors (nicotinic cholinergic receptors) on parasite muscle cells. The excessive nicotinic effect would cause an initial stimulation and spastic contraction of the parasite's muscles, followed by paralysis and death.

The pleasant taste of liquid pyrantel pamoate facilitates giving the oral suspension to animals by the veterinary professional or the client. Because of its safety and pleasant flavor, a large number of OTC pyrantel products are also available to the general public in a wide variety of retail stores. For this reason, many pet owners will choose to "worm" their pets with these products. Because this drug is effective against ascarids (i.e., roundworms) and hookworms but has no activity against whipworms or tapeworms, clients may not understand why their pet has tapeworms or whipworms when they have "dewormed" the dog at home with pyrantel purchased OTC.

Pyrantel products are used in horses on a continuous basis as top dressing on feed or solutions or pastes given by mouth. Other products are available for mixing with feed for other species, like swine.

The liquid suspensions of pyrantel pamoate quickly settle to the bottom of the bottle, requiring these suspensions be thoroughly shaken and mixed before administration to ensure accurate measurement of the medication. Failure to thoroughly mix the suspension before each dose can result in underdosing when using the diluted concentrations at the top of the bottle or overdosing when using the more concentrated drug found at the bottom of the bottle.

Pyrantel pamoate has been incorporated into a number of veterinary products to extend their spectra of activity. Heartgard Plus combines the heartworm preventive ivermectin with pyrantel; Drontal combines the anticestodal praziquantel with pyrantel; and Drontal Plus combines the antinematodal activity of pyrantel and the benzimidazole febantel with the anticestodal activity of praziquantel.

A related compound found in some livestock medications is morantel. Although less used than pyrantel, it is very similar to pyrantel in its spectrum, mechanism of action, and characteristics.

OTHER ANTINEMATODALS

Emodepside

Emodepside (Profender) is a relatively new topically applied antiparasitic developed specifically for cats. It is not marketed as a stand-alone product but packaged instead with praziquantel for its anticestodal properties. Emodepside is the first of this family of antiparasitics to be released, and it works by a mechanism that is different from most of the other antiparasitics. Instead of stimulating or inhibiting a neurotransmitter's postsynaptic (i.e., on the other side of the synapse) receptor located on the parasite's muscle or neuron, it instead stimulates a receptor found on the presynaptic neuron itself that releases an inhibitory neurotransmitter neuropeptide. This released neuropeptide prevents muscles from contracting, resulting in flaccid paralysis of motion muscles, inability to take in food, and death. Although this mechanism sounds similar to those mechanisms involving GABA or glutamate receptors and chloride influx, neither GABA nor glutamate neurotransmitters are the neuropeptide that produces the inhibition.

Emodepside is applied at the base of the skull of cats with a special applicator. Unlike some topical external parasite drugs, emodepside is designed to be absorbed systemically. To avoid contact with children after application, children should not pet or touch the cat in the area of the application site for 24 h. According to the manufacturer's package insert, pregnant women or women who may become pregnant should avoid contact with the drug and should wear disposable gloves when applying. This concern arises from studies done in rats and rabbits that suggest emodepside may interfere with fetal development in those species.

Piperazines

Piperazine is a vermicide found in most of the "once a month" deworming medications sold in grocery stores and pet shops. Piperazine is very safe but has a very narrow spectrum of activity and is only effective against ascarids. Like pyrantel, when pet owners use piperazine products to deworm their pet, they may believe there is no reason to submit their pet's fecal sample to check for parasite eggs. The veterinary technician should inform the client that piperazines do not kill hookworms, tapeworms, whipworms, or protozoa (Coccidia) that commonly infect dogs and cats. Unlike pyrantel, which kills both ascarids and hookworms, piperazine does not kill hookworms, and severe hookworm infestations can kill a young puppy because of blood loss. Thus, the false sense of security puppy owners might get from using a piperazine product is even more dangerous than when they use an OTC pyrantel product.

Piperazine works by stimulating GABA receptors, resulting in opening of chloride channels on the parasite muscle and an influx of chloride, making the inside of the muscle cell more negative (hyperpolarized) and resulting in paralysis because the muscle cannot depolarize and contract when stimulated to do so. For this reason, the drug is considered a vermifuge because it does not directly kill the worms but paralyzes the ascarid adult worm, preventing movement against the normal peristaltic waves of the intestinal tract. The end result of the ascarid paralysis may appear as a wriggling mass of live roundworms passed with the stool. If the worm is only partially paralyzed and is not passed out with the normal movement of feces, the ascarid may survive the dose of piperazine and go on to reinfect the animal.

Piperazine is very safe for the host animal, including puppies, and some sources state that it is for all intents nontoxic under normal circumstances.[3] But piperazine does not kill the migrating larvae of roundworms; thus within a few days to weeks the larvae will return to the GI tract where they will mature into new adults. Hence OTC versions of piperazine require regular retreatment with the drug on a monthly basis to eliminate the newly emerged adult worms. Therefore, although it is very safe, piperazine is not a very effective antiparasitic for eliminating common GI tract parasites.

Levamisole

Levamisole is an antinematodal that has been around for 50 years but, like most older anthelmintics, has fallen out of favor because of its fairly narrow safety margin, its limited effectiveness against migrating larval stages of nematodes, and the development of resistance by many parasites, especially those affecting horses.[3] It is still used for some livestock (e.g., there are swine formulations) and surprisingly this drug has been used in the past as a microfilaricide for heartworm disease. More recently levamisole has been in the literature not as an animal anthelmintic drug but as an adulterant to "cut" cocaine (to cut cocaine with an adulterant means to dilute the cocaine with an additional substance to increase sales profit). It has been speculated that levamisole continues to be preferred because of its increased neurotransmitter effect associated with cocaine. However, levamisole in humans can cause necrotizing lesions in the vasculature and diffuse inflammatory lesions throughout the brain, which is part of the reason why this drug was discontinued for use in human medicine decades ago.

ANTICESTODALS

Anticestodals and cestocides are drugs that are designed to destroy tapeworms. Because the head or scolex of the tapeworm can regenerate a tapeworm if only the segments or proglottids are removed, modern cestocides destroy all of the tapeworm, including the head.[5] Though removal of all tapeworms is the goal in small animal therapy, tapeworms do not have a significant effect on the feed-to-weight conversion in livestock and so are typically not treated with a specific anticestodal. Instead, some of the less expensive antinematodal compounds like the benzimidazoles may have a secondary anticestodal activity. In horses, some tapeworms can cause damage around the ileocecal valve in the GI tract, resulting in intussusception and colic.[5] The removal of tapeworms in dogs and cats is not only preferred by the owner but also is necessary because of the potential for zoonotic disease (i.e., disease transmitted from animal to human). For example, the larvae of the dog tapeworm Echinococcus granulosus can form large cysts within the human liver.

The two major drugs, **praziquantel** and **epsiprantel**, both work by similar mechanisms. Both drugs cause increased permeability the cell membrane to calcium with subsequent loss of intracellular calcium, resulting in paralysis of the parasite. In addition to the paralysis, the protective covering of the tapeworm becomes damaged, resulting in leakage of essential nutrients and unveiling antigens against which the host's body can produce antibodies to help kill the parasite.[1]

Praziquantel

Praziquantel is a veterinary and human anticestodal drug that was the first of its kind to be classified as a modern anticestodal drug. In veterinary medicine, it is marketed in injectable, tablet, and liquid oral forms for use in dogs and cats (Droncit) and combined with other antiparasitics in several antinematodal veterinary products (e.g., Drontal is praziquantel plus pyrantel pamoate). The advantages of praziquantel are its efficacy with a single dose and its activity against a wide range of cestodes, including *E. granulosus*, mentioned earlier.

Because praziquantel results in the entire worm, including the head, disintegrating, owners usually do not see tapeworm proglottids passing in the feces like they might after killing roundworms. Although a single dose of praziquantel is effective against most of the common tapeworms of dogs and cats, elimination of the tapeworm *Dipylidium caninum* requires elimination of fleas from the host and the immediate environment because fleas are involved in that tapeworm's life cycle. Failure to prevent flea infestation is likely to result in reinfection with this tapeworm.

Although praziquantel is effective against the adult tapeworms, it is not ovicidal (i.e., capable of destroying the tapeworm eggs). Therefore, after administration of the drug and the death of the parasite, microscopic tapeworm eggs may continue pass in the feces for a period of time. Because accidental ingestion of tapeworm eggs by human beings poses a potential public health hazard, the veterinary professional should instruct the pet owner to follow proper hygiene procedures (i.e., washing hands) after cleaning a cat litter box or disposing of feces that might be contaminated with tapeworm eggs.

Diarrhea and vomiting are occasional side effects of praziquantel use in dogs and cats. The injectable form of praziquantel has a slightly greater incidence of vomiting than the oral. Pain at the injection site, ataxia, drowsiness, and weakness have been reported in cats and dogs after receiving the injectable form.

Epsiprantel

Epsiprantel (Cestex) was introduced into the veterinary market several years after praziquantel. It is an oral anticestodal effective against *Taenia* and *Dipylidium* tapeworms but, unlike praziquantel, it is not available in an injectable form. The manufacturer does not list epsiprantel as being effective against *Echinococcus* species, which can produce cystic liver disease in humans after the tapeworm eggs are accidentally ingested. Even so, epsiprantel has high efficacy against the *Echinococcus* tapeworm, although there is some evidence that most doses have the potential to leave behind residual worms.[1,5]

Unlike praziquantel, epsiprantel is not absorbed from the GI tract to any significant degree, which minimizes the risk of systemic side effects while still retaining its effective anticestodal activity. Like praziquantel, epsiprantel causes digestion of the entire tapeworm within the bowel, so there is little evidence of the tapeworm in the stool.

ANTIPARASITICS USED IN HEARTWORM TREATMENT

Heartworms are helminths that produce clinical disease in both the dog and the cat. Because this disease is commonly encountered in veterinary medicine and because its treatment is more complex than that for other internal parasites, it is discussed separately from the other internal parasitic worms.

Heartworm infection has been diagnosed all across the world and in all 50 of the United States, including parts of central Alaska.[2] It is transmitted by mosquito from dogs and wild canids that create endemic areas or pockets of infection in each state. Heartworm disease is different from heartworm infection. Heartworm infection refers to the presence of the *Dirofilaria immitis* adult worms in the heart and pulmonary arteries, but heartworm disease does not occur until the infection is significant enough to produce clinical signs. Most of the significant clinical signs are attributed to damage and obstruction of the pulmonary arteries caused by the physical presence of juvenile and adult heartworms. The presence of these worms causes inflammation of the pulmonary intima (i.e., the inner lining of the vessels), resulting in proliferation or thickening of the intima, which narrows the pulmonary blood vessels, further restricting blood flow.

As the worm burden (i.e., the number of heartworms) increases, the adult heartworms will begin to fill the right ventricle, then the right atrium, and finally even the large vena cavae that return blood to the right side of the heart. The worms present in the ventricles and atria can interfere with the closing function of the right atrioventricular valve (AV; the tricuspid valve), resulting in the blood from the ventricle ejecting back up into the atria when the ventricle contracts. This backward flow can increase the pressure inside the right atrium and vena cavae, eventually raising pressure in the capillary beds of the liver and kidney and interfering with normal organ function.[2] Because of these effects, heartworm disease can result in an inability of the heart to adequately pump blood to the lungs, resulting in failure of the right side of the heart (i.e., right-sided congestive heart failure) and, in severe cases, death.

In addition to the damage caused by the presence of the heartworm itself is the damage caused by a Gram-negative intracellular bacteria called *Wolbachia pipientis* that infects heartworms and microfilariae young and contributes to the clinical disease associated with heartworm infections. The relationship between *Wolbachia* and *Dirofilaria* is called *symbiotic* because it appears that each organism benefits from the presence of the other. Similarly, removal of one organism seems to decrease the viability of the other. The damage to the body caused by *Wolbachia* comes from certain proteins found on the *Wolbachia* species bacteria—*Wolbachia* surface protein

(WSP)—that stimulate an inflammatory response, adding to the inflammation and clinical signs caused by the heartworm. Apparently the increased inflammation that occurs at the point the adults or microfilariae are killed is likely due in some significant part to WSP. Therefore, part of the treatment regimen for heartworm disease includes antibiotics to eliminate this bacteria and reduce its effect at the time of killing the heartworm adults.

Although *D. immitis* creates pathology by its irritating physical presence in the pulmonary vasculature, the more severe pathology occurs when the worms die of an adulticide drug or from completion of their life cycle. Dead and dying worms produce severe clinical signs by two mechanisms[1]: the release of inflammation and immune stimulating proteins and[2] the blocking of pulmonary arteries by chunks of dead, decaying worms passing from the heart or larger pulmonary arteries to the smaller arteries where the emboli (i.e., any detached mass or object traveling within the blood vessels) lodge and obstruct blood flow.[6] The increased velocity and turbulence of blood through the heart and vasculature when an animal exercises can "shake loose" larger pieces of worm to form bigger emboli that obstruct more major pulmonary arteries, producing a far greater inflammatory response. Thus, after dogs are treated with an adulticide, exercise restriction is mandatory. In addition to the emboli, the dead worm stimulation of the immune response can result in lung pathology even in areas of the lung not directly affected by the physical presence of worms.[6] Overall, the time of adult heartworm decomposition after treatment is the time of greatest risk of death of the animal from heartworm disease treatment.

The cat is not a natural host for *D. immitis*, and therefore *D. immitis* infective larvae injected into the cat by the mosquito typically do not survive. However, if a sufficient number of infective larvae are injected, some will develop into adult heartworms. The worm burden in cats is typically only around two to five adult worms, and the worms have a shorter lifespan of only 2–3 years. But even a small number of adult heartworms in the cat can produce significant clinical disease because of the much smaller pulmonary vasculature in the cat compared with the dog.

Some cats with adult heartworms living in their pulmonary vasculature may not show clinical signs, which suggests that the live adult heartworm is not the primary source for clinical signs in the cat. Clinical signs tend to appear when the infective larvae first become very young adults and arrive in the pulmonary vasculature, where they produce an inflammatory process in the pulmonary arteries and the lung tissue itself. Many of the arriving immature adult worms die, and their death contributes significantly to the inflammatory process. The inflammatory process in the lungs affects not only the vasculature but also the airways, producing coughing and an asthma-like syndrome called HARD, or heartworm-associated respiratory disease. This acute phase of heartworm disease in the cat is often mistaken for feline asthma.[2]

As the remaining heartworms mature, the inflammatory reaction actually subsides and the clinical signs of HARD begin to lessen or disappear.[2] The adult heartworm may suppress the immune inflammatory response, allowing the cat to tolerate the presence of the few adult heartworms in the pulmonary vasculature. However, once the adult heartworms die at the end of their shortened life cycle, they cause a return of the inflammatory reaction, and the emboli produced by the decaying dead worms can potentially produce severe clinical signs and even death. Thromboemboli (i.e., emboli made of thrombocytes or platelet clots) will spontaneously form and contribute to the occlusion of the pulmonary arteries.

Cats usually are not treated for adult heartworms because the resulting emboli from degenerating dead worms would cause obstruction in the major pulmonary arteries because of their relatively small size and because cat pulmonary arteries have far fewer branches than the dog, with less collateral circulation to compensate for the emboli obstruction. Instead, treatment in the cat focuses on reducing the initial inflammatory reaction from the immature worms, then allowing any adult heartworms to die one at a time on their own and controlling the subsequent inflammatory response and embolic effect from the dead worm.

The pathology of heartworm disease and the protocols needed to treat it are complex and our understanding continues to evolve as we learn more. Likewise, we are still learning how best to treat the complicating factors such as the effects of *Wolbachia* in the dog and the multitude of triggers for immune and inflammatory responses in both the dog and cat. Therefore, the veterinary professional should be familiar with the most recent discoveries and therapeutic advances reported in the current literature and by the American Heartworm Society.

Different Stages, Different Drugs

To effectively eliminate heartworm from the mammalian host, multiple drugs affecting different stages of the life cycle of *Dirofilaria* must be used. An adulticide is a drug used to kill mature (adult) heartworms that live in the pulmonary vasculature and the right chambers of the heart. Female adult heartworms produce microscopic young (larvae) called *microfilariae*, which circulate in the bloodstream of infected dogs and are taken up by mosquitoes when they feed on an infected dog's blood. Microfilaricides are drugs used to kill the circulating microfilariae produced by the adult heartworms.

After the microfilariae have been ingested by a mosquito, they undergo changes to become infective third-stage larvae (L3). These infective larvae migrate to the head and mouth parts of the mosquito, through which they enter another dog's or cat's body the next time the mosquito feeds. The injected infective L3 larvae migrate through the body for several weeks and eventually reach the pulmonary arteries, where they mature to adult worms. Heartworm preventives are drugs given to kill these infective larvae so they do not mature to adults.

Generally, drugs used to treat one stage are less effective or not effective against other stages. For example, the adulticide drug used at the dose to kill adult heartworms is not effective against microfilariae or the infective L3 larvae. Most preventives are not particularly effective against adults although with chronic high-dose therapy they may have some effect.

In addition to the antiparasitic drugs, antibiotics are used to kill the *Wolbachia* bacteria, and antiinflammatory drugs may be used to reduce the body's reaction to the proteins or antigens that produce disease. Successfully treating heartworm disease requires using multiple drugs that are given in a particular order to effectively eliminate all stages of the heartworm from an infected dog.

Heartworm Adulticides

Melarsomine (Immiticide) is the only approved heartworm adulticide for use in the dog since 1996. It is far less reactive to tissue than its predecessor, and even though it is an organic arsenical (arsenic) type of drug, it does not produce toxicity or liver damage to the degree that the previous arsenic adulticide drug did, probably because of the lower dose of arsenic required to kill adult heartworms with melarsomine than the previous drug.[1]

Melarsomine's mode of action against heartworm is unknown, but it is considered to be 92%–98% effective against adult *D. immitis* in the dog.[7,8] Female heartworms are considered to be more resistant to the effects of the adulticide than male adult heartworms, which means fewer treatments of the adulticide will kill off the males and leave a single-sex population of female heartworms. The spacing of the doses of melarsomine is targeted specifically to insure death of the more robust female worms. Although melarsomine is quite effective against adult *D. immitis*, it does not kill young adult heartworms less than 4 months old.[2,7]

Although melarsomine can kill adult heartworms in the cat, melarsomine is not used in the cat because of the risk of emboli and severe inflammation from disintegrating dead adult heartworms thoroughly obstructing the cat's pulmonary arteries. In addition, dogs with a Class 4 level of heartworm disease or caval syndrome should not be treated with melarsomine. Caval syndrome refers to the vena cavae and means the pulmonary vasculature and heart are so physically full of worms that they extend back into the vena cavae. Killing off that mass of adult heartworms at once would most likely result in death when the decaying worms bombard the lungs. Dogs with Class 4 or caval syndrome require surgical removal of the worms from the vena cavae and the right side of the heart by threading a loop down the right jugular vein and into the heart, where worms are snagged and physically removed one or two at a time.

Melarsomine is packaged as an injectable product that comes in a powder that must be reconstituted just before administration. The manufacturer is very specific that the drug must be administered intramuscularly (IM) but can only be injected into the epaxial muscles, which are muscles located dorsally on either side of the spinal column. Specifically, the drug should be injected into the epaxial muscles between the third and fifth lumbar vertebrae, 1–2 in. lateral to the center of the spinal column as marked by the vertebral dorsal spinous process.

Dogs that weigh less than 10 kg (22 lb) should be injected with a 23-gauge, 1-in. needle; larger dogs should be injected with a 22-gauge, 1.5-in. needle. The longer needles are required to place the drug deep within the belly of the epaxial muscles and the small gauge of the needle (small gauge = narrower needle diameter) helps prevent drug leakage from the injection site. Although far fewer side effects occur with melarsomine than the older adulticide it replaced, swelling and pain at the injection

site are frequently reported. It is important to ensure that the entire drug is injected into the site before withdrawing the needle to avoid additional pain and swelling at the injection site.

The manufacturer-recommended dosage regimen is to give two injections of melarsomine in the epaxial muscles separated by a 24-h interval. However, evidence is emerging that a three-injection protocol may be more effective. The 2018 report of the American Heartworm Society stated that the two-injection protocol killed about 90% of the heartworms. This does not mean that 90% of the dogs treated this way were cleared of heartworms, it means that the worm burden was reduced by 90%, leaving approximately 10% of the heartworms in the patient. An alternative protocol gives one injection of melarsomine followed by a month of "rest" and then the two-injection method 24 h apart. This protocol is said to kill 98% of the worms.[2] The three-injection protocol was already part of the approved method for administering melarsomine to small dogs as a means of reducing the risk for serious emboli in their relatively smaller pulmonary arteries. But regardless of the size or severity of the heartworm disease, the American Heartworm Society now recommends the three-injection protocol for all dogs, and has a detailed protocol on their website for treatment. The treatment guidelines clearly state the recommended protocol for treating heartworm disease based on the stage of the disease.

Levamisole is a drug mentioned with the antinematodal drugs that at one time was used as an inexpensive, but less effective, alternative adulticide to the older arsenical drug. Although levamisole did kill adult heartworms to some extent, the inconsistent number of worms killed and the side effects (primarily CNS related) made it a risky drug to use, and today, with the availability of melarsomine, its use is almost nonexistent. However, because levamisole is inexpensive and still available, veterinary technicians may occasionally hear of an animal (typically an economic hardship case) being treated with this drug to reduce (but not eliminate) adult heartworms and clear microfilariae from the blood.

The **macrolide endectocides** discussed previously (e.g., ivermectin, selamectin, milbemycin) have been shown to reduce the number of adult worms when given over several months. It is presumed that exposure to these drugs over prolonged periods reduces the life span of the adult heartworm and can kill infective larvae up to the immature adult stage. However, the American Heartworm Society does not recommend this approach because older adult heartworms are not very susceptible to the macrolides and may take up to 2 years or longer of continuous administration of the drug before 95% of the adult heartworms are eliminated.[2] During this prolonged administration of drug, the pathology in the lungs, pulmonary vasculature, and heart would continue to progress. The American Heartworm Society does recommend this therapy throughout the recommended treatment to prevent further infection during treatment. The animals should be strictly exercise restricted during this entire treatment time to reduce the degree of inflammatory reaction after the worms die. Additionally, the use of the macrolides by themselves has the potential to put selection pressure on the parasites, allowing strains of heartworm resistant to macrolides to emerge.

Heartworm Microfilaricides

As of the writing of this text, there is only one approved microfilaricide and that is the topically applied **moxidectin** found in the product **Advantage Multi**. Moxidectin was mentioned with the antinematodals and is part of the milbemycin branch of the macrolide family of endectocides. All of the macrolides or macrocyclic lactones (the avermectins and milbemycins) have the potential to reduce or eliminate microfilariae produced by the female adult heartworms. In addition to the microfilariae (which would be the larval stage 1 [L1] of the life cycle), macrolides are effective against the L3 and early L4 larval stages before the heartworm arrives in the pulmonary vasculature. Unfortunately there is a period of time in the L4 stage of heartworm where the macrolides may not be effective, but the parasite is still too young to be eliminated by the adulticide melarsomine. Thus, there exists the potential for some L4 stage larvae to survive and grow into new adult heartworms if the macrolides and melarsomine are given close to the same time.[2] The recommended protocol for the American Heartworm Society mentioned at the end of this section is designed to close that gap in treatment.

Macrolides can cause a rapid decrease in the microfilariae, and the sudden mass death of this larval stage has the potential to produce a very strong inflammatory reaction in some dogs. The approved topical moxidectin microfilaricide did not produce any significant adverse reaction in dogs with high microfilaria count according to laboratory studies and field studies conducted to receive FDA approval.[2] However, such reactions have been reported with other macrolides when they were used as microfilaricides. If extra-label avermectins or milbemycin products are used in dogs with high microfilaria counts, it is advisable to pretreat the animals with antihistamines or corticosteroids to reduce the inflammatory reaction set off by the dead microfilariae.

The diluting of large animal ivermectin injectable products for use as microfilaricides in dogs is not recommended because the lack of accuracy of diluting such concentrated products can result in a dose that may be subtherapeutic and ineffective or so high as to be toxic.

Heartworm Preventives

The heartworm preventives are targeted against the mosquito-injected infective L3 larval stage and the L4 stage up to the young adult heartworm. The older daily heartworm preventive drug **diethylcarbamazine** (DEC) that was administered as chewable tablets has been discontinued. Therefore, all current preventives are products that are more conveniently dosed at monthly or 6-month intervals. Table 12.2 shows the heartworm preventives currently available in the United States.

Many of the **macrolide** preventive drugs come in forms that have other anthelmintics added (e.g., pyrantel) to expand the spectra of their approved uses and provide the consumer with products that conveniently control/kill internal parasites (e.g., GI worms) and external parasites (e.g., fleas). Because these products change constantly, it is important that the veterinary professional keep abreast of each new product, or each new approved use of old products, to understand the mechanisms and potential side effects. The individual macrolide products were also discussed in "Antinematodal" section.

Ivermectin is the most widely used macrolide heartworm preventive. The preventive dose of monthly administered ivermectin (Heartgard) is 0.006 mg/kg and is much lower than the dose used for microfilaricidal activity (0.05 mg/kg) and well below the toxic dose mentioned in "Antinematodal" section. Thus, the likelihood of a Collie breed experiencing an adverse reaction to ivermectin used as a heartworm preventive is minimal. Nevertheless, the manufacturer recommends observing the animal for 8 h after administration of the preventive dose

TABLE 12.2 Current (2016) Products for Heartworm Prevention in the United States*

Preventive	Trade Name	Other Ingredients	Route and Frequency	Dogs	Cats
Ivermectin	Heartgard		PO monthly	✓	✓
	Heartgard Plus	Pyrantel	PO monthly	✓	
	Iverhart Plus	Pyrantel	PO monthly	✓	
	Tri-Heart Plus	Pyrantel	PO monthly	✓	
	Iverhart Max	Pyrantel praziquantel	PO monthly	✓	
Milbemycin Oxime	Interceptor		PO monthly	✓	✓
	(Trade Name) Interceptor Plus			✓	
	(Other ingredients) Praziquantel			✓	
	(Route and Frequency) PO monthly			✓	
	Sentinel	Lufenuron	PO monthly	✓	
	Sentinel Spectrum	Lufenuron praziquantel	PO monthly	✓	
	Trifexis	Spinosad	PO monthly	✓	
Selamectin	Revolution		Topically monthly	✓	✓
Moxidectin	Advantage Multi	Imidacloprid	Topically monthly	✓	✓
	ProHeart 6		Injectable 6 months	✓	

PO, By mouth.

*Trade names, species approval, and available dosage forms may be different in Canada, the United Kingdom, or Australia.

of ivermectin. The formulation of ivermectin approved as a preventive for use in cats (Heartgard for Cats) comes in chewable cubes. Both the canine and feline forms are packaged according to weight classes, making it convenient for the owner to dispense the appropriate amount.

Selamectin (Revolution) is a heartworm preventive that uses the topical application as its route of administration. Unlike ivermectin, moxidectin, and milbemycin, selamectin has not been combined with other products to produce a multiuse, broad-spectrum antiparasitic. However, its approved spectrum of use includes hookworms, roundworms, adult fleas, ear mites, ticks, and sarcoptic mange mites. As is true for all macrolides, it is not effective against tapeworms. As mentioned in "Antinematodal" section, the product is absorbed systemically over a period of days after topical application, although it is far better absorbed in the cat than the dog. Once the topical application has dried, it is not adversely affected by bathing or swimming. This product is approved for heartworm prevention in both dogs and cats. MDR1 mutation Collies (and many other breeds) with defective P-gps do now show adverse effects from selamectin administration and even at 10 times the recommended dose, the predominant adverse sign was only hypersalivation.[1]

Milbemycin oxime is the monthly, orally administered heartworm preventive found in Interceptor, Sentinel, and Trifexis. It shares all the characteristics with the avermectins because the milbemycins are also macrolides. It is nontoxic to dogs with the MDR1 mutation when given in doses up to 20 times the recommended dose.[1] One study suggested that milbemycin oxime may help control raccoon roundworms (*Baylisascaris procyonis*).[1] Dogs can acquire the raccoon roundworm by ingesting eggs spread in raccoon scat (i.e., feces) into the water, soil, or on contaminated surfaces. Infected dogs can then shed eggs into the household environment, increasing the potential exposure of humans to accidental ingestion of these eggs. Milbemycin oxime eliminates *B. procyonis* in the dog, reducing the human contact with the eggs in the feces. Accidental ingestion of *B. procyonis* eggs by humans can result in damage to the eyes, organs, and the CNS by migrating larvae that emerge from the ingested eggs. The migration can produce severe disease including liver damage, blindness, coma, and even death.

Moxidectin is available as orally administered, once-monthly combination products like Advantage Multi, as well as the injectable 6- and 12-month formulation (ProHeart 6 and 12). As a milbemycin type of macrolide, it shares the same spectrum as milbemycin oxime. The injectable form is given SQ to dogs only (not cats) that are 6 months of age and older. Reports of injection site granulomas (i.e., reaction to the injection) correlate with the size of the dose used.[1]

After ProHeart 6 was pulled off the market and later returned to the US market, it became the first veterinary drug to be placed under the additional surveillance program called RiskMAP (*Risk Minimization Action Plan*). The plan restricted the use of the drug to dogs less than 7 years of age and required the veterinarian to give information about the drug risks to the pet owner and to obtain written permission from the pet owners before the drug could be administered. In addition, the drug could only be administered by veterinarians and not by

veterinary technicians. Veterinarians could not even buy the drug unless they had registered with the drug company and completed an intensive training program on how to administer the drug. In 2013, these restrictions were lifted so that dogs older than 7 years could now be given the drug, no client consent form was required to be signed, veterinary technicians could administer the drug after they had successfully completed a 20-min online certification, and it became easier to purchase the drug from the manufacturer.

The current RiskMAP still requires that the drug be given only to healthy dogs older than 6 months and to avoid giving vaccinations at the same time as ProHeart 6 or 12 because of reports of anaphylactic (i.e., allergy mediated) reactions that were, in some cases, severe enough to cause death. Since its return to the US market, reported adverse reactions are infrequent and usually not serious.

Doxycycline for Treating *Wolbachia*

Doxycycline is a lipophilic member of the tetracycline group of antibiotics (see Chapter 10). Because of its lipophilic nature, it is able to penetrate heartworm adults and larvae to reach the symbiotic bacteria *Wolbachia* living within *D. immitis*. When doxycycline kills the *Wolbachia* bacteria in L3 and L4 larval stages, the larvae die.[2] The administration of doxycycline also reduces the numbers of microfilariae produced by the adult female heartworms. The microfilariae that were produced appeared normal but were unable to develop into adult worms after they were taken up by the mosquito and molted into the infective L3 larval stage.[2]

Because the WSP is thought to contribute to pulmonary and kidney inflammation, killing the *Wolbachia* with doxycycline before administering the melarsomine adulticide resulted in less pulmonary injury or pathology from the dead adult heartworms.[2] Thus, doxycycline is now part of the American Heartworm Society treatment protocol for canine heartworm disease.

It has been suggested that if a dog with adult heartworms cannot take the arsenical adulticide melarsomine, a combination of monthly heartworm preventive plus 4 weeks of doxycycline (10 mg/kg BID) can reduce, and with repeated treatments, perhaps clear adult heartworms over several months. The disadvantage of this approach using doxycycline is that exercise would need to be restricted for the entire time the animal was taking this drug combination.[2]

Additional Drugs Used in Heartworm Treatment

Glucocorticoids are antiinflammatory drugs that help control the signs associated with inflammation of the pulmonary vasculature and the lungs secondary to the emboli and immune-stimulating proteins. The American Heart Association recommends treating with a glucocorticoid like **prednisone** for initial stabilization if the dog is clinically ill from its heartworm disease. The recommendation is to also administer prednisone at the time of melarsomine treatment to reduce inflammation and help reduce the pain associated with the injection. Antihistamines are also sometimes administered to further reduce the histamine-mediated part of the inflammatory reactions.

American Heartworm Society 2018 Protocol Recommendation

The protocol for heartworm treatment today is very different from the standard protocols traditionally used. This protocol uses the three-injection method for adulticide treatment described previously.

- Step 1 (Day 1)
  - Confirm diagnosis and determine whether microfilaria are present
  - Begin exercise restriction. The more clinical signs, the more strict the restrictions need to be.
  - Stabilize the dog if it has life-threatening clinical signs secondary to heartworm infection.
  - Administer a dose of a monthly heartworm preventive. If microfilaria are detected, pretreat with antihistamine and glucocorticosteroids to reduce risk of anaphylaxis. Monitor patient for at least 8 h to monitor for anaphylaxis.
  - Apply an EPA-registered canine topical product labeled to repel and kill mosquitos
  - Dispense glucocorticosteroids per the guidelines if dog is symptomatic
- Step 2 (Days 1–28)
  - Administer doxycycline (10 mg/kg BID) for 28 days.
- Step 3 (Day 30)
  - Apply an EPA-registered canine topical product labeled to repel and kill mosquitos
  - Administer a dose of a monthly heartworm preventive.
- Step 4 (Days 31–60)
  - A 1-month wait period to allow time for the *Wolbachia* surface proteins and metabolites to dissipate before killing the adult worms.
- Step 5 (Day 60)
  - Administer a dose of a monthly heartworm preventive.
  - Give injection #1 of melarsomine (i.e., adulticide).
  - Begin prednisone on a decreasing dose for 4 weeks.
  - Restrict exercise strictly
- Step 6 (Days 90–91)
  - Administer a dose of a monthly heartworm preventive.
  - Give injection #2 of melarsomine (i.e., adulticide); give injection #3 24 h later.
  - Begin prednisone on a tapering dose for 4 weeks.
  - Continue exercise restriction for 6–8 weeks after last melarsomine injection.
- Step 7 (Day 120)
  - Test for the presence of microfilaria (reference guidelines if positive)
  - Continue a year-round heartworm prevention program
- Step 8 (Day 365)
  - Antigen test 9 months after last melarsomine injection; screen for microfilaria

As more is understood about heartworm disease in both the dog and the cat, new products and protocols will be introduced. The information provided in this section will provide a foundation for understanding not only how current drugs and protocols work but also how new heartworm products or new protocols might be similar or different from established medications and procedures.

ANTIPROTOZOALS

Protozoa are single cellular organisms that most frequently cause GI disease but can also produce disease in almost every other organ system. Antiprotozoal drugs in veterinary medicine are most commonly used against *Coccidia*, *Giardia*, *Toxoplasma* (causes toxoplasmosis), and *Sarcocystis neurona*, the agent of equine protozoal myeloencephalitis (EPM). There are many other protozoa (e.g., *Balantidium*, *Entamoeba*) that are less commonly encountered in veterinary patients, and there are other compounds used to treat those. This is especially true for poultry and avian livestock in which *Coccidia* plays an important economic role in production. But the focus on this section will be on the most commonly used antiprotozoals against the four protozoan groups listed earlier.

Sulfonamides

The sulfonamides are antibiotics discussed in Chapter 10. They were the first drugs used to treat *Coccidia* species that infect the GI tract of both large and small animals and are still one of the main drugs used to control these protozoa. Animals acquire *Coccidia* both by ingestion of food or water contaminated with oocysts (i.e., egg cells) or eating a rodent that is infected with *Coccidia*. Thus, environmental decontamination is often necessary to reduce reinfection with *Coccidia*.

There is one solo sulfonamide product, **sulfadimethoxine** (Albon); two veterinary potentiated sulfonamides, **sulfadimethoxine/ormetoprim** (Primor) and **sulfadiazine/trimethoprim** (Tribrissen); and one human potentiated sulfonamide, **sulfamethoxazole/trimethoprim** (Septra, Bactrim) that have been used to treat *Coccidia*.[9] The sulfonamide and the potentiator compound (trimethoprim or ormetoprim) both work on the same metabolic pathway needed by *Coccidia* to produce folic acid. By working at two different parts of the pathway, the combination products are more coccidiocidal than the sulfonamide might be working alone.

Sulfadimethoxine is the only sulfa approved by the FDA for treating *Coccidia* in dogs and cats, but all of the sulfas are effective against these protozoa. Trimethoprim sulfadiazine was the first potentiated sulfonamide used in veterinary medicine and is the one of the most widely used because of its long history. Trimethoprim sulfamethoxazole is a human potentiated sulfonamide, and therefore any use in veterinary patients would be extra-label. However, because it has a very similar spectrum to the veterinary trimethoprim sulfadiazine and because there are inexpensive generics available, this human drug is being used in veterinary medicine for the treatment of *Coccidia* and other microbes in small animals.

Although these more modern sulfonamides are more soluble in water than the older sulfas and hence less likely to precipitate out of the urine and form crystals in the urine (i.e., crystalluria), it is still recommended that any patient receiving sulfonamides be given free access to water at all times. Veterinary technicians and veterinarians must always be watchful for signs of keratoconjunctivitis sicca (KCS) or dry eye whenever sulfa drugs are used.

A compound related to trimethoprim and ormetoprim called **pyrimethamine** is combined with sulfadiazine to treat the protozoon *Toxoplasma gondii,* the cause of the potentially zoonotic disease toxoplasmosis in dogs and cats, and *S. neurona,* the protozoon that causes EPM.

Amprolium

Amprolium (Corid) is a feed or drinking water additive that is commonly used as an antiprotozoal in calves and avian species to treat *Coccidia.* It is structurally similar to thiamin but does not possess thiamin's intrinsic vitamin activity. Thus, in the presence of amprolium, competitive antagonism between amprolium and thiamin occurs and thiamin absorption into the *Coccidia* is inhibited. The parasite dies from thiamin deficiency. Use of amprolium in large doses for extended periods can also result in thiamin deficiency in the host animal.

Benzimidazoles

The benzimidazoles were discussed with the antinematodal drugs, and, as mentioned previously, some also have antiprotozoal properties. Specifically, the three benzimidazoles **albendazole**, **fenbendazole**, and **febantel** (the prodrug that is converted to fenbendazole) are used primarily against *Giardia. Giardia* is a mobile protozoon that lives in the lumen of the GI tract and moves by use of a long flagellum. It is a problem in dogs, cats, and cattle but also poses a human health hazard via contaminated drinking water supply. *Giardia* is often difficult to diagnose because common fecal examination techniques (e.g., fecal flotation) will not identify the flagellated protozoa. Thus, animals can be undiagnosed shedders of *Giardia* and potential sources for human zoonotic disease.

Albendazole (Valbazen) is a broad-spectrum benzimidazole anthelmintic approved for use on intestinal worms of cattle and sheep but has also been used in an extra-label manner to treat *Coccidia* in these species and dogs and cats. However, albendazole has been shown to be teratogenic (i.e., causing birth defects), so it is not to be administered to pregnant livestock in the first stages of pregnancy. Bone marrow toxicity, lethargy, and loss of appetite have been reported in the dog and the cat from albendazole use, and therefore its use in these species is discouraged but not contraindicated.

Fenbendazole (Panacur, Safe-Guard) is an FDA-approved oral product used to remove intestinal parasites in dogs and some "carnivorous/omnivorous" exotic or zoo animals. A slightly different formulation is also available for similar anthelmintic activity in cattle and horses. Fenbendazole products are not approved for use in treating protozoa, but extra-label use of fenbendazole has shown excellent activity as a multi-day, orally administered antiprotozoal for treatment of *Giardia* in dogs. It appears to be well tolerated by dogs and cats, with only some mild side effects (e.g., vomiting, diarrhea) reported. Although fenbendazole's efficacy against *Giardia* is very good in dogs, it is far less effective in cats, with only 50% of cats treated with fenbendazole being cleared of *Giardia* after 3 weeks of treatment.[9] Fenbendazole is considered to be an effective antiprotozoal for treating *Giardia* in cattle.

Febantel is only available in a combination product with praziquantel and pyrantel (Drontal Plus) that is approved for removal and control of intestinal worms in dogs but not cats. Because the febantel is converted to fenbendazole and oxfendazole, it would be expected to have good activity against *Giardia.* Even though it is an extra-label use, the combination febantel product has been effective against *Giardia* in cats. This product would be too expensive to justify its use to control *Giardia* in livestock species.

Metronidazole

Metronidazole was mentioned with the antimicrobials (Chapter 10) as an oral drug that is bactericidal against anaerobic bacteria in the gut and was sometimes used to treat chronic diarrhea of unknown origin. Because metronidazole is also effective against *Giardia,* as well as other less common protozoa, it is one of the drugs of choice for treatment of giardiasis (i.e., infection with *Giardia*) in dogs and cats. It is protozoacidal by disrupting the helical structure of protozoan deoxyribonucleic acid (DNA) and interfering with other key molecules needed by the protozoa.

Metronidazole eliminates *Giardia* cyst shedding in cats and dogs with 5–8 days of continuous treatment (the length of treatment varies with the dosage used).[10] Although metronidazole is effective at removing *Giardia* in cattle, the family of compounds to which metronidazole belongs has been suspected of producing mutations and being potentially carcinogenic, which means they are strictly prohibited from being used in any animal that could be used for human food consumption.[10]

Oral metronidazole is notoriously bad tasting and readily dissolves in the saliva, making the drug easy to taste and therefore difficult to administer to animals, especially cats.[10] In an attempt to reduce the ability of the metronidazole to dissolve and create an unpleasant taste, it is combined with benzoic acid to create **metronidazole benzoate**. Although cats are susceptible to benzoic acid toxicity, at the dosages used to treat *Giardia* in cats, toxicity is unlikely to occur from the benzoate.

As mentioned with the antimicrobials, metronidazole can produce neurotoxicity manifested as staggering, nystagmus, circling, and seizure-like activity. It is suspected that these neurologic signs are caused by inhibition of the inhibitory neurotransmitter GABA (see benzodiazepines), resulting in overstimulation of the CNS. The signs are temporary and reverse over several days without any long-term after-effects.

Clindamycin

Clindamycin (Antirobe) is an antibiotic belonging to the lincosamide antibiotic group that is usually used for treating anaerobic bacterial infections in small animals. Clindamycin is one of the drugs of choice for treating disseminated toxoplasmosis in dogs and cats.[9] The dose used to treat *Toxoplasma* is higher than the dose cited on the label for use in treating anaerobic bacteria and must be given daily for 4 weeks, but the higher dose and longer duration are apparently tolerated. At the higher doses, clindamycin also becomes coccidiocidal after a few days of treatment. Clindamycin may be combined with potentiated sulfonamides or pyrimethamine to treat other protozoa.

Ionophores

Ionophores were briefly mentioned in Chapter 4 on GI drugs. They are called ionophores because they can combine with selected ions and transport them across biological membranes. Ionophores found their first uses in poultry to treat *Coccidia*, a use that continues today. Because of their unique mechanism of action, resistance has been much slower to develop in ionophores than other antibiotics. Two of the ionophores used as feed additives in veterinary medicine to control *Coccidia* in poultry, cattle, and other small ruminants are **lasalocid** (Bovatec) and **monensin** (Rumensin). It is important that horses not be given access to feed containing monensin because the ionophore will cause degeneration of skeletal and cardiac muscle that could lead to death. In fall of 2014, the accidental addition of monensin and lasalocid to horse feed at an equestrian center in Florida resulted in 22 animals being poisoned; over the course of several weeks, all died because of permanent damage to the heart caused by the ionophores.[11]

Ponazuril

Ponazuril (Marquis) is approved for use to eliminate the protozoa *S. neurona* that causes EPM in horses. *Sarcocystis* is picked up by the horse by drinking water, grass, or feed contaminated by cats, opossum, or other wildlife that can shed the sporocysts of *Sarcocystis*. The protozoa causes damage in the spinal cord or the brain and can produce almost any neurologic sign depending on which area of the spinal cord is affected. Most often signs reflect spinal cord damage and can appear as lameness, staggering, incoordination, ataxia or weakness in one limb or one side, and muscle atrophy of those muscles supplied by damaged nerves. Lesions in the brain cause head tilt, depression, and facial paralysis. Although ponazuril and pyrimethamine can kill the protozoa, the damage caused is often irreversible.

EXTERNAL ANTIPARASITICS

External antiparasitics, or ectoparasiticides, are used to control flies, grubs, and lice on livestock; flies (both bots and maggots) on horses; and fleas, ticks, and mange mites on companion animals. In addition to decreasing skin disease in companion animals or increasing weight gain in livestock by controlling these external parasites, another benefit is the control of diseases such as Lyme disease, bubonic plague, and Rocky Mountain spotted fever that can be transmitted from animals to humans through insects.

As mentioned previously, the EPA is charged with regulating topically applied pesticides or insecticides that are minimally absorbed into the body. However, for any external parasiticide that is administered by mouth or injection into the body, the FDA would have jurisdiction because that compound would be considered a drug. Topically applied products that need to be systemically absorbed to produce their beneficial effect would also be regulated as a drug by the FDA.

Although the word *insecticide* technically applies only to six-legged true insects, it often is extended to cover arachnids (i.e., spiders) and adult ticks and mites (i.e., acarines), which all have eight legs. Insecticides and external antiparasitics are available in many formulations and delivery methods including collars, powders, dips, aerosol sprays, pump sprays, baths, foggers, foams, pour-ons, spot-ons, and even roll-ons. Most of these formulations are designed for the convenience of application for the companion

animal owner, or in some cases they are marketed in a novel delivery system designed to set the product apart from its competitors. Table 12.3 shows a list of the more common or mainstream brands of flea and tick products a veterinary technician is likely to encounter.

In contrast to the individual animal application in companion animals, insecticides and external antiparasitics for livestock are designed for ease of application to large groups or herds of animals; hence the ectoparasiticides may be incorporated into rubbing bars and dust bags that deliver a dusting of the chemical that kills or repels insects. Other formulations for livestock include pour-on products that are absorbed into or through the skin, sprays, dips, impregnated ear tags from which insecticide diffuses into the body, and feed additives. Although products for companion animals are designed to be applied in a carefully controlled manner and dose for each animal, livestock products are formulated based on the "average" amount of insecticide each animal is likely to acquire, but the actual dose varies considerably depending on the length of time or amount of chemical with which the animal comes in contact.

By far, the most common application of external parasiticides in veterinary medicine is for control or elimination of fleas and ticks in the dog and cat. Many of the modern flea products are targeted at specific stages of the flea life cycle, as opposed to the entire life cycle from ova to larva to adult. Therefore, the veterinary technician must understand the flea life cycle and the limitations of flea products so the client can understand the need for the use of other products, repeated treatments, or environmental control measures needed to break the life cycle.

The generic flea's life cycle can be summarized as follows (Fig. 12.1). The female flea feeds on the pet's blood and produces thousands of eggs in a normal lifetime. These eggs fall off the pet and within a few days will hatch larvae in the pet's environment. Flea larvae then create pupae (cocoons) in which they can remain for months. When the environmental conditions are right, the young adult flea will emerge from the cocoon and seek the pet or the pet owner on which to feed and continue the life cycle. Because some flea products only stop one component of the flea life cycle (e.g., just the egg or just the adult), failure to kill the other stages of the life cycle simultaneously will allow adult fleas to continue to plague the pet (in the case of compounds that kill larvae or affect eggs) or will only temporarily eliminate the flea problem until the eggs hatch or the new adults emerge from the pupae. As stated previously, the veterinary technician must thoroughly understand this life cycle and how the individual drugs affect it to provide appropriate advice for the client.

All modern insecticides or ectoparasiticides, regardless of which external parasite they target, are neurotoxins in some manner. Like many of the internal parasiticides and the endectocides, the ectoparasiticides typically do one or more of four different actions[1]: inhibit a neurotransmitter (acetylcholine),[2] enhance a neurotransmitter (GABA),[3] block a neurotransmitter's receptor (cholinergic receptor), or[4] enhance a neurotransmitter's receptor (GABA receptor opens chloride channels, nicotinic cholinergic receptor for acetylcholine). Knowing whether the target receptor or the neurotransmitter of the ectoparasiticide is excitatory or inhibitory and whether the ectoparasiticide enhances or reduces the neurotransmitter effect will

TABLE 12.3   Current (2016) Flea and Tick Products Used in Small Animals (Major US Brands)*

Trade Name	Ingredients	Route and Frequency	APPROVED FOR USE IN	
			Dogs	Cats
Advantage II	Imidacloprid and pyriproxyfen	Topically monthly	✓	✓
K9 Advantix II	Imidacloprid, permethrin, and pyriproxyfen	Topically monthly	✓	Toxic
Advantage Multi	Imidacloprid and moxidectin	Topically monthly	✓	✓
Frontline Spray	Fipronil	Topically monthly	✓	✓
Frontline Top Spot	Fipronil	Topically monthly	✓	
Frontline Plus	Fipronil and methoprene	Topically monthly	✓	✓
Frontline Tritak	Fipronil, cyphenothrin, and methoprene	Topically monthly	✓	✓
Certifect	Fipronil, methoprene, and amitraz	Topically monthly	✓	Toxic
Parastar for Dogs	Fipronil	Topically monthly	✓	
Parastar Plus	Fipronil and cyphenothrin	Topically monthly	✓	
Effitix for Dogs	Fipronil and permethrin	Topically monthly	✓	Toxic
Effipro for Cats	Fipronil	Topically monthly		✓
Revolution	Selamectin	Topically monthly	✓	✓
Activyl	Indoxacarb	Topically monthly	✓	✓
Activyl Plus	Indoxacarb and permethrin	Topically monthly	✓	Toxic
Cheristin for Cats	Spinetoram	Topically monthly		✓
Comfortis	Spinosad	PO monthly	✓	✓
Trifexis	Spinosad and milbemycin oxime	PO monthly	✓	
Sentinel	Lufenuron and milbemycin oxime	PO monthly	✓	
Sentinel Spectrum	Lufenuron, milbemycin oxime, and praziquantel	PO monthly	✓	
Simparica	Sarolaner	PO monthly	✓	
NexGard	Afoxolaner	PO monthly	✓	
Capstar	Nitenpyram	PO as needed	✓	✓
Bravecto	Fluralaner	PO every 12 weeks	✓	
Seresto	Flumethrin and imidacloprid	8-month collar	✓	✓
Preventic Tick Collar	Amitraz	3-month collar	✓	Toxic

PO, By mouth.

*Trade names, species approval, and available dosage forms may be different in Canada, the United Kingdom, or Australia.

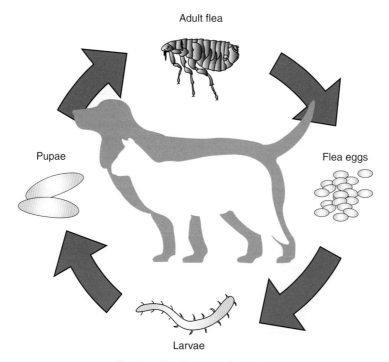

Adult flea

Pupae

Flea eggs

Larvae

Fig. 12.1 The life cycle of the flea.

allow the veterinary technician to understand how the product works and the possible toxicity signs that could be seen in the animal.

Organophosphates and Carbamates

Organophosphates (OPs) and carbamates are considered to be old insecticides once widely used in veterinary medicine but now only occasionally found and more commonly experienced in veterinary medicine as toxicities from exposure to agricultural or garden pesticides. These compounds are still found in a few animal ectoparasiticide products in North America as the OP compounds tetrachlorvinphos (in flea collars); chlorpyrifos, diazinon, coumaphos, and pirimiphos (all found in cattle ear tags); and as the carbamate compound propoxur (e.g., Zodiac tick collars). In the United States, the companies producing propoxur-impregnated flea and tick collars reached an agreement with the EPA in 2014 to stop producing such collars and to terminate sales of existing stock by April 1, 2016. Other OP and carbamate products for animals are found and purchased outside the United States and Canada, where insecticidal use may be less stringently regulated. Thus, it is conceivable that the veterinary technician may encounter OP or carbamate ectoparasiticides.

A more thorough briefing on these compounds can be found in veterinary toxicology resources. OPs and carbamates, which are two chemically different types of insecticides, are usually grouped together because of their similar mechanisms of action, effects on insects, and toxic effects. These products still have several agricultural applications, including use on crops, on garden plants to control aphids and other pests, in the soil to control lawn grubs, and on nursery trees, and can be found in stores where garden supplies are sold.

A tip-off that a product contains OPs or carbamates can be found in a container's warning label to physicians stating that the product "contains a cholinesterase inhibitor" and should be treated as such in cases of accidental contact or ingestion. The term *cholinesterase inhibitor* comes from the way OPs and carbamates bind to acetylcholinesterase, the enzyme that normally breaks down the neurotransmitter acetylcholine to terminate its action at the receptor site. With the acetylcholinesterase inhibited by OPs or carbamates, acetylcholine neurotransmitter released by the axon continues to stimulate muscarinic and nicotinic types of acetylcholine receptor sites. Overstimulation of the muscarinic cholinergic receptors for acetylcholine located in the heart, bronchioles, GI tract, and other organs produce clinical signs associated with parasympathetic nervous system stimulation, which include SLUDDE signs: Salivation, Lacrimation (i.e., tearing), Urination, Defecation, Dyspnea (i.e., difficult breathing because of bronchoconstriction and increased respiratory secretions), and Emesis. Bradycardia and miosis (i.e., pinpoint pupils) are also characteristic signs of overstimulation of the parasympathetic nervous system and are associated with muscarinic receptor overstimulation from the action of OPs or carbamates. Overstimulation of the *nicotinic cholinergic receptors* produces clinical signs related to the neuromuscular junction, or NMJ, where nerve axons contact skeletal muscles. Overstimulation of the nicotinic receptor initially produces muscle tremors that progress in severity until the nicotinic receptor stops responding to the overstimulation, resulting in a block of axonal depolarization waves to the voluntary or skeletal muscles. Thus, toxicity signs associated with nicotinic receptor stimulation appear initially as tremors, progressing to shaking, and then to ataxia and paralysis. Because the diaphragm is a skeletal muscle, the diaphragm and the intercostal muscles that help lift the rib cage during inspiration can also be paralyzed, contributing to respiratory failure. Death in toxicity cases is usually because of hypoxia from being unable to adequately ventilate (i.e., exchange oxygen for carbon dioxide). Pupils in these animals may be dilated (especially in cats).

Treatment of acute OP toxicity consists of removing any insecticide remaining on or in the animal and blocking the parasympathetic effects. **Atropine** at 10 times its typical preanesthetic dose is still the drug of choice for reversing SLUDDE clinical signs because it is a muscarinic cholinergic receptor antagonist (blocker) that decreases the effect of the excessive acetylcholine at the muscarinic receptor site. Atropine does not block nicotinic cholinergic receptor sites except at very high doses, so nicotinic signs of toxicosis may not significantly improve from atropine administration. **Pralidoxime**, also called **2-PAM**, reverses OP toxicosis by separating the OP from the acetylcholinesterase molecule, thereby freeing the enzyme molecule to work again. Pralidoxime only works as long as the bond between the OP and the acetylcholinesterase remains "loose." Once the bond becomes a strong covalent bond or "ages," the pralidoxime can no longer separate the OP from the acetylcholinesterase. 2-PAM can be obtained from human hospitals, emergency centers, and sometimes first-responder centers.

Because OP and carbamates have such a low margin of safety, because there are so many newer and safer external parasiticides, and because the EPA is cracking down on any use of these products in a way potentially harmful to humans (e.g., children coming in contact with flea collars impregnated with these products), it is doubtful these products will continued to be manufactured in the future. But for now, there still exist products available for animal use, and the veterinary technician needs to be aware of their actions and potential toxicity.

Pyrethrins and Pyrethroids

Pyrethrins and pyrethroids constitute the largest group of OTC insecticides marketed for use against external parasites and common household insect pests such as flies and mosquitoes. Unlike OP and carbamate insecticides, most of the pyrethrins and pyrethroids have a large therapeutic index (see Chapter 3) and are **selectively toxic**, meaning that the dose that is effective (i.e., kills the parasite) is much smaller than the dose that produces toxicosis in the animal host.

Pyrethrin in its purest form is considered to be an old insecticide—a natural insecticide derived from chrysanthemum flowers. As an ectoparasite product, pyrethrin has a quick "knockdown" effect, as evidenced by the way flies drop or fleas fall from an animal sprayed with pyrethrins. However, the killing activity of pyrethrins is not as marked as the stunning effect, and the immobilized flies or fleas may recover after several minutes. For that reason, the basic pyrethrin molecule has been modified to enhance the insecticidal effect. These modified pyrethrin-like insecticides are called *pyrethroids.*

There are many **pyrethroids** available for veterinary, agricultural, and household use. A wide variety of pyrethroids can be found in horsefly sprays. Fortunately, most pyrethroids can be recognized by the *-thrin* suffix at the end of the compound name (e.g., permethrin, flumethrin, tetramethrin, deltamethrin, cyfluthrin, cypermethrin, and cyphenothrin). A couple of the exceptions to this rule are **fenvalerate** and **etofenprox**, two pyrethroid ingredients used in some OTC insecticidal applications.

Pyrethrin and pyrethroids are topically applied and are lipophilic, but large, molecules, which mean that they tend to penetrate through the superficial layers of the skin, but cannot penetrate very deeply and hence are not absorbed systemically.[12] Hence, these products are regulated by the EPA and not the FDA, making them available as OTC products.

Although pyrethrin and pyrethroids probably have multiple actions on receptors, the main mechanism of action is by locking open the sodium channels that normally allow sodium ions to move into the neuron to initiate depolarization of the nerve. The duration of this effect is dependent on the type of pyrethroid, with some pyrethroids keeping the channel open for a short period of time and others locking it open for much longer. The difference in effects results in different causes of death signs in the parasite, and different clinical signs of toxicity if it occurs in the host.

By opening the sodium channel, the neuron will depolarize. If the channel is allowed to close again, the cell will be allowed to repolarize, meaning that the effect of the pyrethroid in opening the sodium channel again will produce a rapidly repetitive cycling of depolarization/repolarization. In the parasite or the toxic host animal, this will produce muscle tremors, hyperactivity, and seizure activity. If, however, the sodium channel is opened and then locked open, the neuron or muscle will depolarize once but be unable to repolarize and hence will be nonresponsive to any further stimulation. The net effect in this case is paralysis of muscle and shut-down of neuronal firing. So-called type I pyrethroids (e.g., permethrin, resmethrin) produce the hyperactivity type of response and the type II pyrethroids (e.g., fenvalerate) produce the paralysis type of syndrome.

As mentioned earlier, pyrethrins and pyrethroids for the most part have very selective toxicity because of the poor absorption into the body from the skin, the affinity these compounds have for insect sodium channels vs mammalian sodium channels (said to be 1000 times greater), and because mammals have many enzymes that can break down pyrethrin and most pyrethroids.[12] Although pyrethrins are very safe for mammals, fish readily absorb pyrethrin insecticides through their skin, do not have the same enzymes mammals do to readily break down pyrethroids, and can easily become poisoned and die. Therefore, pyrethrin and pyrethroid use around koi ponds, fish farms, and aquaculture establishments must be carefully controlled to prevent the spray or application from settling into the water. Partially, because of the potential toxicity and effect on fish, some pyrethroids previously found in veterinary products in the past are no longer available because of EPA restrictions (e.g., EPA

stopped all sales and distribution of resmethrin as of December 31, 2015). Fortunately, most pyrethrins and pyrethroids currently in use tend to degrade in the environment fairly quickly, minimizing the effect of these compounds if they are sprayed onto ground water run-off that passes into streams, lakes, or rivers.

Synergists are compounds added to the pyrethrin products to enhance their insecticidal effect. The synergists most commonly used with pyrethrins are **piperonyl butoxide (PBO)** and another called **MGK 264**. These synergists are generally safe, but PBO has been reported to cause neurotoxicity signs in cats licking their treated fur. Because pyrethroids usually have sufficient insecticidal activity by themselves, they are not often combined with a synergist. To enhance the disruption of the flea life cycle, some pyrethrin and pyrethroid flea products now include insect growth regulators (IGRs), which are compounds that retard or stop the development of flea eggs or flea larvae without directly killing the flea. These products are discussed at the end of this chapter.

As stated at the beginning of this section, there are many pyrethroid products, some of which are OTC, some of which are available to veterinarians, and others that are limited to use by licensed pest control operators for premise and environmental use. Veterinary technicians should be aware of the characteristics of a smaller subset of selected pyrethroids of medical or toxic significance encountered in veterinary medicine that are listed later.

Permethrin is a common product in many household fly and insect killer sprays (e.g., Raid), is a component of several OTC horsefly sprays, is used as pour-ons and spot-ons for livestock and horses, is impregnated into cattle ear tags, and is also one of the more widely used pyrethroids in veterinary medicine. In addition to multiple off-brand products, permethrin is found in a few mainstream canine-only products like K9 Advantix II and Activyl Plus. Part of the appeal of permethrin as a topically applied pesticide is that in addition to being an insecticide, it is a repellent that can keep insects from landing on horses, cattle, or small ruminants in the first place. It also has fairly effective tick-repelling action, which reduces the chances of being bitten by a tick and infected with tick-borne diseases like Rocky Mountain spotted fever. Permethrin is incorporated into some materials used to make outdoor clothing so as to have inherent fly- or tick-repelling characteristics and goes by interesting marketing names such as "No Fly Zone" or "Buzz Off" fabric.

The topically applied canine products K9 Advantix II and Activyl Plus contain very high concentrations of permethrin (45%–65%), and if such high concentrations are applied to cats topically and the cat ingests the chemical after grooming the application spot (or the paw that is used to itch the application spot), permethrin toxicosis is possible. As described in Chapter 3, cats are inefficient at metabolizing drugs that depend on drug conjugation with glucuronide, and glucuronide conjugation is one of the main ways in which permethrin is metabolized. Permethrin itself is the toxic element (vs its metabolites), so the slower rate at which permethrin is metabolized in cats predisposes them to toxicity.

There are many reports of permethrin toxicity in cats after application of high-concentration canine products onto the cat. Because permethrin is a type I pyrethroid, the clinical signs reflect multiple, rapid depolarizations manifested as tremors and seizures. A report exists of permethrin toxicosis in a cat occurring 48 h after two large dogs in the cat's household were treated with a concentrated permethrin spot-on product.[13] Even though canine permethrin products clearly state warnings about avoiding exposure of the product to cats, it is the role of the veterinary technician to emphasize to clients and pet owners how important it is to make sure cats are not exposed to the high-concentration permethrin product or to keep the cat from contacting the treated area on the dog for 24 h after the dog's permethrin treatment. Permethrin is very toxic to fish so care must be taken not to contaminate aquariums or koi ponds after application of the permethrin product. Though permethrin is not especially toxic to birds, spray products with permethrins may contain other compounds that can potentially damage the respiratory tract of birds if inhaled. Permethrins are very toxic to honey bees and other beneficial insect pollinators.

Cypermethrin is a type II pyrethroid found in many household insect products and also as an approved product for use in dust bags to apply insecticidal dust to cattle, horses, and small ruminants. It is indicated for use in poultry to control biting lice in chicken, ducks, and turkeys. It is incorporated into insecticide ear tags for use in cattle combined with PBO to increase its insecticidal effect. Cypermethrin has found limited use in small animals.

Fenvalerate, like cypermethrin, is a type II pyrethroid. It was implicated along with the repellent diethyltoluamide (DEET) in the deaths of several cats after treatment with an OTC topical application product (Hartz Blockade for Cats spray). Currently there are no companion animal products that appear to contain fenvalerate, and livestock products are becoming scarcer.

Etofenprox is an ingredient combined with fipronil or other ectoparasiticides in some lesser known brands of topically applied flea and tick products for dogs and cats, as well as some fairly well-known OTC flea sprays (e.g., Adams Plus Flea and Tick Spray). It is also included in some products intended to be used inside a house as a fogger. It is important to read the label of etofenprox products because some packages state clearly that the product containing etofenprox should not be used on or around cats, but others are made especially for cats (e.g., Sentry Fiproguard Max). The difference is likely the amount of etofenprox applied by the product because when used at higher concentrations etofenprox can produce toxicity in cats, similar to permethrin.[14]

Tetramethrin is found in combination with etofenprox in OTC yard sprays to reduce fleas, ticks, ants, and mosquitos (e.g., Adams Plus Premises Protection) and as indoor foggers that claim to control fleas for up to 7 months. It is also sometimes included as one of multiple pyrethroid combinations used to kill and repel flies, gnats, and mosquitos in horse sprays.

Cyfluthrin is considered to be a fourth-generation pyrethroid, meaning it is one of the newest products compared with the others listed here. It is the active ingredient impregnated into cattle ear tags, marketed as a monthly pour-on product for cattle

to control biting and sucking lice and face and horn flies, and used as a premises spray. It is said to have repellent characteristics and therefore of some additional use around horses. There are currently no small animal applications. The closely related compound **flumethrin** is a component, along with imidacloprid, of the 8-month flea collar for dogs and cats called Seresto.

There are dozens of other pyrethroid compounds used in household sprays, premises sprays, horsefly sprays, mosquito foggers, and a variety of livestock products, but the compounds listed here should provide a core of pyrethroids to which any other products can be compared.

Amitraz

Amitraz was one of the first effective agents available for treatment of demodectic mange in dogs. The amitraz formulation for demodectic mange is still available for use in dogs (Mitaban) and comes in a liquid form that is to be used as a dip or sponge-on bath. It is a legend drug and carries the legend label that "Federal (USA) law restricts this drug to use by or on the order of a licensed veterinarian." This is most likely because of the potential toxic nature of the ectoparasiticide if improperly used.

It is not entirely clear by what mechanism amitraz kills ticks or mites; however, it is known that amitraz is an α_2 receptor agonist similar to sedative/tranquilizer drugs like xylazine (Rompun) and detomidine (Dormosedan). Stimulating the α_2 receptor in the brain decreases the release of norepinephrine from axons and thus decreases the excitatory effect on the brain, bringing about sedation. The sedative side effects observed with amitraz are consistent with this α_2 receptor agonist activity.

Amitraz is also known to inhibit monoamine oxidase (MAO), an important enzyme involved in the normal breaking down and recycling of the norepinephrine neurotransmitter. Because many behavior-modifying drugs are also MAO inhibitors (MAOI), the manufacturers of amitraz products strongly recommend against using amitraz on any animals that are being treated with MAOIs, tricyclic antidepressants, or serotonin-reuptake inhibitors. Because of the increased use of psychotropic drugs for behavior modification in veterinary medicine (see Chapter 9), the potential for this interaction is much more likely to occur than might have been the case a few years ago.

Gloves should be worn during application of this product to decrease contact with the skin of the person administering the dip or bath because of the potential for intoxication from topical exposure. The animal must be completely wetted with the mixture and allowed to dry without rinsing or toweling off after treatment. Treatment for demodicosis typically requires three to six treatments 14 days apart.

After the normal dipping procedure, animals may show CNS depression manifested by clinical signs of sedation and incoordination for 24–72 h after treatment. Some depression of the body's thermoregulatory mechanism may cause dogs damp from their dip to become hypothermic (i.e., low body temperature). Therefore, after a dip the animal should be placed in a well-padded cage so it does not lose body heat to the metal surface of the cage. Pruritus (itching) often occurs for several days after treatment and is thought to be caused by death of the mites and the body's subsequent reaction to the mite body as a foreign protein.

Amitraz is not effective in killing fleas; however, it can kill and repel ticks. Amitraz has been impregnated into a tick collar for dogs (Preventic Tick Collar for Dogs); it prevents attachment of ticks, causes detachment of existing ticks within 48 h, and kills ticks for up to 3 months. Amitraz has been combined into another flea and tick collar (Preventic Plus) with an IGR for fleas called *pyriproxyfen*. Formulations of amitraz are marketed all around the world for use to treat mange mites, lice, and ticks in swine and cattle.

Even though some toxic side effects can be observed in many animals after topical treatment with amitraz at label doses, cats are especially sensitive to the toxic effects of amitraz. Products containing amitraz, including some labeled for use in dogs, should never be applied to cats. Clinical signs of profound sedation, ataxia, and death have been reported in cats treated with canine-approved amitraz products. The concentrations found in the large animal products would easily be lethal to cats and likely to cause significant toxicosis to dogs or horses.

Another common source of amitraz toxicosis is ingestion of discarded amitraz tick collars or extra parts of tick collars that are cut off to make the collar fit better. Although cats tend to leave these alone, dogs and children have been known to chew and possibly swallow these, producing severe amitraz toxicosis and death. Therefore, veterinary technicians must caution pet owners that amitraz collars should not be handled by children or be available where children or pets can find, play with, or chew on them. It is also very important that the discarded segments of collars be promptly disposed of so they are not accidentally picked up by children or animals.

If the dog loses the amitraz collar, it should be located and properly disposed of to prevent its becoming a toxic accident. If a dog loses its amitraz collar, it is not located, and the dog begins to appear depressed or sedated, the owner should suspect amitraz toxicity from ingestion and get the dog to a veterinarian as soon as possible. Death from ingestion of amitraz collars has been reported in both the veterinary and human medical literature.

Fortunately, because amitraz is an α_2 agonist, the α_2 antagonist drugs yohimbine (Yobine), tolazoline (Tolazine), and atipamezole (Antisedan) can be used to reverse many of the toxic effects caused by excessive sedation. All of the products listed are only available as veterinary medications. Because the half-life for the reversal agents is very short compared with the half-life for amitraz, multiple dosages of the α_2 antagonists must be administered to maintain the reversal effect.

Macrolides

The macrolides or macrocyclic lactones consist of the avermectin group and the milbemycin group of drugs. They were discussed extensively with the internal parasite medications because these drugs are considered to be endectocides. What follows are selected comments about some of the macrolides relative to their ectoparasite use.

Ivermectin has been used for years in an extra-label manner for a variety of lice and mites in livestock and small animals. It is not effective against fleas and does not kill ticks immediately.

There is an ivermectin-based otic solution for treatment of ear mites in cats (*Otodectes cynotis*). Several ivermectin products are approved for treatment of lice and mites in cattle, and other products are approved to control migrating fly larvae (grubs and warbles) in domestic livestock, horses, bison, and reindeer. Ivermectin is used in horses to kill migrating larvae of *Onchocerca*, biting black flies. The dying larvae often produce an inflammatory reaction in the skin along the ventral midline, resulting in an intense pruritus (i.e., itching) and swelling. The reaction can be dampened by the use of glucocorticoids before the administration of the ivermectin. Because ivermectin has been available for so long, the restriction from the parent drug company on manufacturing the drug has long since expired, meaning that dozens of generic brand products have flooded the market and continued to be released.

Eprinomectin is an avermectin for use exclusively in large animals to treat lice, biting flies, fly larvae, and mites. It is available as a pour-on (Eprinex) and as an extended-release 100- to 150-duration injectable for cattle (LongRange). When used as a pour-on, eprinomectin has no withdrawal time for milk or meat owing to minimal, if any, systemic absorption. However, the extended-release injectable must be administered as an SQ injection in the front of the shoulder and has a 48-day withdrawal time and considerable restrictions because of the systemic nature of this form of the drug. The injectable form is not to be given IM or intravenously (IV), and the manufacturer cautions that underdosing an animal can contribute to emergence of parasite resistance. Note that the manufacturer has been given approval to allow use of this product only on cattle that are on open pasture, and it is not to be used in cattle that are confined to feedlots or on intensive grazing (rotational grazing) programs because the environmental effect of this drug being dumped via the feces into a restricted environment has not been determined.

Doramectin (Dectomax) is another avermectin exclusively for large animal use and has a similar spectrum as eprinomectin. Like eprinomectin, it comes in a pour-on formulation for use in cattle, and an SQ injectable also for cattle, but the injectable is also approved for use in swine. Although there is no label indication for this drug in small animals, it has been used in an extra-label manner for treating demodicosis (*Demodex* mange mite) in one clinical study of 38 dogs despite the manufacturer's warning that this drug has produced severe adverse reactions, including death, when used in dogs. It is assumed that the most severe reactions would be associated with MDR1 (ABCB1) genetic mutation in Collies and other breeds.

Selamectin (Revolution) is an approved topically applied avermectin for monthly use in dogs and cats for treating ear mites and adult fleas and to prevent flea eggs from hatching. In addition, in dogs it is indicated for treating sarcoptic mange and killing ticks. Unlike some of the other avermectins, selamectin has not been particularly successful in treating demodicosis (demodectic mange). The monthly duration of action against ectoparasites is thought to be because of **sequestration** (i.e., taking up and holding) of the selamectin in the sebaceous glands of the skin. This product is not used in large animals either for label or extra-label uses.

Milbemycin oxime is part of the milbemycin macrolides and was originally developed as an agent against agricultural mites. Its only approved use for ectoparasites is for use as an otic preparation against ear mites in the cat (MilbeMite Otic). Although some early studies were done to investigate the possibility of using milbemycin oxime at a high dose to treat tough canine demodicosis cases, the results have been conflicting, with some improvement but in consistent results. Because there are amitraz products and other macrolides that may be more effective, milbemycin is not considered for extra-label use to treat demodicosis.

Moxidectin is the other topically applied milbemycin macrolide and is FDA approved for use in cattle as Cydectin to treat cattle grubs (larvae of flies in the skin), mites, and horn flies, and as the monthly administered Advantage Multi in dogs and cats to treat fleas. In addition, moxidectin is approved for treating ear mites in cats and sarcoptic mange in dogs. The manufacturer advises that the topical application site of Advantage Multi should be isolated from other animals to prevent licking because the oral ingestion of moxidectin can produce severe side effects, including coma and death. Moxidectin can be used in an extra-label manner to treat demodicosis in the dog; however, animals should be evaluated for MDR1 or ABCB1 mutation sensitivity to macrolides before using the recommended dose found in the literature. A weekly topical application of moxidectin is used in some countries outside of the United States to treat demodicosis.

Several extra-label dosages exist for macrolides, especially for exotics or wildlife species. Although the use of macrolides in an extra-label manner may be routine in some practices, it still warrants caution and intensive client education about the potential side effects of the product in that species. In many cases, little information is published regarding potential complications. Therefore, the veterinary professional is always obligated to inform the client that the medication being used is not approved for that species or for that particular use and procure the client's permission to use the product in the prescribed manner. Informing the client of this risk does not protect the veterinarian against litigation if an animal dies or is injured because of the extra-label use of this or any compound, but it does facilitate the communication and partnership between the veterinarian and the client, especially if something does not go as planned.

Fipronil

Fipronil was first marketed in 1996 for control of fleas, ticks, and biting lice in dogs and cats as the Frontline topical application (Frontline Top Spot and Frontline Plus) and as a spray. It has since been incorporated into several other products (e.g., Frontline Tritak, Certifect and Parastar) for monthly topical application and is often combined with the IGR called methoprene to extend fipronil's killing effect on the adult fleas to other stages of the flea life cycle. Methoprene halts flea larval development and kills flea eggs by concentrating in the ovaries of adult fleas at the time the flea eggs are formed.

Fipronil works as a neurotoxin in insects by blocking the chloride channels that normally open when GABA or glutamate receptors attached to the chloride channels are stimulated. By blocking the chloride ion influx, fipronil blocks the normal inhibitory effect the chloride ions would have on the neuron and thus allows the neuron to fire more than normal, resulting in overstimulation of the neuron, hyperexcitability of the nervous system, and subsequent death of the parasite. The safety of fipronil is attributable to fipronil's much higher affinity (i.e., ability of the drug to bind) for combining with the insect's chloride channel on glutamate receptors than the chloride channel on mammalian GABA receptors.

The topical liquid products of fipronil are applied on the back between the shoulder blades; because it is soluble in fat, it dissolves in the skin's oily sebaceous layer and spreads across the skin surface via the animal's movements. Fipronil is stored in the sebaceous glands associated with the hair follicles; apparently this site acts as a depot of the compound that is then exuded back onto the skin surface. The residual effect of fipronil in efficacy trials indicated a residual insecticidal effect of at least 30 days, even if the animal is bathed. Thus, fipronil products are typically marketed as once-a-month products.

The binding of fipronil to the dermis, hair follicles, and sebaceous glands makes toxicity from licking unlikely after 24 h. Clients and veterinary professionals should wear gloves when applying this product to prevent exposure to the drug. Any skin that contacts the fipronil product should be washed thoroughly with soap and water. Bathing, swimming, and contact with water do not diminish the effect of the fipronil products; however, the animal should not be bathed with shampoo until 48 h after the application of the product.

Fipronil is highly toxic to some types of fish and therefore must be used with caution to prevent accidental contamination around aquariums or pools of fish. Fipronil is also known to be toxic to rabbits even though previous publications in the United Kingdom reported successful use of fipronil. Today, it is generally accepted that fipronil poses too great a toxic risk to rabbits to justify its use in that species. Although fipronil itself is well tolerated by cats, some of the combination products are very toxic because of the presence of amitraz or permethrin, which are known to be toxic to cats.

Neonicotinoids: Imidacloprid and Nitenpyram

Hundreds of years ago European farmers were aware that tobacco extracts could be used on plants to kill common pests found in the gardens or on crops. Human medical cures from writings in the mid-1600s describe how tobacco juice could be used to kill lice on children's heads. And in the New World of North America, farmers were aware that tobacco dust or liquid tobacco extracts could be used as insecticides. The active insecticidal ingredient in tobacco is nicotine.

Although tobacco has been used as a crude folk-remedy for removing parasites in livestock, today modification of the basic nicotine molecule provides us with very safe and effective antiparasitics. These "new nicotine" products are called neonicotinoids, the term conveying new as "neo" and "nicotinoids" meaning "nicotine-like." The two compounds used in veterinary medicine are **imidacloprid** products like the Advantage brand (Advantage II, K9 Advantix II, Advantage Multi) and the 8-month flea and tick collar Seresto and **nitenpyram** flea products like the orally administered Capstar.

The name *neonicotinoid* and reference to nicotine also suggest the mechanism by which these antiparasitics work. As mentioned with the OPs, acetylcholine receptors come in slightly different shapes, with one type more likely to combine with nicotine (nicotinic cholinergic receptors) and the other type more likely to combine with a compound called muscarine (muscarinic cholinergic receptors). The nicotinic receptors are found at the junction between motor neurons and skeletal muscles (the NMJ) and also in both the parasympathetic and sympathetic nervous systems. Compounds that mimic acetylcholine and stimulate nicotinic cholinergic receptors, like the neonicotinoid insecticides, have a biphasic response: low doses stimulate the nicotinic receptor repetitively, producing muscle tremors and even convulsions; at higher doses and greater stimulation, neonicotinoids cause the nicotinic receptor to "lock up" and not repolarize again, essentially preventing impulses from traveling from the motor neuron to the skeletal muscle and producing paralysis of the muscle. Because the nicotinic cholinergic receptors are differently shaped in insects than they are in mammals, the neonicotinoids are quite safe because they bind much better to the insect receptor sites.

Imidacloprid (Advantage products and Seresto collar) was first developed for use in agriculture to control insects on crops. It was the first neonicotinoid to be used as a topical spot-on for control of fleas. Today imidacloprid is found in multiple products, some of which are very safe for use in cats and others that have been combined with permethrin for its tick and repellent properties, and therefore are contraindicated for use in cats.

Imidacloprid is applied to the back of the neck in cats or between the shoulder blades in dogs (and over the rump area of large dogs). The drug is disseminated across the skin by the animal's movement. Imidacloprid is poorly absorbed through the skin and kills adult fleas on contact without the flea having to feed on the animal. The manufacturer claims 4 weeks of residual activity in cats, with a slightly longer residual effect in dogs. Some of the topically applied imidacloprid will be shed into the environment with skin, hair, and sebum; if it contacts flea larvae in the environment, it can have a larvicidal effect, helping to break the flea life cycle. Unlike fipronil and pyrethrins, toxicity to fish is low, according to the manufacturer.

Imidacloprid is combined with the pyrethroid flumethrin in the 8-month flea and tick collar called Seresto. The tick-repellent and tick-killing activity comes only from the flumethrin because imidacloprid has poor activity against ticks. The prolonged duration of activity comes from the way the collar releases the ectoparasiticides over an 8-month time period into the lipid layer of the skin. Like the other imidacloprid products, this product can be larvicidal against flea larvae in the environment if the hair, sebum, or skin of the treated animal comes into contact with the flea larvae. Note any ticks that are already attached at the time the collar is applied usually have to be removed manually as they will not die within the 48 h it takes for the flumethrin to begin its repellent and tick-killing activity. As of this writing Seresto was not available in Canada or Puerto Rico.

Nitenpyram (Capstar) is an oral tablet used in dogs and cats to kill adult fleas. Nitenpyram claims to be faster in onset of flea-killing activity (less than 30 min) than fipronil or imidacloprid, although the clinical significance of this difference may be minimal. Unlike imidacloprid that is not absorbed appreciably into the body, nitenpyram is absorbed and works systemically to kill flea adults. Nitenpyram does not accumulate in tissues but is excreted rapidly and would need to be given on a daily basis to kill adult fleas continuously.

One of the common uses for nitenpyram is for animals coming from a potentially flea-populated area that are entering a flea-free home and the owners want to be sure that no adult fleas are brought into the environment. Kennels may use nitenpyram on animals at the time they go home as a means to eliminate any adult fleas the boarding animal may have acquired. An extra-label use of the drug is to kill maggot (i.e., fly larvae) infestation in necrotic wounds, such as those found in older outdoor dogs or cats with severely matted fur.

The manufacturer warns that flea-infested pets treated with nitenpyram may increase their scratching for a short period after drug administration because the initial nicotinic receptor stimulation produces increased nervous system and muscle activity, making the fleas move around a lot on the animal's skin or even have seizure-like activity before they die. The increased flea activity can make the animal very pruritic, but the reaction is usually short-lived because the adult flea dies quickly. However, the veterinary technician should inform the owner of this temporary but common side effect, explain why this effect is occurring, and reassure the owner that it is not a drug reaction to the nitenpyram.

Spinosyns: Spinosad and Spinetoram

Spinosyns are a family of chemicals that were discovered by a scientist from Eli Lilly and Company who took soil samples containing crushed sugar cane from an abandoned rum still while on vacation in the Caribbean. The scientist sent them back to the laboratory as part of the effort to identify new chemical agents from natural sources. A few years later it was found that the fermentation products of the bacteria *Saccharopolyspora spinosa* isolated from the soil samples had insecticidal activity. These isolated fermentation compounds were called *spinosyns* and the natural combination of the two principle spinosyns created the chemical called **spinosad**, which takes its name from *S. spinosa*.

Spinosad was initially marketed as a "natural" and environmentally friendly product for control of insects on turf, ornamental plants, and cotton. A few years later the veterinary spinosad product Comfortis was released as a once-monthly tablet for control of fleas in both dogs and cats. Since then, chemists have modified the original spinosyn isolates to create multiple variations that have been combined together and tested for their insecticidal activity. From two semisynthetic spinosyns,

spinetoram was created that is now available as Cheristin for Cats as a once-monthly topically applied treatment for flea control.

Spinosad and spinetoram act just like the neonicotinoids to overstimulate nicotinic cholinergic receptor sites, producing the biphasic excitatory and paralytic effect that results in the death of the insect or parasite. However, these spinosyns also work at a different site on the nicotinic receptor, and hence they are considered a different compound from the neonicotinoids, although their actions are very similar. Spinosad has a secondary effect as an antagonist on the GABA-linked chloride channels, reducing the inhibitory effect of GABA and increasing the hyperexcitability of the insect's nervous system. The manufacturer contends that the unique location on the nicotinic receptor site for spinosad and spinetoram will reduce the development of resistance to these compounds.

Although side effects from these drugs are mild, there is an interaction between spinosad and ivermectin. When ivermectin is used at higher, extra-label doses to treat demodicosis in dogs, the addition of spinosad has been shown to produce mild to moderate signs of ivermectin toxicity including tremors, ataxia, depression, mydriasis, blindness, and disorientation. Signs of ivermectin toxicity do not appear in animals that are taking ivermectin products for heartworm preventive, so there is no need to avoid the use of spinosad with those products. However, the use of spinosad is likely contraindicated if the dog is receiving higher-than-label doses of ivermectin to treat demodicosis.

Because spinosad is taken orally, it is regulated and approved by the FDA, whereas the topically applied spinetoram is registered only with the EPA as a pesticide. FDA products generally are legend products sold through veterinarians, but EPA products tend to be available through retail outlets.

Isoxazolines: Afoxolaner and Fluralaner

The isoxazolines are a group of insecticidal compounds developed in the early 2000s and released as two veterinary products in 2013: **afoxolaner** (NexGard) and **fluralaner** (Bravecto). Both products work by inhibiting GABA-linked chloride channels, similar to fipronil, resulting in suppression of the inhibitory GABA neurotransmitter effect and resulting in overexcitation of the parasite's nervous system and death. The selective toxicity and wide safety margin are because of the differences in the shape of the insect GABA receptors vs the mammalian GABA receptors that result in isoxazolines combining much more readily with insect GABA receptors than mammalian GABA receptors.

Afoxolaner (NexGard) is a prescription-only, monthly, soft-chewable tablet approved for use in dogs to treat fleas and some ticks. This product is not approved for use in cats. In a field study as part of the approval application process, one dog with a previous history of seizures experienced a seizure on the same day it received a dose of NexGard and again the second time it received a dose of NexGard. It had a seizure a week after its third dose of NexGard. Another dog also with a history of previous seizures had a seizure 19 days after being administered a dose of NexGard. However, a third dog with a previous history of

seizures showed no seizures during the clinical trial. Still, the manufacturer recommends using this product with caution in animals with a previous history of seizure activity. As a veterinary technician, it will be important to make sure that warning is conveyed to an owner of any dog with a history of seizures.

Fluralaner (Bravecto) is also a prescription-only, soft-chewable tablet approved for dogs to treat fleas and ticks. However, instead of being given as a monthly medication, fluralaner lasts for up to 12 weeks for fleas and most ticks. It is only effective for 8 weeks against the Lone Star tick. Unlike afoxolaner, fluralaner does not have the caution about using the product in dogs with a previous history of seizures, even though one dog during the course of clinical trials experienced a seizure 46 days after a second dose of fluralaner.

Note: A new isoxazoline called sarolaner was released in April 2016 as the product Simparica. This product is a PO administered monthly treatment for fleas and ticks for use in dogs only.

Indoxacarb

Indoxacarb was developed for use in agriculture to overcome the resistance developed in crop insects and has also been used as the main insecticide in ant and roach baits. More recently it has been marketed as a prescription-only, monthly, topical spot-on application for dogs and cats (Activyl). It has also been combined with permethrin into a flea and tick spot-on application (Activyl Tick Plus) that is for use in dogs only because the permethrin would be toxic to cats.

The unique feature about indoxacarb is that the compound itself must be converted by enzymes within the insect to the active insecticidal ingredient. Because the enzymes needed for activation of indoxacarb are not found in mammals, the product is safe from being activated in the host animals; instead mammals' enzymes change indoxacarb into nontoxic metabolites.

Like all the other spot-on ectoparasiticides discussed, the product is placed on the skin, where it combines with the skin oils and spreads throughout the skin surface. Medium-sized dogs should have the product placed in two spots (shoulder blades and rump), and large dogs should have the product placed in three spots as directed by the manufacturer's drug insert information.

Like many of the more modern flea products, the flea does not have to ingest a blood meal to absorb the indoxacarb. Instead it is absorbed directly through the flea's cuticle. Once absorbed it targets the sodium channels at a different site than do the pyrethroids. Instead of locking channels open like the pyrethroids, indoxacarb blocks the sodium channels in a manner similar to local anesthetics like lidocaine. The resulting paralysis produces flea death. Flea larvae in the environment that contact indoxacarb will also die.

Applications of indoxacarb retain activity against fleas for at least 4 weeks, and sometimes longer. Because the indoxacarb compounds are applied topically and absorption is minimal, these compounds are registered and regulated as pesticides with the EPA. As such they are available for purchase without a prescription or order by a veterinarian.

INSECT GROWTH REGULATORS: THE INSECT DEVELOPMENT INHIBITORS AND JUVENILE HORMONE ANALOGS

IGRs are a broad group of compounds that inhibit the maturation of the developing larvae of insects and ectoparasites but do not generally affect the adults. Because they target specific metabolic processes only found in insects, they have no effect on mammalian cells. IGRs are broken down into two groups: the insect development inhibitors (IDIs) and juvenile hormone analogs (JHAs).

Lufenuron (a component of Sentinel products) is an IDI available in oral form. Lufenuron is absorbed and distributes throughout an animal's tissue fluids. When the adult flea bites and feeds on the animal, the lufenuron is taken into the adult flea and produces its effect on developing flea eggs and immature fleas. IDIs work by interfering with the deposition of chitin into the flea egg and the exoskeleton of the larva within the egg. Chitin is what accounts for the "crunch" noticed when an insect is crushed and is a key structural component of the exoskeleton. Thus, the larva may die because of the poor construction of the egg, or the larva may be unable to hatch out of the egg because of a lack of an effective egg tooth, which is also composed of chitin. Larvae that do hatch out of the eggs will be smaller and less likely to survive because of poor chitin deposition in their exoskeleton. Although chitin deposition occurs in adult fleas, the concentration of lufenuron achieved in adult fleas is insufficient to significantly affect chitin formation. Therefore, lufenuron is not effective against adult fleas. Because lufenuron targets chitin and because mammals do not have chitin in their bodies, lufenuron is considered a very safe compound.

Because lufenuron affects eggs laid by adult fleas, there is a lag time of up to 2 weeks between when lufenuron treatment is started and when significant changes in flea reproduction are noted. Thus, for lufenuron to be effective to a client's satisfaction, it is highly recommended that a flea adulticide be used simultaneously to reduce the pet's aggravation from adult fleas.

It is interesting to note that the enzyme system needed for chitin deposition that is disrupted by lufenuron is the same system used by some fungal agents for normal function. Thus, lufenuron has been mentioned as a possible treatment for superficial mycoses like ringworm in cats. However, clinical trials have been inconclusive as to whether or not lufenuron actually decreases the incidence or extent of ringworm in cat colonies.

Methoprene and **pyriproxyfen** are two JHAs. These compounds work by mimicking the actions of natural juvenile hormones that retard development into adult insects. By delaying development, the larvae will eventually die. **Methoprene** is incorporated into the monthly topical products Frontline Plus and Frontline Tritak for control of fleas on dogs and cats. Methoprene is also found in the product Certifect for dogs, but Certifect also contains amitraz, which would be toxic if applied to cats. Many premise sprays contain methoprene (e.g., Precor) for treatment of carpets, rugs, and floors. It should be noted that methoprene is somewhat sensitive to direct sunlight, which may shorten its duration of action. Some premise sprays with methoprene claim to work up to 7 months.

Pyriproxyfen, which also goes by the trade name Nylar, is the other JHA most commonly used in veterinary medicine. It is incorporated into spot-on applications like Advantage II, K9 Advantix II, and Bio Spot for Cats, as well as room foggers (e.g., Virbac Knockout Fogger). As mentioned with methoprene combination products, some pyriproxyfen combination products, like K9 Advantix II, contain ingredients that are toxic to cats (e.g., permethrin) and therefore cannot be safely used in cats even though pyriproxyfen by itself is very safe to use in cats.

INSECT REPELLENTS

Insect repellents are used to repel insects and keep them off animals. Repellent formulations include horsefly sprays, cattle or livestock ear tags, and products applied to the tips of dogs' ears. Some of these products are insecticides and repellents. In horses and cattle, repellents prevent flies from laying eggs on the skin, reducing bot and warble infestations in the skin. In outdoor dogs, especially those with upright ears such as German shepherds and Doberman pinschers, flies sometimes continually bite the ear tips, producing oozing wounds and encrustations of black, scabby material (i.e., ear tip fly strike). Application of a repellent to the ears of these dogs reduces fly strike. Keeping ticks off animals or people is important so as to avoid tick bites that may communicate diseases like Lyme disease that are transmitted by arthropods.

- **Permethrin** has natural repellent properties and insecticidal properties and was discussed at length with the pyrethroids.
- **Butoxypolypropylene glycol** is a repellent and a wetting agent and has been incorporated into equine fly repellents because it provides a shine that is of cosmetic value in show animals. Butoxypolypropylene glycol can cause dermal irritation if a harness or collar is applied over the area while the coat is still wet with spray.
- **DEET** is a common ingredient in repellent products formulated and approved for use in people. However, there are no products available for use in pets because toxicity has been reported, especially in cats. DEET was one of the products along with fenvalerate in the Hartz Blockade product that caused the death of several cats. Because DEET is absorbed quickly when applied to the skin, people who use DEET in high-concentration formulations have reported numbness of the lips or tingling associated with repeated use or application of large amounts. People may be tempted to use DEET on their pets, but they should not because of the risk for toxicity.

ANTIPARASITIC DRUGS

Internal Parasite Drugs

Antinematodals
  Avermectins and milbemycins (macrolides)
    Ivermectin
    Selamectin (Revolution)
    Doramectin (Dectomax)
    Eprinomectin (Eprinex, LongRange)
    Milbemycin oxime (Interceptor, Sentinel, Trifexis)
    Moxidectin (Cydectin, Quest, Advantage Multi, ProHeart 6)
  Benzimidazoles
    Thiabendazole
    Fenbendazole (Panacur, Safe-Guard)
    Oxibendazole (Anthelcide EQ)
    Albendazole (Valbazen)
    Febantel (Drontal Plus)
Pyrantel pamoate and pyrantel tartrate
Emodepside
Piperazine
Levamisole
Anticestodals
  Praziquantel
  Epsiprantel
Heartworm medications
  Adulticide
    Melarsomine (Immiticide)
  Microfilaricides
    Moxidectin (Advantage Multi)
  Preventives
    Ivermectin (Heartgard)
    Selamectin (Revolution)
    Milbemycin oxime (Interceptor, Sentinel, Trifexis)
    Moxidectin (Advantage Multi, ProHeart 6)
  Doxycycline
Antiprotozoals
  Sulfonamides
    Sulfadimethoxine (Albon)
    Sulfadimethoxine plus ormetoprim (Primor)
    Sulfadiazine plus trimethoprim (Tribrissen)
    Sulfamethoxazole plus trimethoprim (Septra, Bactrim)
  Amprolium (Corid)
  Benzimidazoles
    Albendazole (Valbazen)
    Fenbendazole (Panacur, Safe-Guard)
    Febantel (Drontal Plus)
  Metronidazole and metronidazole benzoate
  Clindamycin (Antirobe)
  Ionophores
    Lasalocid (Bovatec)
    Monensin (Rumensin)
  Ponazuril (Marquis)

External Parasite Drugs

Organophosphates and carbamates
Antidotes
  Atropine
  Pralidoxime (2-PAM)
Pyrethrins and pyrethroids
  Pyrethrin
  Permethrin
  Cypermethrin
  Fenvalerate
  Etofenprox
  Tetramethrin
  Cyfluthrin
  Flumethrin (Seresto collars)
  Synergists
    Piperonyl butoxide (PBO)
    MGK 264
Amitraz
Macrolides
  Ivermectin
  Eprinomectin (Eprinex, LongRange)
  Doramectin (Dectomax)
  Selamectin (Revolution)
  Milbemycin oxime (MilbeMite Otic)
  Moxidectin (Cydectin)
Fipronil (Frontline products, Certifect, Parastar)
Neonicotinoids
  Imidacloprid (Advantage products, Seresto collar)
  Nitenpyram (Capstar)
Spinosyns
  Spinosad
  Spinetoram
Isoxazoline
  Afoxolaner (NexGard)
  Fluralaner (Bravecto)
  Sarolaner (Simparica)
Indoxacarb (Activyl)

Insect Growth Regulators (IGRs)

Insect development inhibitors (IDIs)
  Lufenuron (Sentinel)
Juvenile hormone analogs (JHAs)
  Methoprene
  Pyriproxyfen (Nylar)

Insect Repellents

Permethrin
Butoxypolypropylene glycol
Diethyltoluamide (DEET)

REFERENCES

1. Coles TB, Lynn RC. Drugs for treatment of helminth infections: anthelmintics. In: Boothe DM, ed. *Small Animal Clinical Pharmacology and Therapeutics*. Philadelphia: Saunders; 2012:451–468.
2. American Heartworm Society. Current Canine Guidelines for the Prevention, Diagnosis, and Management of Heartworm Infection in Dogs. Wilmington, Delaware: American Heartworm Society; 2019.
3. Lanusse CE, et al. Antinematodal drugs. In: Riviere J, Papich M, eds. *Veterinary Pharmacology and Therapeutics*. Ames, Iowa: Wiley-Blackwell; 2009:1053–1094.
4. Campbell WC. Anti-inflammatory and analgesic properties of thiabendazole. *JAMA*. 1971;216(13):2143.

5. Lanusse CE, Virkey GL, Alvarez LI. Anticestodal and antitrematodal drugs. In: Riviere J, Papich M, eds. *Veterinary Pharmacology and Therapeutics.* Ames, Iowa: Wiley-Blackwell; 2009.

6. Guerrero J.G.. Overview of heartworm disease. In *The Merck Veterinary Manual (Online Edition).* http://www.merckvetmanual.com/. Accessed 06.2022.

7. Lanusse CE, Lifschitz AL, Imperiale FA. Macrocyclic lactones: endectocide compounds. In: Riviere J, Papich M, eds. *Veterinary Pharmacology and Therapeutics.* Ames, Iowa: Wiley-Blackwell; 2009:1119–1144.

8. Rawlings CA, McCall JW. Melarsomine: a new heartworm adulticide. *Compend Contin Educ Vet.* 1996;18(4):373–379.

9. Lynn RC, Boothe DM. Drugs for treatment of protozoal infections. In: Boothe DM, ed. *Small Animal Clinical Pharmacology and Therapeutics.* Philadelphia: Saunders; 2012:434–450.

10. Davis JL, Gookin JL. Antiprotozoan drugs. In: Riviere J, Papich M, eds. *Veterinary Pharmacology and Therapeutics.* Ames, Iowa: Wiley-Blackwell; 2009:1145–1180.

11. Scheidegger J. Feed manufacturer settles with horse owners after fatal monensin poisoning. *DVM360 Magazine.* 2015;(January 14):1.

12. Baynes RE. Ectoparasiticides. In: Riviere J, Papich M, eds. *Veterinary Pharmacology and Therapeutics.* Ames, Iowa: Wiley-Blackwell; 2009:1181–1202.

13. Meyer EK. Toxicosis in cats erroneously treated with 45 to 65% permethrin products. *J Am Vet Med Assoc.* 1999;215(2):198–203.

14. Volmer PA. Pyrethrins and pyrethroids. In: Plumlee KH, ed. *Clinical Veterinary Toxicology.* St. Louis, Missouri: Mosby; 2004:188–190.

SELF-ASSESSMENT

1. Fill in the following blanks with the correct item from the Key Terms list.

   A. _____ This agency regulates antiparasitic products that must be taken internally or are absorbed significantly from topical application.

   B. _____ This agency regulates antiparasitic products that are applied topically and not absorbed to any significant extent.

   C. _____ This very general term means "kills parasites."

   D. _____ This term describes the safety of an antiparasitic compound; it means that the product is much more toxic to the parasite than it is to the host.

   E. _____ This term describes any antiparasitic compound that is effective against both internal parasites and external parasites.

   F. _____ This term refers to those parasites that live within the body.

   G. _____ This term refers to those parasites that live on the outside of the body.

   H. _____ This term is used to describe *any* compound that kills internal parasitic worms.

   I. _____ This term describes the characteristics of an anthelmintic in which the compound kills the worms.

   J. _____ This term describes the characteristics of an anthelmintic in which the internal worms are paralyzed and pass out with the feces.

   K. _____ A type of anthelmintic that treats any roundworm (i.e., worms that are round in cross section).

   L. _____ A type of anthelmintic that treats any segmented flatworm or tapeworm.

   M. _____ Two other terms used to describe anticestodals.

   N. _____ A term used to describe any compound that kills flukes.

   O. _____ A term used to describe any compound that kills single-celled parasitic organisms.

   P. _____ A type of antiprotozoal that specifically inhibits the growth of the protozoa *Coccidia.*

   Q. _____ Two terms used to identify the family of antiparasitics that includes avermectins and milbemycins.

   R. _____ The neurotransmitter in insects that opens chloride channels and causes an inhibitory effect on neurons; this neurotransmitter's receptor is the site of action for the macrolide antiparasitics.

   S. _____ The neurotransmitter in mammals that opens chloride channels and causes an inhibitory effect on neurons; this neurotransmitter's receptor is the site of toxicity for ivermectin or any other macrolide used in mammals.

   T. _____ This is the pump in the blood-brain barrier that keeps macrolides from reaching the neurons in the mammalian brain.

   U. _____ Mutation of this gene results in defective formation of P-glycoprotein (P-gp) and susceptibility to macrolide toxicosis. Indicate both names!

   V. _____ This term means "pupillary dilation."

   W. _____ This intracellular structure keeps the cell's shape and functions in cellular division; it is the site of action for benzimidazoles.

   X. _____ This term means that a compound creates birth defects.

   Y. _____ This is the term that refers to the head of the tapeworm.

   Z. _____ This is the term that describes the tapeworm segments.

   AA. _____ This means that the compound kills the eggs of the parasite.

   AB. _____ This is the term that describes the inner lining of the blood vessels; this layer proliferates as part of the pathology of heartworm disease.

AC. _____ Name of the proteins from the bacteria living in Dirofilaria that produces part of the inflammatory reaction associated with heartworm disease.

AD. _____ This is any detached mass or object floating along in the blood that can eventually lodge in a very small blood vessel.

AE. _____ This is the asthma-like syndrome that occurs in cats infected with heartworms.

AF. _____ This describes any drug that kills the adult heartworm parasite.

AG. _____ This describes any drug that kills the young produced by the adult heartworm.

AH. _____ This is the stage of the heartworm life cycle in which the parasite emerges from the mosquito mouth parts and enters a new dog or cat when the mosquito feeds.

AI. _____ This describes any drug that kills the infective L3 larval stage of _D. immitis_.

AJ. _____ This is the bacteria that inhabits _D. immitis_ parasites in a symbiotic relationship with the heartworm.

AK. _____ This is the condition of heartworm that is so severe that the worms fill the right side of the heart and extend to the large vessels that bring blood to the right atrium.

AL. _____ This is a drug surveillance program for monitoring the effects of a drug known to have a previous history of adverse drug effects.

AM. _____ Refers to antiprotozoal drugs that kill Coccidia.

AN. _____ This is the condition of being infected with Giardia.

AO. _____ This is the term for any agent that kills parasites that live exclusively on the outside of the body.

AP. _____ This is the enzyme that breaks down acetylcholine.

AQ. _____ This is the type of acetylcholine receptor that produces SLUDDE signs.

AR. _____ This is the type of acetylcholine receptor found between the motor neuron and the skeletal muscle.

AS. _____ This the junction between the motor neuron and the skeletal muscle.

AT. _____ These types of compounds (not specific drugs) are added to pyrethrin to enhance the killing power of the pyrethrin.

AU. _____ These compounds do not kill insects directly but instead disrupt the flea lifecycle by stopping larval development or egg hatching.

AV. _____ These types of compounds do not kill insects but keep them from landing on the skin or face of animals.

AW. _____ This is the enzyme that is involved in breaking down the norepinephrine neurotransmitter.

AX. _____ This term means "itching."

AY. _____ This term means "to take up and hold something," like a drug is taken up and held within the sebaceous glands.

AZ. _____ Broad term for any type of compound that inhibits the maturation of an insect or parasite by any means.

BA. _____ This is what adds strength to the exoskeleton of the adult insect and comprises the egg tooth that larvae need to hatch out of insect eggs.

BB. _____ Type of insect growth regulator (IGR) that prevents maturation of larvae or hatching of fleas by interference with chitin formation.

BC. _____ Type of IGR that prevents maturation by delaying normal development of larvae, eventually causing their death.

2. Fill in the following blanks with the correct drug from the Antiparasitics list. When practicing these questions, write out the answers on a separate sheet, focusing also on the appropriate spelling of these drug names.

A. _____ This is the group of macrolides that includes ivermectin, selamectin, doramectin, and eprinomectin.

B. _____ Two avermectin compounds developed specifically for livestock.

C. _____ This is a macrolide but not an avermectin; approved for use in the dog and cat as a heartworm preventive and as a treatment for hookworms and roundworms; also found in its own otic treatment for ear mites.

D. _____ This is a macrolide but not an avermectin; approved for use in both large animals and small animals; pour-on in cattle, oral gel in horses, topically applied spot-on in dogs and cats.

E. _____ Ingredient in the 6-month injectable heartworm preventive for dogs only.

F. _____ Prototype drug for group that acts by interfering with β-tubulin in the cell's exoskeleton.

G. _____ This is the group of macrolides that includes milbemycin oxime and moxidectin.

H. _____ Very pleasant-tasting oral liquid antinematodal effective against roundworms and hookworms in dogs and cats but ineffective against whipworms or tapeworms; formulations available for livestock and equine use; suspensions quickly settle out, so must be shaken before each use to assure consistent delivery of drug; many over-the-counter (OTC) versions of this drug are available.

I. _____ The two anticestodal drugs.

J. _____ Large animal avermectin that comes in both a topical application (pour-on) plus a subcutaneous (SQ) injectable form that is good for 100–150 days.

K. _____ Heartworm adulticide.

L. _____ First macrolide available to veterinary medicine; now often combined with other products, like pyrantel, into oral, monthly medications for heartworm preventive and other internal parasite control.

M. _____ Topically applied heartworm preventive that is also an effective endectocide for gastrointestinal (GI) worms and fleas.

N. _____ Topically applied macrolide heartworm preventive but not an avermectin; comes in both monthly topical application and 6-month injectable forms.

O. _____ Large group of antibiotics well known for their activity against protozoa; often are combined with another drug to produce a potentiated form of this antibiotic.

P. _____ Antiprotozoal that is given as feed or water additive to calves and poultry to treat _Coccidia_; structurally similar to the vitamin thiamin.

Q. _____ Pyrethroid that is a repellent; is both in ectoparasiticides and in fabric used in outdoor clothing.

R. _____ Name three benzimidazoles used as antiprotozoals.

S. _____ This antiprotozoan has an extremely unpleasant taste and is combined with benzoate to make it less soluble and have less of a taste.

T. _____ Most widely used macrolide heartworm preventive; used in dogs and cats; orally administered; manufacturer recommends watching Collie breeds closely for 8 h after administration.

U. _____ Macrocyclic lactone compound that is topically applied monthly in dogs and cats; conveys heartworm protection, kills most GI tract worms; is used against fleas, ear mites, sarcoptic mange, and one tick species.

V. _____ Anaerobic antibacterial drug that is also an antiprotozoal; one of the drugs indicated for use to treat toxoplasmosis in dogs and cats; may be combined with sulfas or pyrimethamine to improve activity against other protozoa.

W. _____ OTC antinematodal with limited spectrum of activity; does not kill hookworms, whipworms, or tapeworms; vermifuge for roundworms.

X. _____ Two external parasiticides that have limited use in veterinary medicine but are still found in cattle ear tags, flea collars, and tick collars; work by inhibiting acetylcholinesterase.

Y. _____ This is the cestocide that is listed as being effective against _Echinococcus_ tapeworm that can cause potentially fatal cyst development in the liver of people who ingest the eggs.

Z. _____ Milbemycin compound that is the only Food and Drug Administration (FDA)-approved drug for eliminating heartworm microfilariae.

AA. _____ Two ionophores used as antiprotozoals in cattle and poultry.

AB. _____ Ectoparasiticides that can produce SLUDDE effects in host if given at toxic levels.

AC. _____ Ectoparasiticide derived from chrysanthemum flowers.

AD. _____ Benzimidazole antiprotozoal that is known for being potentially teratogenic, so is not used in animals in the early stages of pregnancy.

AE. _____ Natural ectoparasiticide that works by locking open the sodium channels.

AF. _____ Antibiotic that is also used against protozoa; known for neurologic side effects like nystagmus and circling; neurologic signs are reversible after the drug is stopped.

AG. _____ The two synergists added to pyrethrins or pyrethroids to increase killing activity.

AH. _____ Pyrethroid that is very toxic to cats and should never be used on cats because of their poor ability to conjugate the metabolite to a nontoxic metabolite.

AI. _____ Antiprotozoal used to treat _S. neurona_, the cause of equine protozoal myeloencephalitis (EPM).

AJ. _____ The type II pyrethroid implicated in deaths from a product that incorporated diethyltoluamide (DEET) with this product; few products use this pyrethroid today.

AK. _____ Pyrethroid found in the 8-month flea collar for dogs and cats called Seresto; related to cyfluthrin.

AL. _____ Dip approved for use in dogs that have demodicosis; often produces sedation after dipping as a side effect.

AM. _____ Repellent and wetting agent found in many horsefly sprays because of the shine it produces on the coat; can cause dermal irritation if harness or collar is applied over the area where the product was applied.

AN. _____ Benzimidazole that has antiinflammatory and antifungal activity and therefore is found in some otic products.

AO. _____ External parasiticide that is used in a collar; care must be taken to prevent accidental ingestion of the collar or discarded parts of the collar; has resulted in poisoning and deaths in animals and humans; antidote is yohimbine.

AP. _____ Benzimidazole prodrug that is activated to fenbendazole and oxibendazole for its antiparasitic activities; not used as a standalone product; is combined with praziquantel and pyrantel.

AQ. _____ This pyrethroid is commonly found in combination with etofenprox in OTC yard sprays and indoor foggers; sometimes found with multiple other pyrethroids in horsefly sprays.

AR. _____ Ectoparasiticide incorporated into tick collars because it can kill ticks, repel ticks, and cause attached ticks to detach; very toxic to cats.

AS. _____ Ionophore that if given accidentally to horses can kill them.

AT. _____ Avermectin that has been used as an ectoparasiticide to kill lice, mites, and migrating fly larvae in livestock and horses; causes intense pruritus in horses infected with biting black fly larvae when the larvae die.

AU. _____ Topically applied neonicotinoid that gives 4 weeks of residual flea-killing activity in cats and slightly longer residual effect in dogs; toxicity to fish is considered to be lower than fipronil or pyrethroids; part of 8-month collar Seresto.

AV. _____ GI antibiotic that is also an antiprotozoal particularly known for its activity against Giardia; this drug is only good against anaerobic bacteria; works by disrupting protozoan deoxyribonucleic acid (DNA).

AW. _____ Macrocyclic lactone but not an avermectin; taken by mouth but also available as an otic medication; thought to be effective against demodectic mange, but evidence is conflicting and therefore it is not recommended for this purpose.

AX. _____ Topically administered ectoparasiticide incorporated into multiple other products, often with methoprene; works by blocking chloride channels that normally open when stimulated by gamma-aminobutyric acid (GABA) or glutamate.

AY. _____ Avermectin ectoparasiticide that is used exclusively in large animals for lice, biting flies, fly larvae, and mites; available as a pour-on and a 100- to 150-day injectable.

AZ. _____ Name two isoxazoline compounds used in veterinary medicine.

BA. _____ The two neonicotinoid ectoparasiticides.

BB. _____ Kills _Wolbachia_.

BC. _____ Insecticide found in ant and roach baits; used as a spot-on for dogs and cats, except for the combination product that has permethrin; must be activated to insecticide inside of the flea.

BD. _____ Antiprotozoal that must be converted to other metabolites to be the most effective; is a member of benzimidazole group of drugs.

BE. _____ Oral tablet neonicotinoid; used to kill only adult fleas; dogs become intensely pruritic shortly after drug is given because of dying fleas that are having seizures; extra-label use to kill maggot infestation in the skin.

BF. _____ Name two spinosyns used in veterinary medicine.

BG. _____ Ectoparasiticide that acts like neonicotinoids but works at different location on the nicotinic cholinergic receptor so is not a neonicotinoid; monthly tablet for flea control in dogs and cats.

BH. _____ Arsenical injectable medication; used against _Dirofilaria_ but does not kill microfilariae or L3 larvae.

BI. _____ Pyrethroid combined with fipronil in flea and tick sprays; included in some household foggers and at lower doses in some cat products; high doses can produce premethrin-like toxicity signs.

BJ. _____ Human repellent that should not be used on animals.

BK. _____ Isoxazoline compound that should be used with caution in dogs with a previous history of seizure activity because of some suggestion that the product increases seizure activity in such dogs.

BL. _____ Ectoparasiticide that should not be used when ivermectin is also being used at a high, extra-label dose to treat demodicosis because the combined compounds will produce a mild to moderate ivermectin toxicosis.

BM. _____ Reverses organophosphate (OP) toxicosis by separating the OP molecule from the acetylcholinesterase molecule, allowing the enzyme to begin to work again.

BN. _____ Spinosyn developed from two semisynthetic spinosyns to create a cat-only topically applied flea product.

BO. _____ The only FDA-approved microfilaricide found in Advantage Multi.

BP. _____ Prescription-only isoxazoline tablet for dogs to treat fleas and ticks; lasts for up to 12 weeks for most fleas and ticks but only 8 weeks against the lone star tick.

BQ. _____ Ectoparasiticide family that is the only family that works by blocking sodium channels in the same way local anesthetics do.

BR. _____ Insect development inhibitor; works by interfering with chitin formation.

BS. _____ Name two juvenile hormone analog (JHA) compounds.

BT. _____ The only ectoparasiticide that works by being an α-2 agonist with a similar action to xylazine, detomidine, and medetomidine.

BU. _____ Orally administered monthly heartworm preventive; macrolide but not avermectin; only available as oral form; effective against raccoon roundworms (_Baylisascaris_).

BV. _____ Antidote for OP and carbamate toxicity; reverses SLUDDE signs but not nicotinic cholinergic–related signs.

BW. _____ Pyrethroid repellent.

BX. _____ JHA chemical that goes by the trade name of Nylar; found as component of some Advantage products; not used in premise sprays like the other JHAs.

BY. _____ Antiprotozoal drug that has risk for forming crystalluria and KCS.

3. What do the following abbreviations stand for?
    A. GABA _____
    B. PBO _____
    C. WSP _____
    D. KCS _____
    E. EPM _____
    F. IGR _____
    G. IDI _____
    H. JHA _____
    I. HARD _____

4. Indicate whether each of the following statements is true or false.

    A. Environmental Protection Agency (EPA)-registered antiparasitic products tend to be sold OTC instead of through veterinarians.
    B. If a product is listed as an antitrematode, it means that it is effective against roundworms (i.e., worms that are round in cross section).
    C. A coccidiostat would be an antiprotozoal compound.
    D. Eprinomectin, moxidectin, and milbemycin oxime would all be macrocyclic lactones.
    E. Ivermectin products kill parasites through action on glutamate receptors, but produce toxicity in mammals through GABA receptors.
    F. P-gp metabolizes and breaks down drug molecules that pass through the blood-brain barrier and enter the brain tissue.
    G. If a cardiac drug is used that inhibits the action of P-gp as a side effect, another drug like selamectin would be able to achieve higher than normal concentrations within the brain.
    H. The multiple drug resistance 1 (MDR1) gene defect causes production of P-gp molecules to stop.
    I. Loss of the menace response is characteristic of avermectin toxicosis.
    J. Antidotes for ivermectin toxicosis are readily available and include atropine.
    K. If severe intoxication occurs because of excessive macrolide dose, the clinical signs typically resolve within 24 h or less.
    L. Macrolides are excreted intact by the liver and undergo enterohepatic circulation.
    M. Dogs with the MDR1 mutation tend to show signs of avermectin or milbemycin toxicosis after normal administration of heartworm preventive medications.
    N. Selamectin would be classified as an endectocide.
    O. Milbemycin oxime heartworm preventives are oral and selamectin is topically applied.
    P. The heartworm protection provided by the 6-month moxidectin injectable product lasts longer than the hookworm protection.
    Q. Benzimidazoles typically need to be given a few days in a row to be effective against parasites.
    R. Benzimidazoles work primarily by stimulating glutamate receptors to open chloride channels in the parasite's neurons.
    S. Pyrantel blocks nicotinic cholinergic receptors as its primary means of killing parasites.
    T. Pyrantel is primarily used as a topical spot-on.
    U. Emodepside works by stimulating GABA or glutamate receptors and producing paralysis in the parasite.
    V. The approved adulticide heartworm drug can also kill microfilariae.
    W. *W. pipientis* is a bacteria that infects heartworms, making them weaker; their presence assists the adulticide drugs in eliminating the heartworm adults.
    X. Cats are treated with melarsomine for heartworm, but they require a lower dose than dogs.
    Y. Dogs with caval syndrome (heartworm) should not be treated with melarsomine.
    Z. Heartworm adults give birth to L3 larvae, which are picked up by the mosquito and molt into microfilariae that are then injected into a new animal to produce heartworm disease.
    AA. Penicillin antibiotic kills *Wolbachia.*
    AB. To kill adult heartworms, melarsomine needs to be given as three injections, with one injection every 24 h.
    AC. Milbemycin oxime is the compound approved by the FDA to eliminate heartworm microfilariae.
    AD. Modern heartworm treatment regimens use drugs to eliminate the microfilariae before the dog is treated with the adulticide.
    AE. Doxycycline is used to kill the adult heartworms.
    AF. Glucocorticoids used to decrease heartworm-associated inflammation also increase the ability of the adult heartworm to better survive treatment with melarsomine.
    AG. Aspirin is currently recommended for routine use in heartworm-positive dogs to reduce the thickening of the intima of the pulmonary arteries.
    AH. *Giardia, Toxoplasma,* and *Coccidia* are all protozoa.
    AI. *S. neurona* causes EPM.
    AJ. Amprolium is primarily used to treat *Coccidia.*
    AK. Fenbendazole is the benzimidazole for which there is caution about its potential teratogenic effect.
    AL. Benzoate was added to metronidazole to improve its absorption.
    AM. The antibiotic used for treating anaerobic bacteria that is one of the drugs indicated for treating toxoplasmosis in dogs and cats is clindamycin.
    AN. Monensin works better against *Coccidia* in horses than it does in cattle.
    AO. Ponazuril is the drug of choice for treating the protozoa that cause EPM.
    AP. An ectoparasiticide delivered by a rubbing bar or dust bag would be a product more likely regulated by the EPA than the FDA.
    AQ. Organophosphates (OPs) work by combining with acetylcholine and blocking its activity.
    AR. The paralysis observed with OPs and carbamates is because of overstimulation of the cholinergic muscarinic receptors.
    AS. Atropine is effective in reversing the muscarinic cholinergic signs of OP toxicosis but is not effective in reversing the nicotinic cholinergic signs.

AT. Pyrethrins are known more for their ability to quickly stun insects than their ability to kill them quickly.

AU. Type I pyrethroids cause tremors and signs associated with a hyperactive nervous system, and type II pyrethroids produce signs of paralysis.

AV. Piperonyl butoxide (PBO) is a repellent added to pyrethrin sprays.

AW. MGK 264 is a synergist added to pyrethrin sprays.

AX. Permethrin is one of the few strong repellents that is safe for use in the cat.

AY. Permethrin breaks down quickly when exposed to water and therefore does not pose a threat to fish like some of the other pyrethroids do.

AZ. Etofenprox is a neonicotinoid.

BA. Amitraz increases the activity level of the nervous system.

BB. The antidote for amitraz toxicosis is yohimbine.

BC. Amitraz is great at repelling ticks and fleas, but it is totally ineffective at killing fleas.

BD. Amitraz is safe for use in cats and dogs.

BE. The large animal avermectin that comes in an injectable form approved for use in open pasture cattle every 100–150 days is doramectin.

BF. Fipronil works by blocking the chloride ion influx into the neuron, decreasing the inhibitory effect and increasing neuronal excitability.

BG. Fipronil is highly toxic to fish.

BH. Low-dose stimulation of the nicotinic cholinergic receptor causes paralysis of the muscles, and high-dose stimulation causes tremors and convulsive-like muscle activity.

BI. Imidacloprid and nitenpyram are both neonicotinoids.

BJ. Imidacloprid and flumethrin are the ingredients in the 8-month flea and tick collar (Seresto).

BK. Nitenpyram is quite effective in killing flea larvae, but has little effect on the adult fleas.

BL. A spinosyn is a type of spinosad, and spinetoram is made up of two types of spinosads.

BM. Spinosad acts like a neonicotinoid but is not a neonicotinoid.

BN. Spinetoram is very toxic to cats.

BO. Ivermectin heartworm preventive and spinosad should not be given together because of the high probability of producing ivermectin toxicosis signs.

BP. Afoxolaner and fluralaner are isoxazolines.

BQ. Afoxolaner should be used with caution in dogs with a previous history of seizures.

BR. Indoxacarb must be activated to another compound to be a truly effective insecticide or parasiticide.

BS. Fleas must bite the animal before they absorb enough indoxacarb to be deadly to the flea.

BT. JHAs work by preventing the proper incorporation of chitin into the flea's exoskeleton.

BU. Lufenuron is a repellent.

BV. Methoprene is an insect development inhibitor (IDI).

5. What are the five characteristics of the ideal antiparasitic compound?

6. Which of the following would be characteristic primary clinical signs (not signs caused by a secondary effect of the intoxication) of ivermectin toxicosis?

____ miosis
____ mydriasis
____ agitation
____ depression
____ tachycardia
____ bradycardia
____ seizures
____ coma

7. Why can injectable macrolides not be used in actively milking dairy cattle?

8. Why do OTC dewormer products create a "false sense of security" for pet owners who think they have protected their young puppies from life-threatening worm infestations?

9. An owner complains that the anticestodal drug the veterinarian dispensed did not work because he did not see any worms expelled into the feces. How would you answer this complaint?

10. A dog in surgery needs blood from a donor and the only donor currently available has heartworm disease with circulating microfilariae. If this donor's blood with microfilarial were to be given to the dog in surgery, would the recipient then develop heartworm disease?

11. What do the letters in SLUDDE stand for?
S = _____
L = _____
U = _____
D = _____
D = _____
E = _____

12. The veterinarian is treating an old dog who is somewhat neglected, kept outdoors in a run, and has severely matted hair. Shaving away the clumps of matted hair she reveals a patch of dead skin infected with fly larvae (maggots). She tells you to administer a dose of Capstar to this dog. Why?

Antiinflammatory Drugs

OBJECTIVES

After studying this chapter, the veterinary technician should be able to:

- Describe the difference between mineralocorticoids and glucocorticoids regarding their physiologic effects and the drugs that are classified as each of these.
- Explain the mechanism by which the body maintains levels of cortisol and how use of an exogenous glucocorticoid drug can affect the regulation of natural cortisol.
- Describe which drugs are short-acting, intermediate-acting, and long-acting glucocorticoids; explain why the duration of activity is important in treating veterinary patients.
- Describe the different types of injectable dosage forms for glucocorticoid drugs, how they are identified by their names, and how the form affects the route of administration.
- Explain the difference between a physiologic dose, an antiinflammatory dose, and an immunosuppressive dose of glucocorticoids.
- Describe the effects glucocorticoid drugs have on insulin, blood sugar, skeletal muscle, collagen, hair coat, wound healing, antibody response, cell-mediated immunity response, and lymphocytes (B cell and T cell).
- Explain what a stress leukogram is and what the cellular characteristics are (i.e., what happens to neutrophils, lymphocytes, and monocytes in the dog).
- Explain why glucocorticoids cause polyuria, polydipsia, and polyphagia.
- Explain why glucocorticoids are not to be given in the eye of animals with corneal ulcers.
- Explain the difference between Addison's disease and Cushing's syndrome; which is hyperadrenocorticism and which is hypoadrenocorticism; what signs Cushing's syndrome shows; what it means if the Cushing's syndrome is

iatrogenic; and why glucocorticoids cannot be stopped immediately in cases of iatrogenic Cushing's syndrome.
- Explain the principles of safe use of glucocorticoids.
- Explain the difference between nonselective NSAIDs and selective cyclooxygenase (COX)-2 inhibitor NSAIDs; list what drugs are included in each group; explain how they vary as far as potential toxicity.
- Explain the difference between COX-1 and COX-2 enzymes in what they do for or to the body.
- Explain how NSAIDs can cause gastrointestinal (GI) ulcers, melena, vomiting, and renal papillary necrosis.
- Describe the adverse side effects common to all NSAIDs.
- Explain why hypoproteinemia, or hypoalbuminemia, is such a concern when using most NSAIDs.
- Explain why cats have a harder time handling NSAIDs than dogs or horses.
- Explain why phenylbutazone is a potential human health hazard.
- Describe the key characteristics that denote each classic NSAID and the things that make COX-2 selective NSAIDs different.
- Explain the "real" story behind the public rumors and press regarding carprofen being a deadly drug that kills many animals.
- Explain how dimethyl sulfoxide (DMSO) and acetaminophen are not "antiprostaglandin" drugs; explain how they produce their effect.
- Describe at least four compounds that are considered to be chondroprotective, how they are different from each other, and how they work.
- Explain what makes acetaminophen so deadly to cats; list the clinical signs and the antidote.

KEY TERMS

acetylcysteine	cyclooxygenase-2 (COX-2)	mastitis
Addison's disease	eicosanoids	melena
adrenal cortex	endotoxemia	mineralocorticoids
adrenocorticosteroids	eosinopenia	monocytopenia
adrenocorticotropic hormone (ACTH)	gastritis	neutrophilia
alcohol solution	glucocorticoids	nociceptor
aldosterone	gluconeogenesis	nonselective cyclooxygenase inhibitor
allodynia	humoral immunity	nonsteroidal antiinflammatory drug (NSAID)
alopecia	hydroxyl radicals	nutraceuticals
analgesic	hyperadrenocorticism	phospholipase
antidiuretic hormone (ADH)	hyperalgesia	phospholipid
antipyretic	hyperkalemia	polydipsia
aplastic anemia	hypersensitivity reaction	polyphagia
aqueous solution	hypoadrenocorticism	polyuria
arachidonic acid cascade	hypoalbuminemia	prostaglandins
atrophy	hyponatremia	renal papillae
autoimmune reactions	hypoproteinemia	renal papillary necrosis
B-lymphocytes	hypoxic/hypoxia	renal pelvis
catabolism	iatrogenic	salicylic acid/acetylsalicylic acid
cell-mediated immunity	idiosyncratic	stress leukogram
chondro-	ischemic/ischemia	supraphysiologic
collagenase	laminitis	superoxide radicals
corticotropin-releasing hormone (CRH)	leukogram	suspensions
coxibs	leukotrienes	thromboxanes
Cushing's syndrome	lipoxygenase	T-lymphocytes
cyclooxygenase-1 (COX-1)	lymphopenia	uveitis

Inflammation is a protective mechanism that is designed to remove or neutralize the underlying cause of injury whether it be physical (trauma), chemical (irritant compounds), or biologic (immune responses). The presence of the inflammatory process results in the five cardinal signs of inflammation: redness, heat, swelling/edema, pain, and loss of function. The redness is caused by release of inflammatory mediators that cause local vasodilation to bring more blood to the injury site; increased blood supply makes the overlying skin appear redder as the blood vessels are brought closer to the skin surface. The heat is felt because the body temperature blood is brought closer to the skin surface and so the inflamed area feels warmer than the surrounding normal tissue. Swelling or edema is the result of loss of integrity of the capillaries, allowing protein to leak out into the tissue and pulling water from the blood into the tissues by hydrostatic and osmotic forces. The pain is caused by inflammatory mediators that increase the firing of pain receptors (i.e., nociceptors) and other processes that will be discussed later. Finally, the loss of function is a natural response to the pain and swelling that prevents movement of a joint or makes the animal voluntarily immobilize the area to prevent further pain. All of these responses are designed to protect and stabilize the affected area and improve the healing process.

If inflammation goes beyond its protective function and interferes significantly with the animal's function, then the inflammatory effect needs to be reduced. Or, if the source of the inflammation is an autoimmune reaction wherein the body attacks itself (e.g., allergies, rheumatoid arthritis, donated organ/tissue rejection) the inflammatory process is not serving any truly protective function and should be suppressed. Excessive inflammation creates damage to surrounding normal healthy tissue as a side effect of the inflammatory response, so reducing inflammation also spares surrounding healthy tissue. Therefore in veterinary medicine, drugs need to be used to reduce this response to a tolerable level or eliminate it altogether if possible.

Two large groups of antiinflammatory drugs are used to reduce the pain or discomfort: **steroidal antiinflammatory drugs,** made up mostly of glucocorticosteroids; and nonsteroidal antiinflammatory drugs (NSAIDs). Both of these drug groups relieve pain indirectly by decreasing inflammation in the local tissue and dampening the number of signals ascending through the spinal cord. However, antiinflammatories do not decrease the perception of pain at the uppermost level of the central nervous system (CNS) like the opioid analgesics do (Chapter 8); therefore, antiinflammatories cannot relieve pain to the same degree as the opioid analgesics. Still, the antiinflammatory drugs do reduce the number or intensity of pain signals running up the spinal cord toward the brain, and in that capacity, antiinflammatories do have analgesic properties.[1]

THE INFLAMMATION PATHWAY

The pain pathway involving initiation of painful stimulus at the pain receptor (i.e., the nociceptor) via transduction (i.e., the conversion of physical change into a pain nerve signal), the transmission of the pain sensation along the sensory nerves to the spinal cord, the modification or modulation of the pain sensation as it ascends the spinal cord, and the perception of pain signals in the brain were all discussed in Chapter 8 with the analgesic drugs. Inflammation mostly influences the initiation of the pain signal at the nociceptor, although the pain signals modulated in the spinal cord can also be influenced by antiinflammatory drugs.

Arachidonic Acid Pathway

The translation of the physical insult into the five cardinal signs of inflammation results from the action of dozens of biologic compounds. Some of these compounds are already present inside granules within cells (e.g., histamine, serotonin), waiting to be released immediately after the injury. Other inflammatory mediators are generated by enzymatic processes that are initiated by trauma to cells. One of the principal mechanisms by which inflammatory mediators are generated is via the arachidonic acid cascade or pathway.

The arachidonic acid cascade enzymatically generates prostaglandins, leukotrienes, and other inflammatory mediators collectively called eicosanoids.[2] Antiinflammatory drugs produce their beneficial effects by blocking the arachidonic acid cascade and preventing production of these inflammatory eicosanoid compounds. When inflammation is reduced, the amount of stimulation of the nociceptors surrounding the affected area is reduced, fewer pain signals are sent to the brain, and the animal perceives less pain from the area. To better understand how antiinflammatory drugs work, it is important to illustrate the key steps in the arachidonic acid cascade.

Any time cells are traumatized, a well-described series of steps in the arachidonic acid pathway occurs in sequence, similar to knocking over the first domino in a line of dominos. The sequence starts with trauma to a cell membrane, which activates the enzyme phospholipase (remember -ase at the end of the word indicates an enzyme), which converts phospholipid molecules that make up the cellular membrane into *arachidonic acid*. The arachidonic acid is then acted on by either *cyclooxygenase* (COX) enzymes to produce prostaglandins and thromboxanes, or by the enzyme lipoxygenase, which produces another group of inflammatory mediators called leukotrienes. The prostaglandins, thromboxanes, and leukotrienes produce a variety of physiologic reactions (the next steps in the sequence) that are associated with the inflammatory response. This pathway is shown in Fig. 13.1.

Corticosteroids, specifically the glucocorticoids, reduce inflammation by blocking the action of phospholipase; hence they stabilize the cell's phospholipid membranes. This blocks the early portion of the pathway shown in Fig. 13.1, reducing production of most of the inflammatory mediators. NSAIDs have no significant effect on phospholipase but instead inhibit COX and, to varying degrees, lipoxygenase, which reduces

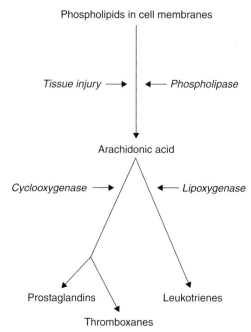

Fig. 13.1 The arachidonic acid cascade for production of inflammatory mediators.

production of prostaglandins, thromboxane, and leukotrienes. Glucocorticoids also depress COX, thus potentially inhibiting the arachidonic acid pathway at two different sites.

When these inflammatory mediators are decreased by corticosteroids or NSAIDs, this decreases the inflammatory effect of other inflammatory mediators like histamine, kinins, substance P, and superoxide radicals, which would normally contribute to the redness, swelling, heat, and pain associated with inflammation.

CORTICOSTEROIDS

The term *corticosteroids* (technically called adrenocorticosteroids) refers to a group of hormones produced by the *cortex* (the outer layer) of the adrenal gland. There are two groups of corticosteroids: mineralocorticoids and *glucocorticoids*. Although both groups of hormones are produced by the same gland, they have very different effects on the body.

Mineralocorticoids

Mineralocorticoids, as the name implies, affect the "minerals" in the body, such as sodium, potassium, and other electrolytes. Mineralocorticoids are involved with water and electrolyte balance in the body but have little or no antiinflammatory effect. Aldosterone is the mineralocorticoid hormone of medical significance in animals with adrenocortical insufficiency. Aldosterone's primary effect is to increase the sodium (Na^+) retained in the body by opening sodium pores in the distal convoluted tubule and collecting ducts of the kidney, allowing sodium to move from the urine back into the cells lining the renal tubules; from there sodium is actively pumped back into the blood. In exchange for the positive Na^+ ion being retained, potassium (K^+) ions pass from the tubular cells into the urine through their own pores in the tubules to balance the electrical charge caused by movement of the charged ions. The same pump that pumps sodium from the tubular cells into the blood also pumps potassium ions from the blood into the tubular cells where they diffuse through the pores into the urine. This balance of sodium and potassium by aldosterone is illustrated by conditions where aldosterone is not adequately produced by the adrenal gland, producing hypoadrenocorticism or Addison's disease. In Addison's disease, animals can suffer from potentially fatal hyperkalemia (i.e., increased blood potassium) and corresponding hyponatremia (i.e., decreased blood sodium) because of a lack of aldosterone driving the retention of sodium and excretion of potassium.[1] Fortunately, there are injectable mineralocorticoid drugs like **desoxycorticosterone pivalate** (Percorten-V) that mimic the effects of aldosterone and can be used to successfully treat animals with Addison's disease signs.

Glucocorticoids

Glucocorticoid receptors are found on all cells in the body, although the liver is the primary systemic target for many of the glucocorticoid effects.[3] The natural glucocorticoids produced by the adrenal glands are cortisol (which when used as a drug is called **hydrocortisone**) and cortisone. Cortisone is really a precursor compound to cortisol, so when we talk about natural glucocorticoid effects, most often we are referring to cortisol.

Control of the release of natural cortisol begins in the hypothalamus where corticotropin-releasing hormone (CRH), sometimes referred to by some older sources as corticotropin-releasing factor (CRF), is secreted; CRH then travels a short way to the anterior pituitary with secreted adrenocorticotropic hormone (ACTH).[3] The ACTH is released into the blood, where it circulates until it reaches the adrenal cortex and stimulates the release of both glucocorticoids and, to a lesser degree, the mineralocorticoid aldosterone. The production of cortisol by the adrenal gland stimulates the negative feedback effect on the hypothalamus and pituitary gland needed to curtail release of CRH and ACTH. Thus, the CRH-ACTH-cortisol negative feedback loop (Fig. 13.2) is similar to the self-regulating mechanisms described for other hormones in Chapter 7.

Cortisol and synthetic glucocorticoid drugs are used primarily for their antiinflammatory effect, although they have some effect on almost every cell in the body.[3,4] All of the other effects unrelated to inflammation suppression constitute the variety of side effects observed with glucocorticoid drug use.

Glucocorticoids produce their antiinflammatory effect by inhibiting phospholipase, the enzyme that converts cell membrane phospholipids to arachidonic acid at the beginning of the cascade. To a lesser degree glucocorticoids also inhibit COX; this action decreases prostaglandin and leukotriene production. The glucocorticoids also appear to inhibit the production of other inflammatory mediators that are involved in toxic and immune-mediated cellular damage, which helps explain corticosteroid's role in controlling allergic reactions. Corticosteroids also reduce production of cell factors that cause increased vascular permeability of the capillaries and in so doing help

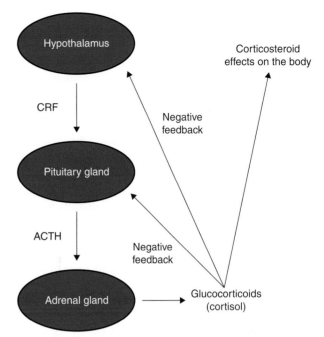

Fig. 13.2 The hypothalamus produces corticotropic-releasing factor (CRF), which stimulates the pituitary gland to release adrenocorticotropic hormone (ACTH). ACTH is what stimulates the adrenal cortex to release cortisol.

maintain the integrity of the capillaries and reduce some of the mechanisms by which swelling occurs in injured tissues.

Exogenous glucocorticoids administered as antiinflammatory drugs (e.g., prednisone, prednisolone, methylprednisolone) have the same negative feedback effect on the hypothalamus and pituitary gland as the natural cortisol. This negative feedback from exogenous corticosteroid drugs can, over time, produce potentially severe side effects because of the continued suppression of the adrenal gland by lack of CRH and ACTH production. This will be discussed more with the glucocorticoid drugs.

Note that use of high dosages of glucocorticoids for shock or trauma in general is no longer considered an effective use for these drugs. Low doses of short-acting glucocorticoids have been shown to improve the survivability of some severely ill or septic patients who are likely to have adrenal gland depletion and for whom the low dose simply replaces the depleted cortisol. However, just using glucocorticoids as a catch-all stabilizing drug for all types of emergencies is no longer considered to be appropriate use of these potent drugs.

Glucocorticoid Drugs

When veterinarians use the terms "cortisone," "corticosteroids," or just "steroids" in general, they are usually referring in a loose way to glucocorticoid drugs. One of the important ways that glucocorticoids are classified is according to their duration of biologic activity or their effect on the body. A glucocorticoid that exerts an antiinflammatory effect for less than 12 h is considered to be a short-acting glucocorticoid. **Hydrocortisone** is a short-acting glucocorticoid drug that is the same as the natural cortisol hormone. It is a common ingredient in topically applied medications for humans to combat inflammation from stings, insect bites, poison ivy, and other common sources of skin irritation. **Cortisone** is another common short-acting glucocorticoid often cited as being the same as hydrocortisone, but it is chemically different and must be converted by the liver to hydrocortisone before it becomes active. Cortisone is not used in veterinary medicine to any appreciable amount even though hydrocortisone is found in a variety of topical veterinary preparations.

Many of the glucocorticoids used systemically in veterinary medicine are classified as intermediate-acting glucocorticoids and exert their biologic activity for 12–36 h. These drugs include the "preds" (e.g., **prednisone, prednisolone,** and **methylprednisolone**) and **triamcinolone**. Although prednisolone and prednisone are often considered to be interchangeable, they are slightly different in that prednisone must be converted by the liver to prednisolone to exert its maximal effect. Although these two drugs are essentially bioequivalent to each other in the dog and other species, in the cat the conversion from prednisone to prednisolone is less efficient, and for that reason some veterinarians prefer to use the active form prednisolone in cats.[5] Because of their intermediate duration of activity, these drugs are ideally suited for alternate-day doses for control of longer term allergic or inflammatory diseases.

The long-acting glucocorticoids, such as **dexamethasone, betamethasone,** and **flumethasone** (the "methasones") and **isoflupredone** (PREDEF for use in cattle) exert their biologic activity for 48 h or longer. This longer duration means there is greater beneficial effect on cells and tissues; however, it also means that suppression of CRH and ACTH release occurs for a longer period, with potential side effects resulting from this effect.

Dosage Formulations of Glucocorticoids

It is not unusual to see that one glucocorticoid drug comes in many different forms. For example, prednisone is available as prednisone sodium phosphate, prednisone acetate, and just plain prednisone. Is there a difference in these drug forms?

Injectable glucocorticoid drugs are available in three forms: aqueous solutions, alcohol solutions, and suspensions. The type of formulation determines the the drug's route of administration and often its clinical use. Glucocorticoids in aqueous solution (i.e., water) are usually combined with a salt such as sodium phosphate or sodium succinate to make them soluble (i.e., dissolvable) in water. Therefore, prednisone sodium phosphate and prednisolone sodium succinate (Solu-Delta-Cortef) are aqueous solutions of glucocorticoids and can be administered intravenously (IV) or put into eye drops. The aqueous forms of glucocorticoids have been used as IV injections in situations where a rapid delivery antiinflammatory or cell-stabilizing effect of the glucocorticoids is needed.

Glucocorticoid molecules dissolved in alcohol do not need to be attached to a salt to dissolve. Thus, if the label on a vial of dexamethasone specifies the active ingredient as "dexamethasone" alone without mention of sodium phosphate salt, it is likely an alcohol solution form of the glucocorticoid drug.

Suspensions of glucocorticoids contain the drug particles floating, but not dissolved, in a liquid vehicle. Hence suspensions are characterized by the need to resuspend the drug by shaking the vial before use; opaque appearance after shaking and resuspension of the drug; and the terms *acetate, diacetate, pivalate, acetonide,* or *valerate* appended to the glucocorticoid drug name. Some glucocorticoids in suspension exist as relatively large crystals that must dissolve before the drug can diffuse away from the site of injection and be absorbed. Because the crystals may dissolve over several days, they release small amounts of glucocorticoid each day and provide prolonged duration of activity. The acetate form of glucocorticoid suspensions is also very lipid soluble and therefore used in topical ophthalmic medications.

Suspensions of glucocorticoids must be stored within a certain temperature range. Extremes of hot or cold temperatures (e.g., being left in the practice truck on a hot day or a very cold night) can cause the crystals to change size or shape, resulting in a change in the ability of the crystal to dissolve, an alteration in the length of absorption, and pain, irritation, or inflammation at the site of injection if the crystals are larger than normal.

Effects of Glucocorticoids and Glucocorticoid Drugs

The effects of glucocorticoids are dose related. This means that at normal, physiologic concentrations produced by the adrenal gland to maintain essential function, cells function in a particular way and the physiologic mechanisms operate for the benefit of the body. However, when glucocorticoid drugs are administered, the dose used results in concentrations that are supraphysiologic, meaning they achieve higher glucocorticoid concentrations than are achieved under normal physiologic conditions. These supraphysiologic levels of glucocorticoid alter or disrupt the normal glucocorticoid physiology and produce a variety of side effects associated with glucocorticoid drug use.

Doses of glucocorticoid drugs are classified as "physiologic," "antiinflammatory," or "immunosuppressive." These doses are not specific doses cited consistently throughout the literature, but reflect general "low, medium, or high" doses, respectively. Physiologic doses are those used to achieve normal physiology in those animals who have hypoadrenocorticism and low natural cortisol production. Antiinflammatory doses are supraphysiologic but are lower than the doses needed to produce immunosuppression. The dose at which an antiinflammatory glucocorticoid dose becomes an immunosuppressive dose is not clearly defined. But the terms are still widely used to suggest a medium vs a high dose of glucocorticoids.

The natural glucocorticoid hormones are first and foremost a stress-related hormone designed to help the body get through periods of crisis or physiologic stress. One function of glucocorticoid hormones is to increase blood glucose (hence the name glucocorticoids) by stimulating the liver to convert amino acids from proteins into new glucose, a process called gluconeogenesis (which translates into "glucose-new-creation"). Normally, this additional glucose dumped into the blood would stimulate the release of insulin that would then stimulate insulin receptors on the peripheral tissues (e.g., skeletal muscle, skin, organs), moving the glucose from the blood into the tissues and keeping the blood glucose levels from increasing.

However, glucocorticoids, in addition to stimulating gluconeogenesis, also alter the insulin receptors on the peripheral tissue, making the receptors unavailable for the increased insulin and thus preventing the blood glucose from moving into the tissues. The rationale for increasing the blood glucose is to provide glucose to the brain and heart, which are two tissues that require a constant supply of glucose and are not dependent on insulin to move the glucose into the tissues. Thus glucocorticoids keep a sufficient supply of blood glucose available to these vital tissues during periods of physiologic stress.

To have a sufficient supply of amino acids to create glucose via gluconeogenesis, glucocorticoids also cause catabolism (i.e., breakdown) of proteins to their amino acid constituents. The source of this protein is skeletal muscle and collagen in skin and healing wounds. Under conditions of elevated glucocorticoids for short periods of time, the increased demand for amino acids to create new glucose molecules does not produce a noticeable change in the skeletal muscle or collagen-rich tissues. However, prolonged uses of glucocorticoid drugs results in thinning of the skin, atrophy (i.e., shrinking) of the skeletal muscles, a pot-bellied or pendulous abdomen appearance caused by thinning of abdominal muscle mass and loss of muscle tone needed to keep the abdomen tucked up, thinning of the hair coat, and slowed wound healing.

Because glucocorticoids cause insulin receptors on the peripheral tissue to become less responsive to the glucose-transporting effect of insulin, diabetic animals who are given high doses of glucocorticoids for a short period of time, or who are put on lower doses of glucocorticoid drugs for an extended period, may require an increase in their insulin doses to compensate for the less responsive insulin receptors. However, if the glucocorticoids are only used for a short period of time, the insulin dose might not be changed because the effort required to balance feeding with the new insulin dose to stabilize the patient's blood sugar again may not be worth it for just a short period of time. Still, the veterinary technician should anticipate higher blood glucose levels and perhaps more glucose spilling into the urine (i.e., glucosuria) when the diabetic animal is on a glucocorticoid drug.

When used at antiinflammatory doses, glucocorticoid drugs decrease inflammation by inhibiting phospholipase and COX enzymes that would form prostaglandins and decrease the ability of monocytes, macrophages, and eosinophils to enter the inflamed area, thus reducing some of the collateral damage these cells cause to normal tissue surrounding the trauma site.

Glucocorticoids stabilize the membranes of lysosomes within cells, preventing release of lytic enzymes that would cause the cells to self-destruct. Glucocorticoids maintain the integrity of capillaries and prevent them from leaking protein and fluid into the tissue by inhibiting the activity of some inflammatory mediators and reducing the release of histamine by basophils. By maintaining the capillary integrity, the degree of swelling is lessened.[4]

Although normal physiologic concentrations of glucocorticoids stimulate fibroblasts to form collagen fibers necessary for connective tissue structure and the wound healing process, supraphysiologic concentrations of glucocorticoids inhibit collagen formation and may catabolize existing collagen, causing delays in wound healing, thin and more fragile skin, and a poor

hair coat as discussed earlier.[3,4] This delayed wound healing might cause a problem in a pet recovering from abdominal surgery if the absorbable sutures holding the deeper layers of the incision together begin to be absorbed and lose their ability to hold the incision closed before the wound healing process has occurred. Without collagen to hold the healing incision together, the animal could dehisce the incision site, meaning the incision site breaks down and the abdominal organs or tissue could poke through the incision site.

Glucocorticoid drugs are often used at supraphysiologic concentrations to decrease the immune system overreaction to its own tissues or cells, known as autoimmune reactions, such as autoimmune hemolytic anemia; supraphysiologic concentrations are also used on hypersensitivity reactions to external antigens or stimuli such as recurrent airway obstruction disease in horses, asthma in people, or systemic allergic reactions to bee stings, drug reactions, or food. Unfortunately, this same glucocorticoid immunosuppression can cause parts of the immune system to lose effectiveness in fighting some invading organisms. At most therapeutic doses, glucocorticoid drugs suppress one type of lymphocyte called the T-lymphocytes. T-lymphocytes, or T cells, are associated with the cell-mediated immunity in which cells like macrophages are attracted to, and engulf, foreign materials or selected disease-causing organisms.

Because the primary defense against fungal disease (e.g., histoplasmosis, blastomycosis, and aspergillosis) is by cell-mediated immunity (vs humoral immunity, which is the production of antibodies by B-lymphocytes), the use of glucocorticoids can increase the risk for severe infections from fungal agents. In addition to suppressing fungi, glucocorticoid drugs suppress the cell-mediated immune response to bacteria. Thus glucocorticoid use in animals with suspected bacterial or fungal infections is a risk and, especially for fungal infections, may be contraindicated. In those situations, the veterinarian has to make a decision whether the animal is more at risk from dying from the infection itself or from the inflammation or immune response associated with the infection. For example, a severe obstructive inflammatory response in the airway secondary to a fungal infection might be an indication for use of glucocorticoids in spite of the fungal disease because the airway obstruction from the inflammation is more likely to kill the patient more quickly than further proliferation of the fungal infection itself.

Generally, at normal therapeutic doses of glucocorticoids, humoral immunity and antibody formation to antigens is not significantly depressed. Thus the process of the body's response to vaccine antigens by production of antibodies is not significantly impaired.[3,4] This is important to remember because of the large number of dogs that may be on glucocorticoid drugs for allergy-related skin inflammation and whose owners want them vaccinated while the animal is still on doses of prednisone or prednisolone. At much higher than normal doses of glucocorticoid drugs some suppression of humoral immunity begins to occur.

Elevated physiologic levels of glucocorticoids or the use of glucocorticoid drugs dramatically alters the leukogram (i.e., the number of different white blood cells counted in the complete blood count, or CBC). Glucocorticoids cause lymphocytes, eosinophils, and monocytes to become sequestered (i.e., taken up or stored) within the lungs, spleen, and other organs, thereby decreasing the number of these cells observed in systemic circulation and resulting in lymphopenia, monocytopenia, and eosinopenia. In contrast, glucocorticoids increase the number of platelets and neutrophils in circulation, giving rise to neutrophilia. The neutrophilia is initially caused by the mobilization of neutrophils that are "parked" along the blood vessel wall (i.e., the "marginated pool" of neutrophils). Thus, although it may appear that the bone marrow is increasing production of neutrophils, the initial increase in observed neutrophils is more of a reflection of neutrophils simply rejoining circulation instead of lingering along the vessel wall. Longer term neutrophilia is caused by increased production of the neutrophils by the bone marrow and a reduced removal of neutrophils from the circulation.

The combination of neutrophilia, lymphopenia, and monocytopenia is considered characteristic of the "stress leukogram" and is attributed to either glucocorticoid drug administration or a physiologic stress response in which endogenous corticosteroids are released. This classic stress leukogram is found in the dog, but it is important to remember that different animal species will vary in the extent to which monocytopenia or eosinopenia may be observed, and therefore interpretation of the stress leukogram will also vary according to species.

Although the short-term lymphopenia seen with the stress leukogram is mostly caused by sequestration of the lymphocytes in tissues outside of the blood, glucocorticoids are also capable of destroying malignant lymphocytes associated with lymphoma, a fairly common cancer involving lymphatic cells in the lymph nodes, or lymph tissue in the gastrointestinal (GI) tract, spleen, bone marrow, skin, or chest of dogs, cats, and cattle. Because lymphocytes are the primary cell type that proliferates in lymphoma, most canine lymphoma protocols feature prednisone as a component.

In the GI tract, glucocorticoids increase gastric acid and gastric enzyme secretion and decrease mucus production, predisposing the patient to hyperacidity, reduced protection against acid and enzymes, and increasing the risk for the stomach tissues to be damaged and inflamed (i.e., gastritis).[3] In addition to the increased risk of injury, glucocorticoids reduce cell growth and renewal of the cells lining the GI tract, decreasing the ability of injured tissue to repair itself. Thus the use of glucocorticoids predisposes an animal to gastric ulcers. Because glucocorticoids and NSAIDs have similar effects on acid, gastric enzymes, and mucus production, the use of these two types of drugs simultaneously would magnify the risk for gastric ulceration and perhaps perforation (i.e., a hole forming in the wall of the GI tract).

Most patients on glucocorticoid drugs exhibit polyuria (i.e., increased volume of urine produced) and polydipsia (i.e., increased drinking) as a side effect of glucocorticoids. Though part of this effect may be caused by the mineralocorticoid effect of the glucocorticoid drug, most of the effect comes from glucocorticoid's inhibition of antidiuretic hormone (ADH). ADH is released from the pituitary gland and causes increased permeability to water of the distal convoluted tubule and the collecting ducts in the kidney. This increased permeability allows more water to move out of the urine and be retained in the body (i.e., antidiuresis). By inhibiting the action of ADH, glucocorticoids reduce the retention of water by the body, increase the water lost into the urine, and create polyuria. The polydipsia is most likely a compensatory mechanism to replace the water lost by the polyuria.

Some forms of ophthalmic medications contain glucocorticoids that are used to relieve inflammation in the eye. Although glucocorticoids play a very important role in preventing eye damage from excessive inflammation and reducing scar formation during healing in an injured cornea, glucocorticoids are contraindicated if corneal ulceration is present. Glucocorticoids in the eye activate an enzyme called collagenase and, as the name implies, this enzyme degrades the collagen protein that forms the middle layers of the cornea, resulting in a deepening ulcer to the point that the cornea ruptures.

There is an additional risk in ophthalmic corticosteroid use in horses because of the suppression of the cell-mediated immunity. Common fungal agents found in barn and stall environments may exist in the normal eye without producing clinical disease. However, if glucocorticoids are used to treat inflammation in the eye, the glucocorticoid's suppression of cell-mediated immunity, the primary defense against fungal infections, may allow a fungal agent to proliferate and establish a clinical infection in the eye. Because many ophthalmic preparations exist in forms with and without glucocorticoids, the veterinary technician should always double-check to be certain that the packaged preparation is exactly what has been prescribed.

As discussed in Chapter 7, exogenous glucocorticoids can induce premature parturition or abortion in cattle and mares in the latter stages of pregnancy.

Disease Caused by Excessive Glucocorticoid Hormone or Glucocorticoid Drugs

Overproduction of glucocorticoids by the tumors of the adrenal cortex or other pathologic conditions results in a condition called hyperadrenocorticism, or Cushing's syndrome. Underproduction of glucocorticoids by the adrenal cortex results in a condition called *hypoadrenocorticism,* or *Addison's disease.*

A state of hyperadrenocorticism can also be produced by overuse of exogenous glucocorticoid drugs, such as might occur with long-term administration of large glucocorticoid doses to control an allergic skin problem in dogs. When a disease is caused by a treatment or action by the veterinarian (or physician), the disease has the word iatrogenic attached to it. Thus *iatrogenic Cushing's* would indicate excessive levels of glucocorticoids caused by drugs prescribed by the veterinarian.

In addition to the poor hair coat, thin skin, muscle *atrophy,* and pot-bellied appearance of the *Cushingoid* patient described previously, these patients also show the "three Ps" of hyperadrenocorticism: polyuria, polydipsia, and polyphagia (i.e., increased eating). The cause of the increased appetite is not clear, but it may have something to do with the protein catabolism caused by the glucocorticoids.

Although the increased water consumption, urination, and appetite become apparent soon after the animal begins receiving glucocorticoid drugs, the signs of alopecia (i.e., hair loss or thin hair coat) and muscle atrophy do not become apparent until the animal has been treated with glucocorticoids for weeks.

Unlike many drugs used in veterinary medicine, cats seem to be more resistant to the beneficial effects and side effects of glucocorticoid drugs than dogs. It has been shown that the cat has fewer glucocorticoid receptors on its tissues than the dog, and the degree to which glucocorticoids readily combine with these receptors (i.e., the receptor affinity) is less in the cat than the dog.[6] Thus the doses required to produce an equivalent beneficial effect in cats may be double that of the dose required in the same-sized dog.[7]

Fortunately, this increased resistance also means that iatrogenic Cushing's is not seen as often in cats as in dogs. However, when clinical signs of hyperadrenocorticism from drugs occur in cats, it includes hair coat changes and fragile skin but also may include more severe signs such as congestive heart failure and increased susceptibility to diabetes mellitus.

It would seem to be common sense that if an animal begins to show signs of iatrogenic hyperadrenocorticism after being treated with glucocorticoids for several weeks, the veterinarian would want to stop the drug immediately. However, stopping the drug abruptly can potentially result in the animal going from hyperadrenocorticism to hypoadrenocorticism. Although hyperadrenocorticism (i.e., Cushing's) makes the animal look awful with the changes in hair coat, muscle loss, and thin skin, an Addison's condition (i.e., hypoadrenocorticism) can result in a crisis that is potentially life threatening. Understanding how this can occur will help the veterinary technician better understand how it is to be prevented.

In an animal that has been receiving glucocorticoid drugs for some time, the supraphysiologic level of glucocorticoids has inhibited the release of CRH and ACTH through the same negative feedback mechanism that natural cortisol would use to regulate its secretion by the adrenal gland. The lack of CRH and ACTH secretion for a long period of time means that the adrenal cortex has not been stimulated to produce cortisol and, like any other tissue in the body, if not stimulated it begins to atrophy. With atrophy the capacity of the adrenal gland to produce natural cortisol is significantly diminished.

If glucocorticoid drug administration is suddenly stopped after weeks of daily use, the levels of glucocorticoid drug in the blood will drop, the negative feedback inhibition on the hypothalamus and pituitary will be removed, and the hypothalamus will begin to release CRH to stimulate the pituitary to release ACTH again. Unfortunately, when the drug levels of glucocorticoids drop low enough that the body needs to begin manufacturing its own natural cortisol, the adrenal cortex is unable to respond to the ACTH because the tissue has atrophied over the time when the glucocorticoid drugs were given. Without the natural cortisol to replace the dropping concentrations of glucocorticoid drugs, the glucocorticoid/cortisol blood levels will drop below the normal level, resulting in an addisonian crisis. Animals with an addisonian crisis show signs of weakness, lethargy, vomiting, and diarrhea. In severe cases the animal will die. Therefore, if an animal has been on glucocorticoid drugs for an extended period of time, the dose of the glucocorticoid drug must be tapered off, over days to weeks if needed, to allow increasing stimulation of the adrenal gland and regeneration of the atrophied adrenal gland to its functional capacity.

Safe Use of Glucocorticoids

As previously described, glucocorticoids have the potential to produce a variety of undesirable side effects in addition to their beneficial effects. The following are guidelines for safe use of these potent drugs:

- The cause of the clinical condition should be identified before the use of glucocorticoids is implemented. Glucocorticoids only control conditions; they typically do not cure the underlying problems. The glucocorticoid antiinflammatory effect may disguise and provide a temporary improvement in clinical signs, only to have the animal's condition decline further if the underlying cause has not been identified and treated.
- If another antiinflammatory drug, such as an NSAID, can accomplish the same result, consider using it rather than the glucocorticoid as long as no contraindications exist for NSAID use.
- Doses are guesses and the recommended glucocorticoid dose is often the estimated starting dose to initially control the inflammation or immune response. The clinical condition should be closely monitored and as the clinical signs begin to subside, the glucocorticoid dose should be decreased to the smallest dose needed to provide control over the clinical condition or to continue to reverse the clinical signs.
- When possible avoid continuous use of glucocorticoids because of the suppression of the hypothalamus-pituitary-adrenal cortex axis and the subsequent atrophy of the adrenal gland. To decrease the risk of adrenal suppression, it is preferable to use an intermediate-acting glucocorticoid such as prednisolone instead of the long-acting glucocorticoids for those animals requiring long-term systemic administration of glucocorticoid.
- If an animal has been receiving glucocorticoids for an extended period and the drug is to be discontinued, the dose should be gradually reduced to allow the adrenal cortex to regain its ability to function normally.

NONSTEROIDAL ANTIINFLAMMATORY DRUGS

NSAIDs are drugs that decrease inflammation like the corticosteroids but do not contain the molecular steroid ring structure and do not have many of the side effects of the glucocorticoid drugs. Many of the veterinary drugs have come from human medicine as a result of human beings being more sensitive to the side effects of glucocorticoids and needing NSAIDs to control chronic inflammation.

Most NSAIDs work by blocking the activity of COX enzymes and thus inhibiting the production of prostaglandins. Although most NSAIDs are not thought to block formation of the leukotriene group of eicosanoids, some NSAIDs such as ketoprofen and ibuprofen may also inhibit lipoxygenase and decrease their production of leukotrienes. Even so, most of the antiinflammatory activity is from COX inhibition.

In the 1990s research showed that COX existed in two forms. COX-1 always exists in the kidney, stomach, and other organs of the body, where it produces prostaglandins that are involved in the normal physiologic regulation of the organ's functions. For example, COX-1 plays a very important role in stimulating secretion of stomach-protective mucus, maintaining blood supply to the stomach, and decreasing acid production. COX-1 also plays a very important role in the kidney where COX-1 prostaglandins counteract vasoconstriction and allow vasodilation of the renal blood supply under conditions where renal blood supply would normally be decreased (e.g., hypotension).

In contrast, COX-2 is an enzyme that is only created when there is trauma or inflammation present in the tissue and it produces the prostaglandins associated with the clinical signs of inflammation. Thus from a simplistic view COX-1 could be said to be the "good guy" and COX-2 the "bad guy."

NSAIDs that selectively inhibit COX-2 without significantly inhibiting COX-1 would theoretically be able to decrease inflammation without decreasing production of the normal, helpful prostaglandins in the kidneys and stomach. This has been the advantage cited for the newer selective COX-2 inhibitory NSAIDs (called "coxibs") used in veterinary medicine since the mid-1990s.

Of course the real story of COX-1 and COX-2 is not as simple as that. For example, it has been found in mice that COX-2 (the "bad" COX) actually helps play some role in healing gastric ulcers in mice. And COX-1 (the "good" COX) produces some prostaglandins that actually enhance the inflammatory reaction. In addition, most of the drugs with selective COX-2 inhibition lose some or all of that selectivity for the COX-2 enzyme as the dose increases, meaning that at higher doses these drugs inhibit as much COX-1 enzyme as they do COX-2. Still, COX-2 selective inhibitor NSAIDs do have advantages over nonselective COX inhibitors at normal therapeutic doses by having fewer (but not totally eliminating) side effects on the stomach and kidney.

COX-2 selective inhibitor drugs approved for use in veterinary medicine include **carprofen** (e.g., Rimadyl, Novox, Quellin, Carpaquin, and other generics), **etodolac, deracoxib** (Deramaxx), **meloxicam** (Metacam and generics), and **robenacoxib** (Onsior). These drugs are discussed in greater detail later.

Nonsteroidal Antiinflammatory Drugs as Analgesics and Antipyretics

Although NSAIDs are, by their definition, antiinflammatory drugs, they also reduce fever (i.e., are antipyretic) and reduce the perception of pain (i.e., are analgesic). The antipyretic effect is not a particularly strong beneficial effect because an increased fever actually increases the ability of the body to fight virus and bacterial infections. However, the analgesic effect of NSAIDs is being used to a greater degree to prevent or diminish postoperative surgical pain.

It is known that when injury occurs (e.g., surgical incision), the initial trauma and pain signals from the nociceptors cause COX-2 enzymes to be produced (i.e., induced) in the spinal cord, leading to the phenomenon mentioned in Chapter 8 as

"wind-up." The spinal cord normally modulates or dampens the impulses of pain through the presence of naturally occurring opioids and by other signal pathways that decrease the ability of the pain-transmitting neurons in the spinal cord to depolarize as readily. However, when pain occurs in the body, the repeated pain signals sent to the spinal cord cause COX-2 enzymes to be generated in the spinal cord, which, in turn, produce prostaglandins that make the transmission of pain signals up the spinal cord more effective so that more pain signals are perceived by the conscious level of the brain. In addition, COX-generated prostaglandins at the injury site itself increase the ability of nociceptors to fire more readily, sending more pain signals to the spinal cord. This state of increased sensitivity or response to pain is called hyperalgesia, and it simply means that the injury hurts more.

COX-generated prostaglandins at the injury site are also involved in allodynia, which is the transmission of pain sensation by sensations or receptors that normally do not transmit pain (e.g., pressure, touch, hot, or cold receptors). You may have experienced this after an injury to a joint or limb wherein after 12 h or so, any touching of the affected area generates pain.

When NSAIDs are used before surgery, they block COX production of these prostaglandins in the spinal cord and at the injury site, which decreases the hyperalgesia and allodynia; reduces the number of pain signals being sent from the nociceptors; diminishes the number of pain nerve impulses successfully reaching the brain; and lessens the perception of pain (even though the injury still exists). By reducing the perception of pain in this manner, NSAIDs can be classified as analgesic drugs.[3]

Even though NSAIDs are effective at preventing hyperalgesia and wind-up, they are not very strong analgesics by themselves and are not very effective for relieving severe visceral pain (i.e., pain associated with organs, such as the intestine in equine colic) or severe somatic pain (i.e., pain associated with the body surface, such as burns or severe abrasions). Therefore, NSAIDs may play a more important role in preventing the wind-up phenomenon vs decreasing the pain after the pain response has begun.

Nonsteroidal Antiinflammatory Drug Precautions and Side Effects

For the most part, NSAIDs are safe drugs when the altered physiology caused by these drugs is understood by the veterinary professionals using them. Veterinary technicians can play an important role in preventing NSAID toxicosis or reducing the risk for significant side effects by ensuring that safeguards are in place for hospitalized animals and effectively communicating with clients whose animals are on NSAIDs at home.

The most common side effects of NSAIDs observed in patients are related to the GI tract. Prostaglandin E (PgE) is one of prostaglandins normally produced by COX-1 all the time to decrease the acidity of gastric secretions released during normal digestion, stimulate secretion of protective gastric mucus, stimulate secretion of sodium bicarbonate to neutralize the acidic stomach contents entering the intestine, increase the perfusion of the gastric mucosa with a healthy blood supply, and stimulate turnover and repair of the GI epithelial cells. The older nonselective COX inhibitor NSAIDs (e.g., aspirin, phenylbutazone) block prostaglandin production by both COX-1 (good) and COX-2 (bad). Without the beneficial COX-1 PgE, the acidity of the stomach increases and the protective mucus is not secreted to an adequate amount to protect the stomach wall; this results in injury to the cells of the stomach, inflammation of the stomach (i.e., gastritis) and, if the superficial cells of the stomach lining are eroded away, GI ulcers. Because of the gastritis, the affected animals lose their appetite, have vomiting and diarrhea, and have evidence of digested blood in the stool from ulcerations. Because the bleeding from these ulcers occurs near the stomach, the blood oozed into the GI tract lumen is digested and turns a dark, tarry black. This is called melena, and when melena appears in the stool, it suggests GI tract hemorrhage far up in the GI tract as opposed to the colon, where hemorrhage would appear as undigested red blood.

Most frequently, ulcerations appear in animals that have received an NSAID overdose (e.g., dog gets access to the tasty chewable NSAID tablets and eats the whole bottle) or have been on nonselective NSAIDs for an extended period of time. If evidence of ulceration appears (i.e., vomiting, melena, appearance of ulcers on an endoscopic examination of the upper GI tract), treatment must be initiated as described in Chapter 4 (antiulcer drugs). Antacids (e.g., H₂ blockers like cimetidine, H⁺ pump blockers like omeprazole), stomach protectants (e.g., sucralfate), and sometimes synthetic prostaglandins (e.g., misoprostol) are used to counteract the antiprostaglandin effect of NSAIDs on the GI tract. It is important to remember that these treatments will not prevent ulcer formation in animals receiving high doses of NSAIDs.

The second, but less frequent, target for NSAID adverse or toxic side effects is the kidney. As mentioned previously, beneficial prostaglandins normally vasodilate the vasculature in the kidney to keep blood flowing under conditions that would normally decrease renal blood flow (e.g., drop in arterial blood pressure, or hypotension). Thus a potential renal problem occurs when an animal has been presurgically medicated with NSAIDs to reduce pain and wind-up from the surgery and then experiences hypotension caused by anesthesia.

As was described in the cardiovascular chapter (Chapter 5), whenever there is a decrease in arterial blood pressure (i.e., hypotension) from any cause (e.g., blood loss, dehydration, drug-induced vasodilation of all arterioles, shock), the baroreceptors in the wall of the large arteries are no longer stretched as much, so they send fewer signals to the brain. These signals normally suppress the sympathetic nervous system; therefore, fewer signals from the baroreceptors means the sympathetic nervous system begins to become activated and sends out signals that, among other things, cause peripheral vasoconstriction (i.e., norepinephrine and epinephrine's effects on α₁ receptors). By reducing blood flow through nonessential tissues and organs not needed for a "fight or flight" situation, there is more blood to go to the brain and skeletal muscles. The kidneys are not considered essential during a fight or flight crisis, and therefore their vessels are also vasoconstricted, reducing blood flow to the kidney tissue.

Normally, when sympathetic nervous system vasoconstriction occurs in the kidney, it is dampened somewhat by COX generation of renal tissue–vasodilating prostaglandins to offset the vasoconstriction; hence, the kidney maintains adequate blood supply. However, if COX is blocked by NSAID treatment, then this vasodilation will not occur and the vasoconstriction will be strong enough to cause some parts of the kidney tissues to become hypoxic (i.e., low oxygen levels in the tissue) from inadequate blood supply (i.e., ischemia). The renal papillae are small projections into the renal pelvis made of collecting ducts from individual nephrons. The papillae dump urine into the open cavity of the renal pelvis, which funnels the urine into the ureters and then onto the bladder. These papillae have a relatively sparse blood supply and hence are very susceptible to the decreased renal blood flow. Thus, under these conditions of poor perfusion caused by systemic hypotension and sympathetic vasoconstriction, the renal papillae die of the tissue **hypoxia**, producing the condition renal papillary necrosis.

Although the newer COX-2 selective NSAIDs have less risk for GI adverse side effects than the nonselective older NSAIDs, in the kidney there is no significant advantage of COX-2 selectives over the older drugs because the COX-2 enzyme also produces renal vasodilating prostaglandins. Hence blocking only COX-2 enzyme would still reduce the compensatory vasodilation that protects the kidney during periods of hypotension.

The lowest incidence of organ/system side effects occurs with the liver. All NSAIDs, including selective COX inhibitors and the older nonselective COX inhibitors, have the potential to produce hepatotoxicity. The effect is considered to be rare compared with the GI and renal toxicity signs. Unlike GI and renal toxicity, which can be predicted based on the dose the animal is given or the conditions under which it is given, the hepatotoxicity is idiosyncratic, meaning that factors that predispose an animal to the hepatotoxicity are unknown, toxicity is not related to dose, and the occurrence of the problem is unpredictable. NSAID hepatotoxicity is not thought to be associated with preexisting liver problems; therefore, the presence of slightly elevated liver enzymes on a blood chemistry profile is not a contraindication to use NSAIDs.

All NSAIDs are tightly bound to plasma proteins (principally the protein albumin) circulating in the blood, and the dosages of NSAIDs take into account that protein-bound drug molecules will be unavailable to enter the target tissues and produce an effect. Thus the dose is formulated based upon the smaller percentage of free drug molecules. Under conditions of hypoproteinemia (i.e., low blood protein concentrations in the blood) or situations where another drug has been given that competes for the same binding site on the protein molecule, there are more NSAID molecules present in the free, nonprotein-bound form, and hence more molecules that can readily distribute from blood to the tissues and produce a greater effect than normal. This effect of hypoalbuminemia (i.e., low albumin protein in the blood) on protein binding and distribution was described in Chapter 3.

There is some debate as to how much clinical significance this increased free drug will actually have. Some experts take the stand that the relative amount of drug entering the tissue is significant enough that the risk for toxic side effects is increased under these conditions. Others say that more free, unbound molecules means more of the drug molecules will be rapidly excreted by renal filtration, reducing the blood concentration of the NSAID and reducing the number of free molecules available to enter the tissues. However, it is generally agreed that NSAIDs that are greater than 90% protein-bound are going to be most affected by hypoproteinemia or drug displacement from albumin because the relatively small fraction of the drug that is free to enter the tissues (10% for a drug that is 90% protein-bound) can be markedly increased by small variations in the number of free drug molecules.

For example, if there is a reduction in protein binding of only 5% of the total drug administered, this means that the total drug binding for a drug normally 90% protein-bound is reduced to 85% protein-bound. Although this does not seem like much, on a relative scale, going from 90% to 85% protein-bound means that the free portion, which is the fraction of the drug dose that is going to actually produce the effect of the NSAID in the tissues, increases from 10% to 15% of the total dose. This additional 5% increase in free drug molecules is an increase in drug mass that is distributing into the tissues by an additional 50%, which could potentially produce toxic concentrations in the tissues.

Contrast this with an NSAID that is normally only 40% protein-bound. In this case 60% of the dose will be in the free form and goes to the tissue to produce the effect. The dose for the drug will take into account that 60% of the dose will be the free form. If protein binding is decreased by 5%, increasing the free form by 5%, this will increase the amount entering the tissue from 60% to 65%, a relative increase of less than 10%. Regardless of to what degree NSAIDs are protein-bound under normal conditions, it is still prudent to carefully monitor any animal that is taking NSAIDs while it is experiencing hypoproteinemia or simultaneously taking another drug that may displace the NSAID molecules from their carrier proteins.

One advantage of this extensive protein binding is that plasma proteins are often exuded into the location of inflammation because of the decreased integrity of the capillaries in the inflamed area, and this exudation of plasma protein into the inflammation site delivers additional NSAID to the site and keeps it there for an extended period of time.

Cats are generally considered to be less tolerant of NSAIDs than most species because of their inherent slower liver metabolism. For this reason NSAIDs persist in the blood in their active forms for longer in cats, and the half-life of elimination for cats is at least twice as long as it is for dogs for the majority of the NSAIDs used in veterinary medicine. Thus the toxicity that cats are "predisposed" to does not necessarily reflect an increased reactivity or sensitivity to the drug itself but more about the accumulation of the drug if administered in a similar manner to dogs. For example, aspirin can be given to dogs on a daily basis, but the equivalent weighted dose in cats would produce toxicity after a few doses because of the slower elimination rate and the accumulation of drug to toxic levels. However, a reduced dose of aspirin given to a cat every 48 h would allow sufficient time for the drug to be eliminated between doses

and prevent the accumulation. The recommended or approved NSAID dosages for cats always take into account this species' limitation on metabolism. Note that acetaminophen, which is not an NSAID but is often thought of as one because of its antipyretic and analgesic effect, is toxic to cats and should not be given at any dosage or dosage interval.

Many of the NSAIDs, especially the newer COX-2 selective NSAIDs, may be eliminated by the liver as intact drug molecules that are reabsorbed into the body after the hepatic bile ducts dump the drug into the GI lumen. This enterohepatic circulation (see Chapter 3) accounts for the longer duration of action in the body by some of these drugs as they are recycled over and over.

The Classic Nonspecific Cyclooxygenase Inhibitor Nonsteroidal Antiinflammatory Drugs

The older NSAIDs include drugs like aspirin, phenylbutazone ("bute"), flunixin meglumine (e.g., the most recognized trade name is Banamine), ibuprofen (e.g., found in human OTC products Advil and Motrin), naproxen (e.g., found in human OTC product Aleve), and diclofenac sodium (e.g., in the topical equine NSAID called Surpass). The systemically absorbed drugs will tend to suppress both COX-1 and COX-2 enzymes and theoretically predispose the patient to more GI side effects than the COX-2 selective NSAIDs. It is important to remember that there is a great deal of interpatient variability for the responsiveness to any of these NSAIDs, which means that the ultimate degree of beneficial effect cannot be predicted. Instead, the dose needs to be adjusted (i.e., titrated) based upon the clinical response, or switched to another drug if it does not produce sufficient antiinflammatory or analgesic benefits.

Aspirin, which is also called salicylic acid or acetylsalicylic acid, is considered to be the prototype NSAID. The salicylates include other aspirin-like compounds such as bismuth subsalicylate, which is found in antidiarrheal preparations such as Pepto-Bismol and Kaopectate (see Chapter 4). In addition to its antiinflammatory effects, aspirin's COX inhibition also blocks formation of the thromboxanes that normally cause platelets to stick together to form a platelet plug, blocking small holes in capillaries or other vessels. Aspirin's inhibitory effect in platelets is considered irreversible, and thus once thromboxanes become inhibited in a platelet, they remain that way for the life of the platelet. The only way the thromboxane inhibition can be reversed is by generation of new platelets. This irreversible binding is characteristic of aspirin but not of other NSAIDs. This feature of aspirin is why aspirin is recommended to be used on a daily basis to reduce risk for spontaneous clot formation and subsequent heart attack caused by obstructed cardiac arteries.

Aspirin is also used to reduce spontaneous clot formation from cats predisposed to formation of aortic emboli from cardiomyopathy (see Chapter 6). Such therapy is designed to reduce the risk for clot formation at the caudal bifurcation (i.e., forking) of the dorsal aorta where it divides to pass into the hind legs. If a clot, usually called a saddle thrombus because of its shape, forms at this point it can markedly reduce or completely obstruct blood flow to the hind legs, resulting in eventual loss of the use of the limbs.

Because of its short half-life and GI side effects in horses, aspirin is not used very often for inflammation control in horses. However, it has been used systemically as part of the long-term treatment protocol for controlling recurring uveitis (i.e., inflammation of the iris and ciliary body of the eye) in the horse.

If aspirin is ever dispensed for use in a veterinary patient, it is extremely important that the veterinary technician thoroughly explain to the client that aspirin is not the same thing as other commonly used OTC human antiinflammatories like ibuprofen (e.g., Advil, Motrin), naproxen (e.g., Aleve), or acetaminophen (e.g., Tylenol), and these other products are never to be used in place of a pure aspirin product. Many clients do not differentiate between these common OTC human products because they may use them interchangeably. However, such interchangeable use with a veterinary patient could produce severe side effects or death of the animal.

Phenylbutazone ("bute") is an older NSAID that is still one of the more commonly used NSAIDs in equine medicine. In horses it is used for relief of musculoskeletal inflammation or decreasing laminitis (i.e., inflammation of the part of the inner hoof tissue that holds the hoof wall to the underlying bone in the horse) by nonselectively inhibiting COX enzymes and decreasing prostaglandin formation. Although it is widely used for musculoskeletal pain, it is not as effective in controlling pain from horse colic as some of the other NSAIDs or the opioid analgesics.

Phenylbutazone is highly protein-bound drug (greater than 99% bound in horses). The relatively small percentage of free drug available for distribution to tissues, and the percentage of the drug upon which the dosage regimen is based, varies considerably if the animal has low blood albumin levels (i.e., hypoalbuminemia) or the NSAID is displaced from the protein by other protein-bound drugs. Under hypoalbuminemic or hypoproteinemic conditions the dose of the phenylbutazone may need to be decreased to compensate for the increased free drug distributing into the tissues.

As mentioned previously, plasma proteins leaking out of damaged capillaries and into inflammation sites allows protein-bound phenylbutazone to enter the site and remain at the site of inflammation for longer than the drug remains in the plasma or blood. Thus, although the half-life of the drug in the blood is fairly short (4–8 h in the horse), in the tissues the half-life is closer to 24 h, reflecting the effect of the plasma proteins being present in the tissue itself.

The adverse effects of phenylbutazone are similar to those of other NSAIDs: risk of GI ulceration, renal papillary necrosis if renal perfusion is decreased, and retention of water and sodium from decreased renal function. Although dosages exist for use of phenylbutazone in dogs, the margin of safety or therapeutic index of phenylbutazone in that species makes it a poor choice given the availability of newer and more COX-2 selective NSAIDs.

Two other adverse effects associated with phenylbutazone include bone marrow suppression, resulting in neutropenia, thrombocytopenia, and anemia, and tissue necrosis; this occurs if an IV phenylbutazone dosage form is accidentally injected intramuscularly (IM) or subcutaneously (SQ). Bone marrow suppression is reported more commonly in people and dogs than horses. Because of the potential for bone marrow suppression and anemia in humans if they ingest this drug, phenylbutazone may not be used in any horses that could potentially be used for human food. In 1975 a jockey died from aplastic anemia (i.e., lack of production of red and white cells from the bone marrow) after taking phenylbutazone about 20 times over the span of 3 years.[8]

Note that the slang designation of "bute" for phenylbutazone can sometimes be confused with the slang "bute" used to indicate butorphanol, the opioid analgesic. Therefore, as a veterinary technician professional it is better to pronounce the whole name of the drug so as to be assured that the correct drug name is being communicated.

Flunixin meglumine (Banamine, Banamine-S) is approved for use in cattle, horses, and swine. Though originally used in horses for treatment of inflammation associated with musculoskeletal injuries and the pain associated with colic, it has found additional approved uses in cattle and swine for reducing fever (i.e., *antipyretic*) associated with respiratory disease, endotoxemia (i.e., a grave condition caused by the presence of bacterial toxins in the blood), and mastitis (i.e., inflammation of the udder or mammary gland). The drug seems to have greater analgesic effects than some of the other nonselective NSAIDs, and in some species it has been shown to decrease adverse effects from specific types of bacterial endotoxins, thus increasing the survivability from endotoxemia. Transdermal formulations for cattle have recently been FDA approved and have improved the ability to administer pain medication to cattle.

Although in dogs flunixin meglumine provides analgesia superior to that of aspirin or phenylbutazone, the sensitivity of the dog to flunixin GI toxicity limits its use to 3 days for visceral pain, postsurgical pain, or endotoxemia. Because of the GI toxicity in dogs, it has fallen out of favor for extra-label use in this species because the toxicity risks are too high compared with the risks from newer approved canine NSAIDs.

Diclofenac sodium (Surpass) is a topically applied NSAID for use in horses with lameness associated with the distal joints in the limbs (e.g., hock, pastern, fetlock, knee joints). When applied topically it penetrates the tissues and establishes therapeutic concentrations for about 6–18 h. Some of the drug is absorbed systemically enough to be detected in circulation; thus, theoretically the application of the drug to multiple sites on all four legs could result in enough systemically absorbed NSAID to produce systemic side effects. Horses seem to tolerate the drug well, but there have been multiple reports of dogs and cats showing signs of NSAID-related toxicity (i.e., GI signs of vomiting, diarrhea, melena) if the product is applied to their skin. Anyone applying the product must wear gloves to avoid absorbing the drug into their own body. Diclofenac is also available in an ophthalmic formulation to treat uveitis inflammation in horses, relieve inflammation in dogs that have had cataract surgery, or reduce allergic conjunctivitis (i.e., inflammation of the tissue of the eye from allergic reaction).

The human OTC NSAIDs ibuprofen (Advil, Motrin) and naproxen (Aleve) share common modes of action and side effects with other nonselective NSAIDs. The equine product of naproxen and another equine product related to ibuprofen called ketoprofen have both been discontinued. Therefore, the veterinary technician is most likely to encounter these drugs in veterinary patients when owners give their pets the same drugs they take for their own headaches, fever, and pain. Though these drugs are well tolerated in humans, both ibuprofen and naproxen consistently produce vomiting in dogs after a few days of treatment (or sooner), and deaths caused by GI bleeding from ulcerations have been reported. There is enough variability from veterinary patient to veterinary patient that is it almost impossible to determine how the animal is going to respond to a dose of these drugs. Therefore, the risk of using these drugs in veterinary patients is far too great to offset the antiinflammatory benefit. Practicing veterinary technicians should recognize the brand names and understand the potential dangers when well-meaning owners indiscriminately give these drugs to their animals.

The Selective Cyclooxygenase-2 Inhibitor Nonsteroidal Antiinflammatory Drugs

COX-2 inhibitors constitute the newest group of NSAIDs in veterinary medicine. Carprofen (Rimadyl) was the first COX-2 selective inhibitor drug released for use in veterinary medicine in the United States. Other COX-2 selective inhibitors include etodolac; deracoxib (Deramaxx), released in 2002; meloxicam (Metacam), released in 2003; firocoxib (Previcox, released for small animals in 2005, and Equioxx, released for horses in 2012); and robenacoxib (Onsior for cats), released in the United States in 2012 (available in Canada and the United Kingdom for dogs also).

The basis for the theoretical benefit of these drugs was previously described, as were some of the limitations of this benefit. It is important to remember that the degree to which each of these drugs is "selective" for COX-2 inhibition over COX-1 is still controversial because laboratory tests do not necessarily translate into a similar effect in the whole, living organism. Even the term "selective" is not used by some references, which prefer to use the term "preferential" COX-2 inhibitors to suggest there is still significant inhibition of both COX-1 and COX-2 enzymes, with slightly more inhibition of the COX-2. Thus claims about selectivity of a particular drug for COX-2 over COX-1 inhibition should not weigh heavily in choosing one selective COX-2 inhibitor NSAID over another.

It is important to remember that the GI side effects seen with the older nonselective COX inhibitor NSAIDs can also occur with the selective COX-2 inhibitors, especially at higher doses when the selectivity for COX-2 over COX-1 becomes less and less. Veterinary professionals should not become complacent and ignore the risk for gastritis and ulceration in animals on these drugs. The use of selective COX-2 inhibitors under conditions of hypotension can still produce renal papillary necrosis because COX-2–generated prostaglandins are the renal vasodilators that keep blood flowing into the kidney. Thus, avoiding

dehydration or any other cause of decreased arterial blood pressure is still important with this class of drugs.

One of the unintended problems arising from some of the oral COX-2 inhibitors comes from the flavoring of the chewable tablets. The flavoring agents added to the soft-chewable tablets have been so effective in encouraging animals to ingest the tablets that there have been several reports of dogs that chewed apart dropped bottles of the flavored formulations of these drugs and ingested large numbers of the flavorful tablets, causing NSAID toxicosis. Clients should be informed that these chewable medications need to be stored safely away from the pet to avoid this overdose situation.

Note that one of the uses for COX-2 selective inhibitor NSAIDs is at very high doses for treating cancer. Although not mentioned specifically with each drug later on, several of these drugs have been used in clinical trials to determine their efficacy for treating cancers like transitional cell carcinoma of the bladder in the dog. Therefore, the veterinary technician should not be surprised to hear of these drugs being part of a cancer chemotherapy protocol.

Carprofen (Rimadyl) was the first selective COX-2 inhibitory drug for dogs. Like the other COX-2 selectives, it is an antiinflammatory with analgesic and antipyretic activity. Unlike the older nonselective NSAIDs, carprofen does not inhibit thromboxane in platelets like aspirin does; hence carprofen does not have the same action to decrease clot formation nor is there a concern about using carprofen with other drugs used to reduce clots (like warfarin).

After its initial release carprofen received a tremendous amount of negative publicity in the popular press regarding unexpected deaths in a few dogs from hepatotoxicity. The facts surrounding these deaths were often not correctly reported, and many clients became fearful of putting their pets on this drug. Therefore, it is important that the veterinary technician be aware of the information surrounding this hepatotoxicity because such a side effect is a rare possibility with any of the COX-2 selective inhibitory NSAIDs.

- The toxicity studies done before carprofen approval showed only mild changes to the liver even at high doses for periods extending up to a year.
- Of 1 million dogs receiving carprofen, the incidence of hepatic-related side effects was 0.02%, or about 200 out of 1,000,000. These 200 reports were not of fatal hepatopathies, but any liver-related side effect, no matter how mild.[1]
- Labrador retrievers were overrepresented in the cases reported, prompting rumors that this breed was predisposed to liver problems. However, liver side effects have been reported in almost every breed of dog over the years, and the initial report did not take into account the popularity of the Labrador retriever and that this breed is one that is prone to arthritic problems, for which carprofen would be prescribed. The consensus is that no particular breed is predisposed.
- In one study of 21 dogs admitted to a veterinary hospital for liver-related disease after treatment with NSAIDs, biopsies of the liver revealed signs consistent with some degree of hepatocellular necrosis; four of these dogs died but the rest recovered.[1]

- No factor related to age, breed, concurrent drug administration, gender, dose, or other variables has ever been consistently and repeatedly identified as a predisposing indicator for hepatocellular damage, although each of these factors was at some point considered to be a possible indicator for risk. This reaction thus appears to be idiosyncratic.

This adverse reaction continues to studied and evaluated. Earlier detection of problems, withdrawal of the drug, and treatment with "hepatoprotective agents" allow greater odds of recovery from liver-related disease associated with this rare, idiosyncratic reaction. It is important to emphasize that in spite of the publicity this hepatotoxicity generated, these newer NSAID drugs are quite safe compared with the older drugs that were used for so many years.

Although carprofen is not approved for use in cats in the United States, it is approved for use in the United Kingdom for cats, horses, and cattle. In cats it is only given once because cats, like dogs, do get GI side effects related to gastric ulceration. As would be expected with a hepatically metabolized drug, carprofen is more slowly eliminated in the cat than the dog, with the elimination half-life in cats being almost double that in dogs (elimination takes twice as long in the cat).[1]

Etodolac was originally approved for use to treat osteoarthritis in the dog. The original compound, EtoGesic, was withdrawn from the market in 2014, but generic compounds are still available as tablets for oral use. There was some suggestion that etodolac had a higher incidence of GI adverse effects than carprofen, but studies were not definitive. Although reports of liver disease have not appeared with etodolac, anecdotal reports have circulated consistently.[1] One of the unique side effects of this drug was the incidence of keratoconjunctivitis sicca (KCS), or dry eye, reported as a side effect. This is similar to the side effect seen with sulfonamide antibiotics (see Chapter 10). The rate of incidence of KCS is unknown. Although etodolac is used less than carprofen, it is still considered to be an effective once-daily drug for reducing pain and inflammation associated with canine hip dysplasia.[1]

Deracoxib (Deramaxx) is a drug approved as a continually administered NSAID for osteoarthritis pain, similar to the indications for carprofen and etodolac. However, deracoxib is also approved at a higher dose (i.e., double the osteoarthritis dose) for treatment of postoperative pain for a maximum of 7 days. Its incidence of GI side effects is about that of the other drugs in this group, but the manufacturer suggests that feeding the animal at the time of the drug administration may reduce some of the incidence of vomiting. Like most of the other NSAIDs in this group, the drug is only approved for use in dogs; information on extra-label use in cats is scarce, and its use is not recommended.

Meloxicam (Metacam) is approved for use in the dog for osteoarthritis, pain, and inflammation and is one of the few NSAIDs approved for use in cats in the United States as a single treatment for pain from orthopedic surgeries or castration. Though the US dosage forms forbid repeated dosages, lower doses of meloxicam are approved for use in a repeating dose manner in other countries outside of the United States. There is a good deal of discussion and argument about how safe the drug is for continued use beyond the single injection in cats, and although evidence exists to suggests its safety, there have been severe side effects reported in cats given more than the single dose of meloxicam.

The drug is approved in the United Kingdom for use in horses to treat pain from colic and for use with antibiotics to treat clinical signs associated with respiratory or GI disease in cattle. Additionally, there are extra-label dosages for swine, ferrets, birds, and reptiles, reflecting its uses in multiple species. Still, incidences of GI toxicity have been reported in dogs, hepatotoxicity has been reported in humans taking the drug, and cases of GI perforation were reported in dogs, raising the question as to whether meloxicam might be more of a GI toxicity risk than some of the other drugs. Generally, this drug is considered to be a good analgesic comparable to other NSAIDs of this class, but does occasionally need opioid analgesia supplementation to achieve desired levels of postsurgical analgesia.

Firocoxib (Previcox, Equioxx) is an NSAID approved for use in dogs and horses to control pain from osteoarthritis and orthopedic surgery. As this is one of the newer drugs in this class, it has not had a long toxicity profile, and therefore most of the adverse effects noted are consistent with those observed with the rest of the drugs of this group. Although not approved for use in the cat in the United States at this time, some preliminary studies have shown favorable results when firocoxib was used in the cat, perhaps foretelling its use in cats in the future.

Robenacoxib (Onsior) is somewhat unique in that is it approved in the United States for cats and not dogs. It is approved for use in dogs in other countries, however. This is the newest NSAID to be added to veterinary medicine, and its uses and expected side effects are similar to other drugs in this group. One difference from the other NSAIDs that are used in cats is that this drug is approved for use for up to 3 days in cats in the United States and for up to 6 days in the United Kingdom. This additional length of time provides for continued analgesia beyond the 24-h postsurgical period a single-injection NSAID cat product would provide. Both robenacoxib and some of the other more recently released NSAIDs include a caution to owners of treated animals to report any decrease in appetite or yellowing of the eyes (i.e., icterus), reflecting the awareness of the potential for hepatotoxicity and educating the owner on signs associated with this rare side effect.

OTHER ANTIINFLAMMATORY DRUGS

Dimethyl sulfoxide (DMSO) is a compound originally developed as an industrial solvent derived from wood pulp that has also found use in the pharmaceutical industry and research as an answer to dissolve drugs that do not readily dissolve in water. DMSO in veterinary medicine is used as an FDA-approved drug for horses and dogs to reduce swelling caused by trauma. It is also included in an otic antiinflammatory product to enhance the absorption of the glucocorticoid antiinflammatory in the product. However, DMSO's extra-label uses are much broader and include stabilizing tissues after ischemic (i.e., low oxygen) conditions; treatment of CNS trauma and edema; treatment of skin wounds and burns; reducing the inflammation of the lining of the uterus (i.e., endometritis); lessening mammary tissue swelling in lactating animals; and decreasing otherwise uncontrollable pain. Unfortunately most of these uses are anecdotal, and controlled clinical studies with effectiveness data are lacking.

DMSO does not produce its antiinflammatory effect through blocking prostaglandin synthesis, even though it does block the production of some prostaglandins. Instead DMSO works mainly by inactivating superoxide radicals ($O_2^{\bullet}$) that are generated by macrophages during cleanup of the inflammatory process. These superoxide radicals can be chemically turned into hydrogen peroxide and then into hydroxyl radicals ($OH^{\bullet}$) (the "dot" on the formula indicates it is a radical), which damage cell membranes, deoxyribonucleic acid (DNA), and other cellular structures. DMSO traps or "scavenges" the hydroxyl radicals, and the metabolite of DMSO called DMS traps superoxide radicals. The combined activity reduces the cellular damage produced secondary to the inflammatory process. DMSO also has a direct analgesic effect by a mechanism that is not understood.

DMSO is best known for its ability to penetrate intact skin and has been used as a vehicle to carry dissolved drugs into the body when applied topically. Unfortunately DMSO can also carry toxins or harmful substances that may be on the skin where the DMSO is applied. Therefore, the skin in the area of application should be thoroughly cleansed to avoid absorption of bacterial toxins or other chemicals such as oil, grease, and insecticides. People applying DMSO as a gel or topical solution should protect themselves by wearing high-quality rubber gloves and applying the medication with swabs and forceps. One DMSO product comes in a spray that can be applied without contacting the drug itself during application.

The smell of DMSO is said to resemble garlic or raw oysters. This odor is evident during topical application, and the drug can sometimes be tasted after it is absorbed into the body. Because of the potent smell, DMSO should only be applied in an open outside area or a well-ventilated indoor area. After DMSO is applied topically, erythema (i.e., redness), edema, and pruritus may develop at the application site. These reactions reflect DMSO's effect on mast cells to release histamine and other vasoactive amines into the skin. Although the localized cutaneous reaction is usually mild, a more severe reaction may occur if the animal has mast cell tumors and the absorbed DMSO causes these large aggregates of mast cells to release huge amounts of histamine.

Although there are no veterinary-approved formulations available for IV use, DMSO has been used for years in horses as an IV product. However, higher concentrations of DMSO administered via IV can cause severe hemolysis, passage of liberated hemoglobin into the urine (i.e., hemoglobinuria), and renal damage from the hemoglobin in the renal tubules. There is also little scientific evidence to demonstrate the effectiveness of IV-administered DMSO over topically applied DMSO because the topical administration is absorbed systemically and distributes to every tissue in the body.

DMSO is very hygroscopic, meaning that it readily absorbs water from the air. Therefore, any container must be tightly capped after use. Also, the solvent quality of DMSO can damage some plastics, fabrics, or other materials.

Chondroprotective agents protect the cartilage (*chondro-*, meaning cartilage) from degradation. There are several products available designed to promote repair of the joint cartilage and slow the degenerative process of arthritis in joints. Some of these compounds are regulated drugs and others are largely unregulated nutraceuticals that are technically classified as food with

health-giving properties. Though there is scientific evidence to indicate that some of these products do help either as sole agents or as adjunct compounds (i.e., secondary to another drug), there are also less rigorous studies cited in newspapers, magazines, and online that show positive "effects" of the compound and improvement in the medical condition. However, without comparing the compound effect to a placebo effect (i.e., a compound without any effect; e.g., sterile water, saline) the reader has no idea whether the observed "effect" from the compound was caused by the product or simply because of the normal healing processes of the body itself. As these types of products and their claims are widely advertised in human medicine, the veterinary technician should be familiar enough with the names of the products, the claims made by the manufacturer, and whether data exist to back the claim so they can more effectively educate an animal owner if asked about such products.

Polysulfated glycosaminoglycans (PSGAGs) are injectable chondroprotective agents that mimic the components of normal joint cartilage. These rather large and complex molecules in joint cartilage trap molecules of water and give cartilage its springy characteristic and ability to tolerate stressful shocks. However, the joint benefit from PSGAGs comes from increased generation of new chondrocytes and the cartilage matrix and simultaneously inhibiting the activity of destructive enzymes in the joint fluid that degrade cartilage. The FDA-approved veterinary product Adequan is approved for use in dogs and horses for injured joints (i.e., either from trauma or surgical intervention) or to decrease degeneration of joints because of conformation problems (e.g., hip dysplasia). They have few side effects; more side effects are related to the injection technique itself than the drug.

Zycosan™ (pentosan polysulfate sodium injection) is a once weekly, for 4 weeks, IM injection approved for horses with osteoarthritis. This medication was approved by the FDA in December, 2022. There is a lot to still learn about this medication; however, it has demonstrated efficacy for the treatment of clinical signs of osteoarthritis with the most common side effect being injection site swelling and pain.

Hyaluronic acid or **hyaluronate sodium** is an essential component of the synovial fluid; it increases the thickness or viscosity of the joint fluid and, in so doing, acts as a lubricant for contact between cartilage surfaces. In addition, hyaluronic acid or hyaluronate sodium acts as an antiinflammatory compound through its suppression of prostaglandin production and by scavenging free radicals that are destructive to the joint cartilage and tissue. The veterinary products Legend, Hyalovet, and others are injected either systemically IV or into the joint space (i.e., intraarticularly) to relieve inflammation of the *synovium* (i.e., tissue surrounding the joint). Although this product has been used in the dog, no controlled studies have demonstrated a beneficial effect in dogs, so its use is not generally recommended in that species. There are many different equine injectable products available, so it is important to read the package insert information on each product because the limitations or different routes of administration by which the compound is to be safely used vary.

Glucosamine and chondroitin sulfate are orally administered OTC products referred to as nutraceuticals because they are used like drugs but are actually food products containing natural compounds found in the body or used by the body for normal healthy function. Nutraceuticals are not regulated by the FDA, and their labels, by law, cannot imply that the compound is to be used as a therapeutic agent.

Though there has been some evidence generated that suggests animals with osteoarthritis improve when given these nutraceuticals, there are no well-controlled clinical studies that demonstrate the effectiveness of these products over placebos. Glucosamine and chondroitin sulfate are actually precursors for PSGAG formation produced by the chondrocytes and for the proteoglycans that are found in cartilage. Chondroitin sulfate binds with collagen fibers in the cartilage and supports the collagen strands. The presence of both chondroitin and glucosamine in the serum increases efficiency of the chondrocytes to repair cartilage, stimulates production of hyaluronic acid (glucosamine's action), and inhibits some of the destructive enzymes found in injured or diseased cartilage (chondroitin's action). The challenge with these products is the variability in the amount of active product because some products are extracts from living organisms (e.g., mussel, sea cucumber, sea algae, shark cartilage) and others are purified extracts (more expensive). Cosequin is perhaps the best known trade name of the glucosamine/chondroitin sulfate nutraceuticals used in veterinary medicine, but there are many other products available OTC to the public.

Acetaminophen is not an antiinflammatory drug. However, because of its analgesic and antipyretic (i.e., fever-reducing) properties, it is often grouped with NSAIDs. Unlike NSAIDs, acetaminophen (Tylenol) does not block prostaglandin formation associated with inflammation but reduces the perception of pain by a mechanism not clearly defined and decreases the effect of endogenous pyrogens (i.e., substances that increase fever).

Acetaminophen does not cause the GI upset, ulcers, or interference with platelet clumping associated with NSAIDs. However, the metabolites of acetaminophen can have other severe side effects, especially in cats. Acetaminophen is normally conjugated with glucuronic acid and sulfate for metabolism and elimination. A small portion of acetaminophen is also metabolized to a toxic metabolite. In most species this toxic metabolite is quickly conjugated with glutathione to form a nontoxic metabolite. Because of the relatively less effective glucuronide and sulfate conjugation in cats, more of the toxic metabolite tends to be produced. Unfortunately, the supply of glutathione needed by the liver to biotransform this toxic metabolite to a nontoxic metabolite is limited in the cat. Therefore, the toxic metabolite accumulates in the liver and other tissues, producing cellular destruction.

In addition to liver damage, the red blood cells are also severely affected. The hemoglobin in red blood cells is converted to methemoglobin, which is much less capable of efficient oxygen transport. Increased red blood cell hemolysis and Heinz bodies are evident on blood smears. Cats with methemoglobinemia have chocolate-colored mucous membranes and dark urine, caused by methemoglobin in the blood and urine.

An acetaminophen dose of 50–60 mg/kg can poison a cat. A single extra-strength acetaminophen tablet (i.e., 500 mg) can kill an average-size cat. In dogs, a higher dose (above 150 mg/kg) is required before signs of hepatic necrosis, weight loss, and icterus (i.e., jaundice) become evident.

Treatment of acetaminophen toxicity focuses on providing sulfhydryl groups of glutathione to convert the toxic metabolite to its nontoxic form. The drug most commonly used to treat acetaminophen toxicity is acetylcysteine (Mucomyst), a mucolytic agent used in treatment of respiratory infections.

ANTIINFLAMMATORY DRUGS

Corticosteroids (Adrenocorticosteroids)
Mineralocorticoids
  Desoxycorticosterone pivalate (Percorten-V)
Glucocorticoids
  Short-acting (<12 h)
  Hydrocortisone
  Cortisone
  Intermediate-acting (12–36 h)
  Prednisone
  Prednisolone
  Methylprednisolone
  Triamcinolone
  Long-acting (≥48 h)
  Dexamethasone
  Betamethasone
  Flumethasone
  Isoflupredone (PREDEF)

NSAIDs
Nonspecific cyclooxygenase (COX) inhibitors
  Aspirin
Phenylbutazone
Flunixin meglumine (Banamine)
Diclofenac sodium (Surpass)
Ibuprofen (Advil, Motrin)
Naproxen (Aleve)
Selective COX-2 inhibitors
  Carprofen (Rimadyl)
  Etodolac
  Deracoxib (Deramaxx)
  Meloxicam (Metacam)
  Firocoxib (Previcox, Equioxx)
  Robenacoxib (Onsior)

Other Antiinflammatory Drugs
Dimethyl sulfoxide (DMSO)
Chondroprotective agents
  Polysulfated glycosaminoglycans (PSGAGs)
  Hyaluronic acid/hyaluronate sodium
  Glucosamine and chondroitin sulfate (Cosequin)
Acetaminophen

REFERENCES

1. Boothe DM. Antiinflammatory drugs. In: *Small Animal Clinical Pharmacology and Therapeutics*. Philadelphia: Saunders; 2012:1045–1118.
2. Adams RH. Prostaglandins, related factors, and cytokines. In: Riviere J, Papich M, eds. *Veterinary Pharmacology and Therapeutics*. Ames, Iowa: Wiley-Blackwell; 2009:439–456.
3. Boothe DM, Mealey KA. Glucocorticoids and mineralocorticoids. In: *Small Animal Clinical Pharmacology and Therapeutics*. Philadelphia: Saunders; 2012:1119–1149.
4. Ferguson DC, Dirikolu L, Hoenig M. Glucocorticoids, mineralocorticoids, and adrenolytic drugs. In: Riviere J, Papich M, eds. *Veterinary Pharmacology and Therapeutics*. Ames, Iowa: Wiley-Blackwell; 2009:771–802.
5. Graham-Mize CA, Rosser EJ, Hauptman J. In: *Absorption, bioavailability and activity of prednisone and prednisolone in cats. Proceedings of the Fifth World Congress Veterinary Dermatology. Philadelphia*; 2005:152–158.
6. van den Broek AH, Stafford WL. Epidermal and hepatic glucocorticoid receptors in cats and dogs. *Res Vet Sci*. 1992;52 (3):312–315.
7. Feldman EC, Nelson RW. Glucocorticoid therapy. In: *Canine and Feline Endocrinology and Reproduction*. 3rd ed. St. Louis, Missouri: WB Saunders; 2004:464–484.
8. Ramsey R, Golde DW. Aplastic anemia from veterinary phenylbutazone. *JAMA*. 1976;236(9):1049.

SELF-ASSESSMENT

1. Fill in the following blanks with the correct item from the Key Terms list.

A. _____ These are the sensory receptors specifically for pain.

B. _____ This is the series of steps that starts with trauma to cell membranes and ends with the production of compounds that produce the clinical signs of inflammation.

C. _____ This is the collective name for inflammatory mediators that includes prostaglandins and leukotrienes.

D. _____ In the arachidonic acid cascade, this is the enzyme that begins the process by breaking down molecules that make up the cell membrane of the traumatized cell.

E. _____ This enzyme converts phospholipids to arachidonic acid.

F. _____ This enzyme converts arachidonic acid to prostaglandins and thromboxanes.

G. _____ This enzyme converts arachidonic acid to leukotrienes.

H. _____ This compound, when activated, causes platelets to adhere to each other to form a platelet plug (i.e., clot).

I. _____ This is the name of the *broad category* of corticosteroid drugs that reduces inflammation.

J. _____ This is the enzyme that is blocked by glucocorticoids in the arachidonic acid cascade.

K. _____ This term describes a collective term for all of the steroid hormones produced by the adrenal cortex.

L. _____ This is the outer layer of the adrenal gland.

M. _____ This is the collective term for adrenocorticosteroids that are involved with the balance of water and electrolytes in the body.

N. _____ This is the principal mineralocorticoid hormone produced by the adrenal gland that causes retention of sodium.

O. _____ This is the other name for Addison's disease that describes the state of the adrenal gland.

P. _____ This means "elevated blood levels of potassium."

Q. _____ This is produced by the hypothalamus and stimulates release of adrenocorticotropic hormone (ACTH).

R. _____ This is released by the pituitary in response to stimulation from corticotropin-releasing hormone (CRH).

S. _____ This refers to the dosage form of glucocorticoid in which the drug is combined with sodium phosphate or sodium succinate to make it water soluble.

T. _____ This refers to the dosage form of glucocorticoid in which the drug is completely dissolved in a liquid medium that is not water based; the label only lists the glucocorticoid name without sodium phosphate, pivalate, or diacetate.

U. _____ This refers to the dosage form of glucocorticoid in which the drug is complexed with diacetate, pivalate, acetonide, or valerate.

V. _____ When higher concentrations of glucocorticoids are achieved in the body than could be produced by natural body processes, the concentrations are said to be this.

W. _____ This is the process by which the liver converts amino acids into glucose.

X. _____ This term means the "breakdown" of tissue such as the breakdown of skeletal muscle protein into amino acids.

Y. _____ This term refers to the shrinking of tissues or organs.

Z. _____ This describes the overreaction of the body to its own tissues in which case it starts attacking its own cells.

AA. _____ This describes the type of immune reaction in which the body overreacts to external antigens in an allergic type of response.

AB. _____ The lymphocytes responsible for cell-mediated immunity.

AC. _____ The type of immunity that produces antibodies.

AD. _____ The type of lymphocyte that produces antibodies.

AE. _____ This term refers specifically to that part of the complete blood count (CBC) analysis that describes the different white blood cell numbers.

AF. _____ This means "decreased lymphocytes in the blood."

AG. _____ This means "decreased monocytes in the blood."

AH. _____ This means "decreased eosinophils in the blood."

AI. _____ This means "increased neutrophils in the blood."

AJ. _____ This term collectively describes the leukogram changes in the previous four questions.

AK. _____ This term means "increased urination volume."

AL. _____ This term means "increased drinking."

AM. _____ This is the natural hormone that prevents excessive loss of water into the urine; it conserves water in the body.

AN. _____ This specific enzyme breaks down the middle protein layer of the cornea under the influence of glucocorticoid eye drops.

AO. _____ This is another name for hyper-adrenocorticism.

AP. _____ This is another name for hypo-adrenocorticism.

AQ. _____ This term means "the doctor caused it."

AR. _____ This term means "increased eating."

AS. _____ This term refers to the loss of hair or a thin hair coat.

AT. _____ This cyclooxygenase (COX) always exists in the tissues and is responsible for normal functioning of the tissue or organ.

AU. _____ This COX becomes activated with trauma and produces prostaglandins responsible for the signs of inflammation.

AV. _____ This single word is a term coined in the 1990s to specifically describe the selective COX-2 inhibitory nonsteroidal antiinflammatory drugs (NSAIDs).

AW. _____ This means "a drug that reduces fever."

AX. _____ This means "a drug that reduces the perception of pain."

AY. _____ This refers to the state of having increased sensitivity or perception of pain.

AZ. _____ This refers to the phenomenon where a few hours after injury to a location, the other sensory receptors (e.g., light touch, pressure, hot, cold) in that area also begin to send signals that are interpreted as pain.

BA. _____ This means "inflammation of the stomach."

BB. _____ This term describes the dark tarry stool that results from digested blood that originated from bleeding in the stomach or duodenum.

BC. _____ This term refers to low levels of oxygen in the tissues.

BD. _____ These anatomic structures in the kidney are where the collecting ducts from the individual nephrons come together and dump urine into the renal pelvis.

BE. _____ This is the cavity in the middle of the kidney that funnels urine into the ureter.

BF. _____ This kidney condition results from having NSAIDs in a patient that becomes hypotensive.

BG. _____ This means "low protein in the blood."

BH. _____ This means "low albumin in the blood."

BI. _____ These are two other names for aspirin.

BJ. _____ This is inflammation of the iris and ciliary body in the eye.

BK. _____ This is inflammation of the tissue that holds the hoof wall to the underlying bone in the foot of the horse.

BL. _____ This is when the bone marrow is unable to produce red or white blood cells.

BM. _____ This term means "reducing fever."

BN. _____ This condition is associated with poisons released from bacteria floating in the bloodstream.

BO. _____ This means inflammation of the udder.

BP. _____ These are two very reactive molecules produced by macrophages during inflammation that are targeted by dimethyl sulfoxide (DMSO).

BQ. _____ Prefix that means "cartilage."

BR. _____ This term describes food-type supplements with health giving properties; they are not regulated by the Food and Drug Administration (FDA).

BS. _____ Term that describes "low sodium in the blood."

2. Fill in the following blanks with the correct drug from the Antiinflammatory Drugs list. When practicing these questions, write out the answers on a separate sheet, focusing also on the appropriate spelling of these drug names.

A. _____ This is salicylic acid.

B. _____ This is the short-acting glucocorticoid made from the precursor cortisone.

C. _____ This old equine NSAID is 99% protein-bound in the horse and produces aplastic anemia in humans.

D. _____ These are the three -pred compounds most commonly used in veterinary medicine.

E. _____ This antiinflammatory is a solvent that easily carries other drugs, chemicals, or poisons through the skin and into the body.

F. _____ This selective COX-2 inhibitor NSAID is approved for two dose levels: one for osteoarthritis and a higher one for postoperative pain.

G. _____ This NSAID produces irreversible inhibition of thromboxane in platelets.

H. _____ This is the mineralocorticoid drug.

I. _____ This antiinflammatory does not work by inhibiting COX but by scavenging reactive radical molecules that damage healthy tissue.

J. _____ This nonselective COX inhibitor NSAID is also thought to be effective for reducing the effects of endotoxins.

K. _____ This is the long-acting glucocorticoid that is not a "methasone" drug.

L. _____ This was the first COX-2 selective inhibitor NSAID in veterinary medicine.

M. _____ Not an antiinflammatory but an antipyretic and analgesic that is very toxic to cats.

N. _____ This selective COX-2 inhibitor NSAID is unique in that it was developed specifically for the cat and is not approved for use in the dog in the United States; can be given for up to 3 days in the cat.

O. _____ Glucocorticoid drug that is most like natural cortisol.

P. _____ This selective COX-2 inhibitor NSAID received a great deal of sometimes inaccurate publicity because of a few reports of hepatotoxicity.

Q. _____ This over-the-counter (OTC) NSAID has been used systemically to decrease inflammation associated with recurrent uveitis in horses.

R. _____ This short-acting glucocorticoid must be activated by the liver to be effective.

S. _____ These are the three commonly used "methasones" used in veterinary medicine.

T. _____ This nonselective COX inhibitor NSAID is applied topically to the legs of horses; do not use in dogs; compound is absorbed through the skin.

U. _____ These are two common OTC human NSAIDs that are not used to treat veterinary patients but can be seen in practice as toxicosis cases from owners using these in place of aspirin or veterinary NSAIDs.

V. _____ This selective COX-2 inhibitor NSAID is still used but produces keratoconjunctivitis sicca (KCS) as one of its side effects.

W. _____ This antiinflammatory is applied topically but causes mast cells to release histamine; should not be used in animals with mast cell tumors.

X. _____ This injectable chondroprotective agent is an essential component of synovial fluid; it provides additional lubrication and has antiinflammatory qualities.

Y. _____ This is the intermediate-acting glucocorticoid whose name does not include "pred."

Z. _____ This selective COX-2 inhibitor NSAID is one of the few for which a single dose is allowed to be used in cats; it is not to be given more than once in cats because of side effects.

AA. _____ This antiinflammatory drug stinks like garlic or oysters; it must be applied topically in a well-ventilated place.

AB. _____ This injectable chondroprotective agent mimics the components of normal joint cartilage but also inhibits destructive enzymes in the joint space.

AC. _____ This NSAID is used to prevent spontaneous clot formation in people and cats with cardiomyopathy.

AD. _____ This orally administered nutraceutical chondroprotective agent is actually a precursor for PSGAG formation by the chondrocytes.

3. What do these abbreviations stand for?

ACTH _____
COX _____
ADH _____
KCS _____
PSGAG _____

4. Indicate whether each of the following statements is true or false.

A. Glucocorticoids decrease inflammation in the arachidonic acid cascade primarily by inhibiting COX.

B. COX and phospholipase are eicosanoids.

C. Lipoxygenase produces leukotrienes.

D. The adrenal cortex is the central core of the adrenal gland.

E. Aldosterone's function is primarily to retain sodium in the body while allowing excretion of potassium.

F. Cushing's disease is hyperadrenocorticism.

G. In hypoadrenocorticism the animals have hyponatremia and hyperkalemia.

H. Hydrocortisone is the precursor drug to cortisone.

I. Increased ACTH would produce increased secretion of CRH.

J. Elevated levels of cortisol decrease release of CRH and ACTH.

K. Triamcinolone has a longer duration of effect than isoflupredone.

L. An every-other-day dose of dexamethasone is more likely to cause atrophy of the adrenal gland over time than an every-other-day dose of prednisolone.

M. Dexamethasone diacetate is more likely to be given intravenously (IV) than dexamethasone sodium phosphate.

N. The antiinflammatory dose of a glucocorticoid is typically lower than the immunosuppressive dose.

O. The doses of glucocorticoid drugs produce supraphysiologic concentrations of glucocorticoids.

P. Gluconeogenesis is the conversion of amino acids into glucose.

Q. Atrophy is the _breakdown_ of structures in the body, and catabolism is the _shrinking_ of structures in the body.

R. If a diabetic patient needed its insulin dose adjusted after being placed on a high dose of dexamethasone, the insulin dose would most likely need to be _decreased_.

S. Hypersensitivity reactions are to _external_ substances, and autoimmune reactions are to _internal_ cells or tissues.

T. T cells produce antibodies.

U. Humoral immunity produces antibodies.

V. The stress leukogram is characterized by neutrophilia, monocytosis, and lymphopenia.

W. Glucocorticoids _inhibit_ the action of antidiuretic hormone (ADH).

X. Idiosyncratic Cushing's means that the Cushing's disease was caused by the veterinarian.

Y. Cats are much more sensitive to the effects of glucocorticoids than dogs.

Z. If an animal is showing signs of hyperadrenocorticism after several weeks of being on glucocorticoid drugs, the drugs should be stopped immediately before further damage occurs.

AA. COX-1 produces the prostaglandins most often associated with inflammation.

AB. An antipyretic drug is one that decreases the perception of pain.

AC. Allodynia is the perception of pain from signals sent by sensory receptors other than the nociceptors.

AD. Opioids are better analgesics than the NSAIDs.

AE. Melena is bright, red blood observed in the feces from intestinal bleeding.

AF. Prostaglandins in the stomach increase mucus production and decrease stomach acid production.

AG. Renal papillary necrosis occurs when an animal becomes hypertensive (i.e., elevated blood pressure) and is on NSAIDs at the same time.

AH. The factors that predispose a dog to NSAID-related hepatotoxicity are well defined and predictable.

AI. Liver toxicity from NSAIDs occurs more frequently than renal toxicity.

AJ. If an animal has a severe hypoproteinemia, the dose of any NSAID given should be *increased* to compensate.

AK. In most circumstances it should be okay to substitute a tablet of ibuprofen for a tablet of aspirin in the dog, but that should not be done in the cat.

AL. Veterinarians and veterinary technicians do not need to bother advising pet owners about looking for signs of gastrointestinal (GI) toxicity when using COX-2 selective NSAIDs; such problems do not occur with these drugs because of their COX-2 selectivity.

AM. Labrador retrievers are much more predisposed to have side effects from carprofen than any other dog breed.

AN. Robenacoxib is approved in the United States for cats but not dogs.

AO. Nutraceuticals must still conform to the same standards set by the Food and Drug Administration (FDA) as other drugs.

AP. Acetaminophen, if used in dogs or people, is much more likely to produce gastritis than aspirin.

AQ. The antidote for acetaminophen toxicosis in cats is acetylcysteine.

AR. Vaccinations should not be given to a dog on an antiinflammatory dose of prednisone because the body will be unable to generate sufficient antibody response.

AS. The two most common organ systems for toxicity from NSAIDs are the kidney and the liver.

AT. NSAIDs should be able to provide enough analgesia to manipulate an animal with a broken leg to obtain a properly positioned radiograph.

AU. The antiinflammatory effects of ocular-applied glucocorticoids speed the healing of corneal ulcers.

AV. As doses of selective COX-2 inhibitors are increased, the selectivity for COX-2 over COX-1 inhibition *decreases*.

5. For each of the following, indicate "decreased" or "increased" for what would be expected after prolonged use of antiinflammatory doses of a glucocorticoid drug.
   - Blood sugar concentrations
   - Insulin dose requirements
   - Number of circulating neutrophils
   - Number of circulating lymphocytes
   - Skeletal muscle mass
   - Urine production
   - Appetite
   - Hair growth
   - Time to heal

6. For each of the following, indicate "decreased" or "increased" for what would be expected during use of antiinflammatory doses of NSAIDs.
   - Gastric acid production
   - Stomach mucus production
   - Secretion of GI sodium bicarbonate
   - Rate of turn-over of GI tract cells
   - Blood supply to the GI tract cells
   - Diameter of renal blood vessels

7. If an animal has an adrenal cortex tumor that is producing glucocorticoids, what would the clinical condition be called? Would levels of natural cortisol be higher or lower than normal? What about CRF and ACTH levels?

8. An animal has been on immunosuppressive doses of dexamethasone tablets for 5 weeks to control an autoimmune reaction. He is showing signs of hyperadrenocorticism. If you were to check concentrations of ACTH, CRF, and natural cortisol, would they be higher or lower than normal? What would this clinical condition be called? Should the dexamethasone be stopped immediately to prevent worsening of clinical signs?

9. The owner of an animal that is being discharged from the hospital after orthopedic surgery wants to know why an "aspirin-like" drug was given for pain before the surgery. "That doesn't make any sense," she says. "And according to the doctor, it was an aspirin-like drug! Who takes aspirin before having bone surgery?" What do you say to explain this?

CHAPTER 1

1. Fill in the following blanks with the correct item from the Key Terms list.
   A. clinical pharmacology or therapeutics
   B. chemical
   C. nonproprietary name, generic name
   D. active ingredient
   E. proprietary name, trade name, brand name
   F. Food and Drug Administration (FDA)
   G. generic equivalent drug
   H. extract
   I. over-the-counter (OTC) drug
   J. legend drugs
   K. veterinarian–client–patient relationship (VCPR)
   L. dosage form
   M. tablets
   N. excipients
   O. caplet
   P. molded tablets
   Q. enteric coating
   R. sustained-release, controlled-release
   S. gel caps, capsules
   T. lozenge or troche
   U. suppositories
   V. medium
   W. suspension
   X. solution
   Y. aqueous solution
   Z. syrup
   AA. xylitol
   AB. tinctures, elixirs
   AC. insoluble
   AD. emulsion
   AE. liniment
   AF. ointment, cream
   AG. paste
   AH. ampule
   AI. repository dosage form, depot form
   AJ. implant
   AK. drug insert, package insert
   AL. label information
   AM. extra-label drug use (ELDU), off-label use
   AN. controlled substances, schedule drugs
   AO. United States Pharmacopeia (USP)
   AP. inert ingredients
   AQ. indication
   AR. side effect, adverse drug reaction (ADR)
   AS. precaution
   AT. warning
   AU. black box warning, boxed warning
   AV. contraindications
   AW. United States Adopted Names (USAN) Council
   AX. bioequivalence
   AY. Animal Medicinal Drug Use Clarification Act of 1994 (AMDUCA)
   AZ. withdrawal time, withdrawal period

2. Identify the meaning of the following acronyms.

ADR	adverse drug reaction
AMDUCA	Animal Medicinal Drug Use Clarification Act of 1994
ELDU	extra-label drug use
EPA	Environmental Protection Agency
FDA	Food and Drug Administration
OTC	over-the-counter
SR	sustained-release
USAN	United States Adopted Names (Council)
USP	United States Pharmacopeia
VCPR	veterinarian–client–patient relationship

3. Indicate whether the following statements are true or false.
   A. True. The veterinarian must adhere to the requirements for ELDU, but such drugs can be safely and legally administered to food-producing animals. The exception would be the drugs on the FDA list that should never be given to food-producing animals because of their risk to humans.
   B. False. The ® indicates that the drug name is registered with the federal government as belonging to one company or individual. Proprietary drug names are often registered (®) or trademarked (™). The trademark indicates that a company has laid claim to the name but has yet to register it with the federal government to obtain the ® symbol.
   C. True. Legend drugs either contain active ingredients that have the potential to produce harm if inappropriately used or have the potential to injure the administrator or the general public. Drugs without the legend rating are OTC drugs.
   D. False. If a topically applied drug works primarily by being absorbed into the body, then it would be considered an "internal" drug and therefore, regulated by the FDA. The EPA regulates drugs or "pesticides" that act topically only (on the surface of the skin).
   E. True. However, dosages suggested in veterinary journals or textbooks may be extra-label dosages and subject to the restrictions of ELDU.
   F. True. ".gov" websites usually indicate a governmental entity like the FDA, EPA, or the Centers for Disease Control and Prevention (CDC).
   G. False. The lower the value of the Roman numeral, the higher the abuse potential of the drug.
   H. False. This would be a contraindication because it is describing a condition in which the drug should

NOT be given. With a warning, a drug may be given if the potential benefit outweighs the potential risk in the veterinarian's judgment.

4. Today's veterinary technician cannot legally make a diagnosis, do surgery, or prescribe treatment or medications, but the veterinary technician needs to understand how the drug works, its uses and contraindications, and the signs of adverse reactions. This is necessary to properly monitor in-hospital patients for early detection of any possible adverse reactions and to educate clients or animal owners about the drug or answer questions.

5. A generic drug is a drug manufactured by a company other than the original parent company. Generic drugs are less expensive because the generic drug company did not have to make the tremendous financial investment required to research, develop, test, and market the original drug. Generic drugs are required to have the same amount and type of active ingredient as the parent brand of drug. They are generally considered to be equivalent to the often better-known parent drug, although minor differences in the types of inert ingredients may affect the drug's performance in the body.

6. The veterinary technician may report the adverse drug reaction to the drug's manufacturing company through their technical veterinarian or technical support services (readily found on the web) or directly to the FDA through its adverse drug reporting service (found on the FDA's website: www.fda.gov).

7. The enteric coating protects the medication from the acid in the stomach. Acid can denature or destroy some types of drugs; thus, the generic coating allows the drug to pass through the stomach to the less-acidic environment of the intestine, where it can dissolve and be absorbed.

8. SR is commonly put on the label of sustained-released oral medications. Sustained release means that the drug is dissolved or released over a longer period of time, thus supplying amounts of drug to be absorbed for a longer duration.

9. It negates the protective enteric coating or disrupts the slow sustained-released rate of the SR medication.

10. Xylitol causes the pancreas to release additional insulin, resulting in the dog's blood glucose (i.e., sugar) plummeting as the additional insulin moves the blood glucose into the cells. This drop in blood glucose can be severe enough to produce a hypoglycemic crisis and death. In addition, xylitol can also cause severe liver damage in the dog.

11. Solutions are safe to be given intravenously. Generally suspensions are not because the drug is not fully dissolved in the liquid medium. Suspensions always need to be shaken (sometimes carefully, as in the case of insulin) to equally disperse the drug within the liquid medium before removal of the drug from the bottle or vial.

12. 48 h. A repository drug is the same as a depot drug. Both are designed to be absorbed over a long period after being injected into the body. Therefore, the dosage interval between drug administration should be longer between injections of a depot or repository drug than it would be for a nondepot or standard drug.

13. An extract is an active ingredient derived from specially processed plant or animal parts. It is relatively cheaper to produce than chemically synthesizing the drug and hence is often less expensive to sell to the consumer. The disadvantage of extracts is that they may be more inconsistent in the amount of active ingredient contained in the drug and, if marketed as a nutraceutical, may not be as tightly regulated for safety and consistency as a synthesized drug regulated by the FDA and the USP manufacturing standards.

14. No. A valid VCPR does not exist in this case. The veterinarian has not seen this animal, does not know what type of medication the animal is currently using for motion sickness, and does not know if there are any physical contraindications that would prevent the safe use of the drug in this animal.

15. Explain whether each of the following situations is considered an appropriate or inappropriate use of drugs in an extra-label manner according to FDA requirements.

A. Not appropriate. A valid VCPR has not been established because the veterinarian has not seen the animal. Also this is poor veterinary practice in many cases because the veterinarian is assuming that the interpretation of the affected animal's behavior by the nonmedically trained client is medically accurate. Though a skillful veterinarian can elicit valuable information from the client's history, the history is always tainted by the client/pet owner's own interpretation of what they are observing.

B. Not appropriate. If there is an FDA-approved drug form for the condition, that drug formulation is the only one that can be used regardless of a cost differential.

C. Not appropriate in most circumstances, especially if it occurs in small animal or equine practice. No VCPR has been established for the other individual animals, plus the veterinarian has transferred the responsibility of diagnosis to the livestock producer. There is a caveat to this for herd treatment, however. In some states or provinces, a VCPR may exist for a herd if the veterinarian has knowledge of the conditions and medical treatments of the herd in general. In those circumstances, a VCPR has been considered to be established for all members of the herd. This VCPR assumes that all members of the herd are mostly housed together, exposed to the same conditions or disease causes, and have enough biologic similarities that a sample animal from the herd represents the health condition of the rest of the herd.

D. Not appropriate. The cow is producing products potentially for human consumption and therefore, by law, there needs to be a withdrawal time between when the last dose is given and the milk can go into the human food supply chain. If no withdrawal time exists on the label and the drug is given extra-label, the veterinarian is still obligated to establish and enforce a withdrawal period based upon what recommendations exist in the veterinary literature, from regulatory agencies, or from the use of similar medications in that species.

E. Possibly appropriate if the vial in which the drug is dispensed is properly labeled according to extra-label use requirements and animal's medical records are accurately maintained. Goats and sheep are minor species and therefore, it is fairly common to use cattle medications in these species because there are very few, if any, medications specifically approved for use in these minor species.

F. This is appropriate use based upon the requirements for extra-label use. The label must also have the veterinarian's name and the active ingredient listed on it.

16. Rule #1: All Drugs Are Poisons. Rule #2: No Drug Is a Silver Bullet. Rule #3: All Doses Are Guesses. Rule #4: Complacency Kills.

CHAPTER 2

1. Fill in the following blanks with the correct item from the Key Terms list.
   A. pharmacy
   B. pharmacology
   C. drug order
   D. prescription
   E. Controlled Substances or Schedule drugs
   F. DEA (Drug Enforcement Administration)
   G. Schedule drugs
   H. dosage regimen
   I. dose
   J. dose interval
   K. dosage
   L. dosage form
   M. dosage range
   N. metric system
   O. apothecary system
   P. household measurement system
   Q. strength of the dosage form or concentration
   R. weight by volume (w/v) percentage solution
   S. volume by volume (v/v) percentage solution
   T. weight by weight (w/w) percentage solution
   U. compounding
   V. veterinarian–client–patient relationship (VCPR)
   W. Poison Prevention Packaging Act of 1970
   X. cytotoxic
   Y. Occupational Safety and Health Administration (OSHA)
   Z. teratogenic and mutagenic
   AA. carcinogenic
   AB. material safety data sheet (MSDS)

2. What do the following abbreviations stand for?

DEA	Drug Enforcement Administration
ELDU	extra-label drug use
FFDCA	Federal Food, Drug and Cosmetic Act
FDA	Food and Drug Administration
MSDS	Material Safety Data Sheet
OSHA	Occupational Safety and Health Administration
VCPR	veterinarian–client–patient relationship

3. What do the following abbreviations from drug orders stand for?

b.i.d.	twice daily
q.i.d.	four times daily
t.i.d.	three times daily
q12h	every 12 hours
PO	per os or by mouth
OD/OS/OU	right eye/left eye/both eyes
IM	intramuscular
IP	intraperitoneal
IV	intravenous
SQ	subcutaneous
PRN	as needed
TBL	tablespoon

4. Filling a drug order is the practice of pharmacy. Pharmacology would be the understanding of how the drug works in the body.

5. It has the notice that: "Federal law restricts this drug to use by or on the order of a licensed veterinarian."

6. A drug order is from a veterinarian to a veterinary technician for in-hospital purposes. A prescription is a drug order to a pharmacist to fill outside of the veterinary hospital. A veterinary technician may not fill a drug order from another hospital not directly affiliated with where he or she works because that would be acting as a pharmacist.

7. The concentration or strength of the drug to be dispensed is missing. We know the drug and the number to be dispensed, but do not know if the 50, 100, or 200 mg tablet strength is supposed to be dispensed.

8. C-II. C-I drugs include illegal drugs like LSD, heroin, and marijuana.

9. "Caution: Federal law prohibits the transfer of this drug to any person other than the [client and] patient for whom it was prescribed."

10. No. The Controlled Substance Log needs to track the individual bottle of drug from the time it arrived at the veterinary hospital until the contents were used. The log needs to identify the specific patients to which the contents of that specific bottle were dispensed and the specific amount used for that patient. In the event of a question regarding the amount of drug used, the data in the log book can be checked against the information written in the patient's medical record. The log is also the document that helps identify where the source of a possible drug diversion may have originated; thus information about the individual administering the drug is also important.

11. Any paper recording method by which a page could be removed from the notebook and replaced by another page containing false information makes it a bad system. A better method is to have a bound "laboratory-style" notebook with numbers imprinted sequentially on each page by the notebook manufacturer so no page can be removed without the record obviously being altered.

12. No. Veterinarians are required to store all C-II through C-V drugs in a "securely locked" and "substantially constructed" cabinet to which few personnel have a key or know the

combination to the lock. A metal box of 1 cubic foot size could easily be picked up and carried off; thus it is not a secure method for storing Controlled Substances. A wooden cabinet with a lock would come closer to meeting the requirements, as long as it was attached to a wall and of substantial construction.

13. Expired, damaged, or otherwise unusable Controlled Substances must be disposed of through authorized *reverse distributors* who have the legal authority to receive and dispose of these drugs.

14. Three years. This may be superseded by state or local regulations in which the length of time is longer.

15. Most abuse to least abuse: C-I, C-II, C-III, C-IV, C-V.

16. Translate the following drug orders:
    50 mg q8h 3d = 50 milligrams every 8 hours for 3 days.
    100 mg PO PRN for pain = 100 milligrams by mouth as needed for pain.
    0.5 mg/lb IV stat = 0.5 milligrams per pound of body weight intravenously immediately.
    3 gtt OD q2h = 3 drops in the right eye every 2 hours.

17. "b.i.d." means twice daily and does not necessarily mean that the doses are evenly spaced at 12-hour intervals. The same is true with "t.i.d.," which means three times daily but does not specify the interval between doses to every 8 hours.

18. Make the following conversions:
    2 g = 2000 mg
    5 mg = 0.005 g
    14 lb = 6.363 kg
    23 kg = 50.6 lb
    83 kg = 83,000,000 mg (8.3×10^7 mg)
    65 kg = 143 lb
    0.4 kg = 400 g
    0.003 lb = 1363.63 mg
    15 lb = 6818.18 g
    0.00043 kg = 430 mg
    25,488 mg = 0.056 lb
    0.0092 lb = 4181.82 mg
    25 mL = 0.025 L
    43 cc = 43 mL
    1.5 L = 1500 mL
    800 cc = 0.8 L
    0.055 L = 55 mL
    0.65 mL = 0.00065 L

19. Given the dosage, determine the dose for the patient:
    10 mg/lb for a 20-lb dog = 200 mg
    2.2 mg/kg for a 35-lb dog = 35 mg
    6 mg/lb for a 15-kg dog = 198 mg
    0.8 mg/kg for a 5-kg cat = 4 mg
    15 mg/kg for a 900-lb horse = 6136 mg
    0.75 mg/lb for a 350-kg steer = 577.5 mg
    10 mg/m^2 for a 1.2-m^2 dog = 12 mg

20. Determine the number of dosage units per dose.
    10 mg/kg, 22-lb dog, 20 mg tablets = 5 tablets
    5 mg/lb, 44-kg pig, 250 mg/mL liquid = 1.9 mL liquid
    50 mg/kg, 1-gram rat, 0.01 mg/mL liquid = 5 mL liquid
    2.5 mg/lb, 5-kg cat, 25 mg tablets = 1.1 tablet = 1 tablet

3 mg/kg, 897-lb horse, 250 mg tablets = 4.89 tablets = 5 tablets
45 mg/kg, 8.1-lb cat, 50 mg tablets = 3.31 tablets = 3.5 tablets

21. Complete the following table of conversions of percentage solutions (w/v, w/w, v/v) and the number of milligrams or milliliters of drug per unit of medium.

Percentage Solution	Milligrams or Milliliters per Unit of Medium
5% solution w/v	5 grams/100 mL = 5000 mg/100 mL = 50 mg/mL
10% solution w/w	10 grams drug/100 grams drug + medium
15% solution v/v	15 mL drug/100 mL drug + medium
20% solution w/v	20 grams/100 mL = 20,000 mg/100 mL = 200 mg/mL
25% solution w/w	25 mg drug/100 mg drug + medium
30% solution w/v	300 mg/mL
4% solution w/v	4000 mg/100 mL
8% solution w/v	160 mg/2 mL
12% solution w/v	36 grams/300 mL

22. Convert 15 lb to kg. First: 15 lb × 1 kg/2.2 lb = 6.82 kg. Now determine how much drug is needed for this sized cat: 6.82 kg × 15 mg/kg = 102.3 mg of drug needed. Now determine what volume of drug you need to inject: 102.3 mg × 1 mL/100 mg = 1.02 mL. Note that when multiplying the dose by the concentration in the bottle, the problem has to be set up so the "mg" in the numerator and denominator cancel each other out, leaving "mL" by itself on top. The 1.02 mL is rounded to the nearest 1/10 mL = 1.0 mL.

23. First convert the dog's weight to kilograms: 55 lb × 1 kg/2.2 lb = 25 kg. Now determine how much drug a 25-kg dog will need: 25 kg × 0.08 mg/kg = 2 mg of drug needed. Now select the tablet size, keeping in mind that you do not want to break a tablet into anything smaller than one half of a tablet. If the 1-mg tablet size is used then we need: 2 mg × 1 tablet/1 mg = 2 tablets per dose. If a 5-mg tablet size is used, it comes out to 2 mg × 1 tablet/5 mg = 0.4 tablet per dose, rounded to 0.5 tablet per dose. This is not as accurate as using the two 1-mg tablets, but it is close enough if this drug is safe. Now determine how many tablets you will need for 5 days of treatment if the drug is to be given q6h (i.e., every 6 h). For the two 1-mg tablet dose, you would need 2 tablets/dose × 4 doses/day ×5 days = 2 × 4 × 5 = 40 tablets for the 5-day period. For the one-half tablet of the 5-mg strength tablets: 0.5 tablet/dose × 4 doses/day × 5 days = 0.5 × 4 × 5 = 10 total for the 5-day period. Cost of the medication: 40 tablets (1-mg tablets) × $0.35/tablet = $14.00, or 10 tablets (5-mg size) × $0.35/tablet = $3.50.

24. 16-lb Chihuahua = 7.27 kg = dose range of 21.8–36.4 mg; use half of a 50-mg tablet. 0.5 tablet/dose × 1 dose/day × 180 days = 90 of the 50-mg tablets needed. 90 tablets at $0.03 per tablet = $2.70 for the 180 days. 27-lb

terrier = 12.3 kg = dose range of 36.8–61.4 mg; use 1 whole 50-mg tablet per dose. 1 tablet/dose × 1 dose/day × 180 days = 180 tablets. 180 tablets × $0.03 per tablet = $5.40 for the 180 days' worth of medication. 66-lb Collie = 30 kg = dose range of 90–150 mg; use either 1 of the 100-mg tablets, 1.5 of the 100-mg tablets, or 0.5 of the 200-mg tablets; costs would be, respectively, $9.00, $13.50, or $6.30.

25. Meters squared (m^2) is used in place of kilograms or pounds of body weight. 0.8 m^2 × 0.22 mg/m^2 = 0.176 mg of drug. 0.176 mg × 1 mL/0.15 mg = 1.17 mL of elixir to be given at full strength. The veterinarian wants you to use 60% of the original dose. Therefore, 60% = 0.60 and 60% of the dose would be 0.60 × 1.17 mL = 0.7 mL of drug. You can also calculate the reduction in dose by taking the calculated dose in mg (0.176 mg) and determining what 60% of that would be—0.1056 mg (0.60 × 0.176 mg = 0.1056 mg)—and then determining the milliliters of elixir to be used: 0.1056 mg × 1 mL/0.15 mg = 0.7 mL.

26. If the total number of tablets dispensed was 115 tablets and they were to be given equally three times a day for 10 days (30 doses total), this means the owner is giving 3.83333 tablets per dose (115 tablets divided by 30 doses = 3.83333 tablets per dose). No client is going to be able to slice off 0.8333 of a tablet to give with the other three whole tablets. The error was from determining total milligrams of drug needed for the whole 10 days dosage regimen instead of determining the number of milligrams needed per dose, then determining the number of tablets needed per dose before determining the total number of tablets that needed to be dispensed. The 19.1-kg dog at a dose of 10 mg/kg needs 190.1 per dose, which translates into 3.8 of the 50-mg tablets per dose. Because tablets cannot be fractionated into anything smaller than a half or whole tablet, round that 3.8 tablets to 4 whole tablets per dose. Now determine how many tablets are needed per day (4 tablets per dose × 3 doses per day = 12 tablets) and how many are needed for 10 days (12 tablets per day × 10 days = 120 tablets total).

27. 8-lb dog = 3.636-kg dog. At a dose of 8 mg/kg, this dog needs a dose of 29.1 mg. Tablets are 15 mg in size so the 29.1 mg dose needs to be rounded to the nearest half or whole tablet. The dog needs gets 2 tablets per dose (29.1 mg rounded to 30 mg per dose). Each tablet costs $0.13 ($130 divided by 1000 tablets) and the dog gets two tablets a day. Therefore, the cost per day of tablets is 2 tablets × $0.13/tablet = $0.26 per day. If the client has only $10, then we divide the $10 by the cost per day to determine how many days of medication the client can have. $10 × day/$0.26 = 38.4 days = 38 days (a partial day does not count).

28. False. Mixing two drugs in a syringe, bottle, or container is considered compounding because you are then administering these as a new combined drug with physical and pharmacologic interactions.

29. No. If the drug exists in an available FDA-approved formulation, the FDA-approved formulation must be used.

30. For food animals, a withdrawal time must be determined for the compounded drug. This is the time between when the drug is last given and the when the animal can be prepared for use as food or its products (e.g., eggs, milk) can be safely put into the human food chain.

31. This would be considered "drug manufacturing" because the repackaging is not being done for a particular patient under a valid VCPR. In effect, the veterinarian is doing what drug manufacturers do when they purchase the "raw" drug in bulk form and then manufacturer the drug under their own label.

32. This would clearly be a violation of the compounding laws because it was not developed for a specific client, and it was sold to another practice, putting that practice in the role of drug manufacturing.

33. False. The Poison Prevention Packaging Act does not apply to veterinarians. However, there is an ethical obligation to warn pet owners of the risk of accidental ingestion of medication in containers that are not childproof and to emphasize keeping the medication out of reach of children.

34. False. "Room temperature" is 59–86°F, whereas a refrigerator would keep drugs cool (46–59°F) to cold (not exceeding 46°F). "Warm" and "excessive heat" also describe specific ranges of temperature.

35. Yes, as long as the packaging does not say, "Do not freeze." Cold temperatures are defined as less than 46°F or 8°C.

36. False. The MSDS notebook must be readily available to all personnel because it contains information the personnel need to know to protect themselves from a drug should it spill or be inappropriately used.

37. No. Surgical masks in one layer are porous enough to allow an aerosolized drug to pass through them. A single pair of latex surgical gloves may not be enough to prevent a drug from getting through.

CHAPTER 3

1. Fill in the following blanks with the correct item from the Key Terms list.
   A. pharmacokinetics
   B. pharmacodynamics
   C. therapeutic range or window
   D. route of administration
   E. loading dose
   F. peak concentration
   G. narrow therapeutic index
   H. parenteral administered drugs
   I. constant rate infusion (CRI)
   J. steady state
   K. extravascular or perivascular injection
   L. subcutaneous (SQ)
   M. intradermal injection
   N. intraperitoneal (IP)
   O. per os (PO)
   P. topically administered drugs

Q. aerosol administration
R. passive diffusion
S. facilitated diffusion
T. active transport
U. absorption
V. bioavailability
W. intravenous (IV)
X. intramuscular (IM)
Y. reabsorption
Z. P-glycoprotein
AA. cytochrome P-450 enzymes
AB. dissolution
AC. gastric motility
AD. intestinal motility
AE. hepatic portal system
AF. first-pass effect
AG. tissue perfusion
AH. distribution
AI. fenestrations
AJ. P-glycoprotein
AK. redistribution
AL. volume of distribution
AM. receptor
AN. affinity
AO. intrinsic activity
AP. agonist
AQ. antagonist
AR. competitive, reversible, surmountable antagonist
AS. partial agonist/partial antagonist
AT. biotransformation or metabolism
AU. induced metabolism
AV. excretion or elimination
AW. filtration
AX. active secretion
AY. glomerulus
AZ. enterohepatic circulation
BA. half-life of elimination
BB. clearance
BC. steady state or plateau
BD. withdrawal time

2. Indicate whether each statement is describing a lipophilic or hydrophilic drug molecule by writing in the appropriate term for each statement.
A. lipophilic
B. hydrophilic
C. lipophilic
D. hydrophilic
E. lipophilic
F. hydrophilic

3. Identify whether each of the following statements is true or false.
A. True. The lower the pH, the more acidic the pH, and the greater the number of free hydrogen ions floating in the liquid, ready to combine with a drug.
B. False. Acid drugs become increasingly ionized as the environment becomes more alkalinized. Thus, a movement of 1 unit of pH (e.g., pH 5 moving to a pH of 6) would result in a 10-fold shift in the direction of the ionized molecules.
C. True. Alkaline drugs are more nonionized in alkaline pH environments and acidic drugs are more nonionized in acidic pH environments.
D. True. Base drugs are more ionized as they are placed into increasingly acidic environments. At a pH of 7 (the pH of the pK_a of 7), the ratio of ionized to nonionized molecules would be 1:1 (equal amounts of both forms). At a pH of 6 (1 pH unit to the acidic side of the pK_a pH of 7), the ratio would be 10 ionized to every 1 nonionized; at a pH of 5 the ratio would be 100 ionized to every 1 nonionized molecule.
E. False. The number of molecules in the ionized and nonionized form is always expressed as a ratio of ionized to nonionized, meaning that some of the molecules are still in the nonionized form, are lipophilic, and can diffuse through cell membranes to leave the compartment. When those nonionized molecules leave, some of the ionized molecules will become nonionized to maintain the ratio of ionized to nonionized within the compartment, thus providing new molecules that can passively diffuse out of the compartment. In this way, the drug can still leave the compartment in which it is "trapped."
F. False. Active skeletal muscle has a much richer blood supply going to it than fat does. Thus, active skeletal muscle is much better perfused than fat.
G. False. A drug that is highly protein-bound usually means that greater than 80% of the drug is bound to blood proteins and is unavailable to passively diffuse through the capillary fenestrations and distribute to the tissues. Only unbound, or free, drug molecules can distribute. Thus, highly bound drugs are far less distributed than unbound drugs.
H. True. A large volume of distribution (V_d) means that the drug is dissolved in a larger amount of bodily fluid. To have a larger volume of fluid, the drug must be able to penetrate more body compartments and thus has a greater distribution than a drug with a lesser volume of distribution.
I. True. Induced metabolism means the rate at which the drug is being broken down has increased, resulting in a more rapid inactivation of the drug. To compensate for the more rapid inactivation, the dose of the drug would need to be increased.
J. False. Cats generally have a lessened capacity to metabolize drugs either because of deficiencies in the enzymes needed for phase I metabolism, or the decreased capacity to conjugate drug molecules to other molecules in phase II metabolism.
K. False. Biliary excretion is via the bile duct in the liver. Renal excretion is via the kidney.
L. True. Drugs bound to protein are stuck in the blood and cannot pass by filtration into the Bowman's capsule. However, if the active transport molecule has a

strong affinity for the drug, the drug molecule can come off the protein to which it is bound and be transported into the urine in the proximal convoluted tubule.

M. True. The longer the half-life, the longer it takes for the drug concentration in the blood to drop by half, thus reflecting a slower rate of elimination. To prevent accumulation of drug, the dose would have to be decreased to compensate for the prolonged half-life.

4. Which one of the following drugs is absorbed in the greatest amount?

A. Bioavailability is the percentage of the drug dose that actually makes it to systemic circulation. Therefore, 100 mg × 0.7 (70%) = 70 mg absorbed, 150 mg × 0.5 = 75 mg, 200 mg × 0.4 = 80 mg, and 250 mg × 0.2 = 50 mg.

5. For each situation or condition, state whether the dose should be *increased* or *decreased* to compensate for the condition and still achieve therapeutic concentrations in the body.

A. Decrease. The half-life is longer, meaning that it takes longer for the drug concentrations to drop by half. Elimination is slower, so the dose must be decreased.

B. Increase. The metabolism/biotransformation has been induced, so active drug is being more quickly converted to inactive drug. More drug (increased dose) is needed to compensate.

C. Decrease. Fewer blood proteins means more drug molecules are in the free unbound form and available to distribute to their site of action. This produces a larger concentration of drug molecules at the target site than normal, requiring a decrease in dose.

D. Decreased, as long as the reduced distribution of drug did not involve reduced distribution to the *target* tissue. Assuming drug in the bloodstream can still reach the target tissues, a decreased V_d results in the absorbed drug being less diluted by a large volume of body fluids; therefore, the drug is more concentrated than normal. Higher concentrations of drug means higher concentrations in the tissues to which the drug can still distribute, with the potential to reach toxic concentrations in the tissues to which it distributes. Dose should be decreased.

E. Decrease. If clearance is decreased that means a smaller volume of blood or plasma is being cleared ("cleaned") of drug than normal in a given period of time. Because elimination is slowed, the dose must be decreased to compensate.

F. Decrease if the drug depends on renal filtration for primary elimination from the body. Decreased blood supply to glomerulus means less blood to filter out drug and a slower rate of elimination unless there are other elimination mechanisms for this drug (e.g., active secretion into the proximal convoluted tubule). The dose needs to be decreased to compensate for the decreased ability to eliminate the drug. Even if the drug is eliminated by active transport from the blood to the renal tubules, the rate of drug elimination would be slowed

because the blood that goes to the glomerulus also continues to the renal tubules and thus blood flow past the active transport sites would also be decreased.

6. Answer the following questions.

A. The half-life is 2 h. Half-life is defined as the amount of time it takes for the drug concentration in the blood/plasma to drop by half. Half of 160 mcg/mL would be 80 mcg/mL, which we do not see on the chart. However, half of 80 mcg/mL is 40 mcg/mL, which we do see. Thus, the amount of time it took for the concentrations to drop from 160 to 40 mcg/mL constituted two half-life periods of time (160 to 80 and 80 to 40). 160 mcg/mL was recorded 1 h postinjection and 40 mcg/mL was recorded at 5 h postinjection. It took 4 h to drop two half-lives, from 160 to 40 mcg/mL, so 1 half-life is 2 h. Thus, every 2 h after the drug is given the concentrations would drop by half.

B. 50 mcg/mL. In the previous question, the half-life was determined to be 2 h. Thus, from any time point on the drug concentration curve, concentrations 2 h later will decrease by half. The data show that at the 2-h postinjection point the concentration was 100 mcg/mL. The 4-h postinjection point occurs 2 h or 1 half-life worth of time from the 100 mcg/mL 2-h postinjection point. Therefore, the concentration at the 4-h postinjection point would be expected to be half of the concentration; 100 divided by 2 = 50 mcg/mL.

C. 20 mcg/mL. The concentration at 7 h postinjection would be expected to be half of the concentration at the 5-h postinjection point because the difference is 2 h, which is 1 half-life for this drug. The concentration at the 5-h postinjection point was shown as 40 mcg/mL, so half of that would be 20 mcg/mL at the 7-h postinjection point.

D. 200 mcg/mL. If the half-life for this drug was determined to be 2 h, then 2 h prior (not after) any time point on the drug concentration would be double the concentration. This question asks what the concentration would have been at 0 h immediately after the drug was pushed as an IV bolus. The concentration at 2 h postinjection was 100 mcg/mL and therefore 2 h before this time point (1 half-life before this time point) the concentration would be expected to be twice what it was at the 2-h postinjection time point. 2 × 100 = 200 mcg/mL.

E. 10 h. Steady state is achieved at approximately five times the time of the half-life of elimination of the drug. Thus, this drug has a half-life of 2 h and the time after multiple administrations of this drug or an IV constant rate infusion to reach steady-state plateau would be 5 × 2 = 10 h.

7. Unless the normal therapeutic range is known for each of the drugs, it is unclear whether the listed concentrations are therapeutic, subtherapeutic, or toxic.

8. The loading dose will establish drug concentrations immediately in the therapeutic range after the first dose. Otherwise, without the loading dose, the drug concentrations will increase a little with each dose until they reach steady state plateau at 5× the drug's half-life.

9. By giving more drug (higher dose) less frequently (q12h instead of q6h), the peak concentration will be higher with the higher dose, and the trough concentration will be lower with the longer dose interval. With the wider swing from peak to trough, it is possible that the concentrations achieved during the dose interval could exceed the therapeutic concentration at the peak and/or drop below therapeutic concentrations at the trough. If the drug has a narrow therapeutic index, such a wide swing is more likely to result in side effects from toxicity or ineffectiveness from subtherapeutic concentrations.

10. An enteric coating is designed to delay dissolution or dissolving of the tablet until it passes safely beyond the acidic environment of the stomach into the more alkaline pH of the small intestine. If the drug itself is very sensitive to being broken down or damaged by the highly acidic contents of the stomach, an enteric coating could protect the drug until it reaches the less-acidic duodenum, where the tablet can dissolve and release the drug for absorption.

11. An alkaline drug is likely to be very ionized in the very acidic environment of the stomach lumen (typically a pH of 2 or 3). Thus, the drug would not be very well absorbed in the stomach. Being trapped in the stomach would delay the ability of the drug to be absorbed and hence would delay the achievement of blood drug concentrations in the therapeutic range. This delay would delay the onset of the beneficial effect of the drug. If the drug was susceptible to acid degrading the drug, the delay in the stomach may actually decrease the total amount of drug that is eventually absorbed into the body and would then result in only subtherapeutic concentrations being achieved.

12. If the diarrhea results in rapid movement of intestinal contents, the tablet might be carried beyond the small intestine (the area of greatest absorption) before the tablet has had the opportunity to fully dissolve small enough to be absorbed. The net effect is drug passing out in the feces.

13. The liver screens all drugs absorbed from the intestinal tract that arrive via the hepatic portal system. The liver may remove much of a drug before it has a chance to enter systemic circulation and distribute to the tissues and organs of the body (the first-pass effect). When a drug is injected, it does not have to pass through the liver first but can enter the systemic circulation from the injection site.

14. On cold days the superficial blood vessels in the subcutaneous tissue vasoconstrict to reduce heat loss through the skin. Thus, under cold conditions the superficial tissues are less perfused with blood. Less perfusion means a drug injected SQ has to travel further to find an open capillary or to be transported away from the SQ injection site by the blood. Thus, absorption from the SQ site is slower on cold days than on warm ones.

15. Fat is very poorly perfused tissue and as such any drug injected into the fat will not be absorbed very well at all. Insulin injected into the fat may remain there for an extended period of time before being absorbed into the body and the disruption of the absorption of the insulin throws off the balance in timing required for insulin to work.

16. The brain is separated from the blood by the blood-brain barrier. This barrier excludes any ionized (hydrophilic) drug molecules from entering. Additionally, P-glycoprotein can actively pump some lipophilic drug molecules that diffuse through the brain capillary wall back into the blood excluding them from entering the brain. If the antibiotic cannot reach the brain in sufficient concentrations to achieve therapeutic concentrations, the antibiotic will not be effective.

17. A drug with a higher volume of distribution (V_d) is a drug that is dissolved in a larger volume of body water. To be dissolved in a larger volume of body water, the drug must be able to penetrate more body compartments. Thus, a larger V_d suggests a greater number of body compartments penetrated. If a drug is dissolved in a larger volume of water, it is going to be more diluted, hence the drug concentrations will be lower. Thus, Drug B will penetrate tissues more, but it will be diluted more than Drug A and hence Drug B will have the lower concentration.

18. A noncompetitive agonist means that the insecticide exerts an effect on the cell (agonist) and that it also binds with the receptor in such a way that it is not easily removed from the receptor (strong affinity, noncompetitive). Thus, if an antidote were to be given that is an antagonist for the same receptor site (combines with the receptor but has no intrinsic activity), the effect of the insecticide is unlikely to be reversed because the insecticide does not move off of the receptor long enough or easily enough to allow the antagonist (antidote) to move onto the receptor and reverse the insecticide's effect.

19. When the strong agonist hydromorphone is given, it exerts its strong pain-killing effect (analgesia) and a respiratory depression side effect. Butorphanol competes for the same receptors as hydromorphone so it would be an antagonist against the hydromorphone. However, butorphanol does produce analgesia of its own but it does not have as strong of an analgesic or respiratory depression effect as hydromorphone. When butorphanol replaces hydromorphone on the receptor, there is a lessening of the analgesia but some analgesia remains. Butorphanol is thus a partial antagonist of hydromorphone. Because butorphanol has some analgesic effect of its own, but not as strong as hydromorphone, it is a partial agonist. Hence, butorphanol is referred to as a partial agonist/partial antagonist drug.

20. A chelating drug produces its effect by directly changing molecules around it without working through a receptor. This is called non–receptor-mediated activity.

21. Young animals and cats of all ages have a reduced capacity to metabolize drugs (i.e., break them down). Hence, a drug that is normally hepatically metabolized will remain in an active state for a longer period of time in a young animal or cats. To prevent too much active drug from accumulating in the blood and tissues, the dose would need to be decreased to compensate. This would not be a problem if the drug were excreted unchanged through the kidneys because the kidneys are capable of filtering drugs even at an early age and cat kidneys are largely as effective as any other species.

22. Phenobarbital is a xenobiotic (i.e., a foreign substance). The liver recognizes it as a "poison" that should be removed,

hence the cytochrome P-450 enzymes in the liver break down the phenobarbital. With repeated exposure to the "poison" phenobarbital, the liver increases the amount of cytochrome P-450 enzymes available and hence is able to inactive the phenobarbital much quicker. This appears clinically as a decreased duration of drug activity or "tolerance." This increased metabolism is referred to an "induced metabolism" and means the biotransformation of the drug has been sped up. To compensate for the accelerated rate at which the drug is broken down, the dose must be increased.

23. Penicillin is actively secreted (active transport) from the blood of the peritubular capillaries in the kidney into the urine. Because this is an active transport process, the penicillin is actively pumped into the urine continuously, regardless of the concentration gradient. Thus, large concentrations of penicillin can be achieved in the urine compared with the blood, whereas other tissues without this active transport process would never achieve concentrations higher than the concentrations found in the blood.

24. Enterohepatic circulation means a compound that is circulating in the blood gets taken out by the liver and excreted into the GI tract without being metabolized. The bile carrying the still active compound delivers it to the GI tract (biliary excretion) where the compound can be reabsorbed through the GI tract wall, reenter the body and go on to poison the animal again. The purpose of the activated charcoal being administered repeatedly is to break the enterohepatic circulation cycle when the compound is excreted into the GI tract and prevent it from being reabsorbed back into the body.

25. When a drug is given repeatedly with multiple doses or is given as a constant rate infusion over time, the drug concentrations build up to the point where the peak and trough concentrations no longer increase. This is steady state. For most drug dosages, steady state should occur within the therapeutic range. The time it takes for the drug to accumulate to the steady-state concentrations is related to the half-life of elimination. Steady state should be mostly achieved after $5\times$ the half-life of the drug in the patient's body. Thus, a drug with a long half-life (say 30-h half-life) could take as long as 150 h or 6 days until concentrations hit steady state. Before that time, the concentrations are likely to be subtherapeutic and thus have little beneficial effect. In the situation where a drug with a long half-life is administered, a loading dose should be given to establish the blood drug concentrations within the therapeutic range and then maintain the therapeutic concentrations with the lower maintenance dose.

26. Drug B, with all other pharmacokinetic factors being equal between Drug A and Drug B. If it takes longer for Drug B to be removed by half than it does Drug A (5 h for Drug B vs only 30 min for Drug A), then Drug B is going to remain in the body longer and requires a longer withdrawal time.

CHAPTER 4

1. Fill in the following blanks with the correct item from the Key Terms list.
   A. enteric
   B. colonic

C. fermentative digestion
D. emetic drug
E. emetic center
F. chemoreceptor trigger zone (CRTZ)
G. neurokinin-1 (NK-1) receptor
H. histamine H_1 receptors
I. α-receptors
J. serotonin receptors
K. vestibular apparatus
L. centrally acting emetics
M. gastritis
N. anticholinergic
O. prokinetic drug
P. relatively contraindicated
Q. absolutely contraindicated
R. secretory diarrhea
S. enterotoxins
T. exudative diarrhea
U. motility diarrhea
V. osmotic or malabsorption diarrhea
W. exocrine pancreatic insufficiency
X. segmental contractions
Y. peristaltic contractions
Z. tenesmus
AA. ileus
AB. melena
AC. mesalamine or 5-aminosalacylic acid
AD. keratoconjunctivitis sicca or dry eye
AE. adsorbent
AF. emollient laxative
AG. bulk laxative
AH. parietal cells or oxyntic cells
AI. chief cells
AJ. histamine, acetylcholine, gastrin
AK. enterochromaffin-like cells
AL. gastrin
AM. mucin
AN. bicarbonate ion
AO. prostaglandins
AP. pepsin
AQ. systemic antacids
AR. ruminatoric
AS. ionophore
AT. bacteremia (i.e., bacteria in blood) or septicemia (i.e., vague term meaning pathogens or poisons in the blood producing sepsis)
AU. motilin

2. Fill in the following blanks with the correct drug from the Gastrointestinal Drug list.
   A. apomorphine
   B. xylazine
   C. hydrogen peroxide
   D. acepromazine
   E. dimenhydrinate (Dramamine) and diphenhydramine (Benadryl)
   F. metoclopramide (Reglan)
   G. ondansetron (Zofran)
   H. maropitant (Cerenia)

I. diphenoxylate (Lomotil) and loperamide (Imodium AD)

J. bismuth subsalicylate (Pepto-Bismol, Kaopectate)

K. ondansetron (Zofran)

L. sulfasalazine (Azulfidine)

M. bismuth

N. activated charcoal

O. mineral oil

P. cod liver oil, white petrolatum

Q. glycerin

R. docusate sodium succinate (DSS, Colace)

S. lactulose

T. castor oil, bisacodyl

U. cimetidine (Tagamet), ranitidine (Zantac), famotidine (Pepcid), nizatidine (Axid)

V. cimetidine (Tagamet)

W. omeprazole (Prilosec, GastroGard, UlcerGard)

X. sucralfate (Carafate)

Y. misoprostol (Cytotec)

Z. neostigmine

AA. monensin (Rumensin)

AB. DSS, dioctyl sodium succinate

AC. tylosin (Tylan)

AD. metronidazole (Flagyl)

AE. erythromycin

AF. pancrelipase (Viokase, Pancrezyme)

3. Indicate whether each effect or structure is associated with the parasympathetic or sympathetic nervous system:

A. parasympathetic

B. sympathetic

C. parasympathetic

D. parasympathetic

E. sympathetic

F. parasympathetic

G. parasympathetic

H. sympathetic

4. Indicate in which of the following situations induction of vomiting would be APPROPRIATE. And if the use of an emetic to induce vomiting is inappropriate, explain why.

A. NOT appropriate. A strong alkali (or acidic) cleaning agent is a corrosive compound and if vomiting is induced will burn the esophagus coming back up because the esophagus is poorly protected from corrosives (unlike the stomach that is well-equipped to handle corrosive compounds, like stomach acid).

B. APPROPRIATE. The medication was only ingested 30 min ago, so is likely still in the stomach; the cat is capable of being induced with xylazine, is not sedated or depressed, and the medication is not corrosive or easily aspirated.

C. NOT appropriate in most cases. Gasoline is easily aspirated if vomiting is induced. Petroleum products can do significant damage to the respiratory tree if aspirated. In this case, the veterinarian would have to evaluate if some tightly controlled means of evacuating the stomach would have greater benefit (by reducing absorption of the petroleum) than the

risk. Also, because it was 2 h ago and the poison ingested was a liquid, it is likely it has passed beyond the stomach and proximal duodenum, thus limiting the effectiveness of induced vomiting to remove the petroleum. Treatment will focus on reducing absorption by use of laxatives or cathartics to move it out of the intestine.

D. NOT appropriate. First, this medication was ingested 4 h ago and thus has likely moved beyond the stomach and proximal duodenum. Obviously the drug has already been absorbed to some degree, and in so doing has depressed the reflexes including, most likely, the gag reflex. Thus, the risk of aspiration in this animal with induced vomiting vs the limited benefit because the drug has moved beyond the stomach or has been largely absorbed makes induction of vomiting not appropriate. Use of drugs to facilitate removal of the drug by laxative effect is more likely. Adsorbents like activated charcoal could be used to adsorb any residual drug not already absorbed into the body.

E. Not appropriate (most likely). In this case, the compound has already been absorbed enough to produce clinical signs. Stimulation of the vomiting, or even manipulation of the patient, is likely to induce further seizure activity. The hyperthermia caused by the severe seizure activity has the potential to pose a very significant risk and further seizure activity must be avoided. In this case, the seizures may be controlled first and then emesis attempted, just in case some of the poison has not yet been absorbed.

F. NOT appropriate. Vomiting is already occurring and likely has already cleared the offending material. Inducing additional vomiting only increases the risk for aspiration without producing any beneficial effect.

G. NOT appropriate. Horses cannot vomit because of the anatomic structure of the connection between the esophagus and the stomach.

5. Indicate whether the following statements are true or false.

A. True. Dogs have more dopamine receptors in their CRTZ and hence dopamine drugs are better able to stimulate the CRTZ in dogs to produce vomiting.

B. False. The nucleus tractus solitarius (NTS) is the part of the brain that contains the pathway that leads to vomiting. Anything that stimulates the NTS produces vomiting. Suppression of the NTS by blocking receptors decreases vomiting.

C. True. The CRTZ of cats is populated with more α-receptors than the CRTZ of dogs. Although drugs with α-receptor stimulation of the CRTZ can cause vomiting in both species, the effect is more dramatic at lower doses in cats.

D. True. Histamine is released with overactivity of the vestibular apparatus (such as in continuous, turning motion) and the released histamine will combine with H_1 receptors on the CRTZ to produce vomiting. Acetylcholine is the other compound released with vestibular apparatus overactivity that produces vomiting associated with motion sickness. Antimotion sickness drugs traditionally use antihistamines and anticholinergic drugs (e.g., scopolamine used as transdermal patches) to reduce vomiting associated with motion sickness.

E. False. Apomorphine needs to be absorbed quickly into the blood to achieve high enough blood concentrations to stimulate the CRTZ before the apomorphine diffuses across the blood–brain barrier and starts to depress the emetic center itself. Giving the drug by IV or SQ injection or by crushing a tablet in saline and dropping it into the conjunctival sac of the eye does this, in contrast to the PO administered tablet, whose blood concentrations rise relatively slowly, resulting in suppression of the emetic center before the CRTZ can be sufficiently stimulated to initiate emesis.

F. False. In addition to blocking dopamine receptors for its antiemetic effect, phenothiazines also block α_1 adrenergic receptors on the smooth muscles of small arterioles that would *normally* increase resistance to arterial blood flow and increase the arterial blood pressure. By blocking these α_1 receptors, arterial blood pressure may actually *decrease* when using phenothiazine tranquilizers. Thus, phenothiazine tranquilizers should not be used in animals with any condition that causes low blood pressure (e.g., dehydration, drugs that drop blood pressure, shock).

G. False. Just the opposite. Antihistamine drugs tend to produce sedation and sleepiness as a side effect.

H. True. Maropitant (Cerenia) competes with Substance P for a position on the NK-1 receptor site in the NTS, and by so doing blocks the emetic effect produced when Substance P stimulates the NK-1 receptor.

I. False. Exocrine pancreatic insufficiency (EPI) results in food being poorly digested; thus the nondigested food particles osmotically hold water in, and may even pull water from the body into, the lumen of the intestine, producing an osmotic or malabsorption diarrhea.

J. True. Segmental contractions are the circular, constrictive contractions that block movement of intestinal contents and peristaltic contractions propel the contents along the intestinal tract.

K. False. In 2002, Kaopectate was reformulated to include bismuth subsalicylate just like Pepto-Bismol. As early as the 1980s the kaolin (kaolinite) had been removed and replaced by another clay-like adsorbent compound.

L. False. Calcium antacids are more prone to gastric acid rebound syndrome. See text to understand how this mechanism occurs.

6. The antihistamine effect of dimenhydrinate or diphenhydramine can decrease the wheal and flare reaction (i.e., swelling and redness) at the site of the skin testing injections, giving inaccurate results.

7. Anticholinergic drugs would be expected to block parasympathetic activity and acetylcholine stimulation of the CRTZ and emetic center. However, because anticholinergics only block one of many receptors in the CRTZ and emetic center that can cause vomiting, and because anticholinergics have so many side effects through their blocking of the parasympathetic nervous system, they are generally not used to control most causes of vomiting.

8. Metoclopramide should be used with extreme caution or not at all in animals with a history of seizure activity.

9. Metoclopramide depends on the activity of acetylcholine to produce the prokinetic effect that keeps the stomach and intestine contracting their contents in the correct direction. Anticholinergics would occupy and block acetylcholine receptors, thus decreasing the prokinetic effect of metoclopramide.

10. Tenesmus is "straining to defecate." The animal postures itself as if defecating and appears to strain and strain with little results. The problem in tenesmus is not the obstruction of the large colon, but the inflammation and irritation of the colon, which stimulates the normal colonic contraction processes even though there is no fecal material to move. Because the owner sees the animal straining but sees no stool produced, they assume it is because the animal is constipated or "blocked" and they may mistakenly use a laxative on the animal, making the situation worse.

11. Anticholinergic drugs block the effects of the acetylcholine neurotransmitter from the parasympathetic nervous system from causing smooth muscle contractions and secretions. Although this will decrease peristalsis, it will also cause the circular segmental contractions to cease, causing the bowel to relax and become flaccid without any resistance to flow of intestinal contents. By blocking segmental contractions, anticholinergics allow fecal contents to flow freely, thus actually increasing the speed with which they pass along the intestinal tract, contributing to the flow of the diarrhea.

12. The atropine is added to the narcotic opioid antidiarrheal drugs to discourage the abuse of these drugs for their narcotic effect. The dose of the atropine is subtherapeutic, but enough to produce some of the annoying effects such as dry mouth and dilated pupils.

13. The opioid antidiarrheal drugs slow the motility of the intestinal contents by increasing segmental contractions. In slowing the progress, they defeat the body's natural mechanism for "flushing out" the offending agents from the intestinal tract. In the case of salmonella bacteria, this slowed transit of intestinal contents means prolonged contact between the disease-causing bacteria and the animal's intestinal tract wall.

14. The oral dose of opioid narcotic antidiarrheals takes into account that much of the PO administered drug will be poorly absorbed because of the P-glycoprotein (P-gp) molecules in the lining of the intestinal tract that pump the opioids back into the lumen of the intestine. Collies and other Collie-like breeds have a genetic defect that renders the P-gp pump less effective, meaning that a "normal" dose of the opioids loperamide and diphenoxylate are likely to be absorbed to a much higher amount than normal and, because the P-gp in the

blood-brain barrier is likewise less effective, more of the opioid will enter the central nervous system, producing narcotic effects (e.g., sedation, ataxia, stupor).

15. The magnesium can be absorbed and the only way magnesium is removed from the body is via the kidneys. If the animal has renal failure or compromised renal function, this decreased elimination can result in accumulation of magnesium and a disruption of the electrolyte balance in the body.

16. Give the antacid no closer than 2 h before the other drug or 3 h after the other drug is given.

17. If the enteric coating of the omeprazole granules is damaged, the hydrochloric acid in the stomach could inactivate the drug.

18. Some studies have demonstrated a potential cancer-causing property of this drug; therefore, use in humans is prohibited.

CHAPTER 5

1. Fill in the following blanks with the correct item from the Key Terms list.
    A. preload
    B. conduction cells
    C. automaticity
    D. sinoatrial (SA) node
    E. P wave
    F. atrioventricular (AV) node
    G. PR interval (P-QRS interval)
    H. QRS complex
    I. T wave
    J. potassium
    K. sodium
    L. sodium-potassium-ATPase pump
    M. calcium
    N. arrhythmia
    O. epinephrine and norepinephrine
    P. β_1
    Q. cholinergic (muscarinic)
    R. β_2
    S. cholinergic (muscarinic)
    T. α_1
    U. tachycardia
    V. ectopic focus (foci = plural)
    W. premature ventricular contraction (PVC)
    X. first-degree AV block
    Y. "-olol"
    Z. upregulation
    AA. baroreceptors
    AB. renin–angiotensin system
    AC. angiotensin II
    AD. aldosterone
    AE. venodilator
    AF. ACE inhibitor
    AG. angiotensin-converting enzyme
    AH. diuretic

2. Fill in the following blanks with the correct drug from the Cardiovascular Drug list.

    A. lidocaine
    B. mexiletine
    C. propranolol
    D. atenolol, esmolol, metoprolol, carvedilol
    E. verapamil, diltiazem
    F. digoxin
    G. dobutamine (epinephrine, norepinephrine)
    H. pimobendan
    I. digoxin
    J. amlodipine
    K. hydralazine
    L. nitroglycerin
    M. enalapril (captopril, benazepril, lisinopril)
    N. furosemide (Lasix)
    O. chlorothiazide (hydrochlorothiazide, thiazides)
    P. spironolactone
    Q. aspirin

3. Anterior vena cava → right atrium → tricuspid valve (right AV valve) → right ventricle → pulmonic valve → pulmonary artery → lungs → pulmonary vein → left atrium → mitral valve (left AV valve) → left ventricle → aortic valve → aorta

4. Right atrium. Left ventricle.

5. The absolute refractory period is when a cell cannot depolarize regardless of the strength of stimulus to make it depolarize; the relative refractory period is the period of time in which a cell may depolarize again if given a sufficiently strong stimulus to depolarize.

6. SA node → atria → AV node → bundle branches → Purkinje fibers → ventricles. The delay in the AV node allows time for blood to move from the atria into the ventricles.

7. Fastest rate of automaticity. The SA node is the leakiest of the heart cells to sodium and thus allows sodium to leak into the cell after repolarization. The sodium leaking in causes the charge to become more positive inside the cell, bringing it closer to threshold. When the charge reaches threshold, the cell spontaneously depolarizes (i.e., fast sodium channels open). Because the SA node does this faster than any other cell in the heart, it is the pacemaker.

8. Sympathetic speeds up the heart through stimulation of β_1-receptors on the SA node. Parasympathetic slows the heart through stimulation of acetylcholine receptors on the SA node.

9. Adrenergic receptors (β_1, β_2, α_1) carry out the actions of the sympathetic nervous system when it releases catecholamines. Cholinergic receptors (i.e., muscarinic and nicotinic) carry out the actions of the parasympathetic nervous system when it releases acetylcholine. See answer to next question for more detailed outward effects.

10. The sympathetic nervous system (epinephrine, norepinephrine) causes an increased heart rate; increased force of contraction; decreased GI tract motility, secretion, and blood flow; increased diameter of bronchioles (i.e., bronchodilation); vasoconstriction of peripheral arterioles; vasodilation of arterioles in the skeletal muscles; dilation of pupils

(i.e., mydriasis). The parasympathetic nervous system slows the heart rate; has no effect on force of heart contraction; increases GI tract motility, secretion, and blood flow; decreases diameter of bronchioles (i.e., bronchoconstriction); has no effect on peripheral or skeletal muscle arterioles; and decreases pupil size (i.e., miosis).

11. Selective adrenergic drugs tend to specifically target one adrenergic receptor (or at least fewer types of receptors than nonselective drugs). Thus, a selective β_1 adrenergic agonist drug will stimulate a β_1 receptor, but is unlikely to stimulate a β_2 adrenergic receptor. A less selective drug would stimulate both and produce effects in another system (cardiac or respiratory) that would be side effects of the drug. For example, a less selective β_2 agonist bronchodilator drug would likely also cause tachycardia as a side effect because of β_1 receptor stimulation.

12. Flutter is multiple, rapid depolarization waves that do have some organization to them. Fibrillation is where depolarization waves are so disrupted that the chamber (atria or ventricles) just quivers instead of fully contracting. Fibrillation is worse. An animal can survive with atrial fibrillation, but ventricular fibrillation is fatal if not corrected quickly. Flutter and fibrillation are both classified as tachyarrhythmias (i.e., faster than normal rate, abnormal rhythms).

13. Classify the following arrhythmias according to heart rate (tachycardia or bradycardia) and the location of the problem (supraventricular or ventricular):
    A. Arrhythmia in a dog with ventricular contraction rate of 200 per minute caused by atrial fibrillation = supraventricular tachycardia (tachyarrhythmia)
    B. Arrhythmia in a dog with a ventricular contraction rate of 40 per minute caused by inability of the SA node to depolarize at its normal rate = supraventricular bradycardia
    C. Arrhythmia in a dog with a series of PVCs that increases the heart rate to 150 beats/min for approximately 30 s = ventricular tachycardia (tachyarrhythmia)

14. First-degree AV block is a slowing of the depolarization wave passing through the AV node, which shows on the ECG as a prolongation of the PR interval. First-degree AV block is common with drugs that increase the effect of the parasympathetic nervous system or decrease the effect of the sympathetic nervous system on the AV node. Second-degree AV block is when the depolarization wave passing through the AV node is slowed so much that it occasionally dies out and does not cause the ventricles to contract. Second-degree AV block appears on the ECG as a P wave (i.e., atrial depolarization) without a corresponding QRS complex (i.e., ventricular depolarization).

15. Animals with congestive heart failure have weak hearts. The sympathetic nervous system is normally activated in animals with congestive heart failure as a means to provide extra force of contraction through sympathetic stimulation (norepinephrine) of β_1 receptors on the heart muscle. β-Blockers block β_1 receptors, preventing norepinephrine from acting and hence blocking the boost the sympathetic nervous system would provide the weakened heart. β-Blocker antiarrhythmics could cause a controlled congestive heart failure patient to decompensate and worsen significantly.

16. This is upregulation of the β_1 receptors because of use of a β-blocker antiarrhythmic drug. In response to the β_1 receptors being blocked, the cell sprouted new β_1 receptors, making it necessary to increase the dose of the β_1-blocking drug to block the additional receptors. Without increasing the dose, the increased sensitivity of the heart cell results in greater responsiveness to the norepinephrine or epinephrine from the sympathetic nervous system and the heart rate slowly increases. If the owner stopped the β-blocker drug immediately, all of the β_1 receptor sites covered by the drug would now be exposed, making the cardiac cells much, much more sensitive to the effects of the sympathetic nervous system. If the dog gets excited, the heart may be stimulated so much that it could have a fatal tachyarrhythmia and die.

17. Digoxin is a poison that is detected by the CRTZ and in so doing causes stimulation of vomiting. At higher dosages signs of cardiac arrhythmias appear, including bradycardia and AV block.

18. Vasoconstriction increases the resistance to blood flowing through the narrowed small arterioles. The heart has to push the blood with greater force to get it through the narrowed openings. Though this narrowing in the arterioles results in an increased arterial blood pressure back upstream from the arterioles, a weakened heart may not be able to summon enough force to successfully push the blood through the vasoconstricted arterioles, causing the animal to go into decompensated heart failure and die.

19. Aldosterone increases the reabsorption of sodium from the urine back into the body. The water in the urine follows the sodium (osmotic effect), causing a more concentrated urine and conserving water in the body. The increased water in the body also adds water to the blood, increasing the blood volume. Increased blood volume = increased arterial blood pressure. The increased blood volume means there is a larger volume of blood that must be pumped by the heart against a higher arterial blood pressure in the arteries. For a weakened heart in congestive heart failure, this increased workload may exceed what the heart is capable of doing, resulting in decompensation of the heart failure.

20. When vasodilator drugs are first used, it is not uncommon for the animal to become hypotensive and possibly faint or act very weak, especially when rising after sleeping or being still for a while. This is part of the reason for starting at a low dose of the vasodilator and slowing increasing so the effect of the drug can be titrated to the particular needs of the patient. Because the sympathetic nervous system is stimulated when arterial blood pressure falls (i.e., baroreceptor stops firing and inhibition on sympathetic nervous system activation is removed), the body uses vasoconstriction and increased heart rate/force of contraction to bring the blood pressure back up to normal. If β-blocker drugs are used, the heart will be less able to increase rate and force of

contraction to bring the arterial blood pressure back up and the animal may remain hypotensive. Because sympathetic vasoconstriction is through stimulation of α_1 receptors, vasoconstriction should still occur in spite of β-blocker antiarrhythmic use, unless, of course, the vasodilating drug used was an α_1 blocker.

21. Vasodilator drugs typically block only one major vasoconstriction mechanism (e.g., α_1 receptor blocking, blocking of angiotensin II formation), leaving the other physiologic mechanisms intact. Over time these other vasoconstricting mechanisms may compensate for the vasodilator effect of the drug, negating the vasodilatory effect.

22. The drop in blood pressure caused by ACE inhibitor vasodilators can further decrease the blood flow and pressure that causes filtration to occur in the kidneys. The net result can be a further decline in kidney function. Blood flow and blood pressure within the renal capillaries (i.e., glomerulus) need to be improved before ACE is used to cause systemic vasodilation. Because angiotensin II stimulates the release of aldosterone, blocking angiotensin II formation with an ACE inhibitor blocks aldosterone release. Less aldosterone means less reclaiming of sodium and water from the forming urine in the kidney and less loss of potassium into the urine (i.e., potassium is normally exchanged into the urine for the sodium that is reabsorbed). Because less potassium is lost, animals with high blood potassium (i.e., hyperkalemia) or on potassium supplementation may further accumulate potassium to a potentially dangerous level.

23. Although ACE inhibitors have a marked beneficial effect in animals with congestive heart failure, normal animals show little response to these drugs because normal animals have not activated the renin–angiotensin system, hence there is no ACE present to inhibit with an ACE inhibitor like enalapril.

24. Because the drug can be absorbed through skin, including the animal owner's skin, clients should be instructed to always wear gloves when applying nitroglycerin. Children and others should be instructed not to pet the animal where the cream or patch has been applied. When the nitroglycerin patch is used, the site of nitroglycerin application by the patch should be changed with each dose.

25. Diuretics promote the excretion of excess body water by enhancing excretion of potassium or sodium in the urine which osmotically carries water with it. Decreasing body water decreases blood volume. Decreased blood volume means lowered pressure in the capillaries and less force pushing water out into the tissues. Net result is less edema formation.

26. Many diuretics produce increased urine flow by inhibiting reuptake of sodium from the forming urine in the renal tubules. More sodium in the urine means more osmotic force holding water in the urine, and the net result is diuresis. Because much of the sodium from the urine is normally reabsorbed in the loop of Henle where furosemide acts, blocking the reuptake at that point means more sodium remains in the urine and holds water in the urine, producing diuresis. Drugs like chlorothiazide block sodium

reuptake at the distal convoluted tubule. However, urine passing into the distal convoluted tubule has already had a significant percentage of the sodium reabsorbed by the normal functions of the loop of Henle. Hence, there is less sodium to block reabsorption in the distal convoluted tubule, less water is retained in the urine, and less diuresis occurs.

27. Furosemide and thiazide diuretics both inhibit reabsorption of sodium from the urine resulting in more sodium remaining in the urine (along with water for the diuretic effect). However, in the distal convoluted tubule the sodium is exchanged for potassium so that sodium is reabsorbed back into the body, but potassium is then excreted in the urine in its place, resulting in potassium loss. Spironolactone works by blocking the effect of aldosterone, the hormone that normally causes more sodium reabsorption from the distal convoluted tubule. Thus, the sodium remains in the urine and is not exchanged for potassium, resulting in a "conserving" of potassium by the body and excretion of sodium.

28. Acetazolamide is used to reduce production of aqueous humor in the globe of the eye. In so doing it reduces the pressure inside the eye and is therefore used to treat glaucoma.

29. Mannitol is an osmotic diuretic that pulls water from the tissues into the blood, and then, as the mannitol is excreted by the kidney, it pulls the water from the blood into the urine. The reason it is not used in congestive heart failure is because when mannitol pulls water from the tissues into the blood, it increases the blood volume temporarily, which increases the workload on a failing heart to pump the extra volume of blood.

30. Aspirin can be used in cats, but it must be used at doses that are lower than those used in dogs. The drug is designed to decrease the stickiness of platelets and therefore reduce spontaneous clot formation often associated with feline cardiomyopathy. See Chapter 13 for further explanation of aspirin.

31. Tranquilizers and sedatives are sometimes used in animals experiencing aerophagia or a sense of inability to oxygenate because of congestive heart failure. Animals can become very stressed, placing an increased sympathetic nervous system workload on the heart that is already in a weakened state. Reducing the fear/anxiety can reduce the sympathetic stimulation and in turn reduce the demand placed upon the weakened heart.

32. Indicate whether the following statements are true or false.
    A. True. Parasympathomimetic means the drug is imitating the parasympathetic nervous system effects.
    B. False. An antagonist blocks the effect. Thus, an adrenergic antagonist would block the effect of the sympathetic nervous system and would cause the heart rate to fall or remain the same (depending on how much parasympathetic effect was occurring at the time).
    C. False. The heart would continue to push blood into the arterial system, but the "exit" at the arteriole end (i.e., going into the capillaries and then onto the venous system) is more narrow so blood will not flow as well out

of the arterial system. The net result is more blood in the arteries pushing against the walls of the arterial system, which is interpreted as elevated arterial blood pressure.

D. False. Deoxygenated blood from the body returns to the heart via the right atrium, then into the right ventricle and is delivered to the lungs via the pulmonary arteries. Thus, the pulmonary arteries contain the least oxygenated blood. The pulmonary veins that return blood to the heart from the lungs contain the most oxygenated blood.

E. True. Parasympathetic input onto the AV node slows conduction of impulses through the AV node resulting in first-degree AV block (i.e., prolonged PR interval) or second-degree AV block (i.e., occasionally loss of the depolarization wave in the AV node, resulting in no QRS complex being generated).

F. False. When a cell is stimulated, the sodium channels open, allowing sodium (Na^+) to move INTO the cell. Potassium (K^+) then moves out of the cell during repolarization to reestablish the proper resting charge within the cell.

G. False. Cats are more sensitive to lidocaine effects than dogs. Cats generally require about one tenth of the dog dose.

H. True. Parasympathetic effects slow the heart rate, but do NOT decrease the force of contraction (only a reduction of sympathetic nervous system stimulation decreases the force of contraction).

I. True. α_1 Receptor stimulation causes peripheral vasoconstriction at the arterioles. Blocking α_1 receptors causes the smooth muscle to relax and the arterioles to dilate. When it is easier for the blood to flow through the arterioles, the pressure in the arterial system decreases (blood is no longer "backing" up waiting to leave the arterial system through constricted arterioles). Blood pressure drops.

J. False. Lidocaine for local anesthesia often contains epinephrine. Epinephrine would stimulate a heart (although the amount of epinephrine is fairly small in local anesthetics). In a heart that already had arrhythmias, the additional epinephrine stimulation could potentially make arrhythmias worse.

K. True. Quinidine blocks acetylcholine effects on the AV node, thereby allowing more impulses from the rapidly depolarizing atria (e.g., atrial fibrillation or flutter) to be more quickly communicated to the ventricles, resulting in a faster ventricular contraction rate.

L. True. Upregulation is the increase of β-receptors on the surface of the cell because of the β-blocker drugs, reducing the sympathetic nervous system's ability to stimulate the cell. β-Agonists, on the other hand, overstimulate the cell, resulting in the cell retracting receptors (i.e., downregulating) and becoming less sensitive to sympathetic nervous system stimulation.

M. True. Digoxin has a parasympathetic-like effect on the SA node, resulting in a slower overall heart rate. It also has a similar effect on the AV node slowing conduction of impulses into the ventricles, further slowing the ventricular contraction rate.

N. False. Negative inotropic means that the drug decreases the force with which the heart contracts. β₁-Blocker drugs are negative inotropic drugs because they block the sympathetic nervous system action on the heart and hence decrease the stimulus for greater force of contraction. Note: Drugs that slow the heart rate are called negative *chronotropic* drugs in reference to time (chronos = time).

O. False. It is the increased availability or increased combining of calcium, not sodium, with the contractile elements of cardiac muscle that produces the positive inotropic effect.

P. False. If β-blockers have been used for a period of time, the body has upregulated in response to the blocking of sympathetic stimulation of the cells. This means the cells are overly sensitive to sympathetic nervous stimulation if the β-blocker drugs are suddenly stopped. This could result in very severe or fatal arrhythmias. If the drug is to be stopped it must be tapered off slowly so that reversal of the upregulation can occur.

Q. True. Pimobendan in a positive inotropic drug and so increases force of contraction that can assist a failing, weak heart in congestive heart failure. However, in hypertrophic cardiomyopathy, the problem is not weak muscle but too much cardiac muscle that crowds the volume of the ventricles and produces a very inefficient contraction. Increasing the force of contraction in an "overmuscled" heart would not make the situation any better and potentially could make it very much worse.

R. False. ACE is angiotensin-converting enzyme. It converts angiotensin I to angiotensin II. The angiotensin II causes vasoconstriction and release of aldosterone for sodium and water retention.

S. False. Baroreceptors normally send signals to the brainstem that dampen or inhibit activation of the sympathetic nervous system. Thus, when arterial blood pressure goes up, stretching the arteries and the baroreceptors, signals are sent from the baroreceptor to inhibit activation of the sympathetic nervous system. The decreased sympathetic nervous system activity slows the heart rate and reduces the force of heart contraction, resulting in less blood being forced into the arterial system and a drop in arterial blood pressure. The opposite is also true in that a drop in arterial blood pressure reduces the arterial stretch, reduces the baroreceptor stimulation, and reduces the inhibitory impulses sent to the brainstem that would normally inhibit sympathetic nervous system stimulation. By reducing the baroreceptor's inhibitory signals, the sympathetic nervous system is activated, which increases the heart rate and force of contraction causing the arterial blood pressure to increase back toward normal.

T. True. Furosemide works in the loop of Henle to block more sodium reabsorption than the distal convoluted tubule where the thiazide diuretics work.

U. False. Mannitol is an osmotic diuretic used to reduce cerebral edema from head trauma.

V. True. However, because cats metabolize it so slowly, it should only be given in low doses every 2 days.

CHAPTER 6

1. Fill in the following blanks with the correct item from the Key Terms list.
   A. nebulization or aerosol therapy
   B. mucociliary apparatus or mucociliary escalator
   C. cor pulmonale
   D. bronchoconstriction
   E. antitussive drugs
   F. mucolytic
   G. expectorant
   H. decongestant
   I. beta-2 (β_2)
   J. alpha-1 (α_1)
   K. beta-1 (β_1)
   L. histamine type 1 (H_1)
   M. dyspnea
   N. inspissated
   O. productive cough
   P. metered dose inhaler
   Q. serotonin
   R. recurrent airway obstruction (RAO)
   S. opioid
   T. cyclic adenosine monophosphate (cAMP)
   U. phosphodiesterase

2. Fill in the following blanks with the correct drug from the Respiratory Drug list.
   A. guaifenesin
   B. butorphanol
   C. aminophylline
   D. glucocorticoids
   E. acetylcysteine (Mucomyst)
   F. antihistamine
   G. hydrocodone
   H. diuretic
   I. dextromethorphan
   J. guaifenesin (glyceryl guaiacolate)
   K. acetylcysteine
   L. theophylline
   M. β_2-agonist drugs: albuterol, terbutaline, metaproterenol
   N. codeine
   O. methylxanthines: theophylline, aminophylline

3. Indicate whether the following statements are true or false.
   A. True. The DNA released after lysis of the inflammatory cells that migrated into the airway and infiltrated the mucus makes the mucus sticky.
   B. False. Labored breathing is called dyspnea. Rapid breathing is called tachypnea. Consider that an animal can be breathing fast, but without excessive labor, after they exercise. Or an animal can be fighting to draw each breath in because of an obstruction, in which case they are dyspneic, but not tachypneic.
   C. True.
   D. True. Diuretics draw water out of the body via the urine and eventually dehydrate tissues. This would decrease the fluidity of the mucus making it more inspissated and thus stickier and less effective.
   E. False. Dextromethorphan is the OTC antitussive and as such is fairly ineffective in veterinary patients, especially compared with the opioids, like butorphanol.
   F. True. In dehydrated animals, the mucus would be less fluid and hence stickier. As the animal coughs, less or no noticeable mucus would be brought up or "produced," making the cough nonproductive.
   G. False. Direct bronchodilators work by stimulating β_2-receptors. If they are not very specific, these same drugs can also stimulate β_1-receptors on the heart as a side effect, producing tachycardia (i.e., increased heart rate), not bradycardia (i.e., slowed heart rate).
   H. False. Though antihistamine drugs can decrease inflammation over time and decrease histamine-mediated bronchoconstriction, in veterinary patients with respiratory distress from bronchoconstriction, a bronchodilator drug would be needed and indicated for a quicker response.
   I. True. Decongestants work by stimulating α_1-receptors that vasoconstrict the small precapillary arterioles in the nasal mucosa.
   J. False. Dextromethorphan is an OTC human antitussive. It is not used in veterinary medicine.
   K. False. Nebulization or aerosolization is the process of delivering a drug in a mist that is inhaled and thereby delivered to the airways of the lungs.
   L. True. Stimulation of the laryngeal area often causes the vocal folds and epiglottis to snap shut, accompanied by a short but gagging type of cough designed to dislodge food or other larger materials from the area around the larynx or upper trachea. Deeper coughs typically are more drawn-out and coordinated inspirations and forceful expirations.
   M. True.
   N. True. Sympathetic stimulation normally bronchodilates to allow for more air to come into the alveoli under fight-or-flight situations. Parasympathetic stimulation, via acetylcholine receptors on the smooth muscles of the bronchioles, causes smooth muscle contraction and bronchoconstriction.
   O. True. Centrally acting antitussives act by suppressing the respiratory center and cough reflex in the brain. Locally acting antitussives sooth inflamed tissues in the respiratory tree that stimulate the cough reflex. Because local antitussives typically are held in the mouth and slowly dissolved, they do not work in veterinary patients.
   P. True.

Q. False. Acetylcholine receptors (i.e., cholinergic receptors) on the smooth muscle surrounding the terminal bronchioles cause contraction of the smooth muscle and bronchoconstriction.

R. True. Histamine type 1 (H_1) receptors on the bronchioles cause bronchoconstriction, and β_2 receptors cause bronchodilation by generating cAMP and allowing the smooth muscles to relax.

S. True.

4. Sympathetic nervous system causes bronchodilation to allow easier flow of air into the alveoli for fight-or-flight situations.

5. Methylxanthines have a CNS stimulatory side effect. Caffeine, for example, is a well-known CNS stimulator and it is also a methylxanthine.

6. Acetylcholine is the neurotransmitter associated with the effects of the parasympathetic nervous system (see Chapter 5 for additional details).

7. Histamine is the major inflammatory mediator released from mast cells.

8. cAMP is the molecular signal generated by stimulating the β_2 receptor that plays the key role in causing the relaxation of smooth muscles.

9. The larynx is designed to keep food and liquids from entering the trachea. Thus, one of its key defenses is to snap shut the opening to the trachea to prevent these from entering. This is associated with a short but violent gagging cough reflex. The upper part of the trachea may produce a similar sort of gagging cough. The mucociliary apparatus will trap dust and other particles that are inhaled and will sweep them up and out of the respiratory tree. Cough reflexes in the lower airways are usually slower and involve a much larger volume of air in a coordinated cough. Bronchoconstriction at the terminal bronchioles is a last ditch attempt to keep things out of the alveoli. It is intended to be a locally protective mechanism to protect individual alveoli. However, when it occurs in large areas of the lungs, the bronchoconstriction can be life threatening. Finally, if particles get into the alveoli, macrophage cells will attempt to neutralize particles. No cough originates from the alveoli as there would be no way to get air "behind" an object in the alveoli to force it out.

10. If an animal is dehydrated, the amount of fluid in the respiratory mucus will be decreased and could mask an excessive amount of mucus production. Once rehydrated, the veterinarian can more accurately assess whether the cough is truly nonproductive or if it was actually very productive but masked by the dehydration.

11. Locally acting antitussives are "cough drops" that are meant to be held in the mouth. No veterinary patient is going to hold a cough drop in its mouth and wait for it to dissolve.

12. Inspissated mucus is sticky and hence the mucociliary apparatus cannot readily move the mucus up and out of the respiratory tree. Sticky balls of mucus can accumulate and obstruct free air flow through the airways. Expectorants add watery secretions to the mucus, making it more liquefied. Mucolytic drugs change the chemical composition of the mucus; specifically they split the sulfhydryl (S–S) bonds from DNA and RNA in cellular debris that make the mucus sticky. In this way, they "lyse" the mucus, making it less sticky and more readily moveable on the mucociliary cilia.

13. Animals that ingest decongestants will experience peripheral vasoconstriction because that is how decongestants reduce edema in the nasal mucosa. This can elevate arterial blood pressure and have a secondary effect of CNS stimulation. Pets may appear anxious or agitated. As long as the hypertension (i.e., elevated arterial blood pressure) is not life threatening, the effects will pass in a few hours.

14. When β_2 receptors are stimulated, they increase the amount of cAMP inside the smooth muscle cells surrounding the terminal bronchioles. cAMP causes the smooth muscles to relax and produce bronchodilation. β-Blocking antiarrhythmic drugs would block this bronchodilating effect and the degree of resulting bronchoconstriction would depend on the degree to which the parasympathetic nervous system or other compounds like histamine were active and attempting to produce bronchoconstriction.

15. Albuterol and terbutaline are more selective β_2-agonist drugs than epinephrine, which has a variety of other autonomic nervous system side effects. Though epinephrine is still used in emergency situations to cause bronchodilation, it is not a drug to be used for long-term control of asthma or bronchoconstriction.

16. Aminophylline and theophylline are both methylxanthines. Theophylline is the active ingredient and aminophylline is a drug that is composed of theophylline and a salt to improve its ability to be used orally without causing too much GI upset.

17. Stopping antibiotic use as soon as the animal "seems" better does not mean that all of the bacteria have been successfully eliminated. Indeed, the bacteria that have survived exposure to the antibiotic for a few days must be the bacteria most resistant to the effects of the antibiotic. If the antibiotic is stopped too quickly, these "selected" resistant bacteria can proliferate and produce a second infection that is not responsive to the same antibiotic that "cured" the animal the first time.

18. Nebulization is indicated for infections that are located on the surface of the lining of the respiratory tract (the airway side). This surface is considered to be "outside" of the body and hence drugs given systemically (PO or parenterally) can have large concentrations in the blood but not be able to reach the airway where the infection lies. Though nebulization works well in humans, the difference is that humans will breathe deeply when instructed to do so to inhale the mist carrying the drug deep into the respiratory tree. Veterinary patients will resist breathing in a mist if it has an odor or taste, and will not breathe deeply, allowing much of the drug to precipitate against the lining of the trachea and the main stem bronchi and not achieving satisfactory delivery of the drug deep into the bronchioles or alveoli. Using metered dose inhalers attached to spacers (i.e., tubes

between the inhaler and where the animal breathes in the mist) allows the drug to be diluted with air first, reducing some of the chemical taste or smell of the mist. The animals will still not breathe deeply, but they will fight the administration of the nebulized drug less.

19. Corticosteroids should be used in situations where the inflammation itself poses a threat to life more than the infectious agent. For example, severe inflammation from chemical or smoke inhalation can kill an animal by causing severe pulmonary edema from the inflammation itself and not involving any infectious agent. Or, if an infectious agent is causing a severe inflammatory reaction, the inflammation itself may end life by causing obstruction of the airways or filling the alveoli with fluid before the infectious agent itself can kill the animal. Thus, the inflammation needs to be controlled, and glucocorticoid drugs can do this. The animal would receive simultaneous treatment with antibiotics or drugs to kill the infection, but the control of the inflammation using corticosteroid drugs would allow the inflammation to subside sufficiently for the animal to live long enough for the antibiotics to work. The disadvantage of using corticosteroids is that they do inhibit the cell-mediated immune response (i.e., killer cells) that plays an important role in eliminating bacterial or fungal infections.

20. Diuretics can be used to decrease pulmonary edema by dehydrating the tissues. Decreasing edema allows better exchange of oxygen between the alveoli and the blood. However, the dehydration reduces the ability of the mucociliary apparatus to work because it causes the mucus to become inspissated and sticky.

21. Oxygen gas by itself does not contain water and thus is very dry. It can dry out the mucous membranes and impair the mucociliary apparatus from working by making the mucus very sticky.

CHAPTER 7

1. Fill in the following blanks with the correct item from the Key Terms list.
   A. negative feedback
   B. thyrotropin-releasing hormone (TRH)
   C. thyroid-stimulating hormone (TSH)
   D. triiodothyronine (T_3)
   E. tetraiodothyronine or thyroxine (T_4)
   F. hypothyroidism
   G. hyperthyroidism
   H. primary hypothyroidism
   I. tertiary hypothyroidism
   J. secondary hypothyroidism
   K. goiter
   L. estrous (not estrus, which is a noun describing the state of heat)
   M. triiodothyronine
   N. tetraiodothyronine or thyroxine
   O. euthyroid
   P. thyroidectomy

   Q. non–insulin-dependent diabetes mellitus (type 2 diabetes)
   R. insulin-dependent diabetes mellitus (type 1 diabetes)
   S. insulin-dependent diabetes mellitus
   T. non–insulin-dependent diabetes mellitus
   U. recombinant human insulin
   V. protamine
   W. U-40
   X. protamine zinc insulin
   Y. hypoglycemic agents
   Z. sulfonylurea
   AA. follicular phase
   AB. luteal phase
   AC. gonadotropin-releasing hormone (GnRH)
   AD. follicle-stimulating hormone
   AE. luteinizing hormone
   AF. oocytes
   AG. estrus (not estrous, which is the adjective that describes a type of cycle)
   AH. inhibin
   AI. progesterone
   AJ. progesterone
   AK. corpus luteum
   AL. myometrium
   AM. adrenocorticotropic hormone (ACTH)
   AN. cortisol
   AO. prostaglandin
   AP. oxytocin
   AQ. oxytocin
   AR. oxytocin
   AS. oxytocin
   AT. gonadotropin-releasing hormone analogs or gonadorelins
   AU. timed artificial insemination (timed AI)
   AV. gonadotropins
   AW. gonadotropins
   AX. human chorionic gonadotropin
   AY. equine chorionic gonadotropin
   AZ. progestins, progestational hormones
   BA. progestogen
   BB. controlled internal drug release
   BC. metritis
   BD. pyometra (or pyometritis)
   BE. carcinogenic
   BF. aplastic anemia
   BG. foal heat
   BH. seasonal anestrus
   BI. dystocia

2. Fill in the following blanks with the correct drug from the Endocrine Drug list.
   A. levothyroxine (synthetic T_4)
   B. liothyronine (synthetic T_3)
   C. methimazole
   D. radioactive iodine (^{131}I)
   E. propranolol or atenolol
   F. amlodipine
   G. crystalline or regular insulin

    H. insulin glargine, insulin detemir
    I. neutral protamine Hagedorn (NPH), lente, porcine insulin zinc suspension
    J. protamine zinc insulin (PZI)
    K. regular (crystalline) insulin
    L. glipizide
    M. gonadorelins (synthetic GnRH analogs)
    N. altrenogest
    O. progesterones, progestogens
    P. melengestrol acetate (MGA)
    Q. estriol
    R. prostaglandin
    S. dinoprost tromethamine and cloprostenol
    T. prostaglandin
    U. prostaglandin
    V. progesterone
    W. progesterone
    X. GnRH analog drugs
    Y. dopamine antagonists
    Z. altrenogest
   AA. megestrol acetate
   AB. mibolerone
   AC. dopamine agonists
   AD. corticosteroids (glucocorticoids)
   AE. oxytocin

3. Hormone B has the effect on the body. Hormone A simply tells gland B that the body needs more of its hormone. Thus, when there is sufficient hormone B, the concentration of hormone B will inhibit gland A production of hormone A, which in turn stops stimulating gland B to produce hormone because the body has enough of hormone B.

4. In primary hypothyroidism, there is a problem with the thyroid gland's ability to produce T_3 and T_4. Thus, T_3/T_4 levels should be lower than normal. Because T_3/T_4 levels are lower than normal, there is not as much negative feedback from T_4 on the hypothalamus and pituitary. Without the negative feedback, the hypothalamus releases TRH, which in turn releases TSH, which is intended to stimulate the thyroid to produce more T_3/T_4 and to bring concentrations of these thyroid gland hormones up to their normal levels. Because the thyroid is incapable of responding, the T_3/T_4 levels stay low. In secondary hypothyroidism, the thyroid is functionally fine but the pituitary gland is diseased or damaged and cannot produce sufficient TSH. Because the pituitary gland cannot produce TSH, the thyroid gland is not stimulated and T_3/T_4 levels would be low. Because T_3/T_4 levels are low, there is no negative feedback so the hypothalamus continues to produce high levels of TRH to try to stimulate the chain of hormones that would restore normal levels of thyroid hormone. In tertiary hypothyroidism, the hypothalamus is not producing TRH and therefore the pituitary gland is not being stimulated to produce TSH. TSH levels from the pituitary would be low and without TSH stimulation. The thyroid would not produce T_3/T_4, so T_3/T_4 levels would be low.

5. Indicate which of the following clinical signs are most often associated with hypothyroidism and which are associated with hyperthyroidism.

Hair loss	Hypothyroidism
Bradycardia	Hypothyroidism
Intolerance of warm environments	Hyperthyroidism
Increased activity, alertness	Hyperthyroidism
Dry, scaly skin	Hypothyroidism
Increased size of thyroid gland or part of thyroid gland	Hyperthyroidism
Heat-seeking behavior	Hypothyroidism
Weight gain in spite of normal food consumption	Hypothyroidism
Polyuria, polydipsia	Hyperthyroidism
Loss of weight in spite of normal or increased appetite	Hyperthyroidism
Tachycardia	Hyperthyroidism

6. Different body tissues have different needs for thyroid hormone. Because of that, enzymes at the tissue sites convert T_4 to the active T_3 form as needed. Using the T_4 form of medication (i.e., levothyroxine) allows the body to convert T_4 to the T_3 form in the amount needed by local tissues. If T_3 (i.e., liothyronine) is used, doses would have to be based on the tissue that needs the most T_3, which means other tissues would receive more T_3 than they needed. The combination drugs of T_3/T_4 are geared toward the ideal T_3/T_4 ratio in human beings, which is quite different from the ratio in dogs. Plus the product is much more expensive than the veterinary T_4 products. For these reasons, combination T_3/T_4 products are rarely used in veterinary medicine.

7. Methimazole blocks T_3 and T_4 formation; only controls the hyperthyroidism.
   ^{131}I (i.e., radioactive iodine) destroys active thyroid cancer cells; cures the hyperthyroidism. Iodine-limited diets deprive the thyroid of the iodine it needs to create T_3 and T_4; only control the hyperthyroidism.

8. In a diabetic hypothyroid dog treated with thyroid supplementation, the increased T_3/T_4 will cause increased gluconeogenesis (i.e., conversion of protein's amino acids to glucose), which increases blood glucose.

9. Hyperthyroid cats are often not presented to the veterinary hospital because they typically have a good or excellent appetite, are drinking sufficiently (actually more than usual and urinating more also), and are very active and often playful. It is not until the signs of diarrhea or unkempt appearance of the cat display that the owner is prompted to take the cat to the veterinarian or to mention these changes during a routine vaccination appointment.

10. Methimazole works by blocking the ability of the thyroid gland to combine iodine onto molecule backbones to form thyroid hormones.

11. Renal disease or failure: the high arterial blood pressure inherent in hyperthyroidism means there is higher pressure in the renal glomerulus where drugs and metabolic wastes (e.g., creatinine, blood urea) are filtered out of the blood and

into the urine. This high pressure filtering can compensate for an overall reduced ability by the kidney to normally filter. Thus, when hyperthyroidism is corrected and arterial blood pressure returns to normal, glomerular filtration of drugs, creatinine, and blood urea in the kidney may decrease, causing these to increase in the blood and show reduced kidney function.

12. Carbimazole is essentially a precursor (i.e., prodrug) for methimazole. It is available in other countries outside of the United States.

13. When a tumor on the thyroid gland produces high levels of T_3 and T_4, the high levels of thyroid hormone produce a large negative feedback effect to shut down production of TRH by the hypothalamus and TSH by the pituitary. Normal thyroid tissue (i.e., the part of the thyroid gland that is not tumorous) is dependent on TSH for normal growth and function; thus the shutdown of TSH means the normal thyroid tissue atrophies. Atrophied thyroid tissue does not take up iodine because it is not creating thyroid hormone. Thus, when radioactive iodine is administered to a cat with a thyroid tumor, only the active, thyroid hormone-producing cells of the tumor take up the radioactive iodine and the atrophied normal thyroid cells do not. The cancer cells exposed to the radiation die, but the normal, atrophied thyroid cells survive. Once the tumor is destroyed and the artificially high levels of thyroid hormones decline, the negative feedback is removed on the hypothalamus and pituitary, allowing TRH and TSH to again be produced, which stimulates the atrophied normal tissue to begin functioning again.

14. In hyperthyroidism, the elevated levels of thyroid hormones produced by the thyroid tumor increase the number of β_1-receptors on cardiac cells, making the heart more sensitive to sympathetic stimulation. Thus, normal sympathetic stimulation produces tachycardia, with heart rates in the cat often exceeding 240 beats/min. β_1 Antagonists (see Chapter 5), such as propranolol or atenolol, decrease the effect of sympathetic stimulation by preventing the normal sympathetic neurotransmitter molecules of epinephrine and norepinephrine from combining with the β_1 receptors. Consequently, the heartbeat slows to a more normal rate.

15. Cats more often have NIDDM than dogs. Sometimes oral hypoglycemic agents, such as glipizide, can be used in cats with NIDDM. IDDM must be treated with injectable insulin. In NIDDM, the hyperglycemia is a problem with the receptor. In IDDM, the problem is insufficient production of insulin. NIDDM receptor problems are caused by alteration of the insulin receptors so they do not accept insulin or respond to insulin as well (such as occurs in overweight human beings). NIDDM can also be because of a lower than required amount of insulin being produced in combination with the less-sensitive receptors. In IDDM, the insulin receptors are fine, but there are not enough functional beta cells left to produce the needed amount of insulin; therefore the insulin must be provided by injection.

16. Insulin used in the dog that originates from another species is not identical to canine or feline insulin and therefore may be viewed by the body's defense mechanisms as foreign; the body attacks the insulin with antibodies, rendering the insulin less effective or ineffective. Fortunately pork insulin is close enough to canine insulin that antibody production is not a significant problem. Human recombinant insulin is not as genetically close, but the extent of antibody development is slow to develop in the dog.

17. The addition of other proteins to the insulin molecule creates crystals or molecular combinations that are slow to dissolve and hence do not release all of the active insulin immediately after being injected. Protamine and zinc are added in different combinations to delay the absorption of insulin, making the insulin intermediate or long acting.

18. Insulin concentration is measured in units and a unit (U) is a measure of the biologic activity of the insulin (as opposed to the mass of insulin, as measured by milligrams and grams). Because insulin in a bottle is measured by units, the syringes used for insulin are marked in units instead of cubic centimeters or milliliters. A bottle of insulin that is listed as a U-40 has 40 U per mL. U-40 bottles need to be used with U-40 syringes so the proper amount of insulin is removed from the bottle. The same applies to U-100 and U-500 designations.

19. Historically resuspension of the insulin crystals was recommended to be done only by rolling the bottle between the palms of the hands instead of vigorously shaking the bottle for fear of physically breaking the insulin molecule and inactivating the drug. However, more recent information provided by the manufacturer of lente insulin and the manufacturer of the porcine insulin zinc suspension (Vetsulin) specifically states that shaking does not negatively affect insulin activity and is required to uniformly resuspend the drug throughout the liquid medium. This constitutes a major change in how veterinarians, veterinary technicians, and human nurses were taught how to resuspend insulin injectables.

20. In order for the insulin to be absorbed consistently from dose to dose, the pet owner must administer the drug in areas that have consistent perfusion. If insulin is injected into a poorly perfused fat pad it may remain at that site for hours beyond what it would if injected subcutaneously (SQ). Thus, proper depth and consistent location of insulin injection are essential for regulation of the diabetic patient by its owner.

21. Cats. Oral hypoglycemic agents like glipizide stimulate the pancreatic beta cells to produce more insulin. Thus, glipizide only works if sufficient beta cells still exist and have not been totally destroyed. Insulin cannot be given by mouth because the stomach acid and digestive enzymes would destroy the insulin molecule; and the molecule is too large to be absorbed across the GI tract wall intact, even if it was not destroyed. Oral hypoglycemics are not used in dogs because diabetic dogs typically do not have sufficient beta cells remaining by the time they show clinical signs of diabetes and they never have non–insulin-dependent diabetes mellitus; dogs require insulin.

22. Progesterone has a negative feedback effect on the release of GnRH from the hypothalamus and FSH/LH from the pituitary. Without the release of FSH during the follicular phase of the estrous cycle, the follicles on the ovaries cannot develop to initiate a new estrous cycle. And if the follicles have already developed, the negative feedback inhibiting LH release will prevent the LH-induced follicular rupture to release the oocytes, allowing the luteal phase to begin.

23. Prostaglandins work by lysing the CL at the end of the luteal phase. Thus, in the follicular phase prostaglandins have nothing to work with and their activity is confined to the latter parts of the luteal phase. When prostaglandins lyse the CL, the CL stops producing progesterone. Progesterone has a negative feedback effect on GnRH release and release of FSH and LH. Removal of the progesterone removes the negative feedback and the hypothalamus releases GnRH and the pituitary releases FSH to begin a new estrous cycle.

24. The developing follicle produces inhibin, which is a hormone that reduces the release of further FSH during the follicular phase when follicles are developing. Those follicles that have developed sufficiently will go on to complete development in spite of the dropping levels of FSH. But those other follicles that have not developed as far will regress because there is insufficient FSH to continue to stimulate their development. This assures that only one or a few (depending on species) follicles develop sufficiently to release an oocyte (i.e., egg).

25. At the end of pregnancy the fetus initiates parturition by producing pituitary ACTH, which stimulates production of cortisol from the adrenal glands of both the fetus and the pregnant female animal. In response to the elevated cortisol levels, the uterus begins to produce estrogens and prostaglandins, both of which make the myometrium more prone to contraction and produce physical changes in the cervix and birth canal that favor passage of the newborn. The prostaglandins produced by the uterus lyse the CL, terminating its production of progesterone and removing the "calming" effect on the myometrium. Estrogen and prostaglandins both make the uterus more prone to contraction, and additionally they increase the number of oxytocin receptors on the myometrial cells, making these smooth muscle cells more sensitive to the powerful contracting effect of oxytocin. Stimulation of the cervix or vagina, such as from entry of the fetus into the birth canal, causes the pituitary gland to release oxytocin, which produces the forceful uterine contractions associated with labor and postpartum contractions. Before parturition, oxytocin would not be able to induce labor because the oxytocin receptors have not emerged on the myometrium and hence there would not be a place for oxytocin to produce its effect.

26. In an animal that is lactating, stimulation of the nipples causes release of oxytocin from the pituitary gland. The smooth muscles surrounding the milk glands in the mammary tissue begin to contract under the influence of oxytocin, forcing milk into the milk chambers where it can be extracted by hand or a milking machine.

27. Timed AI protocols use drugs in a specific, timed order to bring an entire group of cattle into estrus at the same time regardless of where they were in their individual estrous cycles. This eliminates the time-consuming and labor-intensive work of identifying where individual cows are in their cycles.

28. Gonadotropins are FSH- or LH-like compounds. Gonadotropins with LH activity would be able to lyse mature or persistent ovarian follicles. Gonadorelins are synthetic GnRH analog hormone drugs that would cause release of pituitary FSH and LH and theoretically could also lyse mature follicles by secondarily causing release of LH from the pituitary.

29. Human chorionic gonadotropin has primarily an LH-like effect and would be able to lyse mature or persistent ovarian follicles during the follicular phase. It would have no effect during the luteal phase because there are no mature follicles available to lyse during this phase. Equine chorionic gonadotropin has both FSH and LH activities, and has been used to cause superovulation (i.e., development of more than normal ovarian follicles with oocytes because of the FSH effect) during the follicular phase and can also cause ovulation because of its LH effect. This drug would have no real effect in the luteal phase.

30. Altrenogest is a progestogen (i.e., synthetic hormone drug that mimics progesterone) and hence acts like progesterone to maintain the pregnancy. However, altrenogest would only be effective in maintaining pregnancy if the animal was deficient in natural progesterone. It does not appear to provide any significant improvement for maintaining pregnancy in a mare that already has normal levels of progesterone.

31. MGA is an FDA-approved progestogen that is added to cattle feed to suppress the estrous cycle or prolong diestrus by exerting a progesterone-like negative feedback inhibition of the hypothalamic GnRH release and the pituitary FSH/LH release.

32. CIDR apparatus provides a continuous supply of progesterone for several days. The CIDRs are FDA approved for use in cattle and consist of long, slender silicone rubber implants containing progesterone that are inserted vaginally and remain for several days. When the implant is removed it imitates CL lysis and the end of diestrus.

33. Progesterone causes changes in the lining of the uterus that favors survival of a fertilized zygote, but such changes also favor growth of pathogenic bacteria and pyometra if bacteria have gained access to the uterus.

34. Progestin drugs can be well absorbed across the skin of those who handle these drugs. Thus, latex gloves should always be worn when handling a progesterone CIDR and care should be taken not to spill oral progesterone drug on the skin of the person administering the drug. Oil-based progesterone products may penetrate some cheaper, more porous gloves, so good-quality latex gloves should always be used and if there is any suspicion of a tear or puncture, the gloves should be replaced. Absorption of progestins by those administering the drug can

result in changes in the human reproductive tract similar to those observed in veterinary patients: prolonged diestrus, increased uterine lining thickening, increased risk of pyometra, etc.

35. Estrogens are used as estriol for treatment of urinary incontinence in spayed female dogs. DES was found to be a potential carcinogen (i.e., cancer-producing agent) in humans and therefore is completely banned for use in any food-producing animal.

36. Prostaglandins have been used by women to induce their own abortions. Because prostaglandins are readily absorbed through the skin, a veterinary technician who is pregnant could accidentally cause abortion or premature parturition by spilling prostaglandin drugs onto her own skin. Technicians should take precautions such as wearing good-quality latex gloves when handling these drugs. Women of childbearing age and those with asthma should completely avoid handling these drugs at any time.

37. Nymphomania is a term used to describe the behavior associated with persistent follicles and generation of estrogen, producing continuous heat (i.e., estrus). The persistent follicles can be lysed with gonadorelins, which will cause release of LH to lyse the follicles. Theoretically gonadotropins that have LH activity could also be used.

38. Prolactin is a hormone whose natural release has been shown to increase follicle development in transitional anestrus mares. Dopamine from the hypothalamus normally suppresses prolactin release, preventing this. Dopamine antagonist drugs block dopamine, thus allowing release of prolactin and potentially causing follicle development.

39. Megestrol acetate and mibolerone are two hormones that mimic progesterone and testosterone, respectively. Both suppress the estrous cycle by negative feedback on the hypothalamus and pituitary gland. Because mibolerone is a testosterone-like compound, it has the potential for abuse by body builders or those wanting to increase muscle mass (it is a "steroid" as defined in the athletic or sport context) and therefore is prone to abuse. The abuse potential has made it a Controlled Substance.

40. Prolactin is normally released by the hypothalamus to help maintain the CL during pregnancy and thus maintain a critical source of progesterone needed to maintain a pregnancy. Dopamine naturally blocks the release of prolactin. Dopamine agonist drugs mimic the effect of dopamine and therefore block release of prolactin. Without the prolactin, the CL may degenerate, progesterone hormone levels will drop, and this may result in failure of the pregnancy.

41. Glucocorticoids (i.e., corticosteroids) are involved in the first steps of the onset of parturition. By giving an injection of the glucocorticoids the owner may set off the sequence that produces the onset of labor and parturition in an animal that is somewhat near to the end of the pregnancy term.

42. Indicate whether the following statements are true or false.
    A. False.
    B. False. Humans are much more sensitive to excess thyroid hormones than dogs. This is why dogs can be placed on a therapeutic trial of thyroid supplement to

determine whether the animal improves (typically the skin condition improves) with supplementation instead of spending the money to test for thyroid levels first.
    C. False. Radioactive iodine is given by injection, most commonly administered SQ but also given IV.
    D. False. Iodine-limited diets need to be given continuously.
    E. True. Regular insulin can be given IV, IM and SQ, but the others must be given SQ to be consistently absorbed.
    F. False. Estrogen has the potential to have a toxic effect on the bone marrow, suppressing production of all bone marrow cells; this results in a potentially fatal condition called aplastic anemia.

CHAPTER 8

1. Fill in the following blanks with the correct item from the Key Terms list.
    A. nociceptor
    B. transduction
    C. modulation
    D. general anesthesia
    E. hyperalgesia
    F. hyperesthesia
    G. wind-up
    H. opiates
    I. opioids
    J. narcosis
    K. narcotics
    L. neuroleptanalgesic
    M. mu (μ) receptors, kappa (κ) receptors, and delta (δ) receptors
    N. dysphoria
    O. partial agonist/partial antagonist
    P. mixed agonist
    Q. mixed antagonist
    R. mixed agonist/mixed antagonist
    S. μ-receptor
    T. κ-receptor
    U. potency
    V. efficacy
    W. visceral pain
    X. somatic pain
    Y. hyperthermia
    Z. ceiling effect
    AA. tranquilizer
    AB. anxiolytic
    AC. sedative
    AD. phenothiazines
    AE. dopamine
    AF. idiosyncratic reaction
    AG. gamma (γ)-aminobutyric acid (GABA)
    AH. $GABA_A$ receptor
    AI. alpha-2 (α_2)
    AJ. baroreceptors
    AK. anesthesia
    AL. local anesthesia

AM. *N*-methyl-D-aspartate (NMDA) receptors

AN. redistribution

AO. dissociative anesthetic

AP. catalepsy

AQ. tachycardia

AR. apneustic breathing pattern

AS. neurosteroid or neuroactive steroid

AT. minimum alveolar concentration (MAC)

AU. compound A

AV. diffusion hypoxia

AW. bradypnea

AX. apnea

AY. euphoria

2. Fill in the following blanks with the correct drug from the Nervous System Drug list.

A. morphine

B. tramadol

C. methadone

D. diazepam (Valium), zolazepam (component of Telazol), midazolam (Versed), clonazepam (Klonopin)

E. butorphanol

F. isoflurane

G. tramadol

H. xylazine

I. naloxone

J. acepromazine

K. ketamine or tiletamine

L. diazepam

M. acepromazine

N. fentanyl

O. clonazepam

P. isoflurane, desflurane, sevoflurane

Q. buprenorphine, butorphanol

R. ketamine, tiletamine

S. methylxanthines

T. flumazenil

U. acepromazine

V. zolazepam

W. romifidine

X. xylazine

Y. buprenorphine

Z. diazepam

AA. detomidine

AB. propofol

AC. medetomidine

AD. ketamine, tiletamine

AE. yohimbine, atipamezole, tolazoline

AF. xylazine

AG. phenobarbital

AH. propofol

AI. desflurane

AJ. propofol

AK. atipamezole

AL. dexmedetomidine

AM. ketamine, tiletamine

AN. ketamine, tiletamine

AO. tiletamine

AP. ketamine

AQ. alfaxalone

AR. sevoflurane

AS. theobromine

AT. nitrous oxide

AU. hydromorphone

AV. doxapram

3. Indicate whether each of the following statements is true or false.

A. False. The μ-mediated analgesia occurs primarily by decreasing the release of excitatory neurotransmitters (e.g., acetylcholine, dopamine, serotonin) and dampening excitation of the postsynaptic sites where these neurotransmitters would normally act.

B. True. Local anesthetics work by preventing receptor depolarization in response to stimulus, hence they decrease the perception of any sensation including pain (i.e., nociception).

C. False. Wind-up occurs because of changes within the spinal cord when pain signals are being sent up the spinal cord. Whether or not the animal perceives the pain at the highest levels of the brain has no influence on the development of wind-up at the spinal cord level. This is why gas anesthesia by itself would have minimal inhibitory effect on the development of wind-up.

D. True. Narcosis is sedation from which the animal is not readily aroused. Tranquilization means anxiety is decreased but the animal is not necessarily sedate.

E. False. Neuroleptanalgesics are injectable drugs composed of an opioid analgesic and a tranquilizer.

F. False. A partial agonist means that the maximal efficacy (i.e., greatest analgesic effect) is lower than a full agonist.

G. True. μ-Receptor stimulation produces a more profound analgesia than κ-receptor stimulation.

H. True.

I. False. Potency is a relative measure of how much drug it takes to achieve a particular effect. The less drug needed to achieve the effect, the more potent the drug is.

J. False. This is efficacy. Efficacy is the maximum effect achieved by the drug regardless of how high the dose goes. Drug B in this case has lower efficacy than Drug A.

K. False. This is an old misconception carried over from human observations with another phenothiazine drug. There is no evidence that acepromazine makes seizure activity worse or increases the incidence of seizure activity.

L. True. The antidopamine effect of acepromazine blocks dopamine receptors on the chemoreceptor trigger zone (CRTZ) or emetic center reducing vomiting stimulation to some degree.

M. False. Diazepam has no antiemetic activity like acepromazine does.

N. False. Flumazenil is a benzodiazepine reversal agent, not an opioid reversal agent.

O. False. Visceral pain would be like pain associated with GI colic and that type of pain is better controlled than superficial somatic pain from skin receptors that respond to discrete pain stimuli (e.g., a surgical incision in the skin).

P. False. Tranquilizers have no analgesic qualities. The animal appears relaxed because they feel less anxiety but they are fully capable of feeling painful stimuli completely.

Q. False. α_2-Agonist sedatives/analgesics initially cause peripheral arteriole vasoconstriction through stimulation of α_1 receptors, which elevates blood pressure. The elevated arterial blood pressure from the vasoconstriction stimulates baroreceptors, which send signals to the brain to inhibit sympathetic nervous system effects, slowing the heart. In addition, α_2 effects in the brain also directly reduce sympathetic nervous system activity. The net effect is initially bradycardia and hypertension. After a few minutes the α_1 vasoconstriction begins to fade and the vasoconstriction reverses, allowing blood pressure to fall. Normally a falling blood pressure would be compensated for by an increase in heart rate. However, the α_2 suppression of the sympathetic nervous system response in the brain dampens this response and the heart does not respond to the drop in blood pressure. The net effect is bradycardia plus hypotension in phase II.

R. True. Cattle require about one tenth of the dose of an equivalent-sized horse. A horse dose in an equivalent-sized cow may kill the cow. Small ruminants (e.g., goats, sheep) are even more sensitive to xylazine than cows.

S. False. The rapid initial recovery from propofol is from redistribution of the drug from the initial distribution to the brain back into the blood and then to other tissues that are slower to take up the propofol. The initial recovery is because the concentration of propofol in the brain drops as the drug redistributes to other tissues.

T. False. Tiletamine and ketamine both increase the heart rate.

U. False. Doxapram is a CNS stimulant used to stimulate the respiratory centers in animals that have been overmedicated with opioids or other respiratory depressants.

4. Buprenorphine is a partial antagonist and will reverse the respiratory depression of stronger opioids to some degree, but to a lesser degree than naloxone, which is a full antagonist. However, buprenorphine is also a partial agonist, meaning that it has some degree of opioid analgesia of its own that can produce some continued pain relief. Naloxone, as a full antagonist, completely reverses the analgesic effect, also leaving the animal without any pain relief.

5. The opioid depression of the respiratory center is used therapeutically in drugs like butorphanol or codeine to suppress coughing (antitussive effect, see Chapter 6).

6. Opioid drugs increase segmental contractions and decrease intestinal secretions and hence can cause constipation with repeated or long-term use. See Chapter 4 on narcotic antidiarrheal drugs.

7. Pupillary miosis (i.e., constriction) occurs in dogs, rabbits, and rats. Pupillary mydriasis (i.e., dilation) occurs in cats and horses. Because catecholamines (e.g., epinephrine, norepinephrine, or any drugs that act like them) can also be released under stress and cause pupillary dilation, the effect of morphine miosis can be quite variable.

8. Bradycardia occurs by opioid stimulation of μ-receptors centers in the brain that send parasympathetic signals down the vagus nerve to the heart to slow the heart rate. However, in healthy animals the bradycardia does not result in a significant decrease of cardiac output (i.e., the actual amount of blood pumped per minute) because the force of contraction and stroke volume (i.e., amount pumped per beat) compensates to some degree.

9. The dull, aching pain or generalized organ pain of visceral pain is carried through smaller pain fibers than the more discrete and localized perception of pain in the skin that is carried by large, rapidly conducting nerve fibers. Opioids are better at reducing the pain carried by the smaller unmyelinated pain fibers (so-called C-fibers) than the large nerve fibers, meaning that for controlling pain from surgical incisions in the skin, other drugs may have to be used in conjunction to control somatic pain more effectively.

10. Morphine stimulates dopamine receptors in the CRTZ (see Chapter 4) and stimulation of these receptors triggers the vomiting reflex via the emetic center. However, the occurrence of vomiting is determined by how quickly the opioid stimulates the CRTZ before the drug penetrates the blood–brain barrier and begins to depress the emetic center itself. See discussion on apomorphine in Chapter 4 for further details on this phenomenon.

11. Probably not. Evidence seems to point away from cats being more sensitive to the dysphoria (i.e., bad hallucinations) from opioids than other species. See the Myths and Misconceptions box "The myth of morphine mania" in this chapter.

12. Do not cut the patch to a smaller size to accommodate a smaller patient because this disrupts the ability to deliver an accurate amount of drug into the skin. Instead, decrease the surface area of the patch in contact with the skin by covering part of the skin-side of the patch with impervious tape.

13. Fentanyl has a short half-life. It is eliminated quickly, and therefore, to maintain adequate concentrations for analgesia, the drug needs to be given as a constant rate infusion (CRI) or via a depot type of topical application (e.g., patch or long-acting gel).

14. Occasionally the adhesive on the patch irritates the skin, so the owner should monitor the animal at home for any signs

of the patient licking the patch site or trying to remove the patch. The patch is relatively easy to remove, thus it is important that close monitoring prevent the patch from being removed by the patient or by a curious child. Additionally, if the patch falls off by itself, it is important that it be located and disposed of properly to prevent the pet from eating it or children from playing with it and absorbing the drug through their own skin. Finally, narcotic abusers know that fentanyl patches are a source of opioid drug.

15. Fentanyl transdermal solution exists in an FDA-approved product for dogs (Recuvyra by Elanco). The drug is applied onto the skin with a special syringe and needleless syringe adaptor that assures that the drug contacts with the skin surface without having to clip the hair over the application site in any but the most densely coated dogs. Because of the potential danger of this potent opioid being absorbed through the skin of the veterinary professional administering the drug, the manufacturer requires veterinarians to complete an online safety training program before they can order the medication and the drug is not allowed to be administered by anyone but an approved veterinarian. Personal protective equipment should be worn when preparing or administering this drug, including good-quality, impermeable latex or nitrile gloves, eye protection, and a laboratory coat. After application of the transdermal solution, the dog should be isolated from children for 72 h (3 days) and if any adults come into contact with the application site during this time, they should immediately wash the area on their skin that contacted the application site.

16. NDMA receptor inhibition reduces perception of pain in the spinal cord and brain. Some opioids and propofol produce some of their analgesia by blocking this receptor. Blocking the NDMA receptor is thought to reduce wind-up in the spinal cord and is also thought to be involved with the dissociative effect caused by anesthetics like ketamine and tiletamine.

17. Tramadol should not be used with behavioral drugs like tricyclic antidepressants or serotonin reuptake inhibitors (see Chapter 9) because these drugs also inhibit the reuptake of serotonin like tramadol does and can result in an accumulation of serotonin, producing toxic effects associated with serotonin syndrome.

18. Acepromazine has some antihistamine effect and because skin testing is reliant upon a histamine response to those antigens to which the animal is allergic, the acepromazine could dampen the histamine response and produce a false negative response to an antigen to which the animal truly is allergic.

19. Blocking the vasoconstricting effect of α_1-receptors allows vasodilation and a subsequent drop in arterial blood pressure.

20. The $GABA_A$ receptor is linked to chloride channels that open when a drug combines with the GABA receptor. Opening the chloride channels allows chloride to move into the neurons or muscle, causing the inside to become more negatively charged (Cl^- has a negative charge). This more negative charge makes it harder for the neuron or muscle to be stimulated to depolarize, hence it does not fire. The net effect is nervous system depression. Increasing the release of GABA neurotransmitter and subsequent stimulation of the GABA receptor has the same effect.

21. Although these drugs stimulate the appetite center, they also have caused liver failure in cats that were given these drugs on a repeated basis. The risk does not justify the use as an appetite stimulant.

22. α_2 Drugs are analgesic/sedatives. The analgesia can mask the pain from the colic and make the horse appear to be improving because the outward clinical signs of pain associated with the colic decrease.

23. α_2 Drugs, like the μ-opioids, have a ceiling effect. The amount of analgesia obtained with the first dose (provided the correct amount was given) is not likely to deepen with additional drug because of the ceiling effect. The maximum efficacy of the α_2-analgesia cannot be exceeded by giving more of the same drug.

24. The initial hypertension from α_2-agonist drugs is from α_1-receptor stimulation causing vasoconstriction of the peripheral arterioles, which results in increased arterial blood pressure (similar to squeezing the end of a rubber hose through which you are blowing air). The increased arterial blood pressure sends signals to the brain that inhibit the sympathetic nervous system. That combined with the direct suppression of the sympathetic nervous system by α_2-receptor stimulation itself results in a marked decreased of sympathetic stimulation of the heart. The heart slows under the dominance of the parasympathetic nervous system, producing bradycardia. Although bradycardia decreases the amount of blood pumped into the arteries, the effect of the vasoconstriction keeps the arterial blood pressure up.

25. As the effect of α_2-agonist drugs on the α_1 receptors lessens, the vasoconstriction lessens; the arterioles dilate more, allowing blood to pass more readily through; and the arterial blood pressure back upstream drops, producing hypotension. Normally the heart would increase heart rate to try to compensate for the drop in blood pressure, but because the α_2-agonist effect suppresses the release of norepinephrine, the sympathetic response to the drop in blood pressure is dampened and the heart remains bradycardic (i.e., slow beating).

26. Goats and sheep are more sensitive than cattle, but cattle are 10 times more sensitive to xylazine than horses. Swine are the most resistant to the effects of xylazine.

27. α_2-Agonist drugs only prevent further release of norepinephrine (NE). They do nothing about the NE that was previously released from fear or stress. The sympathetic nervous system stimulation effects from previously released NE will have to wear off before the α_2-agonist drug can be observed to have an effect.

28. Cows are 10 times more sensitive to xylazine than horses. Swine are most resistant.

29. Dexmedetomidine contains only one (the "dextro" form) of the two molecular configurations of the drug rather than the older medetomidine that contains both forms. The

"dextro" form has been found to be the major biologically active form; to enhance the effectiveness, dexmedetomidine contains only the dextro form, giving it greater potency than the blended medetomidine.

30. No. As propofol redistributes back out of the brain to other tissues, the concentration drop allows the animal to become more conscious and start breathing again, usually within a couple minutes of administering the drug.

31. Dissociative anesthetics (e.g., ketamine, tiletamine) do not produce good muscle relaxation. Instead, they tend to increase skeletal muscle tone. To manipulate a hip luxation back into the hip socket, the veterinarian has to work against some very strong muscles that are keeping the hip out of the socket. Skeletal muscle relaxation is required to do so.

32. Cats given ketamine tend to keep their eyes open and they do not blink. Therefore the cornea of the eye can dry out and become injured, causing a painful corneal abrasion. Always put ointment in the eyes of cats that are receiving ketamine as an anesthetic agent.

33. There is no significant evidence that compound A poses a serious health risk to veterinary patients.

34. When nitrous oxide is used as an adjunct gas, it readily penetrates all body cavities. At the end of the surgical procedure when anesthetic gas is turned off, the nitrous will fill the alveoli of the lungs crowding out (i.e., lowering the concentration of) oxygen. If the animal is left on room air during this time, the oxygen could be diluted enough by the nitrous oxide coming into the alveoli from the rest of the body that the animal could become hypoxic, a condition called diffusion hypoxia. Therefore pure oxygen must be given during this period of time to increase the oxygen concentration in the alveoli despite this movement of nitrous into the alveoli.

35. For milk chocolate, the type of chocolate typically found in a candy bar, a 10-lb dog would need to ingest a couple of candy bars to produce significant toxicity (depending on the size of the candy bar and the amount that is chocolate). A 65-lb dog eating half a candy bar is not likely to produce significant toxic signs.

CHAPTER 9

1. Fill in the following blanks with the correct item from the Key Terms list.
    A. anticonvulsant
    B. seizures
    C. focal seizures
    D. generalized seizures
    E. convulsions
    F. tonic seizures
    G. clonic seizures
    H. epilepsy
    I. idiopathic epilepsy
    J. status epilepticus
    K. prodrome or prodromal phase
    L. ictus
    M. postictal phase

N. genetic epilepsy
O. structural epilepsy
P. epilepsy of unknown origin
Q. hyperthermia
R. hypoxia
S. gamma (γ)-aminobutyric acid (GABA)
T. mixed-function oxidase (MFO) enzymes
U. cytochrome P450 (CYP)
V. induced
W. polyphagia
X. polydipsia
Y. polyuria
Z. alkaline phosphatase (ALP) and alanine aminotransferase (ALT)
AA. drug-induced hepatopathy
AB. idiosyncratic reaction
AC. grains
AD. adjunct drug
AE. neuropathic pain
AF. major tranquilizers (phenothiazines)
AG. antidepressants
AH. anxiolytic
AI. limbic system
AJ. tricyclic antidepressants (TCAs), selective serotonin reuptake inhibitors (SSRIs), and monoamine oxidase inhibitors (MAOIs)
AK. monoamine oxidase inhibitor
AL. selective serotonin reuptake inhibitor
AM. tricyclic antidepressant
AN. serotonin syndrome
AO. GABA$_A$ receptor
AP. therapeutic monitoring

2. Fill in the following blanks with the correct drug from the Nervous System Drug list.
    A. phenobarbital
    B. diazepam
    C. selegiline or deprenyl
    D. diazepam, clonazepam, clorazepate, lorazepam
    E. phenobarbital
    F. MAOIs and SSRIs
    G. phenobarbital
    H. selegiline (deprenyl) or any MAOI
    I. potassium bromide
    J. acepromazine
    K. phenobarbital
    L. clomipramine
    M. fluoxetine
    N. potassium bromide
    O. phenobarbital
    P. clomipramine (Clomicalm)
    Q. fluoxetine (Reconcile)
    R. selegiline or deprenyl (Anipryl)
    S. phenobarbital
    T. acepromazine
    U. diazepam
    V. selegiline or deprenyl (Anipryl)
    W. phenobarbital

3. Indicate whether each of the following statements is true or false.

  A. False. Other way around. Seizures are changes in electrical activity in the brain and convulsions are the physical manifestation of the seizure activity such as thrashing limbs or vocalization.

  B. True.

  C. True. Idiopathic means "I do not know the disease," which means the origin is unknown.

  D. False. Increased release of GABA neurotransmitter or stimulation of GABA$_A$ receptor results in inhibition of firing of neurons and hence nervous system depression, not stimulation.

  E. True. Phenobarbital induces (i.e., speeds up) metabolism of drugs that use the same CYP enzymes. Thus, if the second drug is being metabolized quicker, it is disappearing from the body quicker and requires an INCREASED dose to compensate.

  F. False. Cats are more sensitive to the effects of phenobarbital and thus require a lower dose.

  G. False. ALP and ALT enzymes are expected to go up in patients on phenobarbital including those patients with normal livers.

  H. False. One grain equals 60 mg (sometimes 65 mg is still used, but most commonly the 60 mg is used today). Thus, one quarter of a grain would be 15 mg (one quarter of 60 mg is 15 mg).

  I. False. Diazepam has a strong first-pass effect when it passes through the liver. Even though some of the diazepam is converted to another active metabolite, much of the drug is rendered less effective. Thus, orally diazepam is much less effective than when given IV because a drug introduced IV goes directly to the target organ (the brain) without first having to go through the liver.

  J. True. When diazepam is mixed with IV fluids, the combination has to be inverted several times to help the diazepam "mix" better with the IV fluids.

  K. False. The half-life of potassium bromide (KBr) in dogs is measured in weeks, not hours. Thus, if a dose is changed, the drug will work its way toward a new steady state, which takes about five times the half-life of the drug to reach steady state (see Chapter 3, steady state). Thus, it will take months for the drug concentrations to level out at the new steady state concentrations. This is why if KBr is overdosed, the animal is going to be profoundly depressed or sedated for days because elimination of the drug is so slow.

  L. True. Increased activity of GABA neurotransmitter means more inhibitory effect on the nervous system.

  M. False. Other way around. Primidone is metabolized to phenobarbital for most of its anticonvulsant activity.

  N. False. Phenothiazine tranquilizers like acepromazine are dopamine antagonists and so they block the effect of dopamine neurotransmitter.

  O. True. SSRI only block the reuptake of serotonin back into the neuron but TCA drugs block serotonin and norepinephrine for a broader effect.

  P. False. The individual patient variable response to TCA drugs means one drug could work very well in Patient A, but have poor results or even adverse effects at the very same dose in Patient B. Often dosages have to be adjusted or drugs changed until the right combination of drug and dose is found for a particular patient.

  Q. True. Fluoxetine is FDA approved for use in dogs as Reconcile.

  R. False. Decreased serotonin levels in the brain lead to depression. This is why SSRIs are antidepressant; they make serotonin released by neurons remain longer in the synapses, where it can stimulate neurons to a greater degree, elevating mood.

  S. True.

  T. True.

  U. False. Most animals develop a significant amount of tolerance to benzodiazepine drugs and their short half-life requires dosing multiple times a day. Thus, benzodiazepines are not used as a sole drug for long-term control of seizures.

  V. False. Phenobarbital induces (i.e., speeds up) its own metabolism. Thus, over time phenobarbital disappears from the body at a quicker rate. To compensate for the quicker metabolism of phenobarbital, more of the drug must be given. The phenobarbital dose needs to be INCREASED after a few weeks.

  W. True. This is a rare idiosyncratic side effect seen in some animals given acepromazine.

  X. True. Phenothiazines alter both normal and abnormal behavior whereas TCA drugs tend to maintain normal behaviors while adjusting abnormal behaviors.

  Y. False. LACK of dopamine neurotransmitter is associated with a senility-like syndrome in dogs.

  Z. False. Benzodiazepines (including diazepam) work by facilitating the effect of GABA neurotransmitter on the GABA$_A$ receptor.

  AA. True. Much of behavior therapy involves behavior modification using techniques as opposed to drugs. Each patient is different.

4. 60 mg = 1 grain so 1.5 grains = 90 mg. 1.5 gr × 60 mg/1 gr = 90 mg

5. This is classic for the idiosyncratic reaction that can occur with phenobarbital in some dogs. Instead of sedation they become anxious. Increasing the dose does not help. The dog needs to be switched to another anticonvulsant.

6. ALT and ALP are normally increased within the liver under the influence of phenobarbital and thus more of these enzymes will leak into the blood (there is always some that leaks into the blood, which is why the reference range or "normal" range is never zero). If the animal is otherwise alert, active, eating, and acting normal then it can be assumed this is just a normal increase that is observed with phenobarbital use.

7. Potassium bromide (KBr) is a salt and as such it can induce gastritis and vomiting. The dose can be divided up into two or three doses per day, the dose can be administered in a

liquid vs a powder (in a capsule), or the dose of KBr can be administered with different foods to reduce the effect of the salt on the gastritis.

8. First, remember that GABA is an inhibitory neurotransmitter. Anything that prolongs or enhances GABA release or time spent in the synapse, or enhances the GABA effect on its receptor, is going to depress the nervous system. If the destruction of GABA is prevented, that means GABA is going to stick around longer and produce more of an inhibitory effect. If a drug occupies the GABA receptor but has no intrinsic activity, it is going to block GABA or other GABA receptor agonists from acting; hence it will block or antagonize the inhibition caused by GABA, producing less inhibition and less nervous system depression.

9. Seizures that lead to convulsions create a tremendous amount of body heat by causing involuntary skeletal muscle contractions. This is like exercising really, really hard. On a hot day the animal can become hyperthermic because of the generation of the excessive body heat from the convulsions and body temperature can get high enough to damage the brain (e.g., heat stroke, heat exhaustion).

10. You need to explain that the liver develops the ability to break down (i.e., metabolize) the phenobarbital much better after a few days, which means the drug is not lasting as long in the body. To compensate for this the dose on almost every animal has to be increased to maintain phenobarbital concentrations within the concentration range (i.e., therapeutic range) needed for the drug to control seizure activity.

11. You need to explain that when diazepam is given by mouth (PO) much of it is removed by the liver before it reaches the bloodstream (first-pass effect and systemic circulation). When giving the drug IV, the drug goes directly to the brain to control the seizure without having to go through the liver and hence the drug works well when given IV. Theoretically a high enough dose of diazepam could be given PO to compensate for the liver metabolism, but the drug would still have to be given three or four times a day, which means long-term client compliance with the drug is likely to be poor.

12. When a drug is first administered, the drug is not totally eliminated by the time the next dose is given. Thus, the second dose of drug is added to whatever remains of the first dose of the drug. This accumulation of drug over subsequent doses results in a gradual increase of concentrations. But because higher concentrations of any drug also means quicker elimination (i.e., drug concentrations in the blood drop quicker from high drug concentrations than they do at low concentrations), the accumulation of drug gets to the point where the amount of drug administered with the dose IS totally eliminated by the time of the next dose. At that point the peak concentrations and trough (low) concentrations no longer increase. This is steady state (see Chapter 3 for more on steady state and elimination half-life). The time to reach steady state after starting a drug regimen is approximately five times the half-life. The phenobarbital half-life of 30 h means it will take 150 h (5 × 30) from when the drug is started until it reaches steady state, or about 6 days. If the drug was dosed properly, the steady state concentrations SHOULD be within the therapeutic range. However, this means that for the first day or so the concentrations may be below the therapeutic range and the animal may experience seizures. Because potassium bromide has a half-life of about 3 weeks, steady state is not going to be achieved until 15 weeks (5 × 3 weeks) or almost 4 months after the dose is started. It can be assumed for the first few weeks the concentrations are likely below the normal therapeutic range and the animal is likely to have breakthrough seizures during that time. A loading dose of KBr is given to boost the first dose much closer to the therapeutic range so that the subsequent maintenance doses can maintain the concentrations within the therapeutic range (see Chapter 3 on loading and maintenance doses).

13. It is important to remember that some tranquilizers, like diazepam, may unmask some learned behaviors. For example, if the animal was normally aggressive, it can be trained (i.e., learned behavior) to control the aggression or direct the aggression toward specific targets (e.g., what a guard dog does). If the tranquilizer suppresses not only abnormal behavior but normal learned behavior, the learned "control" of the aggression may be removed, allowing the more aggressive instinct to reemerge.

14. Both fluoxetine (SSRI drug) and selegiline (MAOI drug) are drugs that enhance the effect of the neurotransmitter serotonin. Although a little increase in serotonin is good for correcting depressant behavior, too much serotonin results in serotonin syndrome, which is characterized as hypertension, hyperthermia, tremors, seizures, and possibly death. SSRIs and MAOIs should not be given together for this reason.

CHAPTER 10

1. Fill in the following blanks with the correct item from the Key Terms list.
   A. antibiotic
   B. antimicrobial
   C. bactericidal
   D. fungicidal
   E. virucidal
   F. bacteriostatic
   G. pathogen
   H. culture and sensitivity test
   I. susceptible
   J. minimum inhibitory concentration (MIC)
   K. maximum tolerated dose (MTD)
   L. resistant
   M. intermediate resistance/susceptibility
   N. susceptible
   O. breakpoints
   P. minimum bactericidal concentration (MBC)
   Q. vertical transmission of resistance
   R. horizontal transmission of resistance
   S. plasmid
   T. selection pressure

U. residue
V. hypersensitivity
W. messenger RNA (m-RNA)
X. transfer RNA (t-RNA)
Y. beta (β)-lactam ring
Z. methicillin-resistant *Staphylococcus aureus* (MRSA)
AA. aerobic
AB. anaerobic
AC. empirical treatment or empirical therapy
AD. porins
AE. beta-lactamase or β-lactamase
AF. penicillinase
AG. cephalosporinase
AH. potentiated
AI. urticaria
AJ. cross-reactivity
AK. superinfection or suprainfection
AL. postantibiotic effect
AM. time-dependent antibiotics
AN. concentration-dependent antibiotics
AO. nephrotoxic
AP. ototoxic
AQ. nystagmus
AR. pyogenic
AS. DNA gyrase (topoisomerase II)
AT. pyoderma
AU. *Wolbachia*
AV. chelates
AW. enterohepatic circulation
AX. enteric sulfonamide
AY. keratoconjunctivitis sicca (KCS)
AZ. thrombocytopenia
BA. leukopenia
BB. crystalluria
BC. aplastic anemia
BD. superficial mycoses
BE. systemic mycoses
BF. liposomal form
BG. teratogenic effects
BH. dermatophyte

2. Fill in the following blanks with the correct drug from the Antimicrobial Drug list.
   A. penicillin G
   B. tetracycline family
   C. ticarcillin, carbenicillin, piperacillin
   D. enrofloxacin
   E. sulfasalazine
   F. florfenicol
   G. ampicillin, amoxicillin
   H. sulfonamides
   I. tetracycline or oxytetracycline
   J. benzathine
   K. cefovecin, cefpodoxime, ceftiofur
   L. doxycycline
   M. sulfasalazine
   N. methicillin
   O. cephalosporins

P. aminoglycosides
Q. chloramphenicol
R. tetracycline and oxytetracycline
S. cefadroxil, cephapirin, cephalexin, cefazolin
T. aminoglycosides
U. fluoroquinolones
V. cephalosporins
W. sulfadiazine, sulfadimethoxine, sulfamethoxazole, sulfasalazine
X. penicillins
Y. enrofloxacin
Z. tetracycline family
AA. cephalosporins
AB. enrofloxacin
AC. trihydrate form
AD. tetracycline family
AE. penicillins, cephalosporins, bacitracin
AF. oxacillin, cloxacillin, dicloxacillin, methicillin
AG. tilmicosin
AH. doxycycline
AI. clavulanic acid and sulbactam
AJ. trimethoprim and ormetoprim
AK. minocycline and doxycycline
AL. clindamycin
AM. tetracycline family
AN. penicillin G
AO. tylosin
AP. erythromycin, azithromycin, tilmicosin, tylosin, tulathromycin
AQ. doxycycline
AR. procaine
AS. metronidazole
AT. tilmicosin
AU. rifampin
AV. amphotericin B
AW. ketoconazole
AX. itraconazole
AY. fluconazole
AZ. clotrimazole and miconazole
BA. fluconazole
BB. griseofulvin
BC. griseofulvin
BD. nystatin

3. Indicate whether each of the following statements is true or false.
   A. True. The MTD is the maximum tolerated dose, which constitutes the upper range of the normal therapeutic range for the drug. The MIC is the minimum inhibitory concentration and constitutes the lower end of the therapeutic range. Therefore, the MIC needs to be lower than the MTD or the drug cannot be used.
   B. False. MBC = minimum bactericidal concentration. The concentrations needed to kill bacteria are typically higher concentrations than those that only inhibit the bacterial growth and replication.
   C. False. Vertical transmission means the transferal of DNA from parent to daughter cells after replication.

Transferal of DNA by physical contact would be an example of horizontal transmission.

D. False. Selection pressure does not increase the mutation rate; it only selects for and eliminates the weakest bacteria, leaving the most resistant bacteria to proliferate.

E. False. Aminoglycosides and fluoroquinolones both are concentration dependent; they must achieve a high peak concentration to be most effective. However, penicillin drugs are time dependent in that they need to be present at the site of infection continuously so as to catch the bacteria when they replicate so they can disrupt new bacterial cell wall formation.

F. True. Bacteriostatic drugs only inhibit replication but do not kill the bacteria outright. They are dependent on the immune system to do this.

G. True. Penicillins are dependent on a replicating bacterial colony to be able to disrupt formation of new bacterial cell walls. After cell walls are formed, penicillins have no effect on that bacterial cell. If a bacteriostatic drug is used with the penicillins, the bacteriostatic drug will inhibit bacterial replication and not allow penicillins the opportunity to disrupt bacterial cell wall formation.

H. False. Amoxicillin, along with most other penicillins, is excreted by the kidney via active secretion that pumps the intact drug into the urine in high concentrations, making it an excellent drug for treating bacterial urinary tract infections.

I. False. Penicillins, except for the extended spectrum penicillins that are called "antipseudomonal penicillins," are mostly ineffective against *Pseudomonas* bacteria.

J. True. The exception is the extended spectrum penicillins (e.g., ticarcillin).

K. True. Oxacillin belongs to that class of penicillins that has natural ability to kill β-lactamase-producing bacteria without having to have clavulanic acid or sulbactam attached to their molecular structure.

L. False. Dicloxacillin and cloxacillin are part of the group that has natural ability to kill β-lactamase–producing bacteria without having to have clavulanic acid or sulbactam attached to their molecular structure. However, this group is less effective against some of the other commonly susceptible bacteria that amoxicillin, ampicillin, or even penicillin G can kill.

M. False. Clavulanic acid does not prolong activity; procaine and benzathine do. Clavulanic acid makes ampicillin and amoxicillin less susceptible to destruction by β-lactamase enzyme produced by *Staphylococcus* bacteria.

N. True. Cross-reactivity to all members of the penicillin drug family should be assumed if an animal appears to be hypersensitive to one penicillin.

O. False. Penicillins can kill Gram-positive bacteria in the GI tract of these species, allowing other pathogenic bacteria to proliferate and produce a suprainfection than can be fatal.

P. False. Procaine penicillin G has a duration of about 24 h but benzathine gives concentrations for about 3–5 days.

Q. True. Penicillin G is unstable in gastric acid whereas amoxicillin is commonly given PO.

R. True.

S. False. Aminoglycosides are dependent on oxygen to be taken up by bacteria. Without oxygen, the transport mechanism does not work and the antibiotics cannot reach their target within the bacteria.

T. False. First, aminoglycosides are concentration dependent, not time dependent, so they do not need to be present constantly. Second, aminoglycosides are very nephrotoxic unless the plasma/blood concentration of the drug is allowed to drop to very low levels between doses. A CRI would not allow that to happen.

U. False. Aminoglycosides are mostly in the ionized hydrophilic form if applied to skin; therefore they will not penetrate the tissue. However, denuded skin that has been traumatized or burned (e.g., the top layer of skin is gone), will absorb the drugs very well because it would be just like injecting them SQ.

V. False. The trough (i.e., low) concentration of the drug must be very low between doses to allow some of the drug to diffuse back out of the cell along a concentration gradient from high concentration within the cell to low concentrations in the plasma or blood surrounding the cell.

W. False. Aminoglycosides can combine with DNA found in cellular debris and not reach the bacteria. Aminoglycosides should not be used in pus-filled lesions or those with lots of cellular debris (e.g., infected dog ears) until the debris has been removed.

X. False. Enrofloxacin interferes with an enzyme involved in the replication of bacterial DNA, not the DNA itself. Enrofloxacin does not interfere with mammalian DNA replication because the enzymes found in mammalian cells are different than the enzymes found in bacterial cells.

Y. True. The phase of rapid bone growth extends longer in large-breed dogs than it does in small- or medium-breed dogs, and enrofloxacin should not be given to dogs during periods of rapid long-bone growth.

Z. False. Enrofloxacin was associated with blindness but it was because of damage to the retina rendering the cat unable to see at all.

AA. True. Because of concerns over development of resistant bacteria, the extra-label use of fluoroquinolones in food animals is prohibited. However, there still are some FDA-approved fluoroquinolones that are labeled for use in some food animals, but extra-label use is prohibited.

AB. True. Although quinolones are not a first drug of choice for CNS infections, they are more lipophilic than aminoglycosides at most body pH and therefore more likely to penetrate barriers.

AC. False. Magnesium also has a similar charge to calcium and can chelate with oxytetracycline or tetracycline very well.

AD. False. Tetracyclines tend to be bacteriostatic at most doses and bacteriostatic antibiotics should not be used with penicillins or cephalosporins, which depend on the bacteria replicating to disrupt the formation of new bacterial cell wall.

AE. True.

AF. False. Both sulfadimethoxine and sulfadiazine are systemic sulfonamides. Sulfasalazine is the enteric sulfonamide intended to work within the GI tract and not be absorbed.

AG. True.

AH. True. Sulfasalazine is metabolized by colonic bacteria to a salicylate compound that can be absorbed and potentially produce salicylate (i.e., aspirin) toxicity in cats if enough of the drug is given.

AI. True. This activity against anaerobic bacteria is one of the characteristics of clindamycin.

AJ. True. This is the most common use for them in veterinary medicine.

AK. False. Though injection of tilmicosin can produce fatal arrhythmias, there are hundreds of reports of accidental injections where no adverse outcome was reported.

AL. False. The neurologic signs associated with high doses or long-term dosing of metronidazole go away after a few days of being off the drug. They are reversible.

AM. False. Amphotericin B is far more nephrotoxic. Fluconazole is actually concentrated in the urine and therefore is used for mycotic cystitis (i.e., fungal infections within the urinary bladder). Though the liposomal amphotericin B is far less nephrotoxic, it is still more nephrotoxic than fluconazole.

AN. True.

AO. False. Amphotericin B begins working right away and the azole antifungals need a few days to begin to produce their fungicidal effect.

AP. False. Just the opposite. Ketoconazole and other azole antifungals can interfere with the cytochrome P450 enzyme that converts progesterone to testosterone, resulting in decreased testosterone levels. Thus, ketoconazole should not be used in male dogs involved in an active breeding program.

AQ. False. Ketoconazole and itraconazole need an acidic pH environment to be absorbed after PO administration.

AR. False. Clotrimazole IS a topically applied drug, but fluconazole is not. Miconazole is the other topically applied antifungal.

AS. False. The smaller the particle size of griseofulvin, the more readily it is absorbed from the GI tract. Thus, if switching from microsized to the smaller ultramicrosized, more of the drug is going to be absorbed and the dose would need to be DECREASED.

4. The bacteria would be classified as being "intermediate" in susceptibility to this drug. Enough drug is going to have to be given to reach a concentration of 10 mcg/mL, but if the bacteria does not respond at that concentration, there is not a lot of hope getting a further response because any concentration of the drug at 16 mcg/mL or higher is an indication that the bacteria are resistant to this drug.

5. Match the mechanism of action with the particular drug.
   A. amoxicillin
   C. minocycline
   E. enrofloxacin
   A. cefovecin
   B. polymyxin B
   D. sulfadiazine
   C. gentamicin
   A. penicillin G
   C. doxycycline
   C. tilmicosin
   E. orbifloxacin
   A. oxacillin
   D. sulfadimethoxine
   C. erythromycin
   C. amikacin

6. remain the same, increased

7. Early signs include increased urine protein and casts.

8. Tetracycline (oxytetracycline and tetracycline) will chelate with calcium in milk, rendering the drug unable to be absorbed.

9. Sucralfate has the ability to chelate with enrofloxacin causing the antibiotic to not be absorbed.

10. Fluoroquinolones have been shown to increase the frequency of seizures in animals predisposed to seizures (e.g., epileptic animals).

11. Doxycycline kills the *Wolbachia* bacteria that exist with, and appear to help, the heartworm parasite.

12. Tetracyclines are able to enter into mammalian cells and accumulate, making them ideal for attacking intracellular organisms like *Chlamydia* species, *Mycoplasma* species, *Rickettsia* species, and spirochete bacteria.

13. Doxycycline (as well as other tablets) can become lodged in the esophagus if the cat does not drink water at the time the tablet is given. The doxycycline can then dissolve and become very ulcerative in the esophagus. Therefore it is important to either avoid the use of oral doxycycline in cats, or to ensure that the cat is given several milliliters of water to drink immediately afterward.

14. Even low doses of doxycycline given IV to horses can produce arrhythmias, collapse, and death. Oral administration does not produce the same effect.

15. Penicillins and sulfonamides are both concentrated in the urine by active transport from blood/plasma into the urine. Thus, very high concentrations of drug (higher than is in the plasma/blood) can be achieved in the urine, making it ideal for treating bacterial infections in the urinary tract.

16. Sulfonamides are known to produce keratoconjunctivitis sicca (KCS) or "dry eye" in which the tear producing gland is damaged and fails to produce adequate tears. The eyes become "goopy" with matter and the animal may squint because of dryness and irritation of the corneal surface. It often is not reversible, but is treatable with a cyclosporin ophthalmic ointment like Optimmune.

17. Lincosamides cause overgrowth of pathogenic bacteria by killing off "good" bacteria in the GI tract and allowing a superinfection/suprainfection of pathogenic bacteria to cause a severe and sometimes fatal diarrhea.

18. Chloramphenicol is totally banned from food animal use because of the ability to cause aplastic anemia in humans who ingest it. Florfenicol was formulated from chloramphenicol but without the key molecular structure that apparently causes the aplastic anemia. Florfenicol is FDA approved for use in treating respiratory disease in food animals.

19. Ketoconazole (and some of the other azole antifungals) inhibit the cytochrome P450 enzyme that converts hormones, including the production of cortisol. In animals with an adrenal tumor that is overproducing cortisol (i.e., Cushing's disease), ketoconazole can be used to disrupt the production of the cortisol by interfering with this cytochrome P450 enzyme and reducing the overall amount of cortisol circulating in the body.

CHAPTER 11

1. Fill in the following blanks with the correct item from the Key Terms list.
   A. nosocomial infections
   B. biofilm
   C. antiseptics
   D. disinfectants
   E. high-level, intermediate-level, low-level disinfectants
   F. vegetative bacteria
   G. enveloped virus
   H. nonenveloped virus
   I. spore form
   J. sterilizer
   K. sanitizer
   L. germicide
   M. bactericidal
   N. virucidal
   O. protozoacidal
   P. fungicidal
   Q. sporicidal
   R. microbicidal
   S. microbiostatic
   T. halogens
   U. iodophor
   V. surfactants
   W. scrub
   X. biguanides
   Y. coagulum
   Z. cytotoxic

2. Fill in the following blanks with the correct drug from the Antiseptics Disinfectants list.
   A. alcohol
   B. chlorine
   C. glutaraldehyde
   D. phenols
   E. alcohol
   F. chlorine bleach (halogen)
   G. chlorhexidine
   H. glutaraldehyde
   I. chlorhexidine
   J. alcohol
   K. chlorine
   L. biguanides
   M. iodine
   N. chlorhexidine
   O. alcohol
   P. iodine
   Q. glutaraldehyde
   R. chlorine
   S. oxidizing compounds
   T. alcohol
   U. phenol
   V. quaternary ammonium compounds

3. Indicate whether each of the following statements is true or false.
   A. False. Biofilm hides the bacteria from the antiseptic or disinfectant.
   B. True. Antiseptics are for living tissue; disinfectants are for inanimate objects.
   C. False. Enveloped viruses are easier to kill or inactivate. The envelope is a thin phospholipid envelope required by the virus to replicate. When it is destroyed, the virus is inactivated.
   D. True. Sterilizer would leave no life left; sanitizer would reduce pathogens to a safe level.
   E. False. The term "germicide" is so nonspecific that it could kill viruses or bacteria or protozoa, or any other organism that could be called a "germ." It is generally a pretty worthless term for describing the spectrum of a product.
   F. False. The spore form is the dormant form. The vegetative form is the actively dividing form.
   G. False. Cleaning is perhaps the most important aspect of disinfecting and antisepsis because it removes organic material, preventing inactivation of some antiseptics from contact with organic material; it likely has some disinfecting properties of its own.
   H. True. This is why cleaning is so important before disinfecting or applying antiseptic.
   I. True.
   J. False. Alcohol does not kill canine parvovirus because it is a nonenveloped virus and therefore resistant to many disinfectants, including alcohol.
   K. False. Increasing the concentration of alcohol in the solution dehydrates the target organism, making it less

susceptible to protein denaturation and death from the alcohol.

L. True. Alcohol has no cleansing ability (i.e., is not soapy) and is greater impaired by the presence of organic material.

M. False. Alcohol needs to remain in contact for 1–3 min to significantly lower the bacterial counts.

N. False. The alcohol denatures the plasma proteins that have oozed onto the surface of the open wound. The denatured proteins now form a solid structure called a coagulum under which bacteria can hide and proliferate, protected against antiseptics or disinfectants.

O. True.

P. False. Color-fast bleaches are typically peroxides (e.g., hydrogen peroxide) in concentrated amounts.

Q. False. The combination of vinegar and chlorine can produce a chlorine gas, which can irritate the eyes, nose, and throat.

R. False. The addition of ammonia to chlorine results in chloramine gas, which is very irritating and quite toxic.

S. False. Chlorine IS effective against canine parvovirus; however, it is readily inactivated by organic material like blood, feces, or dirt. Thorough cleaning is required before applying chlorine.

T. True. Diluted chlorine solutions will evaporate chlorine into the air and break down with exposure to light.

U. True. Free-iodine solutions provide an intermediate level of disinfection but iodophors provide a low to intermediate level. The disadvantage of free iodine is that it was very irritating to tissues and painful to apply on open wounds.

V. False. Povidone-iodine is iodine "captured" within a polyvinylpyrrolidone (PVP) molecule from which it is released over time.

W. False. Scrubs contain detergents or surfactants (i.e., soap) and should not be introduced into a body cavity or area like an abscess. Only the iodine solution should be used.

X. False. A biguanide is chlorhexidine. Iodine is a halogen.

Y. False. Chlorhexidine is not effective against nonenveloped viruses like parvo.

Z. True. Hard water with lots of minerals (e.g., tap water or well water) can inactivate chlorhexidine to some degree.

AA. True. This is why it is a good oral antiseptic agent.

AB. True.

AC. False. One of glutaraldehyde's advantage is being able to penetrate biofilm and reach the bacteria within.

AD. False. Glutaraldehyde is related to formaldehyde and still retains some of the irritation and smell characteristics of this chemical family.

AE. False. Accelerated hydrogen peroxide contains surfactants, wetting agents, and chelators, but not peroxymonosulfate.

AF. False. Trifectant contains potassium peroxymonosulfate, not phenols.

AG. True. Peroxymonosulfate has no residue problems and has low toxicity if contacted topically.

AH. True.

AI. False. Benzalkonium chloride is a quaternary ammonium compound.

AJ. True.

AK. False. Quaternary ammonium compounds are used for disinfection of surfaces, walls, and vehicles.

AL. True.

AM. True.

4. Identify the following viruses as being enveloped or nonenveloped by circling the appropriate term, then identify them as easy to kill or difficult to kill with low- or intermediate-level disinfectants or antiseptics.

Rabies virus	enveloped	easy to kill
Feline calicivirus	nonenveloped	difficult to kill
Canine distemper	enveloped	easy to kill
Canine parvo	nonenveloped	difficult to kill
Feline herpes	enveloped	easy to kill
Cow pox virus	enveloped	easy to kill
Feline panleukopenia	nonenveloped	difficult to kill

5. Soap can inactivate some of the antiseptics so it is important to rinse the site thoroughly to remove soap.

6. Broad spectrum, nonirritating/nontoxic to animals and humans, easily applied without corrosion or stains, stable and not easily inactivated, inexpensive. The ideal disinfectant does not exist.

7. Cytotoxic often refers to being poisonous to cells, and the cells in this case are the cells of the host animal, not the parasite or pathogen. Thus, cytotoxic agents have to be used very carefully so as not to kill healthy mammalian cells.

CHAPTER 12

1. Fill in the following blanks with the correct item from the Key Terms list.
   A. Food and Drug Administration (FDA)
   B. Environmental Protection Agency (EPA)
   C. parasiticide (or antiparasitic)
   D. selective toxicity
   E. endectocide
   F. endoparasites
   G. ectoparasites
   H. anthelmintic
   I. vermicide
   J. vermifuge
   K. antinematodal
   L. anticestodal
   M. cestocide, taeniacide
   N. antitrematodal
   O. antiprotozoal
   P. coccidiostat
   Q. macrolides or macrocyclic lactones

R. glutamate
S. gamma (γ)-aminobutyric acid (GABA)
T. P-glycoprotein (P-gp)
U. MDR1 (Multiple Drug Resistance 1) or ABCB1 (ATP-Binding Cassette type B1)
V. mydriasis
W. beta (β)-tubulin
X. teratogenic
Y. scolex
Z. proglottids
AA. ovicidal
AB. intima
AC. *Wolbachia* surface protein (WSP)
AD. embolus
AE. heartworm-associated respiratory disease (HARD)
AF. adulticide
AG. microfilaricide
AH. infective larvae, infective third-stage larvae (L3)
AI. heartworm preventive
AJ. *Wolbachia*
AK. caval syndrome (Class 4 heartworm disease)
AL. RiskMAP (Risk Minimization Action Plan)
AM. coccidiocidal
AN. giardiasis
AO. ectoparasiticides
AP. acetylcholinesterase
AQ. muscarinic cholinergic receptor
AR. nicotinic cholinergic receptor
AS. neuromuscular junction
AT. synergists
AU. insect growth regulators (IGRs): insect development inhibitors (IDIs), juvenile hormone analogs (JHAs)
AV. repellents
AW. monoamine oxidase (MAO)
AX. pruritus
AY. sequester, sequestration
AZ. IGR
BA. chitin
BB. IDI
BC. JHA

2. Fill in the following blanks with the correct drug from the Antiparasitics list.
   A. avermectins
   B. eprinomectin, doramectin
   C. milbemycin oxime
   D. moxidectin
   E. moxidectin
   F. thiabendazole
   G. milbemycins
   H. pyrantel pamoate
   I. praziquantel, epsiprantel
   J. eprinomectin
   K. melarsomine
   L. ivermectin
   M. selamectin
   N. moxidectin
   O. sulfonamides

P. amprolium
Q. permethrin
R. albendazole, fenbendazole, febantel
S. metronidazole
T. ivermectin
U. selamectin
V. clindamycin
W. piperazine
X. organophosphates and carbamates
Y. praziquantel
Z. moxidectin
AA. monensin, lasalocid
AB. organophosphates, carbamates
AC. pyrethrin
AD. albendazole
AE. pyrethrin
AF. metronidazole
AG. piperonyl butoxide, MGK 264
AH. permethrin
AI. ponazuril
AJ. fenvalerate
AK. flumethrin
AL. amitraz
AM. butoxypolypropylene glycol
AN. thiabendazole
AO. amitraz
AP. febantel
AQ. tetramethrin
AR. amitraz
AS. monensin
AT. ivermectin
AU. imidacloprid
AV. metronidazole
AW. milbemycin oxime
AX. fipronil
AY. eprinomectin
AZ. afoxolaner, fluralaner
BA. imidacloprid, nitenpyram
BB. doxycycline
BC. indoxacarb
BD. febantel
BE. nitenpyram
BF. spinosad, spinetoram
BG. spinosyns: spinosad, spinetoram
BH. melarsomine
BI. etofenprox
BJ. DEET
BK. afoxolaner
BL. spinetoram
BM. pralidoxime, 2-PAM
BN. spinetoram
BO. moxidectin
BP. fluralaner
BQ. indoxacarb
BR. lufenuron
BS. methoprene, pyriproxyfen
BT. amitraz

BU. milbemycin oxime
BV. atropine
BW. permethrin
BX. pyriproxyfen
BY. sulfonamides

3. What do the following abbreviations stand for?

A.	GABA	γ-aminobutyric acid
B.	PBO	piperonyl butoxide
C.	WSP	*Wolbachia* surface protein
D.	KCS	keratoconjunctivitis sicca
E.	EPM	Equine protozoal myeloencephalitis
F.	IGR	insect growth regulator
G.	IDI	insect development inhibitor
H.	JHA	juvenile hormone analog
I.	HARD	heartworm-associated respiratory disease

4. Indicate whether each of the following statements is true or false.

A. True. EPA products are externally applied pesticides, and so are not regulated by the FDA as a drug. This makes them easier to be sold OTC.

B. False. An antitrematodal is effective against flukes. An antinematodal would be effective against roundworms.

C. True. A coccidiostat inhibits the growth of coccidia, which are protozoal organisms.

D. True. Eprinomectin is the avermectin, and milbemycin and moxidectin are milbemycins.

E. True.

F. False. P-glycoprotein is a pump, not an enzyme. P-gp pumps drug molecules out of the brain and back into the blood if they were successful in diffusing through the blood-brain barrier to gain access to the brain in the first place. They do not break down the drug molecule.

G. True. Without P-glycoprotein function, selamectin can diffuse into the brain and not be pumped back out into the blood.

H. False. The MDR1 gene defect causes P-gp molecules to be produced, but the P-gp pump is not fully functional. Hence, the P-gp molecules are not able to pump drug molecules back into the blood as effectively as normal P-gp molecules.

I. True. Loss of menace usually means a loss of vision or a loss of the ability to respond to motion near the eye; and this is common with avermectin toxicosis and the subsequent CNS depression.

J. False. There is no antidote for ivermectin toxicosis. Treatment is to support the animal in a stuporous or comatose state until the body removes the drug.

K. False. Macrolides stick around in the tissue for a long time; thus a severe toxicosis may take days to weeks to resolve completely.

L. True.

M. False. Because the dose of avermectin drug is so low in heartworm preventives, there should not be enough of the drug entering the brain to cause signs of toxicosis. If given a higher dose, however, these animals would be more at risk for developing toxicosis.

N. True. It is effective against both internal and external parasites.

O. True.

P. True. Moxidectin injectable does not prevent reinfection with hookworms for the full 6 months.

Q. True. They require 3 or more days of medication.

R. False. Benzimidazoles disrupt beta-tubulin (β-tubulin) and therefore disrupts the normal cellular shape, motility, cell secretion, and transport of materials within the cell, eventually resulting in death of the parasite.

S. False. Pyrantel stimulates the nicotinic receptors on the muscles involved with motion, causing an initial stimulation of the muscles, followed by the nicotinic receptor ceasing to respond to the stimulation, resulting in paralysis of the muscle (i.e., no nerve impulses can get through to the muscle because the receptor is not responding).

T. False. Pyrantel is a pleasant-tasting oral medication.

U. False. Emodepside works by releasing a different inhibitory neuropeptide than GABA, but produces inhibition of muscle contraction like GABA does.

V. False. Melarsomine (an adulticide) does not kill microfilaria.

W. False. *Wolbachia* has a beneficial effect on heartworms. Killing the *Wolbachia* bacteria weakens the heartworm.

X. False. The adulticide melarsomine is not used in cats because the risk of killing a few adult heartworms and the subsequent obstruction of the pulmonary arteries by decaying dead worm emboli is too great.

Y. True.

Z. False. The L3 larvae are the infective larvae passed by the mosquito into the animal with the mosquito bite; L3 larvae develop into the adults.

AA. False. Doxycycline is the antibiotic used to kill the *Wolbachia* bacteria.

AB. False. The three injection protocol calls for one injection, a wait of 1 month, and then two injections separated by 24 h.

AC. False. Moxidectin is the approved microfilaricide.

AD. True.

AE. False. Doxycycline has little effect directly on the heartworm.

AF. False. This is an old misconception. The use of glucocorticoids does not significantly improve the ability of the heartworm to survive treatment.

AG. False. It used to be recommended several years ago, but aspirin is not recommended for use in heartworm dogs. This is because there is no improvement of survivability of patients treated with aspirin over those not treated; additionally there is the concern that aspirin could cause microhemorrhages because of inhibited platelet adherence (i.e., platelets not sticking together to form a platelet plug).

AH. True.

AI. True.

AJ. True.

AK. False. It is albendazole.

AL. False. Benzoate was added to metronidazole to reduce its ability to dissolve and hence reduce the bad taste that had made this medication difficult to administer PO.

AM. True.

AN. False. Monensin must not be used in horses because it can kill them.

AO. True.

AP. True. EPA regulates pesticides applied topically that do NOT get absorbed significantly into the body.

AQ. False. Organophosphates (OPs) work by combining with acetylcholinesterase, the enzyme that normally breaks down acetylcholine. The net effect is prolongation of the action of acetylcholine.

AR. False. The paralysis observed is because of overstimulation of the nicotinic cholinergic receptors on skeletal muscles. By overstimulating the receptor and causing the receptor to "lock up" and no longer respond to nerve signals, no nerve signals to contract the muscle can get through and the muscle becomes paralyzed.

AS. True. Atropine is a muscarinic cholinergic antagonist.

AT. True. Pyrethrins have quick knockdown but not quick kill.

AU. True.

AV. False. Piperonyl butoxide (PBO) is a synergist that increases the killing activity of the pyrethrin or pyrethroid.

AW. True.

AX. False. Permethrin is the pyrethroid that should NOT be used in cats.

AY. False. Permethrin is very toxic to fish.

AZ. False. Etofenprox is a pyrethroid.

BA. False. Amitraz stimulates α_2 receptors, which decreases further release of norepinephrine, producing sedation and nervous system depression.

BB. True.

BC. False. Amitraz is not effective in killing fleas. It can kill and repel ticks.

BD. False. Amitraz should not be used in or on cats.

BE. False. It is eprinomectin that has a pour-on and 100-to-150-day injectable form.

BF. True.

BG. True.

BH. False. Just the opposite. Low dose stimulation produces tremors, but high dose stimulation locks up the nicotinic receptor so it cannot depolarize again, resulting in paralysis of the muscle to which the nicotinic receptor is attached.

BI. True.

BJ. True.

BK. False. Just the opposite. Nitenpyram only kills adult fleas.

BL. False. Spinosad is a type of spinosyn. Spinetoram is made up of two synthetic spinosyns.

BM. True.

BN. False. Spinetoram was created specifically for cats.

BO. False. It is only the high dose of ivermectin (i.e., the demodectic mange mite dose) given with spinosad that produces increased incidence of ivermectin toxicosis. The dose of ivermectin in preventives is so low that the combination should not produce signs of ivermectin toxicosis.

BP. True.

BQ. True.

BR. True. Indoxacarb is converted into an insecticide within the parasite by the flea's own enzymes.

BS. False. The flea does not have to ingest a blood meal to absorb the indoxacarb.

BT. False. That would be IDIs. JHAs keep the larvae from maturing, eventually causing death.

BU. False. Lufenuron is an IDI that blocks chitin incorporation into the flea egg and larvae.

BV. False. Methoprene is a JHA.

5. Selective toxicity, economical, effective against all stages of parasite life cycle, safe for old, young, pregnant, or debilitated animals, and does not induce resistance.

6. Characteristic primary clinical signs of ivermectin toxicosis:

no	miosis
yes	mydriasis
no	agitation
yes	depression
no	tachycardia
yes	bradycardia
no	seizures
yes	coma

7. The lipophilic nature of macrolides and their penetration into milk means no injectable macrolides can be used in actively milking dairy cattle because of milk contamination for an extended period of time.

8. Some of the OTC internal antiparasitics only kill roundworms (i.e., ascarids) but may not kill dangerous hookworms, whipworms, or tapeworms. The hookworms feed off blood taken from the lining of the GI tract and can potentially cause a young animal to become very anemic from loss of blood.

9. Modern anticestodals typically do not result in passage of tapeworm proglottids because they are digested by the enzymes in the intestine.

10. No. Microfilaria are the young produced by the adult female heartworm and are unable to produce new adult heartworms until they are taken up by a mosquito, go through a molt, and then are reinjected into an animal host.

11. SLUDDE stands for:
    S = salivation
    L = lacrimation (i.e., tearing)

U = urination (i.e., stimulation of muscles that contract bladder)

D = dyspnea (i.e., difficult breathing from bronchoconstriction and excessive respiratory secretions)

D = defecation (i.e., excessive GI secretions and motility)

E = emesis (i.e., vomiting), eructation (i.e., belching in ruminants), erection

12. Nitenpyram can kill the maggots quickly.

CHAPTER 13

1. Fill in the following blanks with the correct item from the Key Terms list.

  A. nociceptors

  B. arachidonic acid cascade or pathway

  C. eicosanoids

  D. phospholipase

  E. phospholipase

  F. cyclooxygenase (COX)

  G. lipoxygenase (LOX)

  H. thromboxanes

  I. glucocorticoids

  J. phospholipase

  K. adrenocorticosteroids

  L. adrenal cortex

  M. mineralocorticoids

  N. aldosterone

  O. hypoadrenocorticism

  P. hyperkalemia

  Q. corticotropin-releasing hormone (CRH) or corticotropin-releasing factor (CRF)

  R. adrenocorticotropic hormone (ACTH)

  S. aqueous solution

  T. alcohol solution

  U. suspension form

  V. supraphysiologic

  W. gluconeogenesis

  X. catabolism

  Y. atrophy

  Z. autoimmune reaction

 AA. hypersensitivity reaction

 AB. T-lymphocyte

 AC. humoral immunity

 AD. B-lymphocyte

 AE. leukogram

 AF. lymphopenia

 AG. monocytopenia

 AH. eosinopenia

 AI. neutrophilia

 AJ. stress leukogram

 AK. polyuria

 AL. polydipsia

 AM. antidiuretic hormone (ADH)

 AN. collagenase

 AO. Cushing's syndrome

 AP. Addison's disease

 AQ. iatrogenic

 AR. polyphagia

 AS. alopecia

 AT. COX-1

 AU. COX-2

 AV. coxib

 AW. antipyretic

 AX. analgesic

 AY. hyperalgesia

 AZ. allodynia

 BA. gastritis

 BB. melena

 BC. hypoxia (low oxygen levels in the tissue) or ischemia (ischemia is decreased blood flow to a tissue that results in low oxygen delivery to the tissue)

 BD. renal papillae

 BE. renal pelvis

 BF. renal papillary necrosis

 BG. hypoproteinemia

 BH. hypoalbuminemia

 BI. salicylic acid or acetylsalicylic acid

 BJ. uveitis

 BK. laminitis

 BL. aplastic anemia

 BM. antipyresis

 BN. endotoxemia

 BO. mastitis

 BP. superoxide radicals, hydroxyl radicals

 BQ. chondro-

 BR. nutraceuticals

 BS. hyponatremia

2. Fill in the following blanks with the correct drug from the Antiinflammatory Drugs list.

  A. aspirin

  B. hydrocortisone

  C. phenylbutazone

  D. prednisone, prednisolone, methylprednisolone

  E. dimethyl sulfoxide (DMSO)

  F. deracoxib

  G. aspirin

  H. desoxycorticosterone pivalate (Percorten-V)

  I. DMSO

  J. flunixin meglumine

  K. isoflupredone

  L. carprofen

  M. acetaminophen

  N. robenacoxib

  O. hydrocortisone

  P. carprofen

  Q. aspirin

  R. cortisone

  S. dexamethasone, betamethasone, flumethasone

  T. diclofenac sodium

  U. ibuprofen, naproxen

  V. etodolac

  W. DMSO

X. hyaluronic acid or hyaluronate sodium

Y. triamcinolone

Z. meloxicam

AA. DMSO

AB. polysulfated glycosaminoglycans (PSGAGs)

AC. aspirin

AD. glucosamine and chondroitin sulfate

3. Abbreviations

CRH	corticotropin-releasing hormone
ACTH	adrenocorticotropic hormone
COX	cyclooxygenase
ADH	antidiuretic hormone
KCS	keratoconjunctivitis sicca
PSGAG	polysulfated glycosaminoglycans

4. Indicate whether each of the following statements is true or false.

A. False. Although they may decrease some of the activity of COX, they primarily inhibit phospholipase.

B. False. Those are enzymes that produce eicosanoids (e.g., prostaglandins, thromboxanes, leukotrienes).

C. True.

D. False. The cortex is the outer layer of the adrenal gland. The medulla is the inner layer.

E. True.

F. True.

G. True. The hyperkalemia can be fatal.

H. False. Cortisone is the precursor to hydrocortisone.

I. False. CRH stimulates the release of ACTH. Increased ACTH causes release of cortisol.

J. True. Release is decreased by the negative feedback mechanism.

K. False. Triamcinolone is an intermediate-acting glucocorticoid and isoflupredone is a long-acting glucocorticoid.

L. True. The suppression of release of CRH and ACTH by supraphysiologic concentrations of glucocorticoids from drugs causes the adrenal cortex to atrophy from lack of stimulation. Dexamethasone has a longer duration of action than prednisolone and hence also has a longer inhibiting effect on the hypothalamic and pituitary release of CRH and ACTH.

M. False. A diacetate form would be a suspension, which is not to be given IV. The sodium phosphate would be an aqueous solution and therefore can be given IV.

N. True. An immunosuppressive dose is higher so as to suppress the body's immune response well beyond what is suppressed at the antiinflammatory dose.

O. True.

P. True.

Q. False. Atrophy is the shrinkage of a gland or tissue and catabolism is the breakdown of tissue such as the catabolism of skeletal muscle for amino acids needed for gluconeogenesis.

R. False. Glucocorticoids increase blood glucose so the dose of insulin would need to be increased to compensate and move the blood glucose into the tissues.

S. True.

T. False. B cells (i.e., lymphocytes) produce antibodies. T-cells are lymphocytes that carry out cell-mediated immune responses.

U. True.

V. False. The stress leukogram is neutrophilia, monocytopenia, and lymphopenia.

W. True. This is how polyuria occurs with glucocorticoids.

X. False. Iatrogenic means that it is caused by the veterinarian. Idiosyncratic means a reaction to a drug that is unpredictable.

Y. False. Cats tolerate glucocorticoids with fewer side effects than dogs.

Z. False. This could kill the animal. If the animal has been on glucocorticoid drugs for a long period of time, the hypothalamus and pituitary have been suppressed by negative feedback and the adrenal gland has not been stimulated. The adrenal cortex has atrophied, and if the glucocorticoid drug is stopped immediately, the adrenal cortex will not be able to respond with sufficient natural cortisol to meet the need of the body (i.e., Addison's disease).

AA. False. That would be COX-2 (although COX-1 enzyme does play a minor role in some inflammation).

AB. False. It is a drug that decreases fever.

AC. True.

AD. True.

AE. False. Melena is digested blood that was leaked into the stomach or upper small intestine by injury or disease. The blood is digested by normal GI enzymes and in so doing the blood turns black and takes on a tarry texture.

AF. True.

AG. False. The renal papillary necrosis occurs when NSAIDs are used in hypotensive animals.

AH. False. The reason is idiosyncratic, meaning the factors that predispose an animal to the problem are unknown and when it will occur is unpredictable.

AI. False. Liver toxicity from NSAIDs is far rarer than renal side effects in hypotensive animals.

AJ. False. If the animal is hypoproteinemic, there is less protein in the blood to bind to the drug molecules, allowing more of the drug molecules to distribute to the target tissues. To compensate for more drug molecules entering the tissue, the dose would need to be decreased.

AK. False. Ibuprofen or naproxen use in the dog produces widely variable responses so it is not as safe to use as aspirin. It should not be used in cats either.

AL. False. COX-2 selective NSAIDs still can reduce the action of COX-1 (i.e., beneficial) prostaglandin production in the GI tract, producing gastritis and ulcerations, especially at higher doses where the selectivity of COX-2 over COX-1 is much less.

AM. False. This is something that was suggested with early adverse effects of carprofen, but did not take into account the number of Labrador retrievers that were put on the drug. Later evaluation did not support that Labrador retrievers were at any greater risk than any other breed.

AN. True.

AO. False. Nutraceuticals are not drugs and therefore do not have to meet FDA requirements.

AP. False. Acetaminophen does not block GI prostaglandins and therefore does not block COX-1 beneficial prostaglandins that could produce gastritis and ulcers. Therefore, acetaminophen is less likely to produce GI signs.

AQ. True.

AR. False. Antiinflammatory (not immunosuppressive) doses will not significantly suppress B-cell production of antibodies in response to vaccines.

AS. False. The GI tract is the most common site for NSAID toxicity, followed by the kidney. The liver idiosyncratic reaction is rare.

AT. False. NSAIDs do not produce as strong analgesia as opioid drugs and should not be used to attempt to control acute pain. Bone pain would not be sufficiently controlled by NSAIDs.

AU. False. Glucocorticoids should not be used in animals with corneal ulcers because of the stimulation of enzymes that digest the center protein layer of the cornea.

AV. True.

5. For each of the following, indicate "decreased" or "increased" for what would be expected after prolonged use of antiinflammatory doses of a glucocorticoid drug.

• Blood sugar concentrations	INCREASED
• Insulin dose requirements	INCREASED
• Number of circulating neutrophils	INCREASED
• Number of circulating lymphocytes	DECREASED
• Skeletal muscle mass	DECREASED
• Urine production	INCREASED

• Appetite	INCREASED
• Hair growth	DECREASED
• Time to heal	INCREASED

6. For each of the following, indicate "decreased" or "increased" for what would be expected during use of antiinflammatory doses of NSAIDs.

• Gastric acid production	INCREASED
• Stomach mucus production	DECREASED
• Secretion of GI sodium bicarbonate	DECREASED
• Rate of turn-over of GI tract cells	DECREASED
• Blood supply to the GI tract cells	DECREASED
• Diameter of renal blood vessels	DECREASED*

* depending on degree of sympathetic tone causing vasoconstriction

7. The condition is hyperadrenocorticism or Cushing's syndrome. Cortisol produced by the tumor would be elevated above normal. CRH and ACTH would both be decreased because of the negative feedback on the hypothalamus and pituitary from the high levels of cortisol.

8. High levels of the drug would have negative feedback suppression on the hypothalamus and pituitary, resulting in decreased CRH, decreased ACTH, and therefore decreased stimulation of the adrenal gland to produce any cortisol, resulting in low cortisol levels. The high glucocorticoid effects from the drug would be classified as iatrogenic hyperadrenocorticism or iatrogenic Cushing's. The dexamethasone must be tapered off to slowly remove the inhibition on the hypothalamus and pituitary while still giving enough drug to provide the glucocorticoid the body needs to survive. This may take weeks of tapering off the drug to safely allow the adrenal gland to get back to producing life-sustaining levels of natural cortisol.

9. You would explain that the "aspirin-like" drug is actually a stronger NSAID that is designed to suppress the development of more painful condition as a result of wind-up, or the ability of the spinal cord to more effectively send pain signals to the brain. The NSAID is not designed to take the place of opioid analgesics needed to produce a stronger level of analgesia needed with bone surgery.

GLOSSARY

A

Absorption The uptake of substances into or across tissues such as the skin, intestine, or renal tubules.

Acetylcholine (ACh) A reversible acetic acid ester of choline; it is a cholinergic agonist and serves as a neurotransmitter at the myoneural junctions of striated muscles, at autonomic effector cells innervated by parasympathetic nerves, at the preganglionic synapses of the sympathetic and parasympathetic nervous systems, and at various sites in the central nervous system. ACh has few therapeutic applications owing to its diffuse action and rapid hydrolysis by acetylcholinesterase (AChE); synthetic derivatives are used for more specific, prolonged action. ACh is used as a vasodilator in pharmacoangiography; it is administered by intraarterial infusion.

Acetylcholinesterase (AChE) An enzyme of the hydrolase class that catalyzes the cleavage of acetylcholine to choline and acetate; it is found in the central nervous system, particularly in gray matter of nerve tissue, in red blood cells, and in motor endplates of skeletal muscle.

Acetylcysteine The *N*-acetyl derivative of L-cysteine used as a mucolytic agent for adjunct therapy in bronchopulmonary disorders to reduce the viscosity of mucus and facilitate its removal, administered by instillation or nebulization; and as an antidote for acetaminophen poisoning, administered orally or intravenously.

Acid drug A drug whose chemical structure causes it to release a hydrogen ion (H^+, or proton) into its liquid environment as the drug is placed into increasingly alkaline environments.

Acidic pH A liquid environment in which many hydrogen ions float freely and are available to react with drug molecules. In an acidic environment, an acid drug will take up a hydrogen ion (i.e., add it to its molecular structure) and shift from an ionized drug molecule to a nonionized molecule.

Active ingredient The component of a drug which produces the intended beneficial effect.

Active secretion (renal) An energy-requiring transport carrier mechanism; the drug movement from the peritubular capillaries into the urine does not depend upon the concentration gradient and can achieve very high concentrations in the urine.

Active transport Cell expends energy to either move the drug molecule across the cell membrane or to "reset" the carrier molecule after transport is completed so that the carrier molecule can transport again. It occurs in only one direction and can actually move drug molecules against the concentration gradient.

Addison's disease Chronic type of adrenocortical insufficiency; characterized by hypotension, weight loss, anorexia, weakness, and a bronzelike hyperpigmentation of the skin. It is caused by tuberculosis- or autoimmune-induced destruction of the adrenal cortex, which results in deficiency of aldosterone and cortisol and is fatal in the absence of replacement therapy.

Adenosine triphosphate (ATP) A nucleotide, the $5'$-triphosphate of adenosine, involved in energy metabolism and required for RNA synthesis; it occurs in all cells and is used to store energy in the form of high-energy phosphate bonds. The free energy derived from hydrolysis of ATP is used to drive metabolic reactions, including the synthesis of nucleic acids and proteins, movement of molecules against concentration gradients (i.e., active transport), and to produce mechanical motion (i.e., contraction of microfibrils and microtubules).

Adjunct drug A drug used in addition to another drug.

Adrenergic Pertaining to sympathetic nerve fibers of the autonomic nervous system that liberate norepinephrine at a synapse where a nerve impulse passes.

Adrenocorticosteroids Also called corticosteroids, a group of hormones produced by the cortex (i.e., the outer layer) of the adrenal gland. There are two groups of corticosteroids: mineralocorticoids and glucocorticoids.

Adrenocorticotropic hormone (ACTH) A hormone of the adenohypophysis that stimulates growth of the adrenal cortex and the synthesis and secretion of corticosteroids. ACTH secretion, regulated by corticotropin-releasing hormone from the hypothalamus, increases in response to a low level of circulating cortisol and to stress.

Adsorbents Drug molecules that cause other molecules to adhere to their outer surfaces.

Adulticide A drug used to kill mature (i.e., adult) heartworms that live in the pulmonary vasculature and the right chambers of the heart.

Adverse drug reaction (ADR) A broader term that includes any adverse reaction either within the therapeutic range (i.e., side effect) or as the result of toxic accumulation of drug.

Aerobic Requires oxygen.

Aerosol administration The drug is delivered into the lungs by air or gas solution.

Aerosol therapy Also called aerosolization; the process of administering a drug as a fine mist that the animal inhales into the airways.

Afferent renal arteriole The incoming renal arteriole.

Affinity A special attraction for a specific element, organ, or structure.

Afterload Refers to the tension or pressure the ventricles must create to eject blood out of the ventricles and into the aorta and pulmonary arteries.

Agonist A drug with both a good affinity for the receptor and the ability to produce intrinsic activity.

Alanine aminotransferase (ALT) An enzyme of the transferase class that catalyzes the reversible transfer of an amino group from alanine to α-ketoglutarate to form glutamate and pyruvate, with pyridoxal phosphate as a cofactor. The reaction transfers nitrogen for excretion or for incorporation into other compounds. The enzyme is found in serum and body tissues, especially in the liver.

Aldosterone The mineralocorticoid hormone of medical significance in animals with adrenocortical insufficiency. Aldosterone's primary effect is to increase the sodium retained in the body by opening sodium pores in the distal convoluted tubule and collecting ducts of the kidney, allowing sodium to move from the urine back into the cells lining the renal tubules; from there they are actively pumped back into the blood.

Alkaline phosphatase (ALP) An enzyme of the hydrolase class that catalyzes the cleavage of orthophosphate from orthophosphoric monoesters under alkaline conditions. Differing forms of the enzyme occur in normal and malignant tissues.

Allodynia The transmission of pain sensation by sensations or receptors that normally do not transmit pain (e.g., pressure, touch, hot, or cold receptors).

Alopecia Deficiency of the hair or wool coat.

Alpha-1(α1) receptor An adrenergic receptor that causes smooth muscle surrounding the small arteriole blood vessels in the skin and intestinal tract to contract (i.e., vasoconstriction), decreasing blood flow to these tissues.

Ampules Dosage forms in which the drug is contained within a small, airtight, thin glass bottle that is opened by snapping the narrow neck of the ampule bottle.

Anaerobic Pertaining to the absence of air or oxygen.

Analgesic A pain relief drug that does not limit sensation.

Anesthesia/anesthetic A pain relief drug that limits sensation.

Anestrus The period of time in which little or no estrous cycling activity is occurring and hormone levels in general are very low.

Angiotensin-converting enzyme (ACE) inhibitor A protease inhibitor found in serum that promotes vasodilation by blocking the formation of angiotensin II and slowing the degradation of bradykinin and other kinins. It decreases sodium retention, water retention, blood pressure, and heart size and increases cardiac output.

Animal Medicinal Drug Use Clarification Act (AMDUCA) Gives the veterinarian the opportunity for off-label or extra-label drug use (often abbreviated as ELDU) under certain conditions. These conditions are listed in Box 1.1.

Antacids: systemic, nonsystemic Decrease stomach acidity by either chemically combining with the hydrochloric acid to make a less acidic molecule or by decreasing acid production. Antacids are classified as systemic (i.e., must be absorbed, circulate, and attach to receptors on

337

the cells of the stomach to produce their effect) or nonsystemic (i.e., given by mouth, but are not absorbed systemically and instead chemically neutralize acid molecules in the stomach or rumen).

Antagonist   A drug with good affinity, but little or no intrinsic activity.

Anthelmintic   A general term used to describe compounds that kill various types of helminths, or internal parasitic worms.

Anticestodal   Compounds or cestocides treat infections of cestodes, which are tapeworms or segmented flatworms.

Anticholinergic drugs   Block the effect of the acetylcholine neurotransmitter on acetylcholine receptors.

Anticonvulsant   Pertaining to a substance or procedure that prevents or reduces the severity of epileptic or other convulsive seizures.

Antidepressant   Mood-elevating drugs used in human therapy. In veterinary medicine, antidepressants are used for a number of behaviors in pets that are not necessarily associated with what we would call "depressed" behaviors.

Antidiuretic hormone (ADH)   Released from the pituitary gland; causes increased permeability to water of the distal convoluted tubule and the collecting ducts in the kidney. This increased permeability allows more water to move out of the urine and be retained in the body (i.e., antidiuresis).

Antipyretic/antipyrexia   Reduces fever.

Antiseptics   Chemical agents that kill or prevent the growth of microorganisms on living tissues.

Antitrematodal   Compounds treat infections of trematodes, flukes, or unsegmented flatworms.

Antitussive drugs   Any of a large group of opioid and nonopioid drugs that act on the central and peripheral nervous systems to suppress the cough reflex.

Anxiolytic   Literally "breaks apart anxiety"; a drug used to calm a patient.

Aorta   The main trunk from which the systemic arterial system proceeds. It arises from the left ventricle of the heart; passes upward (ascending aorta), bends over (aortic arch), and then proceeds downward (descending aorta); the latter is divided into an upper, thoracic part and a lower abdominal part.

Aortic valve   A valve in the heart between the left ventricle and the aorta.

Aplastic anemia   Usually appears 2–8 weeks after estrogen administration and is manifested as low platelet counts (i.e., thrombocytopenia), pinpoint hemorrhages in the skin or mucous membranes (caused by low platelet levels), evidence of bruising, leukopenia (i.e., low white blood cell count), and severe anemia.

Apnea   Cessation of breathing.

Apneustic breathing pattern   An abnormal respiratory rhythm.

Aqueous solution   A water medium in which the drug has been dissolved.

Arrhythmia   Irregular heartbeats or abnormal rhythms.

Arteries   Vessels through which the blood passes away from the heart to the various parts of the body.

Arterioles   Small artery blood vessels.

Arteritis   Inflammation of arterial walls.

ATP-Binding Cassette type B1 (ABCB1)   Also known as MDR1 (Multiple Drug Resistance 1), this gene produces the P-glycoprotein (P-gp) found on the surface of cancer cells that pumps out any antineoplastic drug that makes it into the cancer cell, making the cancer cell resistant to the drugs.

Automaticity   The capacity of a cell to initiate an impulse, such as depolarization, without an external stimulus.

Autonomic nervous system   Regulates bodily functions without involving conscious thought.

B

Bacteremia   The presence of bacteria in the blood.

Bacteriostatic   Temporarily inhibits the growth of bacteria, but once the drug is removed, the organism can begin to multiply again.

Baroreceptors   A type of interoceptor that is stimulated by changes in pressure, particularly one located in the wall of a blood vessel.

Basal metabolic rate   The rate at which cellular functions occur.

Base drug   A drug that becomes more ionized when it acquires a hydrogen ion from an acidic pH environment (acid drugs become more nonionized) and becomes more nonionized when it releases a H^+ ion into the liquid of an alkaline pH environment (acid drugs become more ionized).

Beta-1 (β1) receptor   An adrenergic receptor located primarily in the heart that increases the heart rate, the strength of contraction by the cardiac muscle, and the speed that the depolarization wave passes through the heart's conduction system when stimulated.

Beta-2 (β2) receptor   An adrenergic receptor found on the smooth muscle cells surrounding the arterioles that supply the heart muscle and skeletal muscles, and also surrounding the terminal bronchioles (i.e., smallest bronchioles) in the airway of the lungs. When stimulated, β_2-adrenergic receptors cause smooth muscle that is surrounding blood vessels or bronchioles to relax, causing dilation.

β-Lactam   Describes antibiotics that contain a β-lactam ring.

β-Lactam ring   A ringlike structure in the chemical composition of some antibiotics.

β-Lactamase   Any of a group of bacterial enzymes of the hydrolase class, produced by almost all gram-negative species, that catalyze the cleavage of β-lactam rings.

β-Lactamase resistant   Bacterial enzymes that cause resistance to β-lactam.

β-Tubulin   The subunit from which microtubules are assembled.

Biguanides   Any of a group of substituted derivatives of biguanide, which are used as oral antihyperglycemic agents; they increase insulin action in peripheral tissues; by inhibiting gluconeogenesis, they decrease hepatic glucose production.

Biliary excretion   Elimination of drugs by the liver.

Bioavailability   Measure of how effectively an administered drug is absorbed.

Bioequivalence   An equivalent amount of generic drug is absorbed and delivered to the target site within the body compared with the original brand or parent drug.

Biofilm   Generated by bacteria when they attach to a surface and develop a glycocalyx "shell" around themselves.

Biotransformation   Process of enzymes chemically altering the drug structure in the liver.

Black box warning   Warning that contains adverse effects that have a significant risk for severe or life-threatening effects.

Blood-brain barrier   An anatomical–physiological feature of the brain thought to consist of walls of capillaries in the central nervous system and surrounding astrocytic glial membranes. The barrier separates the parenchyma of the central nervous system from blood. The blood–brain barrier prevents or slows the passage of some drugs and other chemical compounds, radioactive ions, and disease-causing organisms such as viruses from the blood into the central nervous system.

Bowman's Capsule   The cup-shaped end of a renal tubule or nephron enclosing a glomerulus. With the glomerulus, it is the site of filtration in the kidney.

Bradycardia/bradyarrhythmia   Slowing of the heart rate.

Bradypnea   Slow breathing.

Breakpoints   Points that mark a drug's minimum inhibitory concentration (MIC); differentiates between when a bacterial strain is considered susceptible, intermediate susceptible, or resistant to that particular drug.

C

Caplet   A solid dosage form that is elongated to facilitate easy swallowing.

Capsules   Powdered drug surrounded by a capsule made of gelatin, modified starch, or cellulose.

Carcinogenic effect   Increases the risk for development of cancer or preneoplastic changes.

Cardiomyopathy   General diagnostic term designating primary noninflammatory disease of the heart muscle, often of obscure or unknown etiology and not the result of ischemic, hypertensive, congenital, valvular, or pericardial disease.

Catabolism   Any destructive process by which complex substances are converted by living cells into simpler compounds, with release of energy.

Catalepsis   Characterized by an appearance of being awake, but being unable to respond to external stimuli.

Caval syndrome   Refers to the vena cavae and means the pulmonary vasculature and heart are so physically full of worms that they extend back into the vena cavae.

Centrally acting antitussive   Reduces coughing by suppressing the cough center neurons in the brainstem.

Centrally acting emetic   Acts by stimulating the emetic center or the chemoreceptor trigger zone (CRTZ) in the central nervous system; includes drugs such as apomorphine and α_2-agonists such as xylazine.

Cephalosporinase   Bacterial β-lactamases specific for cephalosporins more than penicillins.

Cestocides   *see* Anticestodal

Chelate   To bind to and precipitate out of solution.

Chemical name   Description of the chemical composition or molecular structure of a drug as determined by the rules of accepted nomenclature.

Chemoreceptor trigger zone (CRTZ)   A specialized cluster of receptors that constantly monitor the blood and the cerebrospinal fluid for chemicals that can stimulate vomiting.

Chief cells   Produce an enzyme precursor called pepsinogen.

Chitin   A compound found in the exoskeleton of insects, the egg-tooth of flea larva, and in the cell wall of fungal elements.

Clearance   The rate at which drugs leave the body.

Clinical pharmacology   Applying pharmacology to specific treatments.

Clonic seizures   Seizures in which rapid contraction and relaxation of muscles occurs.

Coagulum   A coagulated mass or clot.

Coccidiostats   Antiprotozoal drugs that specifically inhibit the growth of coccidia.

Collagenase   In reference to corneal ulcers: the enzyme that degrades the collagen protein that forms the middle layers of the cornea, resulting in a deepening ulcer to the point that the cornea ruptures.

Colonic   Related to the large intestine or colon.

Compounding   Any manipulation of a drug product to produce a different dosage form other than what is approved by the Food and Drug Administration (FDA).

Concentration   The ratio of the mass or volume of a solute to the mass or volume of the solution or solvent.

Concentration gradient   Movement of drug molecules from an area of high concentration of drug to an area of lower concentration or vice versa.

Conduction cells   Type of cardiac muscle cells that conducts waves of depolarization from the SA node to the atria, to the AV node, and then to the ventricles.

Congestive heart failure   Weakening of the heart muscle.

Constant rate infusion (CRI)   Slowly injected or "dripped" into a vein over a period of several seconds, minutes, or even hours.

Contractile cells   Type of cardiac muscle cell that actually pumps the blood.

Contraindication   Circumstances or conditions in which the drug should not be used.

Controlled-release coatings   Slow the rate at which the tablet dissolves as the tablet moves along the intestinal tract, resulting in a more gradual and sustained release of the active ingredient as opposed to being released all at once.

Controlled Substance   Drugs like narcotics, strong sedatives, analgesics, or hallucinogenic drugs that have the potential for abuse.

Convulsions   Seizures that manifest themselves as spastic muscle movement caused by stimulation of motor nerves in the brain or spinal cord.

Corticotropin-releasing hormone   A neuropeptide elaborated by the median eminence of the hypothalamus, the pancreas, and the brain; it binds to specific receptors on the corticotrophs of the adenohypophysis and stimulates production of corticotropin.

Cortisol   The major natural glucocorticoid synthesized in the zona fasciculata of the adrenal cortex; it affects the metabolism of glucose, protein, and fats and has appreciable mineralocorticoid activity. It also regulates the immune system and affects many other functions.

Coxibs   Cyclooxygenase (COX)-2 inhibitory nonsteroidal antiinflammatory drugs (NSAIDs).

Crystalluria   Crystals in the urine.

Culture and sensitivity testing   Testing that can determine the susceptibility of a bacterial strain to certain drugs by determining how much drug it takes to inhibit or kill the bacteria.

Cushing's syndrome   Overproduction of glucocorticoids by the tumors of the adrenal cortex or other pathologic conditions; also called hyperadrenocorticism.

Cytochrome P-450 (CYP)   Particular mixedfunction oxidase (MFO) enzyme involved with phenobarbital metabolism.

Cytotoxic   Causes cell destruction.

D

Decongestant   Reduce congestion (i.e, vascular engorgement) of swollen nasal tissues by stimulating the sympathetic nervous system's α_1-receptors on smooth muscle of blood vessels in the skin and mucous membranes.

Deep/systemic mycoses   Fungal infections within the body.

Depolarization wave   "Firing" of cells through the heart.

Depolarize   To reduce toward a nonpolarized condition; to deprive of polarity.

Depot form   Dosage form formulated to allow a slow absorption of the drug from the administration site, providing more sustained drug concentrations in the body over time.

Dermatophyte   Any of various imperfect fungi that cause superficial infections on keratinized tissue of animals (e.g., skin, nails, or hair).

Dirofilaria immitis   The worms of canine heartworm disease.

Disinfectants   Chemical agents that kill or prevent growth of microorganisms on inanimate objects.

Dissolution   Process of breaking down the size to the individual molecules.

Distal convoluted tubule   The portion of the nephron lying between the nephric (Henle's) loop and the collecting duct in the kidney.

DNA gyrase   Also called topoisomerase type II; facilitates the unwinding of DNA strands so they can be re-coiled into tight supercoils.

Dosage   An estimation of the actual amount of drug a specific patient will need for a particular disease.

Dosage form   The description of a drug's physical appearance; is typically included in the drug's description in the package insert and the drug label.

Dosage regimen   The complete information needed to determine the mass of drug to be given to the animal, the route by which the drug is to be given, how often it is to be given, and for how long the drug is to be administered.

Dose   The amount of drug to be given to a specific patient.

Dose interval   The number of times per day medicine is administered.

Downregulation   Controlled decrease. Particularly the attenuation of expression of a gene in response to cellular or environmental factors, as by a decrease in transcription of the gene or by destabilization of mRNA; or the reduction in responsiveness of a cell to stimulatory factors after a first exposure, as by decrease in the number of receptors expressed on the cell surface.

Drug Enforcement Administration (DEA)   A federal law enforcement agency that enforces controlled substances laws and regulations.

Drug formulary   A collection of recipes, formulas, and prescriptions.

Drug insert   The drug manufacturer's documentation inserted into or attached to the side of each bottle, package, or box of medication. The drug insert will contain the information that is mandated by FDA regulations for veterinary drugs, but will only contain that information for which the manufacturer has done the mandated testing or otherwise documented in compliance with FDA requirements.

Drug order   A request by a veterinarian to dispense or administer a drug within a hospital.

Dysphoria   Hallucinations or bad effects from opioids.

Dyspnea   Difficult breathing.

E

Ectoparasites   Externally living parasites.

Ectopic focus   Abnormal site of depolarization.

Eicosanoids   A family of compounds derived from C20 polyunsaturated fatty acids. Includes prostaglandins, prostacyclins, leukotrienes, lipoxins and thromboxanes, the principal mediators of inflammation.

Elixir   Alcohol-based solutions used for oral or topical (i.e., on the surface of the skin) application.

Emboli   Any detached mass or object traveling within the blood vessels.

Emetic center   Group of special neurons located in the medullary structure of the brainstem that produces the physiologic actions associated with the period just before vomiting and the actual act of vomiting itself.

Empirical therapy   The selection of a particular antimicrobial drug before the results of a culture and sensitivity test are returned.

Emulsion   Liquid suspension composed of two liquids that do not readily mix together.

Endectocides   Compounds that kill internal and external parasites.

Endocytosis   Small invagination forming in the cell membrane that surrounds the drug molecule and brings it into the cell.

Endogenous   Produced within or caused by factors within the organism.

Endotoxemia   Grave condition caused by the presence of bacterial toxins in the blood.

Enteric coating   Coating designed to protect the active ingredient from the harsh acidic environment of the stomach by not allowing the tablet to dissolve until it reaches the more alkaline environment of the small intestine.

Enterohepatic circulation   Movement of drug from liver to intestinal tract and back to the liver.

Enterotoxins Toxins produced by intestinal bacteria.

Environmental Protection Agency (EPA) Federal agency dedicated to protecting human health and the environment.

Eosinopenia Abnormal deficiency of eosinophils in the blood.

Epilepsy Recurrent seizures originating from the brain.

Epinephrine Potent vasoconstrictor; epinephrine and norepinephrine are adrenal gland hormones and neurotransmitters that cause peripheral superficial blood vessels to constrict to compensate for a drop in blood pressure from shock or blood loss.

Erosions Gastric ulcers.

Eructation Normal rumen and reticulum contractions allow partially digested plant food (i.e., the cud) to be regurgitated to the esophagus, where it is chewed and reswallowed (i.e., rumination); expelling built-up carbon dioxide or methane gas from the rumen.

Estrogen Generic term for any estrus-producing steroid responsible for the development of the female secondary sex characteristics; during the menstrual cycle they act on the female genitalia to produce an environment suitable for the fertilization, implantation, and nutrition of the early embryo.

Estrous cycle The type of sexual cycle seen in most adult female mammals, with recurring periods that include estrus and the correlated changes in the reproductive tract from one period to the next. The stages are proestrus, estrus, metestrus, and diestrus (the latter sometimes including anestrus of varying lengths of time).

Euphoria Pleasant hallucinatory effect.

Euthyroid Pertaining to a normal thyroid gland and normal thyroid gland function.

Excipient An inert substance added to a prescription to affect texture.

Exogenous Compound that originates outside the body.

Extracellular fluid Fluid/water outside the cells.

Extract A therapeutic agent composed of prepared plant or animal parts rather than synthesized chemicals in a laboratory.

Extra-label drug use (ELDU) Use of a drug in an animal in a manner that is not in accordance with the approved labeling.

Extravascular injection Accidental injection of an intravenous (IV) drug outside the vein.

Exudative diarrhea Occurs when the inflammation or damage to the intestinal wall is significant enough to allow leakage of electrolytes, plasma proteins from the blood, or even blood itself into the intestinal tract.

F

Facilitated diffusion Uses a special "carrier molecule" located in the cellular membrane to move the drug molecule across the membrane. The carrier molecule, usually a protein floating among the phospholipid molecules in the cell membrane, has a specific site to which a drug molecule can attach. When a drug molecule combines with the carrier, the carrier molecule changes its configuration or shape, allowing the drug molecule to be carried through the cell membrane at that point without having to dissolve into the cell membrane like in passive diffusion.

Federal Food, Drug, and Cosmetic Act (FFDCA) A set of laws allowing the US Food and Drug Administration to regulate food, drug and cosmetics safety.

Fenestrations Small holes within the cell that allow water and small drug molecules to move readily back and forth between the blood and the surrounding tissue, but keep larger molecules, proteins, and red blood cells within the capillary.

Fibrillation Uncoordinated muscle contractions.

First-pass effect The phenomenon by which the liver removes so much of the drug that little reaches the systemic circulation.

Follicle-stimulating hormone (FSH) A glycopeptide of about 30,000 Da that stimulates the growth and maturation of ovarian follicles, stimulates estrogen secretion, promotes the endometrial changes characteristic of the first portion (i.e., proliferative phase) of the mammalian menstrual cycle, and stimulates spermatogenesis in the male.

Food and Drug Administration (FDA) The federal agency responsible for protecting public health by controlling and supervising safety standards for food, drug and cosmetic products that are either administered internally (i.e., orally, injectables) or are absorbed significantly into the body if administered topically.

G

Gamma (γ)-aminobutyric acid (GABA) An inhibitory neurotransmitter found in the central nervous system of mammals

Gastric motility Refers to stomach contractions that mix stomach contents and move the contents from the stomach into the small intestine.

Gastrin Hormone produced by gastrin cells (G cells) located in the distal part of the stomach and proximal duodenum. Signals relaxation of the stomach wall so more food can be stored; increases stomach acid production to begin the breakdown of food in the stomach.

Gastritis Inflammation of the stomach.

G cell Cells in the stomach and duodenum that secrete gastrin.

Generalized seizure Seizures that involve all of the body and often are associated with a loss of consciousness.

Generic equivalent Drugs produced or marketed by companies other than the original "brand" developer.

Generic name Also called a nonproprietary name; a more concise name given to the specific chemical compound.

Genetic epilepsy A term now preferred by some veterinarians to describe animals whose epilepsy is most likely traced to a breed or genetic predisposition.

Glomerulus Specialized tuft of capillaries in the kidney.

Glucocorticoids Hormones that increase blood glucose.

Gluconeogenesis The process through which glucocorticoids stimulate the liver and convert amino acids from proteins into new glucose.

Goiter Hypothyroid condition that results from a lack of iodine needed to manufacture triiodothyronine (T_3) or thyroxine (T_4) hormones.

Gonadorelin A synthetic luteinizing hormone–releasing hormone, structurally identical to the natural hormone.

Gonadotropin Any hormone that stimulates the gonads, especially follicle-stimulating hormone and luteinizing hormone.

Gonadotropin-releasing hormone (GnRH) A decapeptide hypophysiotropic hormone secreted by the hypothalamus. It stimulates the release of luteinizing hormone and follicle-stimulating hormone by the anterior pituitary.

Grain (measurement) The smallest unit of weight in the apothecary and avoirdupois systems; equivalent to 64.8 mg.

H

Halogen An element of group VII of the periodic table, the members of which form similar (salt-like) compounds in combination with sodium. The halogens are bromine, chlorine, fluorine, iodine and astatine.

Hepatic portal system The system of blood vessels that conducts the blood from the capillaries of the gastrointestinal (GI) tract to the liver and allows the liver to remove potential poisons, toxins, and other potentially dangerous substances absorbed from the GI tract before they reach systemic circulation.

Hepatocyte One of the polyhedral epithelial cells that constitute the substance of a liver acinus.

Household measuring system A system of measurement common in US households which includes teaspoons, cups, pints, quarts, and gallons.

Human chorionic gonadotropin A hormone produced by the human placenta and has luteinizing hormone (LH)-like effects with few or no follicle-stimulating hormone (FSH) effects.

Humoral immunity The production of antibodies by B-lymphocytes.

Hydrophilic Readily absorbing moisture; hygroscopic; having strongly polar groups that readily interact with water.

Hyperadrenocorticism Abnormally increased secretion of adrenocortical hormones.

Hyperalgesia Abnormally increased nociception (i.e., pain sense).

Hyperkalemia Abnormally high potassium concentration in the blood, most often because of defective renal excretion. It is characterized clinically by electrocardiographic abnormalities (e.g., elevated T waves, depressed P waves, and wide QRS complexes, eventually with atrial asystole).

Hypersensitivity State of altered reactivity in which the body reacts with an exaggerated or inappropriate immune response to what is perceived to be a foreign substance.

Hypertension High arterial blood pressure.

Hyperthermia Elevation of core body temperature.

Hyperthyroidism Condition caused by excessive production of iodinated thyroid hormones. Characteristics include goiter; tachycardia or atrial fibrillation; widened pulse pressure; palpitations; fatigability; nervousness and tremor; heat intolerance and excessive sweating; warm, smooth, moist skin; weight loss; muscular weakness;

excessive defecation; emotional lability; and ocular signs such as a stare, slowing of eyelid movements, photophobia, and sometimes exophthalmos.

Hypertonic salts   Osmotic or saline cathartics.

Hypoadrenocorticism   Abnormally diminished secretion of corticosteroids by the adrenal cortex.

Hypoalbuminemia   An abnormally low albumin content of the blood.

Hyponatremia   Deficiency of sodium in the blood.

Hypoproteinemia   Abnormally decreased levels of protein in the blood, sometimes resulting in edema and fluid accumulation in serous cavities.

Hypothyroidism   Deficiency of thyroid activity; characterized by decrease in basal metabolic rate, fatigue, and lethargy; if untreated, it progresses to myxedema.

Hypoxia   Reduction of oxygen supply to tissue below physiologic levels despite adequate perfusion of the tissue by blood.

I

Iatrogenic   Resulting from the activity of physicians.

Ictus   A seizure, stroke, blow, or sudden attack.

Ileus   Intestinal obstruction that is caused by a nonmechanical cause, such as paralysis of intestinal movement or lack of peristalsis.

Implants   An object or material, such as an alloplastic or radioactive material or tissue, partially or totally inserted or grafted into the body for prosthetic, therapeutic, diagnostic, or experimental purposes.

Indication   A sign or circumstance that points to or shows the cause, pathology, treatment, or issue of an attack of disease; something that points out, or serves as a guide or warning.

Induced   Produced artificially.

Inert ingredient   Any preservatives, stabilizers, liquid media, or other additives that make up the dosage form.

Inhibin   Either of two glycoproteins, A and B; each is composed of a common α-subunit and one of two β-subunits; they are secreted by the gonads and found in seminal plasma and follicular fluid, and inhibit pituitary production of follicle-stimulating hormone. They also contribute to the control of gametogenesis, embryonic and fetal development, and hematopoiesis. They are members of the transforming growth factor-β superfamily of proteins, and their actions are opposed by activins, which share the same β-subunits.

Inhibitors   Any substance that interferes with a chemical reaction, growth, or other biologic activity.

Inodilators   An agent that has both positive inotropic and vasodilator effects.

Insoluble   Not susceptible of being dissolved.

Inspissated   Being thickened, dried, or rendered with less fluid.

Intrinsic activity   The ability of a drug molecule to produce a cellular effect when it combines with the receptor.

Iodophor   Name given to any product in which surfaceacting agents, such as nonoxynol, act as carriers and solubilizing agents for iodine. Used as skin disinfectants, especially as teat dips in mastitis control.

Ionized/nonionized   Separated into ions; contains a net positive or a net negative charge.

Ionophore   Any molecule, as of a drug, that increases the permeability of cell membranes to transport a specific ion.

Ischemic/ischemia   Low oxygen levels in the tissue.

K

Kaolin/kaolinite and pectin   A claylike substance thought to be able to adsorb bacteria and their enterotoxins, thereby reducing their hypersecretory effect on the intestinal tract.

Keratoconjunctivitis sicca/dry eye   Inflammation of the cornea and conjunctiva.

L

Laminitis   Inflammation, congestion, and ischemia of the laminae of a hoof, with breakdown of the union between the horny and sensitive layers; it usually occurs in overweight, overfed animals.

Left atrium   The atrium of the left side of the heart; it receives blood from the pulmonary veins and delivers it to the left ventricle.

Left ventricle   The lower chamber of the left side of the heart, which pumps oxygenated blood out through the aorta into the systemic arteries.

Legend drug   Drugs limited to dispensing by or upon the order of a licensed prescriber (i.e., veterinarian or physician). Legend drugs contain ingredients that require greater control of dispensing either because of their toxic effects, potential to be abused or diverted as an illegal substance, or their potential to do harm to the patient or the person handling the drug.

Leukogram   The number of different white blood cells counted in the complete blood count or CBC.

Leukopenia   Decreased overall white cell count.

Leukotrienes   Any of a group of biologically active compounds consisting of straight chain, 20-carbon carboxylic acids with one or two oxygen substituents and three or more conjugated double bonds.

Limbic system   Pertaining to a limbus, or margin; forming a border around something.

Liniments   An oily liquid preparation to be used on the skin.

Lipophilic   Having an affinity for fat; pertaining to or characterized by lipophilia.

Lipoxygenase   An enzyme of the oxidoreductase class that catalyzes the oxidation of linoleate and related polyunsaturated fatty acids to their hydroperoxide forms.

Loop of Henle   A long, U-shaped part of the renal tubule; extends through the medulla from the end of the proximal convoluted tubule to the beginning of the distal convoluted tubule.

Luteal phase   A phase of the estrous cycle in which hormones of the corpus luteum on the ovary predominate, focusing on sustaining a fertilized egg.

Lymphopenia   Reduction in the number of lymphocytes in the blood.

M

Macrolides   A chemical compound characterized by a large lactone ring containing multiple keto and hydroxyl groups.

Maintenance dose   A dose that is smaller and is given at an amount and rate that matches the amount eliminated by the body.

Maldigestion/malabsorption   Inadequate digestion.

Mastitis   Inflammation of the udder or mammary gland.

Material safety data sheet (MSDS)   Contains guidelines for protective precautions, clean-up procedures, and first aid for accidental exposure.

Maximum effective concentration   Top concentration of the normal therapeutic range.

Maximum tolerated dose (MTD)   The highest concentration of drug tolerated by the animal before significant toxicity signs or adverse effects occur.

Melena   The passage of dark-colored feces stained with blood pigments or with altered blood.

Mesalamine   An active metabolite of sulfasalazine, used in the prophylaxis and treatment of inflammatory bowel disease and ulcerative proctitis; administered orally or rectally.

Metabolism   The sum of all the physical and chemical processes by which living organized substance is produced and maintained (i.e., anabolism), and also the transformation by which energy is made available for the uses of the organism.

Metabolite   Any substance produced by metabolism or by a metabolic process.

Metric system   A standard of measurement commonly used in veterinary medicine (e.g., meters, grams, liters).

Metritis   Inflammation of the uterus.

Microfilaricide   Drugs used to kill the circulating microfilariae produced by the adult heartworms.

Mineralocorticoids   Any of the group of C21 corticosteroids that are involved in the regulation of electrolyte and water balance through their effects on ion transport in epithelial cells; the most important one is aldosterone. They promote retention of sodium, loss of potassium, and the secondary retention of water; some also have varying degrees of glucocorticoid activity.

Miosis (pupils)   Contraction of the pupil.

Monoamine oxidase inhibitors (MAOI)   A family of drugs that works by inhibiting the enzyme monoamine oxidase, whose purpose is to catabolize (i.e., break apart) serotonin, dopamine, and norepinephrine. By inhibiting the enzyme, MAOI drugs allow additional production of these neurotransmitters, stimulating the central nervous system (CNS) in general.

Monocytopenia   Abnormal decrease in the proportion of monocytes in the blood.

Monogastric   Having just one stomach, as opposed to ruminants and certain other animals.

Motilin   A compound found in the intestinal tract that stimulates intestinal motility.

Motility diarrhea   Results when rapid movement of the intestinal contents prevents proper digestion of food or absorption of fluids before the contents are expelled as feces.

Methicillin-resistant *Staphylococcus aureus* (MRSA) A bacterial strain found on the skin that has acquired resistance to all penicillins, including the extended spectrum penicillin called methicillin.

Mucin Complex molecules produced by the mucus-producing cells in the gastric glands; the main constituent of the mucus coating.

Mucolytic Capable of reducing the viscosity of mucus.

Mucous cells Cells that produce the protective mucus layer.

Mucus The free slime of the mucous membranes; composed of secretions of the glands, various inorganic salts, desquamated cells, and leukocytes.

Multidose vials Vials in which multiple doses can be withdrawn over time.

Mutagenic Inducing genetic mutation.

Mydriasis Physiologic dilatation of the pupil.

Myometrium The smooth muscle coat of the uterus.

N

Narcotics An agent that produces insensibility or stupor; applied especially to the opioids.

Narrow therapeutic index The dose that causes the beneficial effect is close to the dose that produces toxic side effects.

Narrow therapeutic range Drugs in which the maximum effective dose and the minimal effective dose are very close to each other.

Nebulization The inhalation of a fine mist containing the drug.

Negative inotropic effect Cause a decreased force of contraction.

Nephrotoxic Poisonous to the kidney.

Neuroleptanalgesic Opioid drugs combined with a tranquilizer or sedative (e.g., butorphanol opioid with a diazepam tranquilizer). The intent of these combination drugs is to use the tranquilizer effects to decrease some of the adverse effects of the opioids.

Neuromuscular junction (NMJ) Where nerve axons contact skeletal muscles.

Neurosteroid/neuroactive steroid A steroid produced in the brain.

Neutrophilia Increase in the number of neutrophils in the blood; it is the most common form of leukocytosis and can have any of numerous causes, including acute infections, intoxications, hemorrhage, and rapidly growing malignant neoplasms.

Nociceptor A receptor for pain caused by injury to body tissues; the injury may be from physical stimuli such as mechanical, thermal, or electrical stimuli, or from chemical stimuli such as the presence of a toxin or an excess of a nontoxic substance.

Nonproductive cough Dry and hacking cough.

Nonproprietary name The official generic name assigned to a drug that is no longer subject to trademark rights.

Norepinephrine One of the naturally occurring catecholamines; a neurohormone released by the postganglionic adrenergic nerves and some brain neurons. It is a major neurotransmitter that acts on α- and β_1-adrenergic receptors. It is also secreted by the adrenal medulla in response to

splanchnic stimulation and is stored in the chromaffin granules. It is a powerful vasopressor and is released in the body usually in response to hypotension or stress.

Nosocomial Pertaining to or originating in the hospital, usually referring to a disease or other pathologic condition.

Nucleus tractus solitarius (NTS) A set of neurons that has many receptors for drugs or compounds that can stimulate vomiting and thus can also be a site of action for drugs that suppress vomiting by blocking these receptors.

Nutraceuticals Foods and food supplements marketed for presumed health benefits, such as vitamin supplements and certain herbs.

Nystagmus An involuntary, rapid, rhythmic movement of the eyeball, which may be horizontal, vertical, rotatory, or mixed (i.e., of two varieties).

O

Ointment A semisolid preparation for external application to the skin or mucous membranes, usually containing a medicinal substance.

Oocyte The immature female reproductive cell before fertilization; derived from an oogonium and occurring in two stages: primary and secondary oocytes.

Opiate A drug derived from opium, or a semisynthetic drug derived from an opium component.

Opioid Any synthetic narcotic that has opiate-like analgesic activity but is not derived from opium.

Ototoxic Causing damage to the vestibulocochlear nerve or the organs of hearing and balance.

Ovicidal An agent destructive to the eggs of certain organisms.

Oxytocin A nonapeptide secreted by the magnocellular neurons of the hypothalamus and stored as a posterior pituitary hormone along with vasopressin. It promotes uterine contractions and milk ejection and contributes to the second stage of labor.

P

Pacemaker An object or substance that influences the rate at which a certain phenomenon occurs.

Parasiticide An agent that destroys parasites.

Parasympathetic nervous system The craniosacral division of the autonomic nervous system. It slows heart rate, increases intestinal peristalsis and gland activity, and relaxes sphincters.

parietal cells The cells on the periphery of the gastric glands of the stomach. They are located on the basement membrane beneath the chief cells and secrete hydrochloric acid.

Paroxysm A sudden recurrence or intensification of symptoms.

Parturition The birth process.

Passive diffusion The random movement of drug molecules "down the concentration gradient" from an area of high concentration of drug to an area of lower concentration.

Pastes A semisolid preparation containing one or more drug substances for topical application. The two classes comprise the fatty pastes, thick, stiff ointments that do not flow at body temperature; and those made from a single phase aqueous gel.

Pathogens Any disease-producing agent or microorganism, such as a bacterium, fungus, protozoon, or virus.

Peak concentration Highest drug concentration.

Pepsin/pepsinogen An enzyme precursor produced by the chief cells in the stomach.

Per os (PO) Drugs given by mouth.

Perfusion The act of pouring over or through, especially the passage of a fluid through the vessels of a specific organ.

Peristaltic contractions Contractions which move in waves to propel the food along the tract.

Peritubular capillaries The continuation of the efferent renal arteriole by which blood exits the glomerulus.

P-glycoprotein (P-gp) An active transport pump is found in the cells making up the barrier lining the intestinal tract (i.e., enterocytes). Its purpose is to actively transport selected molecules out of the cell and back into the lumen of the intestine, preventing their absorption.

Phagocytosis Endocytosis of particulate material, such as microorganisms or cell fragments. The material is taken into the cell in membrane-bound vesicles (i.e., phagosomes) that originate as pinched-off invaginations of the plasma membrane.

Pharmacodynamics The study of the biochemical and physiologic effects of drugs and the mechanisms of their actions, including the correlation of actions and effects of drugs with their chemical structure; also, such effects on the actions of a particular drug or drugs.

Pharmacokinetics The activity or fate of drugs in the body over a period of time, including the processes of absorption, distribution, localization in tissues, biotransformation, and excretion.

Pharmacology The science that deals with the origin, nature, chemistry, effects, and uses of drugs; it includes pharmacognosy, pharmacokinetics, pharmacodynamics, pharmacotherapeutics, and toxicology.

Pharmacy The branch of the health sciences dealing with the preparation, dispensing, and proper utilization of drugs.

Phenothiazine A greenish, tasteless, tricyclic organic compound prepared by fusing diphenylamine with sulfur; used as a veterinary anthelmintic. Called also dibenzothiazine and thiodiphenylamine. Any of a group of antipsychotic agents derived from this structure (i.e., all sharing a three-ring structure in which two benzene rings are joined by a sulfur and a nitrogen atom). They are potent α-adrenergic and dopaminergic blocking agents; their pharmacologic actions include central nervous system depression, prolongation and potentiation of the effects of narcotic and hypnotic drugs, hypotensive activity, and antispasmodic, antihistaminic, analgesic, sedative, and antiemetic activity.

Phosphodiesterase Bronchodilator that works by inhibiting phosphodiesterase.

Phospholipase Converts phospholipid molecules that make up the cellular membrane into arachidonic acid.

Phospholipid Any lipid that contains phosphorus, including those with a glycerol backbone (e.g., phosphoglycerides and plasmalogens) or a backbone of sphingosine or related substance (e.g., sphingomyelins). Phospholipids are the major form of lipid in all cell membranes.

Pinocytosis The cellular uptake of extracellular fluid and its contents by enclosing them in vesicles derived from the plasma membrane; it serves as a method of transport for macromolecules.

pKa The negative logarithm of the ionization constant of an acid (Ka); the buffering power of a buffer system is greatest when its pKa equals the pH.

Plasmid An extrachromosomal self-replicating structure found in bacterial cells that carries genes for a variety of functions not essential for cell growth. Plasmids consist of cyclic double-stranded DNA molecules, replicating independently of the chromosomes and transmitting through successive cell divisions genes specifying such functions as antibiotic resistance (i.e., R plasmid); conjugation (i.e., F plasmid); the production of enzymes, toxins, and antigens; and the metabolism of sugars and other organic compounds. Plasmids can be transferred from one cell to another by conjugation and by transduction.

Poison Prevention Packaging Act of 1970 Enabled the FDA to require special packaging for drugs that may be dangerous to children.

Polarized Contains positive and negative charges at the ends of the molecule.

Polydipsia Chronic excessive thirst and intake of fluid.

Polyphagia Excessive eating.

Polyuria Increased volume of urine produced.

Porins Porelike openings.

Positive inotropic drug Increases the strength of contraction of a weakened heart.

Postictal phase This phase occurs after the seizure activity has subsided. The animal may appear tired, confused, anxious, or even blind depending on the nature and location of the seizure activity within the CNS and the type of seizure experienced.

Potency The relationship between the therapeutic effect of a drug and the dose necessary to achieve that effect; a drug with a higher potency will require a smaller dose to produce a given effect.

Potentiated The increasing of potency; particularly, the synergistic action of two drugs, so that their effect together is greater than the sum of the effects that each one has alone.

Precaution A protective measure taken in advance.

Preload Refers to the pressure exerted on the myocytes (i.e., muscle cells) within the walls of the ventricles by the "load" or volume of blood in the ventricles just before ventricular contraction.

Premature ventricular contractions (PVC) Wave pattern seen on the electrocardiogram (ECG) that occurs during arrhythmias caused by ectopic foci or other abnormalities.

Prescription A written direction for the preparation and administration of a remedy. A prescription consists of the heading or superscription (i.e., the symbol ℞ or the word *Recipe*, meaning "take"; the inscription, which contains the names and quantities of the ingredients; the subscription,

or directions for compounding; and the signature, usually introduced by the abbreviation S. for signa, "mark," which gives the directions for the patient that are to be marked on the receptacle.

Primary hypothyroidism A disease of the thyroid gland itself that results in lower T_3 and T_4 hormones.

Prodromal phase Refers to the signs that appear before the actual seizures. In human medicine this may be referred to as the aura because the patient feels or "foresees" that they are about to experience a seizure. Animals may experience an aura or prodrome in which they seek out their owners, appear anxious, pace, or whine.

Prodrug A compound that, on administration, must undergo chemical conversion by metabolic processes before becoming an active pharmacologic agent; a precursor of a drug.

Productive cough Coughing that produces mucus.

Progestogen Any natural or synthetic progestational hormone.

Progestational hormone Synonymous with progestins.

Progesterone The principal progestational hormone of the body, liberated by the corpus luteum, placenta, and in minute amounts by the adrenal cortex; it prepares the uterus for the reception and development of the fertilized oocyte by transforming the endometrium from the proliferative to the secretory stage and maintains an optimal intrauterine environment for sustaining pregnancy.

Progestin Refers to the group of progesterone-like hormones.

Proglottids The segments making up the body of a tapeworm.

Prokinetic drugs Stimulating movement or motility, such as drugs that promote gastrointestinal motility.

Proprietary name Trade name or brand name; a unique name a manufacturer gives its particular brand of a drug.

Prostaglandin Any of a group of components derived from unsaturated 20-carbon fatty acids, primarily arachidonic acid, via the cyclooxygenase pathway. Prostaglandins act in the cells in which they are synthesized and on surrounding cells, and their actions and effects vary with concentration, hormonal environment, and cell type.

Protamine Any of a class of basic proteins of low molecular weight, occurring in combination with nucleic acids in the sperm of salmon and certain other fish and having the property of neutralizing heparin.

Protamine zinc insulins (PZI) A long-acting insulin with time of onset about 7 h after injection and duration of action of 36 h, consisting of bovine or porcine insulin reacted with zinc chloride and protamine to form a protein complex from which insulin is slowly released. It is unpredictable and is no longer used in the United States.

Proton pump Molecular structure in the cell membrane of parietal cells that pumps the hydrogen ion into the lumen of the stomach.

Protozoacidal Chemicals that kill protozoa.

Proximal convoluted tubule A twisted (i.e., convoluted) tubular segment in a nephron that contains many active transport mechanisms for moving electrolytes, glucose, selected drug molecules, and other essential molecules back and forth between the urine and the renal tubular cell, and the renal tubular cell and the peritubular capillaries that surround the renal tubule. The peritubular capillaries are the continuation of the efferent renal arteriole by which blood exits the glomerulus.

Pruritus An unpleasant cutaneous sensation that provokes the desire to rub or scratch the skin to obtain relief.

Purkinje fibers Modified cardiac fibers composed of Purkinje cells, occurring as an interlaced network in the subendocardial tissue and constituting the terminal ramifications of the conducting system of the heart. The term is sometimes used loosely to denote the entire system of conducting fibers.

Pyoderma Infection of the skin involving pus.

Pyogenic Pus-producing infections.

Pyometra An infection of the uterus in which a great deal of pus is produced.

R

Reabsorption The act or process of absorbing again.

Receptor Molecular structure within a cell or on the cell surface and characterized by (1) selective binding of a specific substance and (2) a specific physiologic effect that accompanies the binding (e.g., membrane receptors for peptide hormones, neurotransmitters, antigens, complement fragments, and immunoglobulins, and nuclear receptors for steroid hormones).

Recombinant human insulin Insulins created by bringing together (i.e., recombining) genetic material from different sources and producing DNA sequences that are capable of producing these insulins that would not be otherwise produced by biologic organisms.

Recurrent airway obstruction (RAO) An asthma syndrome in horses.

Redistribution Relocating the drug to an area of the body that is less likely to produce adverse reactions.

Refractory period The time in the depolarization/repolarization cycle when the cardiac cell cannot again depolarize.

Renal papillae Small projections into the renal pelvis made of collecting ducts from individual nephrons.

Renal papillary necrosis A condition resulting from the death of renal papillae because of tissue ischemia.

Renin–angiotensin–aldosterone system The system that controls the production of angiotensin II and aldosterone.

Repellent Able to repel or drive off; also, an agent so acting.

Repository dosage form Refers to the injection, usually intramuscularly, of a long-acting drug, which is slowly absorbed and is therefore prolonged in its action.

Residue A remainder; that which remains after the removal of other substances.

Reversal agent An inhibitor.

Ribosome A large molecular structure, approximately 12 nm wide and 25 nm long, that has two dissociable subunits and is the site of protein synthesis.

Right atrium The atrium of the right side of the heart; it receives blood from the superior and the inferior venae cavae, and delivers it to the right ventricle.

Right ventricle The lower chamber of the right side of the heart, which pumps venous blood through the pulmonary trunk and arteries to the capillaries of the lungs.

Risk Minimization Action Plan (Route of administration) The way by which the drug dose is to be administered.

Ruminant Mammal with four-chambered stomach.

Rumination The casting up of food (called cud) out of the rumen and chewing it a second time; called also cudding.

Ruminatorics Prokinetic drugs that stimulate an atonic (i.e., no muscle tone) or flaccid rumen.

Rx Symbol (℞) From the Latin, meaning "take thou of."

S

Salicylic acid/acetylsalicylic acid Chemical name for aspirin.

Sanitizers Chemical agents that reduce the number of microorganisms to a "safe" level without eliminating all microorganisms.

Saturated Containing as much solute as may be dissolved under stated conditions.

Schedule drug A controlled substance.

Scolex The head of a tapeworm.

Scrubs Compounds designed to clean dirty surgical sites by solubilizing dirt and organic material and providing some low-level disinfection.

Seasonal anestrus A period of the estrous cycle during which there is no ovarian activity; in cats, horses, sheep, goats, and certain other species this occurs annually for periods of weeks to months.

Sedative Makes an animal sleepy but really does not reduce the patient's anxiety or agitation.

Segmental contractions Circular contractions around a small segment of intestine that mix the contents of the bowel.

Selective toxicity/selectively toxic An occurrence in which antiparasitic compound should be highly toxic to the parasite but should have little adverse effect on the host's tissue and the person applying or administering the product.

Septicemia *see* Bacteremia

Sequestration Taking up and holding.

Serotonin A monoamine vasoconstrictor that is synthesized in the intestinal chromaffin cells or in central or peripheral neurons and found in high concentrations in many body tissues, including the intestinal mucosa, pineal body, and central nervous system. Produced enzymatically from tryptophan by hydroxylation and decarboxylation, it has many physiologic properties, such as inhibition of gastric secretion, stimulation of smooth muscle, serving as a central neurotransmitter, and being a precursor of melatonin.

Serotonin syndrome A serotonin toxicity induced by the combination of excessive production and release of serotonin by monoamine oxidase inhibitors (MAOI) drugs, and inhibition of serotonin removal from the synapse by selective serotonin reuptake inhibitors (SSRIs).

Side effect A consequence other than the one(s) for which an agent or measure is used; the adverse effects produced by a drug, especially on a tissue or organ system other than the one sought to be benefited by its administration.

Single-dose vials Vial in which all the drug is used at once.

Sinoatrial (SA) node A group of cells that sets the pace for the heart rate.

Sinusoids (hepatic) Specialized liver blood cavities.

SLUDDE Signs associated with parasympathetic nervous system stimulation, which include Salivation, Lacrimation (i.e., tearing), Urination, Defecation, Dyspnea (i.e., difficult breathing because of bronchoconstriction and increased respiratory secretions), and Emesis.

Soluble Able to be dissolved.

Solution A drug completely dissolved in a liquid medium.

Somatic pain Pain associated with the body surface, such as burns or severe abrasions.

Spore form A refractile, oval body formed within bacteria, especially genera of the family *Bacillaceae* (e.g., *Bacillus, Clostridium, Desulfotomaculum, Sporolactobacillus,* and *Sporosarcina*), which is regarded as a resting stage during the life history of the cell, and is characterized by its resistance to environmental change.

Sporicidal Destroying spores.

Status epilepticus Refers to the state of being in the seizure activity; often is used to describe the condition of animals with prolonged seizure activity.

Steady state/plateau A condition in which opposing forces exactly counteract each other.

Sterilizer An apparatus used for the destruction of microorganisms.

Stress leukogram The number of different white blood cells, specifically the combination of neutrophilia, lymphopenia, and monocytopenia, counted in the complete blood count or CBC.

Subcutaneous (SQ) Beneath the skin.

Substance P A polypeptide neurotransmitter that stimulates vasodilation and contraction of intestinal and other smooth muscles. It also plays a part in salivary secretion, diuresis, natriuresis, and pain sensation. It has been isolated from certain cells of the GI and biliary tracts.

Subtherapeutic concentrations Drug concentrations below the minimum effective concentration.

Sulfonylurea compound The hypoglycemic drug for which the most experience has been gained.

Superficial mycoses Fungal skin infections.

Superinfection A new infection occurring in a patient having a preexisting one.

Suppositories Dosage forms designed to be placed in the rectum, where they dissolve and release drug that is then absorbed across the intestinal wall of the rectum.

Suprainfection *see* Superinfection

Supraphysiologic Pertaining to an abnormal or artificially created state in which a naturally occurring substance is at a concentration greater than that occurring naturally.

Supraventricular arrhythmia/tachycardia Excessive rapidity in the action of the heart; the term is usually applied to a heart rate above 100 beats per minute in an adult and is often qualified by the locus of origin and by whether it is paroxysmal or nonparoxysmal.

Surfactants Soaplike compounds that break the surface tension of water and allow easier interactions between organic material and chemicals.

Susceptibility The state of being readily affected or acted upon.

Suspension A liquid preparation consisting of solid particles dispersed throughout a liquid medium in which they are not soluble.

Sustained-release (SR) drugs Controlled-release, coated drugs.

Sympathetic nervous system The division of the autonomic nervous system that accelerates heart rate, constricts blood vessels, and raises blood pressure.

Synergist Compounds added to pyrethrin products to enhance their insecticidal effects.

Syrup Drugs dissolved in a liquid sugar solution.

T

T₃ (triiodothyronine) The hormone that produces the physiologic effect of thyroid hormones.

T₄ (tetraiodothyronine) The major hormone elaborated by the thyroid follicular cells, formed from thyroglobulin and transported mainly in the blood serum thyroxine-binding globulin. Its chief function is to increase the rate of cell metabolism. It is also essential for central nervous system maturation and regulates a number of other functions.

Tablets Solid dosage form of a medicinal substance, of varying weight, size, and shape, which may be molded or compressed.

Tachycardia/tachyarrhythmia Faster than normal heart rate.

Tachypnea Excessive rapidity of breathing.

Taeniacide *see* Anticestodal

Tenesmus Straining, especially ineffectual and painful straining at stool or in urination.

Teratogenic Tending to produce congenital anomalies.

Teratogenic effects appearance of birth defects due to exposure to a teratogenic substance during fetal development.

Tertiary hypothyroidism A decrease of thyroid hormones due to a disease or malfunction of the hypothalamus.

Therapeutic monitoring Evaluating the adequacy of a dosage regimen by checking blood concentrations of drug.

Therapeutic range/window Desirable range of drug concentrations.

Therapeutics The branch of medical science concerned with the treatment of disease.

Threshold The minimum level of input required to cause some event to occur.

Thrombocytopenia Decreased platelets.

Thromboxanes Either of two compounds related to prostaglandins and derived from arachidonic acid. Thromboxane A2 (TXA2) is an extremely potent inducer of platelet aggregation and platelet release reactions and is also a vasoconstrictor; it is thus a physiologic antagonist of prostacyclin. It is synthesized by platelets and is very unstable, with a half-life of 30 s, undergoing nonenzymatic hydrolysis to thromboxane B2 (TXB2), which is inactive.

Thyroidectomy Surgical removal of the thyroid tumor.

Thyroid-stimulating hormone (TSH) Stimulates the follicular cells of the thyroid gland to absorb iodine and incorporate it into tyrosine molecules to produce two thyroid hormones: triiodothyronine (T_3) and tetraiodothyronine, or thyroxine (T_4).

Thyrotoxicosis The condition caused by excessive quantities of thyroid hormones.

Thyrotropin-releasing hormone (TRH) A stimulating hormone whose function is to stimulate the pituitary gland to release thyroid-stimulating hormone (TSH) into the blood.

Thyroxine A hormone of the thyroid gland that contains iodine and is a derivative of the amino acid tyrosine. Thyroxine acts as a catalyst in the body and influences a great variety of effects, including metabolic rate (oxygen consumption); growth and development; metabolism of carbohydrates, fats, proteins, electrolytes and water; vitamin requirements; reproduction; and resistance to infection. Thyroxine can be extracted from animals or made synthetically; it is used in the treatment of hypothyroidism and some types of goiter. *See* T_4

Timed–artificial insemination (timed–AI) Protocols where the use of drugs in a specific, timed order brings the entire group of cattle into estrus at the same time regardless of where they were in their estrous cycle and thus eliminates the time-consuming and labor-intensive work of identifying where individual cows are in their cycles.

Tinctures An alcoholic or hydroalcoholic solution prepared from vegetable materials or from chemical substances.

T-lymphocytes The cells primarily responsible for cell-mediated immunity; they originate from lymphoid stem cells that migrate from the bone marrow to the thymus and differentiate under the influence of the thymic hormones thymopoietin and thymosin.

t-max (transportation maximum) The drug molecule transport system is working at its maximum speed.

Tolerance Diminution of response to a stimulus after prolonged exposure.

Tonic seizures Seizure convulsions characterized by increased skeletal muscle tone, resulting in stiffening of limbs.

Tonic–clonic seizures Used to be called "grand mal" seizures; consist of an initial tonic seizure followed shortly by clonic seizures.

Topically administered drugs Pertaining to a particular surface area, such as a topical antiinfective applied to a certain area of the skin and affecting only the area to which it is applied.

Total daily dose The combined amount of drug (i.e., mass) times the number of doses administered in a given day (i.e., dose interval).

Trade name *see* Proprietary name

Trademark (™) A symbol (i.e., ™) that indicates that the name is a registered trademark owned by the company and, like the copyrighted brand name, cannot be used by other manufacturers.

Tranquilizer A drug with a calming, soothing effect.

Transduction The transforming of one form of energy into another, such as by the sensory mechanisms of the body.

Transfer RNA (t-RNA) Small RNA molecules that carries a specific amino acid to the ribosome where the amino acid is attached to a chain of other amino acids to produce a protein in a ribosome.

Tricuspid valve The valve between the right atrium and right ventricle of the heart; it usually has three cusps (i.e., anterior, posterior, and septal).

Tricyclic antidepressants (TCA) Drugs that have been used to decrease excessive arousal and reduce anxiety and thus are used to treat generalized anxiety and separation anxiety behaviors in dogs and cats; to decrease inappropriate spraying and excessive grooming in cats; and to reduce excessive feather plucking in birds.

Triiodothyronine *see* T_3.

Troche Dosage form incorporating drug into a hard, candylike tablet or lozenge.

Trough concentration Lowest drug concentration.

Type 1 diabetes One of the two major types of diabetes mellitus: an autoimmune disease that results in the destruction of β-cells of the pancreas, leading to loss of the ability to secrete insulin.

Type 2 diabetes One of the two major types of diabetes mellitus. Diagnosis is based on laboratory tests indicating glucose intolerance. Basal insulin secretion is maintained at normal or reduced levels, but insulin release in response to a glucose load is delayed or reduced. Defective glucose receptors on the β-cells of the pancreas may be involved.

U

U-40 and U-100 insulin The bottle contains 40 or 100 insulin units per milliliter.

Unbound fraction Drug molecules not attached to the blood protein.

United States Adopted Names (USAN) Council The body that selects generic drug names.

United States Pharmacopeia (USP) A nongovernmental organization that sets the standards for drug manufacturing quality, purity, and consistency for any drugs sold in the United States.

Upregulation The number of $β_1$-adrenergic receptors on the cardiac cells has increased, making the cell more sensitive to the effects of natural sympathetic nervous system catecholamines or to sympathomimetic drugs.

Urticaria A vascular reaction in the upper dermis, usually transient, consisting of localized edema caused by dilatation and increased capillary permeability with wheals. Most types are named for the causative stimulus or mechanism, such as physical urticaria and contact urticaria. Also called hives.

Uveitis An inflammation of part or all of the uvea, commonly involving the other tunics of the eye (i.e., sclera, cornea, and retina).

V

Vagus nerve (CN X) The tenth cranial nerve. It originates by numerous rootlets from the lateral side of the medulla oblongata in the groove between the olive and the inferior cerebellar peduncle. Its branches are the superior and recurrent laryngeal nerves; meningeal, auricular, pharyngeal, cardiac, bronchial, gastric, hepatic, celiac, and renal rami; pharyngeal, pulmonary, and esophageal plexuses; and anterior and posterior trunks. Its distribution: Descending through the jugular foramen, it presents as a superior and an inferior ganglion, and continues through the neck and thorax into the abdomen. It supplies sensory fibers to the ear, tongue, pharynx, and larynx; motor fibers to the pharynx, larynx, and esophagus; and parasympathetic and visceral afferent fibers to the thoracic and abdominal viscera.

Vasoconstriction The diminution of the caliber of vessels, especially constriction of arterioles, leading to decreased blood flow to a part.

Vasodilation Dilation of a vessel, especially dilation of arterioles, leading to increased blood flow to a part.

Vagus Nerve Either of the longest pair of cranial nerves mainly responsible for parasympathetic control over the heart and many other internal organs, including thoracic and abdominal viscera. The vagus nerves communicate through 13 main branches, connecting to four areas in the brain.

Vegetative form Concerned with growth and with nutrition, as opposed to reproduction.

Vena cava Vessels returning blood to the right side of the heart.

Venodilator Dilates the veins.

Ventricular arrhythmia *see* Tachycardia

Vermicide An agent lethal to worms or intestinal animal parasites.

Vermifuge *see* Anthelmintic

Vertical transmission of resistance When a resistant bacterium spreads the resistance genetically to all daughter cells and all subsequent generations of bacteria that originate from this one resistant bacterium.

Vestibular apparatus In the inner ear, this is the organ responsible for balance.

Veterinarian–client–patient relationship (VCPR) The veterinarian has examined or has adequate medical knowledge of the patient and has agreed to assume responsibility for veterinary care of the patient.

Virucidal An agent that neutralizes or destroys a virus.

Visceral pain Pain associated with organs.

Volume of distribution (Vd) A pharmacokinetic value that provides an approximation of the extent to which a drug is distributed throughout the body. The Vd is determined by looking at the concentration of a drug in the blood shortly after an intravenous bolus is given, and assumes that the drug concentration in the blood equals the concentration of the drug equally distributed throughout every compartment of the body.

W

Warning   More serious or frequent side effects than those found in the precautions section. These constitute adverse drug effects that could potentially do significant harm to the patient.

Wind-up (pain)   Process of increasing ease with which pain signals can be sent up the spinal cord to the brain.

Withdrawal time   Time between last dose and when the animal can be slaughtered for meat or food products.

Wolbachia   A gram-negative, intracellular organism that lives symbiotically within, and is dependent upon, the worms of canine heartworm disease.

Wolbachia **surface protein (WSP)**   Proteins found on the *Wolbachia* species of bacteria, which stimulate an inflammatory response, adding to the inflammation and clinical signs caused by the heartworm.

X

Xenobiotic   A chemical foreign to a given biologic system.

Xylitol   An artificial sweetener that in dogs causes massive release of insulin, causing hypoglycemia and liver necrosis.

INDEX

Note: Page numbers followed by *f* indicate figures, *t* indicate tables, and *b* indicate boxes.